FOURTH EDITION

The Massachusetts General Hospital Handbook of Pain Management

Gary J. Brenner, MD, PhD

Associate Professor
Department of Anesthesia
Harvard Medical School
Chief, Division of Pain Medicine
Department of Anesthesia, Critical Care and Pain Medicine
Massachusetts General Hospital
Boston, Massachusetts

James P. Rathmell, MD

Leroy V. Vandam Professor of Anaesthesia
Harvard Medical School
Chair
Department of Anesthesiology, Perioperative and Pain Medicine
Brigham and Women's Hospital
Boston, Massachusetts

Wolters Kluwer

Philadelphia • Baltimore • New York • London
Buenos Aires • Hong Kong • Sydney • Tokyo

Acquisitions Editor: Keith Donnellan
Senior Development Editor: Ashley Fischer
Editorial Coordinator: Ashley Pfeiffer
Marketing Manager: Phyllis Hitner
Production Project Manager: Sadie Buckallew
Design Coordinator: Holly McLaughlin
Manufacturing Coordinator: Beth Welsh
Prepress Vendor: SPi Global

Fourth Edition

9 8 7 6 5 4 3 2 1

Printed in China

Cataloging-in-Publication Data available on request from the Publisher

ISBN: 978-1-4963-4778-7

shop.lww.com

CCS0820

CONTRIBUTING AUTHORS

Gregory Acampora, MD
Psychiatrist
Pain Management Center at MGH
MGH/Harvard Center for Addiction Medicine
MGH/Charlestown Community Health Center
MGH HOME BASE Veteran's and Family Program
Massachusetts General Hospital
Harvard Medical School
Boston, Massachusetts

Alexandra R. Adler, MD
Staff in Anesthesia and Pain Medicine
Good Samaritan Medical Center
Brockton, Massachusetts

Lucien C. Alexandre, MD, PhD
Interventional Pain Specialist
Pain Management
Mount Sinai Medical Center
Miami Beach, Florida

Chantal Berna, MD, PhD
Director, Center for Integrative and Complementary Medicine
Associate Professor
University of Lausanne
Division of Anesthesiology
Lausanne University Hospital
Lausanne, Switzerland

Mark C. Bicket, MD, PhD
Assistant Professor
Department of Anesthesiology and Critical Care Medicine
Johns Hopkins University School of Medicine
Baltimore, Maryland

Jori F. Bogetz, MD
Attending, Pediatric Palliative Care Team
Acting Assistant Professor
Division of Bioethics and Palliative Care
Department of Pediatrics
University of Washington School of Medicine
Seattle Children's Hospital
Seattle, Washington

Gary J. Brenner, MD, PhD
Associate Professor
Department of Anesthesia
Harvard Medical School
Chief, Division of Pain Medicine
Department of Anesthesia, Critical Care and Pain Medicine
Massachusetts General Hospital
Boston, Massachusetts

Emily J. Burress
Clinical Supervisor
OccMed Consulting and Injury Care
Boston, Massachusetts

John W. Burress, MD, MPH, FACOEM
Assistant Professor of Family Medicine
Boston University Medical Center
Principal, OccMed Consulting and Injury Care
LLC
Boston, Massachusetts

Adam J. Carinci, MD
Chief, Division of Pain Medicine
Director, Pain Treatment Center
Department of Anesthesiology and Perioperative Medicine
University of Rochester Medical Center
Rochester, New York

Lucy Chen, MD
Associate Professor
MGH Center for Pain Medicine
MGH Center for Translational Pain Research
Department of Anesthesia, Critical Care and Pain Medicine
Massachusetts General Hospital
Harvard Medical School
Boston, Massachusetts

Divya Chirumamilla, MD
Interventional Pain Medicine Specialist
Clinical Assistant Professor
Vivian L. Smith Department of Neurosurgery
Memorial Hermann Medical Center
UT Health/McGovern Medical School
The Woodlands, Texas

Steven P. Cohen, MD
Chief of Pain Medicine and Director of Clinical Operations
Johns Hopkins Medical Institutions
Director of Pain Research
Walter Reed National Military Medical Center
Professor of Anesthesiology, Physical Medicine & Rehabilitation, and Neurology
Johns Hopkins School of Medicine
Uniformed Services University of the Health Sciences
Johns Hopkins Hospital
Bethesda, Maryland

Lane C. Crawford, MD
Assistant Professor of Clinical Anesthesiology
Department of Anesthesiology
Vanderbilt University Medical Center
Vanderbilt University School of Medicine
Nashville, Tennessee

Bethany-Rose Daubman, MD
Instructor in Medicine
Harvard Medical School
Director of Continuing Medical Education
Division of Palliative Care and Geriatrics
Massachusetts General Hospital
Boston, Massachusetts

Daniel M. DuBreuil, PhD
Research Fellow
Department of Neurology
Massachusetts General Hospital
Harvard Medical School
Boston, Massachusetts

David A. Edwards, MD, PhD
Chief, Division of Pain Medicine
Associate Professor
Departments of Anesthesiology & Neurological Surgery
Vanderbilt University Medical Center
Nashville, Tennessee

Christopher Gilligan, MD, MBA
Chief, Division of Pain Medicine
Vice Chair for Strategy
Department of Anesthesiology, Perioperative and Pain Medicine
Brigham & Women's Hospital
Assistant Professor of Anaesthesia
Harvard Medical School
Boston, Massachusetts

Richard D. Goldstein, MD
Director
Robert's Program on Sudden Unexpected Death in Pediatrics
Assistant Professor
Department of Pediatrics
Division of General Pediatrics
Boston Children's Hospital
Harvard Medical School
Boston, Massachusetts

Benjamin L. Grannan, MD
Resident
Department of Neurosurgery
Massachusetts General Hospital
Harvard Medical School
Boston, Massachusetts

Robert Griffin, MD, PhD
Clinical Assistant Professor of Anesthesiology
Department of Anesthesiology, Critical Care, and Pain Management
Hospital for Special Surgery
Weill Cornell Medical College
New York, New York

Paul Guillod, MD
Anesthesia Resident
Department of Anesthesia, Critical Care and Pain Medicine
Massachusetts General Hospital
Boston, Massachusetts

Asteghik Hacobian, MD, MA, FIPP, DABIPP
Interventional Spine Medicine
Rye Surgical Center
Rye, New Hampshire
Interventional Spine Medicine
Plaistow, New Hampshire
Portsmouth Hospital
Portsmouth, New Hampshire

George Hanna, MD
Director of Pain Management
VIP Medical Group–Pain Treatment Specialists
New York, New York

Michael Hermann, MD
Specialists in Pain Management
Chattanooga, Tennessee

María F. Hernández-Nuño de la Rosa, DDS, MS
Resident, Orofacial Pain Training Program
Division of Oral and Maxillofacial Pain
Department of Oral and Maxillofacial Surgery
Massachusetts General Hospital
Boston, Massachusetts

Mark A. Hoeft, MD
Assistant Professor
Department of Anesthesiology
Larner College of Medicine
University of Vermont
Burlington, Vermont

Eugenia-Daniela Hord, MD
SSM Agnesian Healthcare
Department of Pain Medicine
Fond du Lac, Wisconsin

Shawn G. Hughes, DO
White-Wilson Pain Management Clinic
Fort Walton Beach, Florida

David E. Jamison, MD
Associate Professor
Department of Anesthesiology
Walter Reed National Military Medical Center
Uniformed Services University
Bethesda, Maryland

Susie S. Jang, MD
Director, Resident Education in Pain Medicine
Instructor
Department of Anesthesia, Critical Care, and Pain Medicine
Beth Israel Deaconess Medical Center
Harvard Medical School
Boston, Massachusetts

Ping Jin, MD, PhD
Department of Anesthesia, Critical Care and Pain Medicine
Massachusetts General Hospital
Harvard Medical School
Boston, Massachusetts

Mihir M. Kamdar, MD
Associate Director, Division of Palliative Care
Instructor
Department of Anesthesia, Critical Care and Pain Medicine
Division of Palliative Care & Geriatrics
Department of Medicine
Massachusetts General Hospital
Harvard Medical School
Boston, Massachusetts

David A. Keith, BDS, FDSRCS, DMD
Professor, Oral and Maxillofacial Surgery
Harvard School of Dental Medicine
Visiting Oral and Maxillofacial Surgeon
Massachusetts General Hospital
Boston, Massachusetts

Shehryar N. Khawaja, BDS, MSc, DABOP
Consultant, Orofacial Pain Medicine
Department of Internal Medicine
Shaukat Khanum Memorial Cancer Hospital and Research Centre
Lahore, Punjab, Pakistan

M. Alexander Kiefer, MD
Assistant Professor
Department of Anesthesiology
Georgetown University School of Medicine
Attending Physician
Georgetown Pain Management
Washington, District of Columbia

Karsten Kueppenbender, MD
Instructor, Part Time
Department of Psychiatry
Harvard Medical School
Boston, Massachusetts
Attending Psychiatrist
The Pavilion Center
McLean Hospital
Belmont, Massachusetts

Ronald J. Kulich, PhD
Professor
Diagnostic Sciences
Tufts School of Dental Medicine
Lecturer
Department of Anesthesia, Critical Care and Pain Medicine
Massachusetts General Hospital
Harvard Medicine School
Boston, Massachusetts

Alyssa A. Lebel, MD, FAHS
Director, BCH Chronic Headache Program
Department of Anesthesiology, Critical Care, and Pain Management
Boston Children's Hospital
Associate Professor, Anesthesiology
Harvard Medical School
Boston, Massachusetts

Richard E. Leiter, MD, MA
Instructor
Harvard Medical School
Attending Physician
Department of Psychosocial Oncology and Palliative Medicine
Dana-Farber Cancer Institute
Department of Medicine
Brigham and Women's Hospital
Boston, Massachusetts

Kevin Madden, MD
Assistant Professor
Department of Palliative, Rehabilitation, and Integrative Medicine
University of Texas MD Anderson Cancer Center
Houston, Texas

Dermot P. Maher, MD, MS, MHS
Assistant Professor
Chronic Pain Division
Department of Anesthesia and Critical Care Medicine
Johns Hopkins Hospital & Sibley Memorial Hospital
Baltimore, Maryland

Amir Mian, MBBS
Beltway Anesthesiology Group, PA
Senior Partner
Kingwood, Texas
Department of Anesthesiology
HCA Healthcare Houston Southeast
Pasadena, Texas

Saad Mohammad, MD
Attending Anesthesiologist
Westchester Anesthesiologists
White Plains Hospital
White Plains, New York

Ellen S. Patterson, MD, MA
Assistant Professor and Director of Behavioral Science Education
Department of Comprehensive Care
Tufts University School of Dental Medicine
Boston, Massachusetts

Gary I. Polykoff, MD
Clinical Instructor
Department of Physical Medicine and Rehabilitation
Massachusetts General Hospital
Harvard Medical School
Boston, Massachusetts

Rene Przkora, MD, PhD
Department of Anesthesiology
University of Florida College of Medicine
Gainesville, Florida

James P. Rathmell, MD
Leroy V. Vandam Professor of Anaesthesia
Harvard Medical School
Chair
Department of Anesthesiology, Perioperative and Pain Medicine
Brigham and Women's Hospital
Boston, Massachusetts

Matthew A. Roselli, MSW
Licensed Clinical Social Worker
Department of Anesthesiology and Pain Medicine
University of California, Davis
Sacramento, California

Leah B. Rosenberg, MD
Assistant Professor
Division of Palliative Care and Geriatric Medicine
Massachusetts General Hospital
Harvard Medical School
Boston, Massachusetts

Danielle L. Sarno, MD
Instructor of Physical Medicine and Rehabilitation
Harvard Medical School
Director of Interventional Pain Management
Department of Neurosurgery
Brigham and Women's Hospital
Boston, Massachusetts

Pascal Scemama de Gialluly, MD, MBA
Assistant Professor
Department of Anesthesia & Perioperative Medicine
Umass Memorial Medical Center
University of Massachusetts Medical School
Worcester, Massachusetts

Michael E. Schatman, PhD
Affiliate Clinical Associate
Department of Diagnostic Sciences
Tufts University School of Dental Medicine
Adjunct Clinical Assistant Professor
Department of Public Health and Community Medicine
Tufts University School of Medicine
Boston, Massachusetts

Nathaniel M. Schuster, MD
Associate Clinic Director
Assistant Professor
Center for Pain Medicine
Department of Anesthesiology
University of California, San Diego Health System
San Diego, California

Erin Scott, MD
Director
The Ohio State University Palliative Medicine Fellowship
Assistant Professor
The Ohio State University Medical School
Division of Palliative Medicine
The Ohio State University Wexner Medical Center
Columbus, Ohio

Steven J. Scrivani, DDS, DMedSc
Former Chief, Division of Oral and Maxillofacial Pain
Former Director, Orofacial Pain Residency Program
Department of Oral and Maxillofacial Surgery
Massachusetts General Hospital
Boston, Massachusetts

Shiqian Shen, MD
Assistant Professor
Department of Anesthesia, Critical Care and Pain Medicine
Massachusetts General Hospital
Harvard Medical School
Boston, Massachusetts

Moises A. Sidransky, MD
Department of Pain Management
UT Health East Texas
Tyler, Texas

Jan Slezak, MD
Interventional Spine Medicine
Barrington, New Hampshire
Frisbie Memorial Hospital
Rochester, New Hampshire
Portsmouth Regional Hospital
Portsmouth, New Hampshire

Boris Spektor, MD
Program Director, Emory Pain Fellowship
Assistant Professor
Department of Anesthesiology
Emory University School of Medicine
Atlanta, Georgia

Erin Stevens, DO
Attending Physician
The Ohio State University Wexner Medical Center
Division of Palliative Care
The James Cancer Hospital
Assistant Professor–Clinical
McCampbell Hall
Columbus, Ohio

Mark J. Stoltenberg, MD, MPH, MA
Clinical Instructor
Division of Palliative Care and Geriatrics
Department of Medicine
Massachusetts General Hospital
Harvard Medical School
Boston, Massachusetts

Kenneth S. Tseng, MD, MPH
Assistant Professor
Virginia Commonwealth University School of Medicine
Anesthesiologist
Department of Anesthesiology
INOVA-Fairfax Hospital
Falls Church, Virginia

M. Alice Vijjeswarapu, MD
Associate Program Director, Pain Medicine Fellowship
Assistant Professor of Anesthesiology
Cedars-Sinai Medical Center
Los Angeles, California

Brian J. Wainger, MD, PhD
Assistant Professor
Departments of Anesthesia, Critical Care and Pain Medicine and Neurology
Massachusetts General Hospital
Harvard Medical School
Boston, Massachusetts

Jingping Wang, MD, PhD, FASA
Associate Professor, Harvard Medical School
Director, Oral & Maxillofacial Surgery
Director, In Vitro Fertilization Anesthesia
Department of Anesthesia, Critical Care and Pain Medicine
Massachusetts General Hospital
Boston, Massachusetts

Kelly M. Wawrzyniak, PsyD
Assistant Professor
Department of Diagnostic Sciences
Craniofacial Pain Center
Tufts University School of Dental Medicine
Boston, Massachusetts

Rebecca L. Wu, MD
Instructor and Staff Anesthesiologist
Department of Anesthesia, Critical Care and Pain Medicine
Massachusetts General Hospital
Harvard Medical School
Boston, Massachusetts

Qing Yang, MD, PhD
Anesthesiologist
HSHS Medical Group
St. John's Hospital
Springfield, Illinois

Andrew C. Young, MD
Clinical Fellow
Department of Anesthesia, Critical Care and Pain Medicine
Massachusetts General Hospital
Harvard Medical School
Boston, Massachusetts

Mark J. Young, MD
Clinical Assistant Professor
Department of Anesthesiology and Perioperative Medicine
Tufts University School of Medicine
Boston, Massachusetts
Anesthesiologist
Department of Anesthesiology
Newton-Wellesley Hospital
Newton, Massachusetts

April Zehm, MD
Assistant Professor of Medicine
Division of Hematology and Oncology—Palliative Care Program
Department of Medicine
Froedtert Hospital
Medical College of Wisconsin
Milwaukee, Wisconsin

PREFACE

The fourth edition of the *Massachusetts General Hospital Handbook of Pain Management* represents a major update of the prior edition. This edition contains an extensive new section on interventional approaches to pain management as well as substantial updating of content related to the use of opioids for chronic pain. The appendices have been updated and among other topics provide useful information on medications commonly used in pain treatment. For the first time, the *Handbook* will have full-color images and will be available in e-book format that can be read on computer, tablet, or smartphone and easily converts to audiobook.

The intent of the handbook is to provide a focused coverage of the key topics required pain management with a bias toward the treatment of chronic pain. We wish to extend our gratitude to all contributors to the current and past editions of this text.

Gary J. Brenner, MD, PhD
James P. Rathmell, MD

CONTENTS

SECTION I

General Considerations

1 Neurophysiologic Basis of Pain

Robert Griffin and Gary J. Brenner

Pain is a complex subjective experience that most commonly involves a central nervous system (CNS) response to a peripheral nociceptive stimulus. Sir Charles Sherrington defined nociception as the sensory nervous system's detection of a noxious event or potentially harmful environmental stimulus. The state of the peripheral nociceptive system is plastic, and in addition to the type, pattern, and intensity of a sensory stimulus, the peripheral nervous system response depends on the prior history of sensory stimuli, nerve injury, and tissue trauma. These events may cause extensive alterations in the state of the sensory system such that normally innocuous stimuli evoke a response of the peripheral nervous system that is perceived as pain. In addition, the state of the patient's CNS including both biological and psychosocial parameters may affect the patient's subjective pain response.

At the outset, we will discuss several important clinically observable phenomena that occur in chronic pain conditions. "Ordinary" or nociceptive pain appears to be a relatively simple stimulus-response relationship; for example, a pinprick produces an immediate sensation of sharp pain. Most chronic pain states involve one or more forms of pain hypersensitivity. **Hyperalgesia** describes a painful condition in which the response to a nociceptive stimulus is enhanced; for example, a pinprick produces an immediate sensation of extreme pain. **Primary hyperalgesia** describes hyperalgesia occurring at the immediate location of tissue injury, for example the skin at the site of a bee sting. **Secondary hyperalgesia** refers to enhanced nociceptive responses in the surrounding area of uninjured tissue. Primary hyperalgesia is thought to involve sensitization at the level of the primary sensory neurons, spinal cord, and brain processing. Secondary hyperalgesia is thought to involve sensitization at the spinal cord and brain levels. **Allodynia** refers to a nociceptive response produced by a normally nonnociceptive stimulus, for example the sensation of pain produced by lightly brushing an area of sunburn or the sensation of pain classically produced by wind on the face of a patient with severe trigeminal neuralgia.

Inflammation and nerve injury result in alterations in nervous system function that can produce these phenomena. This chapter will focus on predominantly the anatomic structures involved in nociception.

The peripheral nervous system pain response involves several components.

- **Nociceptors.** Primary sensory neurons with peripheral terminals responsive to noxious mechanical, thermal, or chemical stimuli conduct action potentials along axons arranged into peripheral nerves from peripheral sites to the CNS. The subset of primary sensory neurons that respond to high-threshold pain-inducing mechanical, thermal, or chemical stimuli is termed nociceptors, or primary nociceptive afferents.
- **Spinal cord synaptic transmission.** Most peripheral sensory afferents either synapse in the spinal cord dorsal horn, transmitting information to secondary projection neurons that form ascending fiber tracts, or directly enter an ascending fiber tract and synapse in the brainstem. Nociceptors predominantly synapse in the spinal cord dorsal horn, while nonnociceptive afferents predominantly synapse in the brainstem.
- **Supraspinal pain processing.** The spinothalamic and spinohypothalamic tracts convey nociceptive information from the spinal cord to the brain. Higher brain centers including brainstem, thalamus, basal ganglia, and cerebral cortex are important for pain processing. The brain mediates between nociceptive information and the subjective experience of pain.
- **Descending projections.** Descending efferent projections from the brain to the spinal cord can alter the parameters of spinal cord synaptic transmission of nociceptive information.

I. PRIMARY SOMATOSENSORY NEURONS

A. Definitions

Peripheral nerves carry sensory information from visceral organs, muscle, bone, and skin, among other structures. Peripheral nerves are composed of the axons of primary sensory neurons, which have cell bodies that reside in the dorsal root ganglia of the spinal cord. These peripheral nerves may either be cranial nerves, carrying sensory information to the brainstem, or may form spinal nerves, carrying information to the spinal cord. Spinal nerves are mixed nerves, with an afferent component that may include both somatic and visceral afferent fibers. The cell bodies for both somatic and visceral afferent fibers of spinal nerves are located in the dorsal root ganglia, while those for cranial nerves may be found in the brainstem cranial nerve nuclei.

B. Nerve Fiber Types

Within the dorsal root ganglion, several neuronal populations may be identified according to axon diameter, axon myelination, and expression of biochemical markers (Table 1.1). A-beta fibers are large myelinated fibers that conduct action potentials rapidly and respond predominantly to low-energy mechanical stimuli that in states of normal nervous system function are generally perceived as nonpainful. A delta fibers are moderately small in diameter, are thinly myelinated, and respond to high-threshold stimuli. Small, unmyelinated C fibers respond to multimodal stimuli including chemical, thermal, and high-threshold mechanical stimuli.

C. Nociceptors

1. Nociceptors are largely A delta and C fibers. Not all C-fiber neurons are nociceptors, given that some transmit information about light touch or

TABLE 1.1 Classification of Fibers in Peripheral Nerves

Fiber Group	Innervation	Mean Diameter (μm)	Mean Conduction Velocity (m/s)
A-α	Primary muscle spindle motor to skeletal muscle	15	100
A-β	Cutaneous touch and pressure afferent fibers	8	50
A-γ	Motor to muscle spindle	6	20
A-δ	Mechanoreceptors, nociceptors, thermoreceptors	<3	15
B	Sympathetic preganglionic	3	7
C	Mechanoreceptors, nociceptors, thermoreceptors, sympathetic postganglionic	1	1

From Wainger BJ and Brenner GJ. Mechanisms of Chronic Pain. In: Longnecker DE, Mackey SC, Newman MF, et al., eds. *Anesthesiology*. 3rd ed. New York, NY: McGraw-Hill Education;2017:1443.

itch. C fibers may be subdivided according to biochemical markers. One subgroup expresses the glial-derived neurotrophic factor c-ret and binds to the isolectin IB4. The other subgroup expresses TrkA, the receptor for nerve growth factor, and produces neuropeptides substance P and calcitonin gene–related peptide (CGRP). The functional implications of these chemically defined subpopulations of nociceptor are not yet well understood.

2. Nociceptive peripheral terminals may be specialized to respond to thermal, mechanical, or chemical energy, or a combination of these. Thermosensation relies on transient receptor potential family channels, predominantly TRPV1 and TRPV2. Mechanosensation likely depends on mechanosensitive ion channels, but the identity of the ion channel is yet to be determined. Numerous chemical mediators have been shown to produce pain by activating peripheral nociceptive terminals vis specific receptors, and may be either endogenous chemical mediators typically associated with tissue inflammation, such as ATP, or may be exogenous chemical mediators that are perceived as painful, such as capsaicin or bee venom.

D. Peripheral Sensitization

1. Sensitization of the primary afferent somatosensory system is likely to underlie many pain hypersensitivity states. The phenomenon of peripheral sensitization describes a state in which primary afferent fibers, particularly nociceptive fibers, respond to stimuli at a lower intensity threshold than their baseline state. Peripheral sensitization is thought to result from second messenger pathways triggered by extracellular sensitizing agents acting on membrane receptors. Second messenger signaling can result in phosphorylation of transductive receptor proteins such as TRPV1, reducing activation threshold, or in the phosphorylation of voltage sensitive ion channels, reducing the threshold for action potential generation. Many of the identified peripheral sensitizing agents are cytokines or inflammatory mediators such as bradykinin or histamine, released in the context of an inflammatory response.

Peripheral sensitization may have a protective function in terms of causing the organism to avoid physical contact of an acutely inflamed body part, but can also result in pathologic pain, for example pain associated with chronic inflammation. Primary hyperalgesia can be explained mechanistically by the biochemical changes associated with primary sensitization.

2. Head and neck pain sensation is similar in many respects to pain sensation elsewhere in the body, with primary afferent fibers carried either by upper cervical spinal nerves or by cranial nerves. The ophthalmic, maxillary, and mandibular divisions of the trigeminal nerve carry the primary afferent nociceptive fibers receiving stimulation from the face, as well as the dura and the vascular supply to the anterior brain. These primary afferent fibers have cell bodies in the brainstem trigeminal nuclei. The glossopharyngeal nerve and the vagus nerve also carry primary afferent sensory information about pain from their innervation areas.

II. SPINAL CORD AND DORSAL HORN SYNAPTIC TRANSMISSION

A. Dorsal Horn Laminar Organization

1. Primary afferent fibers enter the spinal cord via Lissauer tract, a fiber bundle consisting predominantly of A delta and C afferent fibers that penetrates the spinal cord en route to the dorsal horn (Fig. 1.1). Upon entering the spinal cord, the primary afferent A delta and C fibers run up or down one to two spinal segments before synapsing onto second-order neurons located in the spinal cord dorsal horn.
2. The target for innervation of most nociceptive peripheral afferent neurons may be found within the spinal cord dorsal horn. The spinal cord gray matter may be divided into 10 laminae, with laminae I-V within the dorsal horn (Fig. 1.2). C-fiber neurons predominantly synapse onto secondary neurons located in laminae I and II of the dorsal horn, with

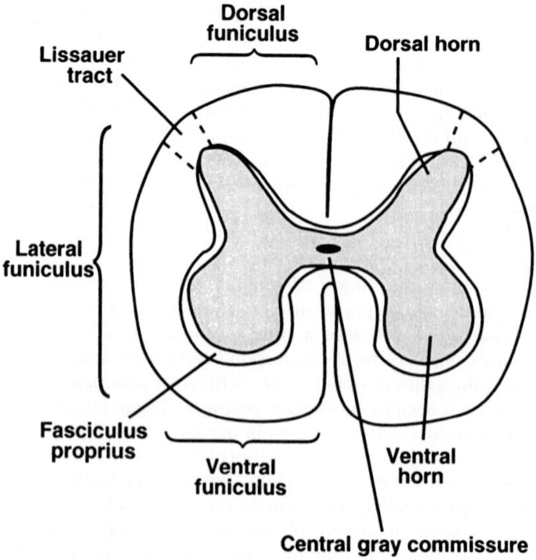

FIGURE 1.1 Diagrammatic cross section of the spinal cord.

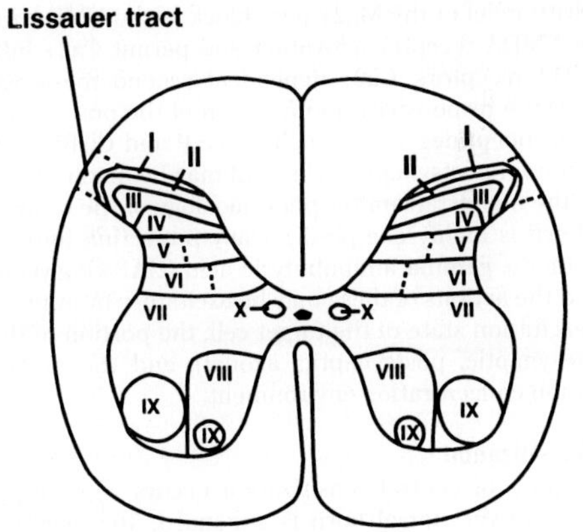

FIGURE 1.2 Laminae of Rexed I through X of the spinal cord.

lamina II referred to as the substantia gelatinosa. Second-order projection neurons then send axons that cross the spinal cord central commissure and ascend to the brain in the spinothalamic tract. A-delta neurons predominantly project to lamina I and lamina V. While most A-beta neurons project predominantly to the brainstem via the ipsilateral dorsal column pathway, some A-beta neurons also project to the deep dorsal horn (lamina III-V). In addition to the primary afferent fibers synapsing onto secondary projection neurons, several other cell types are important for dorsal horn nociceptive information processing and transmission. Large numbers of locally projecting interneurons are present within the dorsal horn of the spinal cord that receive afferent information from nociceptors and/or nonnociceptive afferents, and synapse locally. Both excitatory and inhibitory interneurons are present. These interneurons likely have roles in early sensory processing and sensory integration. In addition to the interneurons, nonneuronal supporting cell types including astrocytes and microglia are important for maintaining the CNS microenvironment appropriate for normal synaptic transmission. Secondary neurons, both projection neurons and locally synapsing interneurons, may be classified by their stimulus responsivity. There are both nociceptive-specific dorsal horn neurons and neurons that respond to a wide range of stimulus intensity, termed wide dynamic range neurons.

B. Dorsal Horn Neurotransmission

A wide range of neurotransmitters, neuropeptides, and other biochemical mediators are released in the dorsal horn by these cell types: primary sensory neurons, neurons with descending projections from the brain to the spinal cord, interneurons, microglia, and astrocytes. Both nociceptive and nonnociceptive primary sensory neurons rely on glutamate as the principal excitatory neurotransmitter for activation of secondary projection neurons and locally projecting interneurons. Glutamate acts on multiple postsynaptic receptor proteins to excite and/or modulate the responsiveness of secondary neurons; these receptors include AMPA- and NMDA-type ionotropic receptors, as well as several types of metabotropic glutamate receptor. Brief postsynaptic activation will be mediated primarily via AMPA glutamate receptor activation, while prolonged postsynaptic activation associated with relief of the Mg2+ pore block of the NMDA receptors will also involve NMDA receptor activation and permit Ca2+ influx into the cell via NMDA receptors. Ca2+ dependent second messenger cascades can then alter the responsivity and function of the postsynaptic neurons. Release of neuropeptides such as substance P and CGRP appear to have a slower action on postsynaptic cells, and may be involved in modulating excitability. The neurotransmitter pharmacology of the other cell types in the dorsal horn is highly complex. Locally projecting interneurons may release glutamate, gamma aminobutyric acid (GABA), glycine, or neuropeptides, and the actions of these may be excitatory or inhibitory depending on the excitation state of the target cell, the portion of the target cell affected (presynaptic, postsynaptic, axonal), and the extracellular and intracellular ion concentration environment.

C. Central Sensitization

The phenomenon of central sensitization occurs when excitatory neurotransmission in the dorsal horn is enhanced. This may occur due to high-intensity peripheral stimulation, or may occur in association with the extensive biochemical changes occurring in the context of peripheral nerve injury. In central sensitization, it is thought that NMDA receptor–dependent postsynaptic events lead to long-term potentiation of central synapses, resulting in increased neurotransmission. Central sensitization is thought to mediate the phenomenon of secondary hyperalgesia, in which an apparently unaffected area of tissue surrounding an area of injury becomes hypersensitive to noxious stimuli.

III. SUPRASPINAL PAIN PROCESSING

A. Ascending Nociceptive Tracts

Second-order projection neurons located in the spinal cord dorsal horn give rise to axons that form ascending tracts to the brain (Fig. 1.3). The predominant ascending pathway for nociceptive information is the spinothalamic tract. The spinothalamic tract consists of axons projecting from the dorsal horn that cross midline in the spinal cord at the same spinal segmental level as the incoming primary sensory neuron. Spinothalamic tract axons originate from both superficial and deep dorsal horn laminae, and carry information about both nociceptive stimuli and nonpainful thermal stimuli. After crossing midline, the spinothalamic tract axons ascend in the anterolateral white matter of the spinal cord. The ascending spinothalamic tract axons then form synapses in the ventral posteromedial and ventral posterolateral thalamic nuclei. Ascending transmission of nociceptive information from structures in the head and neck is mediated by the projection targets of cervical spinal nerves and cranial nerves (V, VII, IX, X). Cervical spinal nerves transmitting via the cervical spinal cord dorsal horn, while cranial nerves transmit via secondary neurons located in brainstem cranial nerve nuclei.

B. Brain Centers

1. Incoming information about painful stimuli primarily targets neurons located in the thalamus. Ascending nociceptive projection neurons also target, to a lesser extent, several brainstem nuclei. The thalamus functions as a relay for many different types of afferent sensory information. Nociceptive secondary projection neurons primarily target neurons located in the ventral posterolateral and ventral posteromedial nuclei of the thalamus. Thalamic projection neurons then transmit nociceptive information in turn to the primary somatosensory cortex.

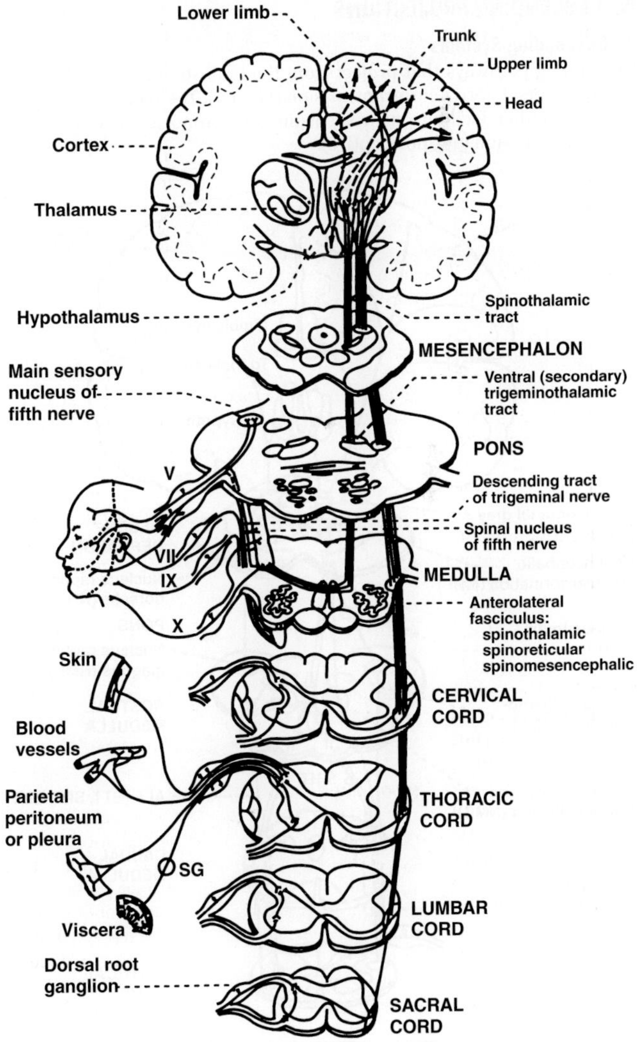

FIGURE 1.3 Ascending pain pathways. (Reprinted with permission from Bonica JJ, ed. *The Management of Pain*, vol. 1. Philadelphia, PA: Lea & Febiger; 1990:29.)

2. Processing of painful information by the brain is highly complex. Localization of painful stimuli, also described as the discriminative component of pain, likely relies on the somatosensory cortex, which receives topographically organized information from the thalamus. The affective response to pain likely involves brain structures that are involved in other affective responses such as the limbic system, cingulate cortex, and amygdala.

IV. DESCENDING PROJECTIONS

A. Descending Systems

Descending pathways that project from the brainstem to the spinal cord can alter dorsal horn neurotransmission (Fig. 1.4). These descending pathways can either facilitate neurotransmission (pronociceptive) or inhibit neurotransmission (antinociceptive).

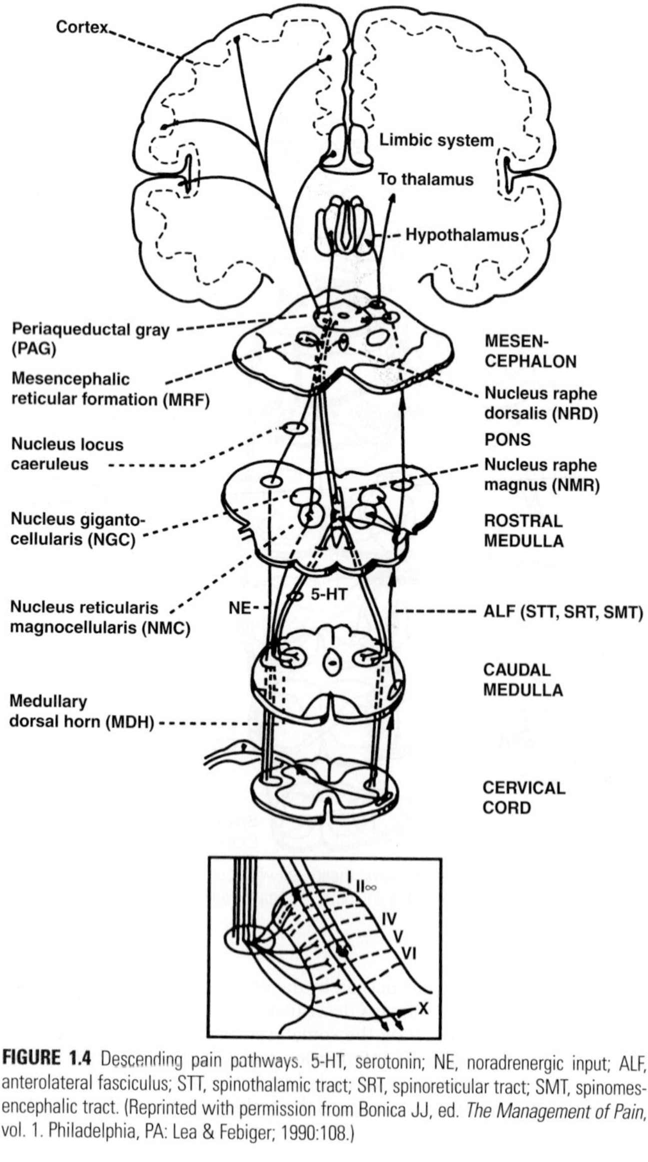

FIGURE 1.4 Descending pain pathways. 5-HT, serotonin; NE, noradrenergic input; ALF, anterolateral fasciculus; STT, spinothalamic tract; SRT, spinoreticular tract; SMT, spinomesencephalic tract. (Reprinted with permission from Bonica JJ, ed. *The Management of Pain*, vol. 1. Philadelphia, PA: Lea & Febiger; 1990:108.)

B. Neurotransmitters Involved in Descending Modulation

Descending pronociception appears to depend on serotonin activity, while descending antinociception appears to depend on the spinal cord action of norepinephrine. Serotonin may have either a facilitatory or inhibitory effect depending on the specific receptor subtypes involved. Endogenous opioid transmission acting on opioid receptors in the dorsal horn is likely also involved in descending inhibition. Mu opioid receptors can mediate inhibition of neurotransmission via both presynaptic and postsynaptic inhibition. Endogenous opioid pathways in the brainstem regulate the activation and inhibition of descending pathway activity.

V. CONCLUSION

The sensation of pain depends on complex behavior of neural systems that extend from the affected body structure to the brain, involving multiple modulatory effects. Nociception is influenced not just by the stimulus type, location, and intensity but also by the duration and timing of the pain stimulus, the prior history of nociceptive stimuli affecting the transducing and transmitting neurons, and the prior history of nerve injury or inflammation affecting those neurons. In addition, pain is affected at the level of the brain by the individual's affective and motivational state. Current diagnostic tools are unable to access this host of electrophysiological and molecular events as they occur in the nervous system, and much of clinical pain pharmacology in practice must treat this as a "black box" relying on patient subjective reports of symptoms and correlative diagnostic testing such as electrodiagnostic testing and magnetic resonance imaging (MRI).

Selected Readings

Bourinet E, Altier C, Hildebrand ME, et al. Calcium-permeable ion channels in pain signaling. *Physiol Rev.* 2014;94:81-140.

Braz J, Solorzano C, Wang X, Basbaum AI. Transmitting pain and itch messages: a contemporary view of the spinal cord circuits that generate gate control. *Neuron.* 2014;82(3):522-536.

Denk, F, McMahon SB, Tracey I. Pain vulnerability: a neurobiological perspective. *Nat Neurosci.* 2014;17:192-200.

Fields HL. *Pain: Mechanisms and Management.* 2nd ed. New York, NY: McGraw-Hill; 2002.

Fishman SM, Ballantyne JC, Rathmell JP, eds. *Bonica's Management of Pain.* 4th ed. Philadelphia, PA: Wolters Kluwer; 2010.

Nolte J. *The Human Brain: An Introduction to Its Functional Anatomy.* 6th ed. Philadelphia, PA: Mosby Elsevier; 2009.

Ossipov MH, Morimura K, Porreca F. Descending pain modulation and the chronification of pain. *Curr Opin Support Palliat Care.* 2014;8(2):143-151.

Sherrington CS. *The Integrative Action of the Nervous System.* New York, NY: Scribner; 1906.

Vardeh D, Mannion RJ, Woolf CJ. Toward a mechanism-based approach to pain diagnosis. *J Pain.* 2016;17(9 suppl 2):T50-T69.

2 Pain Mechanisms and Their Importance in Clinical Practice and Research

Daniel M. DuBreuil and Brian J. Wainger

Clinical and preclinical studies have demonstrated that multiple mechanisms generate chronic, pathological pain across a broad span of diseases. Primary disease factors initiate a range of specific pain mechanisms that induce molecular amplification and structural reorganization of pain circuitry. This reorganization is the primary contributor to pain chronification, and pain therapies should focus on pain-specific mechanisms and processes. In particular, pain mechanisms within a disease may vary across patients, reducing the efficacy of disease-based treatment approaches, but patient-specific pain symptoms may provide valuable insight into active pain mechanisms on an individual basis. Complicating therapy selection further, individual symptoms may result from the activation of multiple mechanisms, which may respond to different treatments, and clinical manifestations of the same mechanisms may vary based on underlying genetic background or epigenetic events that affect pain susceptibility. The best prospect for effective treatment of pain is to improve our understanding of how current therapies impinge on validated pain mechanisms for developing new therapies aimed at mechanisms that are poorly targeted and standardizing diagnostic protocols for assessing pain mechanisms that are activated within individual patients. In the future, classification of pain phenotypes may receive support from molecular, genetic, and imaging biomarkers.

In this chapter, we describe broad pain mechanisms that contribute to pathological pain. We also describe how understanding these mechanisms may lead to more targeted analgesic development pipelines and improved pain management in the clinic.

I. CANONICAL NOCICEPTION PATHWAY

Acute pain is initiated by a subset of highly specialized primary neurons—nociceptors—and the peripheral tissues that they innervate (eg, skin, muscle, bone, and viscera). Nociceptors reside in dorsal root ganglia and are pseudounipolar: they extend a single bifurcating axon innervating both peripheral tissues and spinal cord. Nociceptor fibers are either unmyelinated C fibers or thinly myelinated A-δ fibers and are physically and functionally distinct from the more thickly myelinated low-threshold sensory A-β fibers. Activation of nociceptor-specific ion channel transducers in peripheral nociceptor terminals leads to action potential generation, conduction from the periphery to the spinal cord, and synaptic activation. Action potentials reaching central axon terminals of nociceptor afferents in the superficial dorsal horn generate an inrush of calcium and release into the synaptic cleft of the excitatory neurotransmitter glutamate. Glutamate generates fast synaptic potentials in second-order dorsal horn neurons via α-amino-3-hydroxy-5-methyl-4-isoxazoleproprionic acid (AMPA) and kainate subtypes of ionotropic glutamate receptors. The pattern of synaptic input to the second-order neurons within the dorsal horn encodes information about the onset, intensity, quality, location, and duration of the peripheral noxious stimulus. The input is conveyed, after considerable excitatory and inhibitory processing in the dorsal horn, via projection neurons to higher centers where it is integrated in the cortex into an acute pain sensation. Such pain has an adaptive protective role, both warning of potential tissue damage and eliciting strong reflex and behavioral avoidance responses. Through physiological modifications along this neural path, normal nociceptive pain can be transitioned to pathological pain.

II. PAIN ONTOLOGY AND PATIENT SYMPTOMOLOGY

A number of key terms are used to describe pain in both research and clinical settings, including nociceptive pain, inflammatory pain, neuropathic pain, and dysfunctional pain, although the particular usage can vary. Typically, nociceptive pain refers to pain resulting from a high-threshold stimulus acting on a basal or unenhanced nervous system. Nociceptive pain begins with the noxious stimulus and ends with the termination of the stimulus.

In contrast, amplified or enhanced pain results from changes in the peripheral or central nervous systems that promote pain sensory transduction. This amplification can serve a protective role, for example, when increased skin sensitivity to temperature following a sunburn helps prevent further injury. However, pain amplification persisting without a physiological benefit is considered chronic pathological pain.

Prior to discussing mechanisms leading to pathological pain, it is important to provide a brief overview of the core symptomology of amplified pain. Some components of these may be present in physiologically amplified pain, as in the case of a sunburn, but are generally features of chronic pain patients, particularly those suffering from neuropathic pain: (1) hyperalgesia, perception of exaggerated pain in response to a painful stimulus; (2) allodynia, perception of pain in response to a nonnoxious, low-intensity stimulus such as light touch; and (3) spontaneous pain, ongoing pain in the absence of noxious stimuli. These three manifestations constitute the trinity of pathological pain, but other features, including pain quality and localization, may provide additional information. Correlating these features and the core symptomology with specific neural mechanisms remains difficult as many features are not amenable to modeling in rodents. Furthermore, due to the subjective nature of pain perception, self-reported pain measurements are common in human studies but have no direct surrogate in basic rodent literature.

Pathological pain, especially in the laboratory environment, can be further subdivided into inflammatory pain—pain resulting from experimental injection of inflammatory substances or from an underlying inflammatory condition—or neuropathic pain, pain resulting from nerve injury or damage or dysfunction of the nervous system. In the clinic, this dichotomy is less strict, as some diseases, such as inflammatory neuropathies, blur these distinctions. Finally, dysfunctional pain is often used to describe pain without a specific identifiable causative locus; however, in many cases, this classification may simply reflect insufficient mechanistic knowledge, as suggested by some cases of fibromyalgia with small fiber neuropathy.

III. MECHANISMS OF PATHOLOGICAL PAIN

The core mechanism underlying pathological pain is increased gain of the nociceptive system. Many cellular and circuit-based mechanisms have been identified that contribute to pain amplification and can largely be grouped into peripheral and central types. Peripheral mechanisms occur within primary sensory neurons and facilitate the detection and transmission of noxious sensory stimuli. They tend to involve posttranslational modification in the phosphorylation states and intracellular trafficking of proteins, without changes in circuit structure. By contrast, central mechanisms occur within the central nervous system and usually involve new gene transcription and protein assembly, as well as changes in the synaptic connections among neurons that result in significant reorganization of neural circuitry. Peripheral and central mechanisms are not mutually exclusive and generally act on different timescales on account of different mechanisms. Typically, peripheral mechanisms activate and resolve rapidly to modify sensory processing specifically during tissue injury; central mechanisms act on longer timescales to more permanently modify nervous system form and function. Implications of these mechanisms, which are responsible for the so-called pain chronification, are guiding the development of the next generation of pain therapies and may be useful for assessing and treating pain in the clinic.

A. Peripheral Sensitization

Action potential firing in nociceptors fundamentally underlies neuronal signaling, and regulation of action potential firing is a primary method by which disease modifies pain perception. Increasing action potential firing will increase the synaptic input to central pain-processing centers and amplify pain. Increased excitability can manifest as reduced activation threshold—and thereby allodynia—or by increased output, and thereby hyperalgesia. Furthermore, spontaneous pain may result from sufficiently increased nociceptor excitability alone or from inflammatory mediators attaining the ability to activate sensitized nociceptors without any peripheral stimulus. The positioning of nociceptor excitability to influence all three major pain phenotypes has led to intense interest in reversing nociceptor hyperexcitability in chronic pain.

Nociceptor hyperexcitability has been observed in rodent models of both inflammation and painful neuropathy. Hyperexcitability can occur in response to direct activation of transduction channels, through autosensitization, and by extrinsic sensitizing stimuli. One example of autosensitization is the activity-dependent phosphorylation of TRPV1, via calcium-dependent protein kinase C activation, which leads to reduction of the activation threshold from 43°C to 38°C. In this instance, activation of TRPV1 channels through a normal thermosensation is sufficient to increase the activity of TRPV1 channels, albeit through a second-messenger signaling cascade. By contrast, heterosensitization requires input from a distinct set of signal detection molecules. A classic example of heterosensitization is the phosphorylation of Na_V channels elicited by activation of prostaglandin, bradykinin, serotonin, and nerve growth factor receptors. Activation of these G-protein–coupled and tyrosine kinase receptors synergistically activates intracellular kinases and increases current flow through nociceptor-specific Na_V channels. Although the distinction between these mechanisms may seem minor, there are substantial implications for therapy development. An analgesic that inhibits a self-sensitizing channel may be effective at reducing both the development and expression of pathological pain, whereas the effect of a heterosensitization inhibitor will depend on the specific molecular target.

B. Peripheral Respecification

Nociceptor respecification—modifying the sensitivity of individual sensory neurons to specific stimulus types—can be thought of as a specific form of hyperexcitability in which "silent" or previously nonnociceptive afferents gain either sensitivity to novel stimuli or the capacity to activate downstream pain signaling pathways. Increasing the number of neurons that respond to a given stimulus may increase overall perception, manifesting as hyperalgesia, and may recruit additional CNS structures to pain processing, potentially manifesting as allodynia. The evidence for mechanically and thermally insensitive afferent fibers and their recruitment by inflammatory stimuli is strong; however, the broad involvement of this mechanism in other painful diseases is less clear. The specific cellular mechanisms that drive this process are likely highly overlapping with heterosensitization mechanisms described earlier; thus, therapeutic strategies that reduce hyperexcitability may also effectively mitigate nociceptor respecification.

C. Synaptic Potentiation

Synaptic plasticity—involving postsynaptic *N*-methyl-D-aspartate (NMDA)–type ionotropic glutamate receptors—is a fundamental process by which the activity regulates nervous system function, and a long-standing hypothesis in chronic pain is that synaptic plasticity is fundamental to pain chronification. NMDA-type glutamate receptors conduct substantially more calcium than most AMPA-type glutamate receptors and contribute to calcium-mediated gene expression changes promoting pain. Potentiation of synaptic input from nociceptors to the spinal cord dorsal horn increases activation of central pain-processing pathways and manifests as hyperalgesia. Furthermore, a combination of increased spontaneous transmission and increased postsynaptic sensitivity (as well as reduction in inhibitory inputs onto pronociceptive dorsal horn neurons, as we described later) could manifest as spontaneous pain. The relationship between nociceptor hyperexcitability and synaptic potentiation is complex. Synaptic transmission necessarily depends on action potential firing, and synaptic plasticity can either positively or negatively regulate synaptic glutamate release. When action potentials reach central, presynaptic nociceptor terminals, voltage-dependent calcium entry elicits vesicle fusion and release of synaptic glutamate. Increasing the rate at which action potentials arrive at the terminal increases glutamate release and synaptic signaling. From here, either neurons can homeostatically depress synapses in a compensatory manner to restore normal synaptic activity in the context of nociceptor hyperexcitability or they can lock in the synaptic potentiation to permanently boost the synaptic response for each invading action potential. These processes—synaptic depression and facilitation—are common throughout the nervous system, and targets that are specific to nociceptors are rare. Several common therapies, including opioids and gabapentinoids, aim to reduce synaptic transmission by reducing voltage-dependent calcium influx at nociceptor terminals.

D. Synaptic Sprouting

Synaptic sprouting—generation of new synaptic contacts between primary and secondary neurons—has a long history as a potential contributor to mechanical allodynia. This mechanism may parallel synaptic activity changes or function in concert, but the cellular mechanisms are likely distinct. The core hypothesis is that activity changes in nonnociceptive A-β fiber low-threshold mechanoreceptors resulting from injury or inflammation induce formation of new synapses with superficial dorsal horn neurons that normally receive nociceptor input specifically. Transmission of nonnociceptive information to pain-processing pathways in the spinal cord would lead to perception of light touch as painful, the classic definition of allodynia. Synaptic sprouting has been observed in models of spinal cord injury, peripheral nerve injury, and cancer pain, but specific protein targets have not been identified, and no current therapies are thought to act by preventing sprouting or specifically silencing sprouted synapses.

E. Opening the Gate

In addition to primary sensory neurons, secondary neurons in the spinal cord dorsal horn are key components of the pain sensory transduction pathway and major contributors to pathological pain. When sensory information enters the spinal cord, signals are relayed to multiple populations of inhibitory and excitatory interneurons as well as projection neurons. Ongoing efforts seek to classify spinal cord interneuron populations—based on input selectivity, morphology, excitability, firing pattern, anatomical location, and connectivity—and understand how such complex circuitry impacts sensory processing. These efforts were inspired by the formulation of the gate theory by Melzack and Wall in the early 1960s. The gate theory, in essence, combines labeled line and pattern theory and identifies gates that function to maintain separation between noxious and nonnoxious stimuli while allowing for circuit interactions. Biologically, these gates are now understood to be at least partially made of interneuron populations, some of which have been identified. The basal activity of inhibitory neurons can restrict the amplification and transmission of nociceptive signaling to the brain. For example, parvalbumin-expressing inhibitory interneurons act as a gate to prevent the spread of light-touch information to pain processing areas, and neuropeptide Y–expressing inhibitory interneurons gate mechanical itch. Modification of these gates has powerful effects on sensory processing and contributes significantly to pathological pain. Two cellular mechanisms have been identified that modify gate function, both reducing inhibition in the spinal cord dorsal horn.

1. Inhibitory Interneuron Death

One mechanism by which inhibitory gates can be opened is by the death of inhibitory interneurons. Inhibitory interneuron loss has been observed in cancer pain and nerve injury models of pain. Inhibitory interneuron death may be due to inflammatory activation and migration of immune cells into the spinal cord or may be due to excitotoxic stress. Loss of inhibitory interneurons could manifest in many ways, from increased spontaneous pain to allodynia to hyperalgesia. Several therapeutic strategies are being pursued to restore inhibition, including transplantation of new inhibitory neurons to restore gate function and potentiation of inhibitory synapses from remaining inhibitory neurons. It should be noted that studies directly measuring apoptosis of spinal inhibitory interneurons following nerve injury failed to observe significant cell death, even in the presence of clear tactile allodynia. Thus, perhaps a more nuanced view of inhibitory interneuron loss, in which merely their function is inhibited, may be required.

2. Modification of Chloride Gradient

The second mechanism by which inhibitory gates may be opened is by decreasing the efficacy of inhibitory synapses. GABA and glycine are the primary inhibitory neurotransmitters in the spinal cord, and both act through chloride ion channels. Chloride ion flow through GABA-A and glycine receptors, under physiological conditions of low intracellular and high extracellular concentration, hyperpolarizes postsynaptic membranes, decreasing the probability of action potential firing; however, under conditions of high intracellular chloride, for example, early in development, ion flow reverses direction and can actually mediate membrane depolarization and promote action potential firing. In mature neurons, including neurons in the nociceptive sensory transduction pathway, the chloride gradient is maintained by the potassium-chloride exchanger KCC2. However, KCC2 levels are decreased by inflammation and spinal cord injury. The effect of disrupting the chloride gradient is to broadly disrupt inhibition and induce symptoms similar to death of inhibitory interneurons. The implications of this mechanism for therapeutic strategy are critical: pharmacological potentiation of GABA and glycine receptor–mediated inhibition and transplantation of new inhibitory interneurons both would be ineffective. Rather, the optimal treatment would be to restore the chloride gradient in order to increase the efficacy of endogenous inhibitory circuits. Specific targets within the spinal cord that maintain the chloride gradient have not been identified, and global manipulation of chloride via KCC2 may be limited.

F. Descending Pain Control

Several discrete brain areas send descending projections to the spinal cord and modulate sensory signaling via adrenergic, dopaminergic, serotonergic, and endogenous opioid signaling. The best studied examples of descending pain control involve opioid-rich regions in the brain stem, such as the periaqueductal gray. Electrical stimulation of such regions yields analgesia that is at least partially reversed by opioid inhibitors. Under physiological conditions, descending projections primarily inhibit pain transmission but, in the context of central sensitization, may transition to pain-promoting signals, at least partially due to changes in the chloride gradient.

G. Encoding Pain in the Brain

The existence of central pain syndromes, that is, pain resulting from central injury such as occurs in thalamic pain syndrome, has led some researchers to focus on the encoding of pain at the brain level, rather than the spinal or peripheral levels. Many functional MRI and PET studies show differences between pain regions activated in acute nociceptive pain vs chronic pain. As might be expected, noxious stimuli in healthy controls primarily result in activation of the thalamic termini of the spinothalamic tract—the ventral posterolateral and posteromedial nuclei—as well as the primary and associated sensory cortices. By contrast, for patients experiencing pathological pain, noxious and allodynic stimuli recruit broad regions of the limbic system including the medial prefrontal cortex, amygdala, and insula.

IV. TOWARD MECHANISM-BASED DIAGNOSIS AND THERAPY

The current clinical evaluation of pain uses an etiologic or disease-based approach. We advocate that this approach be modified to incorporate mechanism- and genetic-based diagnosis and therapy selection. There is no doubt that identifying a causative disease is essential, particularly where disease-modifying treatment is required. However, in many patients with persistent pain, for example, those with major nerve or spinal cord injury, the disease or pathology may be untreatable. In such cases, it is helpful to consider pain as the disease and to attempt to identify the mechanisms responsible for the pain, rather than categorizing the patient only by disease or symptomology.

The conventional assessment of pain syndromes includes identifying the causative disease, anatomical referral pattern of pain, and some quantitative global evaluation (such as the visual analog scale [VAS]). This approach groups patients into categories or syndromes such as neuropathic pain, headache, osteoarthritic pain, or cancer pain. Ideally, patients within these categories would preferentially respond to a particular analgesic, many of which have identified mechanisms of action; however, this is not the case, and there is poor correlation between the efficacy of such analgesics and pain syndromes in clinical practice.

The goal of a mechanism-based assessment of pain is to provide an improved classification system that will aid the rational diagnosis and treatment of pain. Some components may come from an assessment of basal pain sensitivity and key aspects of the nature of the patient's symptoms. Another will come from genetic analysis that may reveal both proclivities for pain in specific individuals and pharmacokinetic differences that would render one treatment ineffective but another beneficial. Unbiased sensory threshold testing and functional imaging may each add additional information to help improve classification and infer the main mechanism responsible for pain. This strategy will produce a new clinical pain record based on the nature of the reported pain to supplement the standard history and physical as well as additional unbiased characterization. We believe that breaking down pain into components that reflect some of the major mechanisms may help identify how and why certain treatments work and direct therapeutic development to connect pain mechanisms and effective treatments.

A. Genetics of Pain Mechanisms

Although pain genetics, similar to pain symptomology, is distinct from pain mechanisms, there is great value in understanding how genetic differences affect pain pathology. Genetic haplotypes may predispose individuals to activation of specific pain mechanisms, and use of genetic testing may be useful for developing a refined mechanism-based approach to diagnosis and treatment. Modern genetic studies, such as the human genome project as well as other large-scale genomic analyses specific to pain, have enabled substantial progress in identifying genetic risk variants as well as novel protein targets for analgesic development. Many risk genes encode proteins involved in neurotransmission and neuronal signaling. Most strikingly, mutations in SCN9A, which encodes the sensory neuron–specific sodium channel $Na_V1.7$, can induce congenital insensitivity to pain (CIP), familial erythromelalgia (FE), or paroxysmal extreme pain syndrome

(PEPS). CIP patients experience little or no pain due to homozygous mutations in SCN9A that prevent channel formation. Affected children have been known to walk on coals or stick knives through their arms as pranks; unfortunately, the lack of pain leads to shortened lives, underscoring the evolutionary importance of pain. By contrast, FE and PEPS, characterized by episodes of red, swollen, hot, and painful extremities, are caused by mutations that increase the activity of $Na_V1.7$ channels. Although these disorders are extremely uncommon, genetic analysis of more common syndromes, such as small fiber neuropathy, has revealed relatively common haplotypes in genes such as SCN9A, SCN10A, and SCN11A that may contribute to pathological pain. Our understanding of how specific genetic haplotypes—or multifactorial genetic risks—correlate with particular pain mechanisms is still in its infancy, but it is an important area of ongoing study.

V. IMPLICATIONS FOR EVALUATION OF NEW THERAPIES

A major problem in clinical studies of pain is the high intra- and interpatient variability in pain scoring using global outcome measures and, therefore, the enormous difficulty in evaluating the efficacy of novel analgesics. The usual explanations for the variability are the complexity of pain mechanisms, changes in the primary disease, and psychologic factors. We think another approach is therefore called for, one that leverages mechanism-specific patient assessment and unbiased biomarkers of pain state as well as drug activity.

If a new therapy is selected only on the basis of a heterogeneous individual disease (eg, diabetic neuropathy) or as often happens simply broad neuropathic pain, and the clinical outcome measure is a simple global pain measure (eg, a VAS score of pain at rest), it is simply not possible to assess whether or not the treatment acts on a particular mechanism and reduces a particular symptom (eg, tactile or cold allodynia). The degree and different mechanistic components may differ considerably within this cohort of patients, and any treatment under investigation will produce highly varied responses across the population. Once drugs are available that act specifically on validated pharmacologic targets such as $Na_V1.7$, patients will need to be selected to reduce heterogeneity. The outcome measures, both clinical and biomarker, must be designed to reflect the modulation of the specific target. For example, because TRPV1 is involved in encoding heat pain, a TRPV1 antagonist might not be expected to have a large effect on a patient with tactile allodynia. The selection of patients based on current categories, because they are not mechanism-based, is likely to include patients with quite different mechanisms. In this case, patient nonresponders may produce a negative study by diluting out the benefit in a subgroup with the targeted mechanism.

VI. CONCLUSION

Pathological pain results from the complex interplay of disease factors and pain mechanisms. Pain mechanisms act on multiple timescales and at multiple anatomical sites to produce specific symptoms. Correlation between current diagnostic classifications and identified pain mechanisms is poor, resulting in ineffective therapy selection and misalignment of patient populations and therapeutic target for clinical studies. We propose that by aligning diagnosis with validated pain mechanisms, therapy selection will improve and development of new analgesics will become more successful.

Selected Readings

Decosterd I, Allchrone AJ, Woolf CJ. Differential analgesic sensitivity of two distinct neuropathic pain models. *Anesth Analg.* 2004;99:457-463.
Jordt SE, McKemy DD, Julius D. Lessons from peppers and peppermint: the molecular logic of thermosensation. *Curr Opin Neurobiol.* 2003;13:487-492.
Siddall PJ, Cousins MJ. Persistent pain as a disease entity: implications for clinical management. *Anesth Analg.* 2004;99:510-520.
Sindrup SH, Jensen TS. Efficacy of pharmacological treatments of neuropathic pain: an update and effect related to mechanism of drug action. *Pain.* 1999;83:389-400.
Scholz J, Woolf CJ. Can we conquer pain? *Nat Neurosci.* 2002;(suppl 5):1062-1067.
Woolf CJ, Decosterd I. Implication for recent advances in the understanding of pain pathophysiology for the assessment of pain in patients. *Pain.* 1999;6:S141-S147.
Woolf CJ, Salter MW. Neuronal plasticity: increasing the gain in pain. *Science.* 2000;288:1765-1769.

3 Ethics of Pain Management

Mark C. Bicket

Clinicians have encountered ethical issues since time immemorial, and today's practice of pain medicine stands as no exception. Modern-day ethical teachings build on a lengthy history that includes the 5th century's *Formula Comitis Archiatrorum*, the first code of medical ethics, and al-Rohawi's *Ethics of a Physician*, the first medical ethics book published in the 9th century. A considerable growth in medical ethics as a field over the past century has accompanied the acknowledgment of highly publicized cases involving physicians and patients such as the Nuremberg Doctors' Trial in the 1940s, Henry Beecher's exposé on clinical research ethics in 1966, the Tuskegee syphilis experiment termination in 1972 followed by the seminal publication of the Belmont Report later that decade, and renewed interest in the story of Henrietta Lacks' HeLa immortal cell line.

Most modern practitioners of pain medicine have trained in environments emphasizing formal didactics on ethics during medical school. Vowing to uphold the Hippocratic Oath represents a standard component of many medical school commencement exercises. However, both clinicians individually and the specialties at large face challenges that act to displace the primacy of patient-centered care. The list of ethical challenges related to research is easy to enumerate. However, the desire to maximize financial compensation for individual pain physicians, group practices, or larger health care organizations represents perhaps the most significant ethical challenge confronting pain medicine today. In addition to improper pharmacologic management (via "pill mills"), the excessive use of interventional procedures represents clear violations of ethical behavior for pain physicians. Although egregious unethical behavior may be easy to identify, pain medicine as a specialty also presents more subtle and nuanced clinical challenges of an inherently ethical nature.

I. ETHICAL FRAMEWORKS

Ethical issues may be approached in a deliberate manner using the perspective of an ethical framework. The *four principles*, perhaps the most popular and well-known contemporary approach, offer an abstract and theoretical viewpoint to frame challenging clinical situations. This *traditional approach* builds on a principled-based foundation of ethical reasoning, which readily addresses unique or unusual clinical situations. Other examples of traditional frameworks include the *four-quadrant approach* and *CARE*. However, clinicians also find ethical challenges embedded within otherwise "routine" clinical encounters and need an ethical approach to their everyday clinical practice. Finally, *microethics* provides a complementary perspective to traditional approaches by focusing on the patient-clinician interaction.

A. Four Principles

Since its creation in 1985, Beauchamp and Childress' *four principles* serve as canon within any medical ethics curriculum. The principles include the following:

1. Nonmaleficence

The prevention and relief of pain fall within this principle, often described in the dictum "first, do no harm." We should not cause avoidable or preventable harm to a patient. Consequently, heroic interventions that incur a significant risk out of proportion to the benefit to the patient should be avoided.

2. Beneficence

Clinicians help patients and act in their best interest. We have a fiduciary responsibility, meaning we place and honor their interests above those of other competing entities (financial or professional self-interest, third-party interests such as insurance, pharmaceutical, or device companies).

3. Autonomy

Personal decision-making by the patient, including the provision of complete information regarding treatment options (such as risks and benefits, both known and unknown) should be preserved.

4. Justice

Synonymous with fairness, justice covers both the need to strive to eliminate treatment disparities among diverse patient populations and the need to distribute resources equitably in society.

B. Four-Quadrant Approach

An ordered series of clinical questions serves as a more specific guide to ethics in the *four-quadrant* approach by Jonsen (2010). Each quadrant blends different combinations of Beauchamp and Childress' four principles.

1. Indications for Medical Intervention

What is the patient's medical problem/diagnosis? What are the options and goals of treatment? What is the prognosis for each of those options?

2. Patient Preferences

If the patient is competent, what does she want? If not, then what is in the patient's best interest?

3. Quality of Life

What change in quality of life can the patient anticipate from the treatment? Will it improve quality of life?

4. Contextual Features

What religious, cultural, legal, and societal factors impact this decision?

C. CARE

This four-question approach by Schneider and Snell (2000) strives to acknowledge both individual and collective factors that enter into ethical decisions in the clinical environment. Thoughts and concepts represent interior factors while actions and knowledge exterior.

1. Core Beliefs: Interior Individual

What are my core beliefs and how do they relate to this situation?

2. Actions: Exterior Individual

What are my actions in the past when faced with similar situations? What do I like about what I have done? What do I not like?

3. Reasons: Interior Collective

What are the reasons others have for their opinions about similar situations? What does our culture seem to say about the situation?

4. Experience: Exterior Collective

What has been the experience of others in the past when faced with similar situations? What do I like about what they have done? What do I not like?

D. Microethics

Everyday clinical practice involves ethical issues between clinicians and patients from the standpoint of *microethics*. The spectrum of ethical considerations involves even those clinical decisions that appear to be straightforward at face value. Because a patient's values and preferences may differ based on how a clinician frames a problem, maintaining self-awareness and managing biases assume greater importance from this standpoint for the clinician. Three themes emerge in clinically focused applications of microethics:

1. Respecting and Constructing Patient Values and Preferences

Unlike a recipe in which clinicians provide facts, patients provide values, and medical decisions emerge, the clinician-patient interaction should help a patient to identify and understand her value system in the process of making a medical decision.

2. Self-awareness and Management of Clinician Values and Biases

A clinician's biases and value set should be acknowledged to the patient, even if they are not perceived to be influential in the patient's decision-making. This includes recognition that conscious and unconscious biases may be present.

3. Managing Medical Information

The unique needs of each patient may be best served by tailoring the medical information provided to the patient. The amount of information, as well as the context of information, needed may vary depending on the patient (Table 3.1).

II. EXAMPLES OF ETHICAL APPLICATIONS IN PAIN MEDICINE

A. Nonopioid Pharmacologic Options

1. Case

A 48-year-old man presents to the pain clinic for initial evaluation at a pain center with a chief complaint of chronic testicular pain. For the past 8 years, sharp and lancinating pains involving the left testicle have been present. Besides avoidance of sexual activity due to pain, he denies the presence of other concerning genitourinary symptoms. Over a 6-year period, he has seen various specialists, including at least four other pain

TABLE 3.1 Ethical Frameworks and Descriptions of Underlying Concepts

Framework	Description
Four Principles	
Nonmaleficence	• A physician should not intentionally inflict harm.
Beneficence	• Patient welfare should take a physician's precedence.
Autonomy	• A patient should make decisions for his or herself using complete information.
Justice	• Patients with similar circumstances or conditions should be treated alike.
Four-Quadrant Approach	
Medical indications	• What are the patient's medical background, current problem, and leading diagnosis? • What treatment goals are present and what is the likelihood of success? • What benefit can be anticipated? What harm can be avoided?
Patient preferences	• Is the patient competent? If so, what preferences exist? If not, how will surrogacy be established and built on existing patient preferences? • Is patient choice being upheld and maximized as much as possible?
Quality of life (QOL)	• What outcomes could be anticipated from care, both good and bad? • What physician biases may be present regarding QOL? • What role might palliation or no treatment play?
Contextual features	• How do family, financial, spiritual, legal, institutional, and health care system factors impact care decisions? • What research, teaching, or factors are present?
CARE	
Core beliefs	• What main convictions do I hold, and how do they apply to this scenario?
Actions	• When faced with a similar scenario in the past, how have I acted? How do I feel about that?
Reasons	• What is the basis for the beliefs of other people or communities about a similar scenario?
Experience	• What has the past involvement in similar scenarios revealed? How do I feel about that?
Microethics	
Respect for patients	• As medical decisions are made, physicians should help patients identify their value systems.
Self-awareness	• Physician biases should be acknowledged to patients, even if not believed to be influencing decision-making.
Information management	• Physicians should give patients personalized amounts of information for decision-making.

clinics, in attempts to address this pain. Documentation of a urological workup with unrevealing testicular examination and imaging was present. He noted no trials of neuropathic pain medications at any previous point in time.

Because the persistent testicular pain appeared to have a neuropathic character, after a discussion of treatment considerations, gabapentin was initiated. After 4 weeks of therapy, the patient returned to the clinic noting amelioration of pain and return to functioning from use of the single neuropathic agent.

2. Discussion

If an inexpensive medication with a low-risk to high-benefit profile has an unknown but likely low probably to confer benefit, why had no prior clinician prescribed trial of the therapy? Perhaps, some physicians were unaware of the role for neuropathic pain medicine, but the clinicians at the pain clinics should have had the requisite knowledge for that decision. An argument may be made that some chronic pain patients have characteristics similar to other vulnerable treatment populations given the degree of suffering experienced by the patient in combination with a willingness to trial therapies that have unclear or little formal evidence base. It is not in the role of the clinician to punish patients by withholding therapy.

B. Opioids and Interventions

1. Case

A 24-year-old man presents to the pain clinic for initial evaluation at a pain center with a chief complaint of chronic axial low back pain for 1 year. He has been maintained on long-acting opioid therapy for the past year, previously prescribed by a pain physician. During that time, he received a series of six interventions to address his chronic axial low back pain. None of the interventions provided significant analgesia, and the pain physician has indicated an unwillingness to continue prescriptions of opioid medications. Today, the patient requests continuation of opioid therapy.

2. Discussion

Controversy exists regarding the role of chronic opioid therapy for persistent nonterminal pain. A decision to prescribe opioids for chronic noncancer pain may be made on an individual basis when considering the clinical risk and benefit, as well as the ethical considerations of such medication, when recognizing the current levels of evidence for its use. If the decision to taper opioid medications is made, there should be a specific effort to ensure that patient abandonment does not occur. Although opioid medications may not be appropriate in some clinical cases, clinicians still have an obligation to engage in non–opioid-based alternative treatments.

Another separate issue related to opioid prescribing is whether a clinician chooses to implement or defer the use of an opioid contract or agreement. Some clinics may uniformly implement agreements for all patients to ensure equality. This decision will inadvertently expose some patients who do not require such agreements to inappropriate anxiety and the possibility of an antagonistic patient-clinician relationship related to opioid prescribing. On the other hand, implementing opioid prescribing agreements for only a select group of patients may contribute to biased treatment of patients with lower socioeconomic status, minority race, and less literate backgrounds.

Finally, this case presents the unethical behavior in which one treatment potentially desired by the patient (opioid prescription) is directly linked to a financially lucrative treatment for the physician (interventional therapy).

III. CONCLUSIONS

Most physicians strive to uphold the principles of medical ethics in their everyday practice of medicine, and pain medicine as a specialty is no exception. As a field, pain medicine does encounter a unique combination of ethical challenges due to the combination of a vulnerable population (patients with persistent pain) and significant financial incentives that emphasize inappropriate types of care (the overutilization of procedures and overprescribing of opioid medications). To preserve the integrity of the field, pain medicine must maintain an ethical environment by safeguarding the patient-centered perspective of care and mitigate the misaligned monetary motivations.

Selected Readings

Beauchamp TL, Childress JF. *Principles of Biomedical Ethics.* 3rd ed. New York, NY: Oxford University Press; 1989.

Beecher HK. Ethics and clinical research. 1966. *Bull World Health Organ.* 2001;79(4): 367-372.

Brenner GJ, Kueppenbender K, Mao J, Spike J. Ethical challenges and interventional pain medicine. *Curr Pain Headache Rep.* 2012;16(1):1-8.

Jonsen AR, Siegler M, Winslade WJ. *Clinical Ethics: A Practical Approach to Ethical Decisions in Clinical Medicine.* 7th ed. New York, NY: McGraw-Hill Medical; 2010.

Markel H. "I swear by Apollo"—on taking the Hippocratic oath. *N Engl J Med.* 2004;350(20):2026-2029.

Payne R, Anderson E, Arnold R, et al. A rose by any other name: pain contracts/agreements. *Am J Bioeth.* 2010;10(11):5-12.

Relman AS. Medical professionalism in a commercialized health care market. *JAMA.* 2007;298(22):2668-2670.

Schneider GW, Snell L. C.A.R.E.: an approach for teaching ethics in medicine. *Soc Sci Med.* 2000;51(10):1563-1567.

Skloot R. *The Immortal life of Henrietta Lacks.* New York, NY: Broadway Paperbacks; 2011.

Truog RD, Brown SD, Browning D, et al. Microethics: the ethics of everyday clinical practice. *Hastings Cent Rep.* 2015;45(1):11-17.

SECTION II

Diagnosis of Pain

4 The History and Clinical Examination

Jan Slezak and Asteghik Hacobian

The key to accurate diagnosis is a comprehensive history and detailed physical examination. Combined with a review of the patient's previous records and diagnostic studies, the findings from these steps lead to a differential diagnosis and appropriate treatment. In pain medicine, most patients have seen multiple providers, have had various diagnostic tests and unsuccessful treatments, and are finally referred to the pain clinic as a last resort. With advances in research and better education of primary care providers, this trend is beginning to change, and more patients are being referred to pain management specialists at an earlier stage, with better outcomes as a result.

I. PATIENT INTERVIEW

A. Pain History

1. Development and Timing

The pain history should reveal the pain location, time of onset, intensity, character, associated symptoms, and factors aggravating and relieving the pain.

It is important to know when and how the pain started. The pain onset should be described and recorded (eg, sudden, gradual, or rapid). If the pain started gradually, identifying an exact time of onset may be difficult. In the case of a clear inciting event, the date and circumstances of the pain onset may help determine its cause. The condition of the patient at the onset of pain should be noted if possible. In cases of injuries from motor vehicle crashes or work-related injuries, the state of the patient before and at the time of the injury should be clearly understood and documented.

The time of onset of the pain can be important. If the pain event is of short duration, as in acute pain, the treatment should focus on the underlying cause. In chronic pain, the underlying cause has usually resolved, and the treatment should focus on optimal long-term pain management.

2. Intensity

The various methods used to measure pain intensity are described in Chapter 6. Because the complaint of pain is purely subjective, it can only be compared to the individual's own pain over a period; it cannot be compared to another individual's report of pain. Several scales are used for reporting the so-called level of pain. The most commonly used scale is the visual analog scale (VAS) of pain intensity. Patients using this scale are instructed to place a marker on a 100-mm continuous line between "no pain" and "worst pain imaginable." The mark is measured using a standard ruler and recorded as a numeric value between 0 and 100. An alternative method of reporting the intensity of pain is by using a verbal numeric rating scale. The patient directly assigns a number between 0 (no pain) and 10 (the worst pain imaginable). The verbal numeric rating scale is frequently used in clinical practice. Another commonly used method is a verbal categorical scale, with intensity ranging from no pain through mild, moderate, and severe to the worst possible pain.

3. Character

The patient's description of the character of pain is quite helpful in distinguishing between the different types of pain. For example, burning or "electric shocks" often describe neuropathic pain, whereas cramping usually represents nociceptive visceral pain (eg, spasm, stenosis, or obstruction). Pain described as throbbing or pounding suggests vascular involvement.

4. Evolution

The pattern of pain spread from the onset should also be noted. Some types of pain change location or spread farther out from the original area of insult or injury. The direction of the spread also provides important clues to the etiology and, ultimately, the diagnosis and treatment of the condition. An example of this is the complex regional pain syndrome (CRPS), which can start in a limited area such as a distal extremity and then spread proximally and, in some instances, even to the contralateral side.

5. Associated Symptoms

The examiner should ask about the presence of associated symptoms, including numbness, weakness, bowel and/or bladder dysfunction, edema, cold sensation, and/or loss of use of the extremity because of pain.

6. Aggravating and Relieving Factors

Aggravating factors should be elicited because they sometimes explain the pathophysiologic mechanisms of pain. Various stimuli can exacerbate pain. Exacerbating mechanical factors such as different positions or activities such as sitting, standing, walking, bending, and lifting may help differentiate one cause of pain from another. Biochemical changes (eg, glucose and electrolyte levels and hormonal imbalance), psychological factors (eg, depression, stress, and other emotional problems), and environmental triggers (eg, dietary influences and weather changes, including barometric pressure changes) may surface as important diagnostic clues. Relieving factors are also important. Certain positions will alleviate pain better than others (eg, in most cases of neurogenic claudication, sitting is a relieving factor, whereas standing or walking worsens the pain). History, physical examination, pharmacologic therapies, and "nerve blocks" and other diagnostic tests all help the clinician determine the diagnosis and select the appropriate treatment.

7. Previous Treatment

The patient should be asked about previous treatment attempts. Knowing the degree of pain relief, the duration of treatment, and the dosages and adverse reactions of medications helps avoid repeating procedures or using pharmacologic management that has not helped in the past. The list should include all treatment modalities, including physical therapy, occupational therapy, chiropractic manipulation, acupuncture, reiki, massage, psychological interventions, and visits to other pain clinics.

B. Medical History

1. Review of Systems

A review of systems is an integral part of comprehensive evaluation for chronic and acute pain. Some systems could be directly or indirectly related to the patient's presenting symptoms, whereas others are important in the management or treatment of the painful condition. Examples are the patient with a history of bleeding problems, who may not be a suitable candidate for certain injection therapies, or someone with impaired renal or hepatic function, who may need adjustments in their medication dosage.

2. Past Medical History

Past medical problems, including conditions that have resolved, should be reviewed. Previous trauma and any past or present psychological or behavioral issues should be recorded.

3. Past Surgical History

A list of operations and complications should be made, preferably in chronologic order. Because some painful chronic conditions are sequelae of surgical procedures, this information is important for diagnosis and management.

C. Drug History

1. Current Medications

The practitioner must prescribe and intervene based on medications the patient is currently taking because complications, interactions, and side effects need to be considered. A list should be made of all medications, including pain medications. The list should include nonprescription and alternative medications (eg, acetaminophen, aspirin, ibuprofen, and vitamins and other supplements).

2. Allergies

Allergies, both to medications and nonmedications (eg, latex, contrast, preservatives, food, and environmental factors), should be noted. The nature of a specific allergic reaction with each medication or agent should be clearly explored and documented.

D. Social History

1. General Social History

Understanding the patient's social structure, support systems, and motivation is essential in analyzing psychosocial factors. Whether a patient is married, has children, and works makes a difference. Level of education, job satisfaction, and general attitude toward life are important. Smoking and a history of drug or alcohol abuse are important in evaluating and designing treatment strategies. Lifestyle questions about how much time is taken for vacation or is spent in front of a television, favorite recreations and hobbies, exercise, and sleep give the practitioner a more comprehensive overview of the patient.

2. Family History

A complete family history, including health status of the patient's parents, siblings, and offspring, offers important clues for understanding a patient's biologic and genetic profile. The existence of unusual diseases should be noted. A history of chronic pain, substance abuse, and disability in family members (including the spouse) should be ascertained. Even clues that have no direct genetic or biologic basis may help by revealing coping mechanisms and codependent behavior.

3. Occupational History

The highest level of education completed by the patient and the degrees obtained should be identified. The specifics of the present job and previous employment should be noted. The amount of time spent in each job, reasons for leaving, any previous history of litigation, job satisfaction, and whether the patient works full-time or part-time are important in establishing the occupational framework. Whether the patient has undergone disability evaluation, functional capacity assessment, or vocational rehabilitation is also relevant.

II. PATIENT EXAMINATION

The clinical examination is a fundamental and valuable diagnostic tool. Over the past few decades, advances in medicine and technology and a better understanding of the pathophysiology of pain have dramatically improved the evaluation process. The lack of exact diagnosis in most patients presenting to the pain clinic underscores the need for detail-oriented examinations.

Improper coding and inadequate documentation to support charges billed to carriers for evaluation and management services incur various sanctions. Complying with regulations using appropriate documentation will not only result in proper reimbursement but also provide protection against fraud and abuse. The level of evaluation and management services that can be coded depends partly on the complexity of examination, which in turn reflects the nature of the presenting problem and the clinical judgment of the provider. Types of examinations include either general multisystem (10 organ systems—musculoskeletal, nervous, cardiovascular, respiratory, ear/nose/mouth/throat, eyes, genitourinary, hematologic/lymphatic/immune, psychiatric, and integumentary) or single-organ system examinations. In pain medicine, the most commonly examined systems are the musculoskeletal and nervous systems.

If interventions are a part of a diagnostic or therapeutic plan, the evaluation should reveal whether the patient has risk factors for the procedure being considered. Coagulopathy, untreated infection, history of MRSA, and preexisting neurologic dysfunction should be documented before placement of the needle or the catheter or before implantation of a device. Extra caution is needed when administering medications such as (1) local anesthetics to a patient with seizure disorder, (2) neuraxial anesthetics to a patient who may tolerate vasodilatation poorly, or (3) glucocorticoids to patients with diabetes. Preanesthetic evaluation should assess the patient's ability to tolerate sedation or anesthesia if indicated for a procedure.

The following sections outline a physical examination that incorporates the musculoskeletal and neurologic assessments relevant to pain practice. The examination starts with the evaluation of single systems and commonly proceeds from head to toe.

A. General Examination

1. Constitutional Factors

Height, weight, and vital signs (ie, blood pressure, heart rate, respiratory rate, body temperature, and pain level) should be measured and recorded. Appearance, development, deformities, nutrition, and grooming are noted. The room should be scanned for the presence of assistive devices brought by the patient. Patients who smoke or drink heavily may carry an odor. Observing a patient who is unaware of being watched may detect discrepancies that were not seen during the evaluation.

2. Pain Behavior

Note facial expression, color, and grimacing. Speech patterns suggest emotional factors as well as intoxication with alcohol, and with prescription or nonprescription drugs. Some patients attempt to convince the practitioner that they are suffering a great deal of pain by augmenting their verbal presentation with grunting, moaning, twitching, grabbing the painful area, exaggerating the antalgic gait or posture, or tightening muscle groups. This, unfortunately, makes the objective examination more difficult.

3. Skin

Evaluate for color, temperature, rash, and soft tissue edema. Trophic changes of the skin, nails, and hair are frequently seen in advanced stages of CRPS. In patients with diabetes, vascular disease, and peripheral neuropathy, search for defects that might be a chronic source of bacteremia requiring treatment before hardware implantation (ie, spinal cord stimulator or an infusion pump device). Psoriatic lesions may be associated with painful arthropathy.

B. System Examination

1. Cardiovascular System

A systolic murmur with propagation suggests aortic stenosis, and the patient may not tolerate the hypovolemia and tachycardia that accompany rapid vasodilatation (eg, after administration of neuraxial local anesthetics and sympathetic or celiac plexus blockade). The patient with irregular rhythm may have atrial fibrillation and may be treated with anticoagulants. The pulsation of arteries (diabetes, CRPS, and thoracic outlet syndrome), venous filling, presence of varicosities, and capillary return must be checked. Vascular claudication must be distinguished from neurogenic claudication in patients referred with a diagnosis of lumbar spinal stenosis. Growth in utilization of interventional cardiology procedures, such as coronary artery stenting, has increased the population of younger patients on many new anticoagulants.

2. Lungs

Examination of the lungs may reveal abnormal breath sounds such as crackles, which may be a sign of congestive heart failure and low cardiac reserve. Rhonchi and wheezes are signs of chronic obstructive pulmonary disease. Caution in performing injections around the chest cavity is advised because there may be an increased risk of causing pneumothorax.

3. Musculoskeletal System

The musculoskeletal system examination includes inspection of gait and posture. Deformities and deviations from symmetry are observed. After taking the history, the examiner usually has an idea about the body part from which the symptoms originate. If this is not the case, a brief survey of structures in the relevant region might be necessary. Positive tests warrant further and more rigorous evaluation of the affected segment. Palpation of soft tissues, bony structures, and stationary or moving joints may reveal temperature differences, presence of edema, fluid collections, gaps, crepitus, clicks, and tenderness. Functional comparison of left and right side, checking for normal curvature of the spine, and provocation of usual symptoms with maneuvers can help identify the mechanisms and location of the pathologic process. Examination of the range of motion may demonstrate hyper- or hypomobility of the joint. Testing active movement will determine range, muscle strength, and willingness of the patient to cooperate. Passive movements, on the other hand, when performed properly, test for pain, range, and end-feel. Most difficulties arise when examining patients who are in constant pain, because these patients tend to respond to most maneuvers positively, therefore making the specificity of tests low.

C. Specific Tests

1. Straight Leg Raising (SLR, Lasègue)

SLR tests the mobility of dura and dural sleeves from L4 to S2. The sensitivity of this test to diagnose lumbar disc herniation ranges between 0.6 and 0.97, with a specificity of 0.1-0.6. Tension on the sciatic nerve begins at 15- to 30-degree elevation in supine position. This puts traction on the nerve roots L4-S2 and on the dura. End of range is normally restricted by hamstring muscle tension at 60-120 degrees. More than 60 degrees of elevation causes movement in the sacroiliac joint and, therefore, may be painful in sacroiliac joint disorders.

2. Basic Sacroiliac Tests

Basic sacroiliac tests causing pain in the buttock: Sacroiliac tests are performed to determine when pain occurs in the buttock:

- **a.** Pushing the ilia outward and downward in supine position, with the examiner's arms crossed. If gluteal pain results, the test is repeated with the patient's forearm placed under the lumbar spine to stabilize the lumbar joints.
- **b.** Forcibly compressing the ilia to the midline with the patient lying on the painless side stretches posterior sacroiliac ligaments.
- **c.** Exert forward pressure on the center of the sacrum in a prone patient.
- **d.** Patrick or FABER test (pain due to ligamentous strain)—flexion, abduction, and external rotation of the femur in the hip joint while holding down the anterosuperior iliac spine on the contralateral side provides stretching of the anterior sacroiliac ligament.
- **e.** Force lateral rotation in the hip joint with the knee held in 90-degree flexion in a supine position.

3. Spinal Flexibility

Spinal flexion, extension, lateral bending, and rotation may be limited and/or painful in zygapophyseal joint, discogenic, muscular, and ligamentous pain.

4. Adson Test

Adson test has been used for diagnosis of thoracic outlet syndrome. The examiner evaluates the change of radial artery pulsation in a standing patient with arms resting at the side. Ipsilateral head rotation during inspiration may cause vascular compression by the anterior scalene muscle. During *modified Adson test*, the patient's head is rotated to the contralateral side. Pulse change suggests compression by the middle scalene muscle. Both tests are considered unreliable by some because the findings may be found positive in ~50% of the healthy population.

a. Tinel test: Tinel test involves percussion of the carpal tunnel. If positive, it gives rise to distal paresthesias. It can be performed at other locations (eg, cubital or tarsal tunnel), where it might be suggestive of nerve entrapment. **Phalen test** is positive for carpal tunnel syndrome when a passive flexion in the wrist for 1 minute followed by sudden extension results in sensation of paresthesias.

5. Neurologic Examination

The integrity of **cranial nerve function** is tested by the examination of visual fields, pupils and eye movement, facial sensation, facial symmetry and strength, hearing (eg, use tuning fork, whisper voice, or finger rub), spontaneous and reflex palate movement, and tongue protrusion.

The **motor system** evaluation starts with observation of **muscle** bulk, tone, and presence of spasm. Muscle strength is tested in upper and lower extremities. Weakness might be caused by unwillingness of the patient to cooperate, fear of pain provocation, poor effort, reflex neural inhibition in the painful limb, or an organic lesion. Table 4.1 summarizes the localization of cervical and lumbar radicular nerves.

Further information is obtained by examination of **deep tendon reflexes**, clonus, and pathologic reflexes such as the Babinski reflex. Evaluation of **coordination** and fine motor skills may reveal associated dysfunction.

a. Sensation is tested to light touch (Aδ fibers), pinprick (Aδ fibers), and hot and cold stimuli (Aδ and C fibers). Tactile sensation can be evaluated quantitatively with von Frey filaments. We have found the end of a broken wooden cotton-tipped swab or a toothpick, rather than safety pins, needles, or pinwheels, to be a convenient and safe tool for testing sensation to pinprick. The following are often observed in neuropathic pain conditions:

b. Hyperesthesia—Increased sensitivity to stimulation, excluding the special senses

c. Dysesthesia—An unpleasant abnormal sensation, either spontaneous or evoked

d. Allodynia—Pain caused by stimulus that normally does not provoke pain

e. Hyperalgesia—An increased response to a stimulus that is normally painful

f. Hyperpathia—A painful syndrome characterized by an abnormally painful reaction to stimulus (especially a repetitive one) and a reduced threshold

g. Summation—A repetitive pinprick stimulus applied in intervals of more than 3 seconds, with a gradually increasing sensation of pain with each subsequent stimulus

6. Mental Status Examination

The mental status examination is a part of the neuropsychiatric assessment. Examine the level of consciousness, orientation, speech, mood, affect, attitude, and thought content. The **Mini-Mental Status Exam** (MMSE) of Folstein is a useful guide for documenting a level of mental function. Five areas of mental status are tested: orientation, registration, attention and calculation, recall, and language. Each correct answer is given 1 point. A maximum score on the Folstein is 30. A score of <23 is abnormal and suggests cognitive impairment.

TABLE 4.1 Cervical and Lumbar Radicular Localization

	Spinal Nerve					
	C5	**C6**	**C7**	**L4**	**L5**	**S1**
Disc Level	**C4/5**	**C5/6**	**C6/7**	**L3/4 (L4/5)**	**L4/5 (L5/1)**	**L5/1**
Sensory changes	Lateral upper arm	Lateral forearm and first, second, and half of third digits	Third digit	Medial shin and medial foot	Lateral calf and dorsal foot	Lateral foot
Deep tendon reflex	Biceps	Brachioradialis	Triceps	Patellar	None	Achilles
Muscle tested	Deltoid and biceps	Wrist extensors	Triceps, wrist, and finger extensors	Foot inversion	Dorsiflexion of toes and foot	Plantar flexion and eversion

III. INCONSISTENCIES IN THE HISTORY AND PHYSICAL EXAMINATION

Inconsistencies in the history and physical examination, vague description of symptoms, and evidence of intense suffering, together with inappropriate pain behavior, may suggest symptom exaggeration, malingering for compensation and other gains, or psychogenic pain. The frequently cited Waddell nonorganic signs may raise suspicion in patients with lower back pain. It may be warranted to proceed with the SF-36 Health Survey or other instruments designed to identify underlying problems or issues. The Waddell nonorganic signs are grouped into five categories: tenderness, simulation, distraction, regional disturbance, and overreaction.

A. Tenderness
  1. Widespread superficial sensitivity to light touch over the lumbar spine
  2. Bone tenderness over a large lumbar area

B. Simulation
  1. Axial loading, during which light pressure is applied to the skull in the upright position
  2. Simulated rotation of the lumbar spine with the shoulders and pelvis remaining in the same plane

C. Distraction
  1. >40-degree difference in sitting vs supine SLR

D. Regional disturbance
  1. Motor—Generalized giving way or cogwheeling resistance in manual muscle testing of lower extremities
  2. Sensory—Nondermatomal loss of sensation to pinprick in lower extremities

E. Overreaction
  1. Disproportionate pain response to testing (eg, pain behavior with assisted movement using cane or walker, rigid or slow movement, rubbing or grasping the affected area for more than 3 seconds, grimacing, and sighing with shoulders rising and falling).

IV. CONCLUSION

The history and physical examinations are the foundations for pain evaluation and treatment and are essential elements of good pain management. They need to be tailored to the individual patient, the complexity of the pain problem, and the medical condition of the patient. This chapter outlines a standard history and physical examination that can be applied to most patients presenting in the pain clinic.

Selected Readings

Bogduk N. *International Spine Intervention Society Practice Guidelines for Spinal Diagnostic and Treatment Procedures.* San Francisco, CA: International Spine Intervention Society; 2013.

Benzon H. *Essentials of Pain Medicine and Regional Anesthesia.* Philadelphia, PA: Churchill Livingstone; 2005.

Kanner R. *Pain Management Secrets.* Philadelphia, PA: Hanley & Belfus; 1997.

Ombregt L. *A System of Orthopaedic Medicine.* London, UK: WB Saunders; 1997.

Raj P. *Pain Medicine: A Comprehensive Review.* St. Louis, MO: Mosby-Year Book; 1996.

Tollison D. *Handbook of Pain Management.* Philadelphia, PA: JB Lippincott; 1994.

5 Assessment of Pain

Alyssa A. Lebel

Pain is a complex multidimensional symptom determined not only by tissue injury and nociception but also by previous pain experience, personal beliefs, affect, motivation, environment, and, at times, pending litigation. **There is no objective measurement of pain.** Self-report is the most valid measure of the individual experience of pain. The pain history is key to the assessment of pain and includes the patient's description of pain intensity, quality, location, timing, and duration, as well as ameliorating and exacerbating conditions. Frequently, pain cannot be seen, defined, or felt by the physician, and the physician must assess the pain from a combination of factors. The most important of these factors is the patient's report of the pain, but other factors such as personality and culture, psychological status, the existence of secondary gain, and the possibility of drug-seeking behavior should also be considered. Reports of pain may not correlate with the degree of disability or findings on physical examination. However, it is important to remember that to the patients and their families, distress, suffering, and pain behaviors are often not distinguished from the pain itself.

Diagnosis and measurement of acute pain require frequent and consistent assessment as part of daily clinical care to ensure rapid titration of therapy and preemptive interventions. Chronic pain is often more diagnostically challenging than acute pain, but no less compelling. Application of a structured history and comprehensive physical examination will define treatable problems and identify complicating factors. Somatic, visceral, neuropathic, or combined pain problems suggest specific diagnoses and interventions. An understanding of pain pathophysiology guides rational and appropriate treatment.

I. PAIN HISTORY

The general medical history may contribute considerably and is always included as part of the pain assessment. This is described in Chapter 4. The specific pain history includes three main issues—intensity, location, and pathophysiology. The following questions help define these issues:

- What is the time course of the pain?
- Where is the pain?

- What is the intensity of the pain?
- What factors relieve or exacerbate the pain?
- What are the possible generators of the pain?

A. Pain Assessment Tools

As previously stated, pain cannot be objectively measured. The intensity of pain is one of the most difficult and perhaps frustrating characteristics of pain to pinpoint. Several tests and scales are available. Some of the more commonly used tools are the following:

1. Unidimensional Self-report Scales

In practice, self-report scales serve as very simple, useful, and valid methods for assessing and monitoring patients' pain.

a. **Verbal descriptor scales.** The patient is asked to describe his or her pain by choosing from a list of adjectives that reflect gradations of pain intensity. The five-word scale consists of *mild, discomforting, distressing, horrible*, and *excruciating*. Disadvantages of this scale include limited selection of descriptors and the fact that patients tend to select moderate descriptors rather than the extremes.

b. **Verbal numeric rating scales.** These are the simplest and most frequently used scales. On a numeric scale (most commonly 0-10, with 0 being "no pain" and 10 "the worst pain imaginable"), the patient picks a number to describe the pain. Advantages of numeric scales are their simplicity, reproducibility, easy comprehensibility, and sensitivity to small changes in pain. Children as young as 5 years old, who can count and have some concept of numbers (eg, "8 is larger than 4"), can use this scale.

c. **Visual analog scales.** Visual analog scales (VAS) are similar to the verbal numeric rating scales, except that the patient marks on a measured line, one end of which is labeled "no pain" and the other end "worst pain imaginable," where the pain falls. Visual scales are more valid for research purposes but are used less clinically because they are more time-consuming to conduct than verbal scales and require motor control.

d. **Faces pain rating scale.** Evaluating pain in children can be very difficult because of the child's inability to describe pain or to understand pain assessment forms. This scale depicts six sketches of facial features, each with a numeric value, 0-5, ranging from a happy, smiling face to a sad, teary face (see Fig. 5.1). To extrapolate this scale to the VAS, the

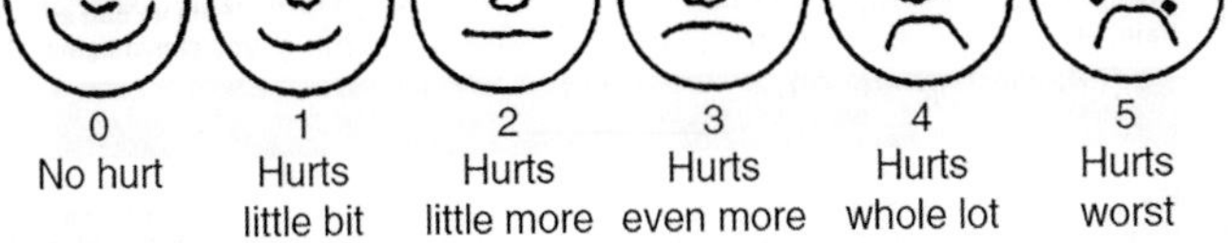

FIGURE 5.1 Wong-Baker Faces Pain Rating Scale. Explain to the person undergoing the rating that each face depicts a person who feels happy because he has no pain (hurt) or who feels sad because he has some or a lot of pain. Face 0 is very happy because he does not hurt at all. Face 1 hurts just a little bit. Face 2 hurts a little more. Face 3 hurts even more. Face 4 hurts a whole lot. Face 5 hurts as much as you can imagine, although you do not have to be crying to feel this bad. Copyright © 1983 Wong-Baker Faces Foundation. www.WongBakerFACES.org. Used with permission.

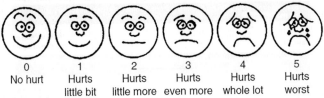

value chosen is multiplied by two. This scale may also be beneficial for intellectually impaired patients. Average children as young as 3 years can reliably use this scale.

2. Multiple Dimension Instruments

These instruments provide more complex information about the patient's pain. They are especially useful for assessment of chronic pain. Because they are time-consuming, they are most frequently used in outpatient and research settings.

STUDY ID# ________ **HOSPITAL#** ________

DO NOT WRITE ABOVE THIS LINE

Brief Pain Inventory (Short Form)

Date: __/__/__ **Time:** ________

Name: ________ ________ ________
Last **First** **Middle Initial**

1) Throughout our lives, most of us have had pain from time to time (such as minor headaches, sprains, and toothaches). Have you had pain other than these everyday kinds of pain today?

1. Yes **2. No**

2) On the diagram, shade in the areas where you feel pain. Put an X on the area that hurts the most.

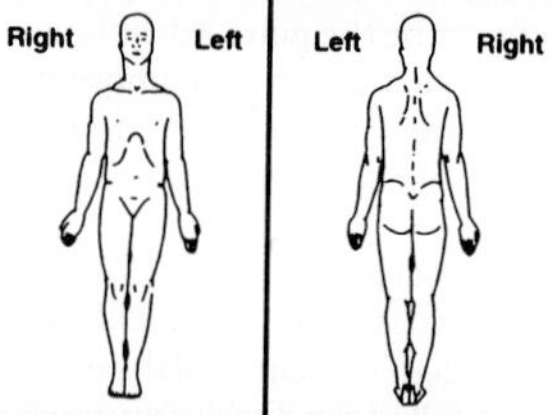

3) Please rate your pain by circling the one number that best describes your pain at its worst in the last 24 hours.

0	1	2	3	4	5	6	7	8	9	10
No Pain										Pain as bad as you can imagine

4) Please rate your pain by circling the one number that best describes your pain at its least in the last 24 hours.

0	1	2	3	4	5	6	7	8	9	10
No Pain										Pain as bad as you can imagine

5) Please rate your pain by circling the one number that best describes your pain on the average.

0	1	2	3	4	5	6	7	8	9	10
No Pain										Pain as bad as you can imagine

6) Please rate your pain by circling the one number that tells how much pain you have right now.

0	1	2	3	4	5	6	7	8	9	10
No Pain										Pain as bad as you can imagine

FIGURE 5.2 A, B. Brief pain inventory (see text). (Adapted from Zempsky WT, Schecter NL. What's new in the management of pain in children. *Ped Clin North Am.* 1989;36:823–836. Copyright © 1989 Elsevier. With permission.) **C.** The Pain Quality Assessment Scale© (PQAS-R©). This assessment tool combines some questions from the validated neuropathic pain scale with additional items that address common pain variables for several chronic pain disorders. (© Galer, Gammaitoni, & Jensen, 2010. All Rights Reserved.)

7) What treatments or medications are you receiving for your pain?

8) In the last 24 hours, how much relief have pain treatments or medications provided? Please circle the one percentage that most shows how much relief you have received.

0% No Relief	10%	20%	30%	40%	50%	60%	70%	80%	90%	100% Complete Relief

9) Circle the one number that describes how, during the past 24 hours, pain has interfered with your:

A. General activity

0 Does not interfere	1	2	3	4	5	6	7	8	9	10 Completely Interferes

B. Mood

0 Does not interfere	1	2	3	4	5	6	7	8	9	10 Completely Interferes

C. Walking ability

0 Does not interfere	1	2	3	4	5	6	7	8	9	10 Completely Interferes

D. Normal work (includes both work outside the home and housework)

0 Does not interfere	1	2	3	4	5	6	7	8	9	10 Completely Interferes

E. Relations with other people

0 Does not interfere	1	2	3	4	5	6	7	8	9	10 Completely Interferes

F. Sleep

0 Does not interfere	1	2	3	4	5	6	7	8	9	10 Completely Interferes

G. Enjoyment of life

0 Does not interfere	1	2	3	4	5	6	7	8	9	10 Completely Interferes

Pain Research Group • Department of Neurology • University of Wisconsin-Madison

FIGURE 5.2 *(Continued)*

PAIN QUALITY ASSESSMENT SCALE© (PQAS©)

Instructions: There are different aspects and types of pain that patients experience and that we are interested in measuring. Pain can feel sharp, hot, cold, dull, and achy. Some pains may feel like they are very superficial (at skin-level), or they may feel like they are from deep inside your body. Pain can also be described as unpleasant.

The Pain Quality Assessment Scale helps us measure these and other different aspects of your pain. For one patient, a pain might feel extremely hot and burning, but not at all dull, while another patient may not experience any burning pain, but feel like their pain is very dull and achy. Therefore, we expect you to rate very high on some of the scales below and very low on others.

Please use the 19 rating scales below to rate how much of each different pain quality and type you may or may not have felt *OVER THE PAST WEEK, ON AVERAGE*.

Place an "X" through the number that best describes your pain. For example:

0	1	2	3	4	5	6	7	8	9	~~10~~ (X)

1. Please use the scale below to tell us how **intense** your pain has been over the past week, on average.

No pain	0	1	2	3	4	5	6	7	8	9	10	The most **intense** pain sensation imaginable

2. Please use the scale below to tell us how **sharp** your pain has felt over the past week. Words used to describe sharp feelings include "like a knife", "like a spike", or "piercing".

Not sharp	0	1	2	3	4	5	6	7	8	9	10	The most **sharp** sensation imaginable ("like a knife")

3. Please use the scale below to tell us how **hot** your pain has felt over the past week. Words used to describe very hot pain include "burning" and "on fire".

Not hot	0	1	2	3	4	5	6	7	8	9	10	The most **hot** sensation imaginable ("burning")

4. Please use the scale below to tell us how **dull** your pain has felt over the past week.

Not dull	0	1	2	3	4	5	6	7	8	9	10	The most **dull** sensation imaginable

5. Please use the scale below to tell us how **cold** your pain has felt over the past week. Words used to describe very cold pain include "like ice" and "freezing".

Not cold	0	1	2	3	4	5	6	7	8	9	10	The most **cold** sensation imaginable ("freezing")

6. Please use the scale below to tell us how **sensitive** your skin has been to light touch or clothing rubbing against it over the past week. Words used to describe sensitive skin include "like sunburned skin" and "raw skin".

Not sensitive	0	1	2	3	4	5	6	7	8	9	10	The most **sensitive** sensation imaginable ("raw skin")

FIGURE 5.2 *(Continued)*

7. Please use the scale below to tell us how **tender** your pain is when something has pressed against it over the past week. Another word used to describe tender pain is "like a bruise".

Not tender	0	1	2	3	4	5	6	7	8	9	10	The most **tender** sensation imaginable ("like a bruise")

8. Please use the scale below to tell us how **itchy** your pain has felt over the past week. Words used to describe itchy pain include "like poison ivy" and "like a mosquito bite".

Not itchy	0	1	2	3	4	5	6	7	8	9	10	The most **itchy** sensation imaginable ("like poison ivy")

9. Please use the scale below to tell us how much your pain has felt like it has been **shooting** over the past week. Another word used to describe shooting pain is "zapping".

Not shooting	0	1	2	3	4	5	6	7	8	9	10	The most **shooting** sensation imaginable ("zapping")

10. Please use the scale below to tell us how **numb** your pain has felt over the past week. A phrase that can be used to describe numb pain is "like it is asleep".

Not numb	0	1	2	3	4	5	6	7	8	9	10	The most **numb** sensation imaginable ("asleep")

11. Please use the scale below to tell us how much your pain sensations have felt **electrical** over the past week. Words used to describe electrical pain include "shocks", "lightning", and "sparking".

Not electrical	0	1	2	3	4	5	6	7	8	9	10	The most **electrical** sensation imaginable ("shocks")

12. Please use the scale below to tell us how **tingling** your pain has felt over the past week. Words used to describe tingling pain include "like pins and needles" and "prickling".

Not tingling	0	1	2	3	4	5	6	7	8	9	10	The most **tingling** sensation imaginable ("pins and needles")

13. Please use the scale below to tell us how **cramping** your pain has felt over the past week. Words used to describe cramping pain include "squeezing" and "tight".

Not cramping	0	1	2	3	4	5	6	7	8	9	10	The most **cramping** sensation imaginable ("squeezing")

14. Please use the scale below to tell us how **radiating** your pain has felt over the past week. Another word used to describe radiating pain is "spreading".

Not radiating	0	1	2	3	4	5	6	7	8	9	10	The most **radiating** sensation imaginable ("spreading")

15. Please use the scale below to tell us how **throbbing** your pain has felt over the past week. Another word used to describe throbbing pain is "pounding".

Not throbbing	0	1	2	3	4	5	6	7	8	9	10	The most **throbbing** sensation imaginable ("pounding")

FIGURE 5.2 *(Continued)*

16. Please use the scale below to tell us how **aching** your pain has felt over the past week. Another word used to describe aching pain is "like a toothache".

Not aching	0	1	2	3	4	5	6	7	8	9	10	The most **aching** sensation imaginable ("like a toothache")

17. Please use the scale below to tell us how **heavy** your pain has felt over the past week. Other words used to describe heavy pain are "pressure" and "weighted down".

Not heavy	0	1	2	3	4	5	6	7	8	9	10	The most **heavy** sensation imaginable ("weighted down")

18. Now that you have told us the different types of pain sensations you have felt, we want you to tell us overall how **unpleasant** your pain has been to you over the past week. Words used to describe very unpleasant pain include "annoying," "bothersome," "miserable," and "intolerable". Remember, pain can have a low intensity but still feel extremely unpleasant, and some kinds of pain can have a high intensity but be very tolerable. With this scale, please tell us how **unpleasant** your pain feels.

Not unpleasant	0	1	2	3	4	5	6	7	8	9	10	The most **unpleasant** sensation imaginable ("intolerable")

19. Finally, we want you to give us an estimate of the severity of your deep versus surface pain over the past week. We want you to rate each location of pain separately. We realize that it can be difficult to make these estimates, and most likely it will be a "best guess," but please give us your best estimate.

HOW INTENSE IS YOUR *DEEP* PAIN?

No **deep** pain	0	1	2	3	4	5	6	7	8	9	10	The most **intense** **deep** pain sensation imaginable

HOW INTENSE IS YOUR *SURFACE* PAIN?

No **surface** pain	0	1	2	3	4	5	6	7	8	9	10	The most **intense** **surface** pain sensation imaginable

20. Pain can also have different time qualities. For some people, the pain comes and goes and so they have some moments that are completely without pain; in other words the pain "comes and goes". This is called **intermittent** pain. Others are never pain free, but their pain types and pain severity can vary from one moment to the next. This is called **variable** pain. For these people, the increases can be severe, so that they feel they have moments of very intense pain ("breakthrough" pain), but at other times they can feel lower levels of pain ("background" pain). Still, they are never pain free. Other people have pain that really does not change that much from one moment to another. This is called **stable** pain. Which of these best describes the time pattern of your pain (please select only one):

( ) I have **intermittent** pain (I feel pain sometimes but I am pain-free at other times).
( ) I have **variable** pain ("background" pain all the time, but also moments of more pain, or even severe "breakthrough pain or varying types of pain).
( ) I have **stable** pain (constant pain that does not change very much from one moment to another, and no pain-free periods).

FIGURE 5.2 *(Continued)*

a. **McGill pain questionnaire.** McGill pain questionnaire (MPQ) is the most frequently used multidimensional test. Descriptive words from 3 major dimensions of pain (ie, sensory, affective, and evaluative) are further subdivided into 20 subclasses, each containing words of varying degrees. Three scores are obtained, one for each dimension, and a total score is calculated. Studies have shown the MPQ to be a reliable instrument in clinical research.

b. **Brief pain inventory.** In brief pain inventory (BPI), patients are asked to rate the severity of their pain at its "worst," "least," or "average," within the past 24 hours and at the time the rating is done. The inventory also requires the patients to represent the location of their pain on a schematic diagram of the body. The BPI correlates with the scores of activity, sleep, and social interactions. It is cross-cultural and a useful method for clinical studies (see Figs. 5.2 and 5.3).

M.G.H. PAIN CENTER
PAIN ASSESSMENT FORM

Information About the Pain

1. What is the problem you would like us to help you with?

2. Please mark the event or events that led to your present pain: (If you experience more than one kind of pain, please write in separate sets of answers for each type of pain you have.)

___ Accident ___ Cancer

___ Other injury ___ ___ No obvious cause

___ Following an operation ___ Other disease ___

___ Other ___

3. For how long have you had this pain?

4. How often does the pain occur?

___ Continuously (nonstop)

___ Several times a day

___ Once or twice a day

___ Several times a week

___ Less than 3 or 4 times per month

5. How has the *intensity* of the pain changed throughout the time you have had it?

___ Increased ___ Decreased ___ Stayed the same

6. The following five words represent pain of increasing intensity:

1 Mild 2 Discomforting 3 Distressing

4 Horrible 5 Excruciating

To answer each question below, write the *number* of the most appropriate word in the space beside the question.

a. Which word describes your pain at its worst? ___

b. Which word describes your pain at its least? ___

c. Which word describes your pain right now? ___

d. Which word describes how your pain is most of the time? ___

7. Location of the Pain
(please shadow in the affected areas).

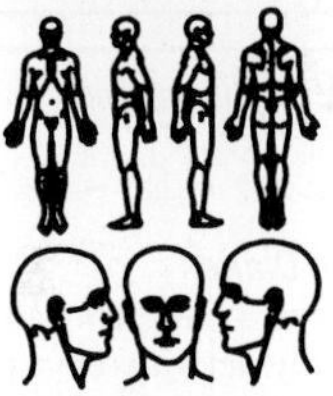

8. Quality of the Pain

Below is list of words that are often used to describe pain. After each descriptive word, indicate with a checkmark whether this word describes a particular quality of your pain and, if it does, the intensity of that quality.

	None (not at all)	Mild	Moderate	Severe
Throbbing	0)	1)	2)	3)
Shooting	0)	1)	2)	3)
Stabbing	0)	1)	2)	3)
Sharp	0)	1)	2)	3)
Cramping	0)	1)	2)	3)
Gnawing	0)	1)	2)	3)
Hot-Burning	0)	1)	2)	3)
Aching	0)	1)	2)	3)
Heavy	0)	1)	2)	3)
Tender	0)	1)	2)	3)
Splitting	0)	1)	2)	3)
Tiring/Exhausting	0)	1)	2)	3)
Sickening	0)	1)	2)	3)
Fearful	0)	1)	2)	3)
Punishing/Cruel	0)	1)	2)	3)

9. Which of the following have an effect on your pain? Please indicate whether it makes the pain *better*, *worse*, or has *no effect*.

___ Heat ___ Cold ___ Noise

___ Sitting ___ Standing ___ Lying down

___ Walking ___ Fatigue ___ Particular position or movement explain: ___

___ Coughing ___ Anxiety/emotions

___ Vibration ___ Massage/rubbing ___ Caffeinated drinks (coffee, tea, colas)

___ Climate ___ Alcoholic beverages

10. How does the pain affect your activity in these different areas:

Work-school–
Household chores–
Social interactions–
Leisure–
Sexual activity–

11. What is your current employment status?

12. Do you have pending a settlement about disability, workers' compensation, or a legal matter?

___ yes ___ no

If yes, briefly explain: ___

13. What treatments have you tried for your pain?

___ Surgery ___ TENS unit

___ Nerve block ___ Exercise program

___ Brace ___ Trigger point injection

___ Physical therapy ___ Acupuncture

___ Relaxation training ___ Chiropractic therapy

___ Biofeedback ___ Psychotherapy/counseling

___ Hypnosis

Other ___ ___ Massage

14. What specialists have you seen for your pain (e.g., orthopedic surgeon, neurologist, neurosurgeon, psychiatrist)?

15. Pain Medications and Other Treatments

A. What are the medications you are currently taking for pain?

	Drug	*Dose*	*Frequency*
1.			
2.			
3.			
4.			

B. What other medications have you taken in the past for pain?

	Drug	*Effect on Pain*
1.		
2.		
3.		
4.		

FIGURE 5.3 The Center for Pain Medicine at MGH's pain assessment form (From www.massgeneral.org).

C. Are you allergic to any medications (including local anesthetics)?

Drug *Type of Reaction*

D. What other medications are you currently taking?

16. Name, address, and phone number of your primary care physician:

____

____

____

____

17. Name, address, and phone number of the physician who referred you to us:

____

____

____

____

FIGURE 5.3 *(Continued)*

3. Pain Diaries

A diary of a patient's pain is useful in evaluating the relation between pain and daily activity. Pain can be described using the numeric rating scale, during activities such as walking, standing, sitting, and routine chores. The evaluation can be done on an hourly basis. Use of medication and alcohol, and emotional responses of the patient and family may also be recorded. Pain diaries may reflect a patient's pain more accurately than a retrospective description that may significantly over- or underestimate pain. Multiple phone applications are available to facilitate this task, such as "My **Pain Diary**: Chronic **Pain** & **Symptom** Tracker" and "PainScale: **Pain** Tracker **Diary**."

B. Pain Location

The location and distribution of pain are extremely important characteristics that help in understanding the pathophysiology of the pain complaint. Body diagrams, found in some of the assessment instruments, can prove very useful. Although the clinician can view the patient's perception of the topographic area of pain, the patient may show psychological distress either by poorly localizing the pain or by magnifying the pain to other areas of the body:

1. **Is the pain localized or referred?** Localized pain is pain confined to its site of origin, without radiation or migration. Referred pain usually arises from visceral or deep structures and radiates to other areas of the body. A classic example of referred pain is shoulder pain from phrenic nerve irritation (causes include liver metastases from pancreatic cancer) (see Table 5.1).
2. **Is pain superficial/peripheral or visceral?** Superficial pain, arising from tissues rich in nociceptors, such as the skin, teeth, and mucous membranes, is easily localized and limited to the affected part of the body. Visceral pain arises from internal organs, which contain relatively few nociceptors. Visceral afferent information may converge with superficial afferent input at the spinal level, referring the perception of visceral pain to a distant dermatome. Visceral pain is diffuse and often poorly localized. In addition, it often has associated autonomic components such as diaphoresis, capillary vasodilatation, hypertension, or tachycardia.

TABLE 5.1 Examples of Referred Pain

Origin of Pain	Region of Pain Referral
Head (dura mater or vessels)	
Anterior cranial fossa	Ipsilateral forehead
Middle cranial fossa	Ipsilateral supraorbital region, temples
Posterior cranial fossa	Ipsilateral ear, postauricular region, occiput
Pharynx	Ipsilateral ear
Chest	
Esophagus	Substernal region
Heart	Left arm, epigastric
Abdomen	
Visceral pain	Segmental muscle spasms
Cholecystitis	Upper abdominal muscles
Appendicitis	Lower abdominal muscles
Renal colic	L2-L3 segments
Subphrenic region	Shoulder pain
Liver	Right phrenic region
Kidney	Lower thorax and back
Ureter	
Upper (renal pelvis)	Groin, testis, or ovary
Terminal	Scrotum/labia
Pelvis	
Prostate	Lower back
Uterus	Lower back
Ovary	Anterior thigh
Lower extremity	
Peroneal entrapment at the fibula	Dorsum of the foot
Other	
Unilateral cordotomy	Pain applied to analgesic side produces pain in symmetrical contralateral body part

Reprinted from Brass LM, Stys K. *Handbook of Neurological Lists.* New York, NY: Churchill-Livingstone; 1991. Copyright © 1991 Elsevier. With permission.

C. Pain Etiology

By taking a complete history and by answering the two questions described in the preceding text (Is pain superficial/peripheral or visceral? Is the pain localized or referred?), the clinician can begin to formulate the etiology of the pain complaint. By doing so, the rest of the history, as well as the physical examination, can be tailored to systematically explore the aspects of pain, such as symptoms and physical signs, common to the form of pain in question.

1. Types of Pain

Pain may be generally divided into three categories nociceptive, inflammatory, and pathological pain (Woolf, 2010):

a. Nociceptive—This high-threshold pain is protective and occurs in the setting of an intense stimulus that is potentially tissue-injuring, including heat, cold, mechanical, and chemical exposures. Such pain is often accompanied by emotional distress and autonomic nervous system activation. It overrides other less intense stimuli to warn of impending injury. Nociceptive activation is present in the fetus and manifests as withdrawal.

b. **Inflammatory pain**—This low-threshold pain is also protective, is present following tissue injury or infection, and is associated with activation of the immune system, including peripheral mast cells, granulocytes, macrophages, and neutrophils and the release of excitatory cytokines, ions, growth factors, and neurotransmitters. Acute inflammatory activation produces local tenderness, allowing for tissue healing and helping to prevent further damage. However, this immune response requires attenuation in the setting of chronic inflammation and can facilitate pathological pain in syndromes such as rheumatoid arthritis and persistent pancreatitis.

c. **Pathological pain**—This type of pain is differentiated from nociceptive and inflammatory pain as it results from activation of a maladaptive vs functional peripheral and central nervous system and is nonprotective. It includes two broad subcategories: **neuropathic pain and dysfunctional pain**. Low-threshold neuropathic pain arises from a lesion or disease of the somatosensory system, such as stroke, vasculitis, diabetic neuropathy, complex regional pain syndrome, and trigeminal neuralgia. Dysfunctional pain is also associated with abnormal central nervous system processing but is not defined by a specific neural lesion. It includes the generally clinically described and probably pathophysiologically complex disorders including somatic symptom disorder and fibromyalgia. In some cases, the classification of pain as dysfunctional may simply reflect the inability of clinicians and scientists to identify a defined causative etiology

II. PHYSICAL EXAMINATION

A complete examination is required, including a general physical examination followed by a specific pain evaluation and neurologic, musculoskeletal, and mental status assessments. It is important not to limit the examination to the painful location and surrounding tissues and structures.

A. General Physical Examination

This physical examination consists of the usual head-to-toe examination, as described in Chapter 4. The important points to note are:

- Appearance—obese, emaciated, histrionic, and flat affect
- Posture—splinting, scoliosis, and kyphosis
- Gait—antalgic, hemiparetic, and using assistive devices
- Expression—grimacing, tense, diaphoretic, and anxious
- Vital signs—sympathetic overactivity (eg, tachycardia, hypertension) and temperature asymmetries.

It is also important to watch how a patient dresses and moves. Favoring an extremity or protecting a part of the body is not advisable unless the relevant movements are elicited despite these drawbacks. Some elements of the comprehensive examination may be missed if a clinician is fearful of invading the patient's privacy.

B. Specific Pain Evaluation

Following general examination, the clinician evaluates the painful areas(s) of the body. The history will often direct the search for physical findings. Inspection of the skin may reveal changes in color, flushing, edema, hair loss, presence or absence of sweat, atrophy, or muscle spasm. Inspection of nails may show dystrophic changes. Nerve root injury may be manifested as goose flesh (cutis anserina) in the affected dermatome. Palpation allows mapping of the painful area and detection of any change in pain intensity within the area during the examination and helps define the pain type and trigger points. Patient responses, both verbal and nonverbal, should be noted, as well as the appropriateness of the responses and their correlation with affect. Factors that reproduce, worsen, or decrease the pain are sought.

While conducting the physical examination, it is important to identify any changes in sensory modalities and pain processing that may have occurred. These changes may be manifest as anesthesia, hypoesthesia, hyperesthesia, analgesia, hypoalgesia, allodynia, hyperalgesia, or hyperpathia. Please refer to Appendix VI: Definitions and Abbreviations for definitions of these terms.

C. Neurologic Examination

Subtle physical findings are often found only during the neurologic examination. It is essential to conduct a comprehensive neurologic examination when first assessing a patient with pain to identify associated, and possibly treatable, neurologic disease. The examination can be performed in 5-10 minutes. Later in the course of treatment, the neurologic examination can be more focused and briefer.

1. **Mental function** is assessed by evaluating the patient's arousal and orientation to person, place, and time; attention is particularly relevant to evaluating delirium; short-term and long-term memory; choice of words used to describe symptoms and to answer questions; and educational background.
2. The **cranial nerves** should be examined, especially in patients complaining of head, neck, and shoulder pain symptoms. Table 5.2 lists the function of each cranial nerve.
3. The **motor examination** should include the assessment of bulk and tone, confrontational strength testing, and abnormal movements such as myoclonus, asterixis, and tremor. Table 5.3 lists the motor and sensory manifestations of common nerve root syndromes.
4. **Coordination** is assessed by testing balance, rapid hand movement, finger-to-nose motion, and toe-to-heel motion.
5. Like the bulk and tone components of the motor examination, **reflexes** are important in distinguishing upper motor neuron from lower motor neuron etiology.
   a. Signs of upper motor neuron dysfunction:
      i. Hyperactive reflexes
      ii. Spasticity
      iii. Present Babinski reflex
   b. Signs of lower motor neuron dysfunction
      i. Absent or hypoactive reflexes
      ii. Muscle tone reduced or normal
      iii. Absent Babinski reflex
6. Table 5.4 lists pain disturbances due to various disease processes that can affect gait.

D. Sensory Testing

1. **Dynamic allodynia**: lightly rub the fingertip, foam, or cotton swab across the skin.

TABLE 5.2 Neurologic Examination of Cranial Nerves

Cranial Nerves		Function
I	—Olfactory nerve	Smell
II	—Optic	Vision
III	—Oculomotor	
	Parasympathetic	Sphincter muscle of the iris, ciliary muscle
	Motor	Superior, inferior, and medial rectus muscles; inferior oblique and levator palpebrae superioris muscle
IV	—Trochlear	Superior oblique
V	—Trigeminal	
	Motor	Muscles of mastication
	Sensory	Face, mucosa of the nose, mouth, dura, and cornea
VI	—Abducens	Lateral rectus muscle
VII	—Facial	
	Motor	Muscles of expression
	Parasympathetic	Lacrimal gland, salivary glands, and mucous membranes of the mouth
	Sensory	Sensation to parts of the external ear, auditory canal, and tympanic membrane Taste to anterior two-thirds of the tongue
VIII	—Vestibulocochlear	Equilibrium and hearing
IX	—Glossopharyngeal	
	Parasympathetic	Parotid gland
	Motor	Stylopharyngeal muscle
	Sensory	Sensation to posterior one-third of the tongue, pharynx, middle ear, and dura
X	—Vagus	
	Parasympathetic	Viscera of the thorax and abdomen
	Motor	Muscles of the pharynx and larynx
	Sensory somatic	Dura and auditory canal
	Sensory visceral	Viscera of the thorax and abdomen
XI	—Accessory	
	Motor	Muscles of the larynx, sternocleidomastoid, and trapezius
XII	—Hypoglossal	Intrinsic muscles of the tongue, genioglossus, hypoglossus, and styloglossus

Sensory examination in the patient with neuropathic pain extends beyond routine discrimination of sharp and dull sensations and requires testing for mechanical and thermal allodynia, summation and aftersensation, hyperalgesia, and hyperpathia.

2. **Static allodynia:** slowly apply perpendicular pressure to blunt device (cotton swab).
3. The sensory examination should include a separate assessment of predominantly large fiber (vibration, proprioception) and small fiber (pinprick, temperature) modalities. The Romberg sign, that is, impaired balance that develops when visual cues are removed, reflects impaired proprioception. Potentially painful peripheral neuropathies are listed in Table 5.5.

TABLE 5.3 Pain-Induced Disturbances of Gait

Diagnosis	Symptoms
Intermittent claudication	Pain on walking a specific distance, arterial insufficiency
	Pain appears sooner with increasing intensity of work
	Pain disappears after rest
	Pain localized to calf
Cauda equina (neurogenic claudication, spinal stenosis)	Urinary retention
	Pain on walking after varying distances
	Patient usually older
	Pain usually bilateral
	Radicular in character
	Pain localized to saddle area, upper thigh, and calf
	Pain in the back on sneezing
	Pain does not usually disappear on cessation of walking
	Pain improves when leaning forward
Hip disease	Pain worsens with first few steps
Inguinal region	Pain increases on prolonged standing
	Usually after appendectomy, hernia repair
Meralgia paresthetica	Pain in the lateral aspect of the thigh
Long bones	Localized pain
	Evidence of tumor/osteoporosis, Paget disease, pathologic fracture
	After surgical procedure—anterior compartment syndrome
Feet	
Foot deformities	Pain after walking or standing
Calcaneal spur	Pain in the plantar aspect of the foot (prevents walking)
Achilles tendinitis	
Tarsal tunnel syndrome	

From Mumenthaler M. *Neurologic Differential Diagnosis.* New York, NY: Thieme-Stratton; 1985: 118-119, with permission.

4. **Gait** is assessed by watching the patient walk, and the observed movement should include a turn. A common term to describe gait is antalgic, which refers to as abnormal due to pain.
5. Pain of psychogenic origin will usually result in a neurologic examination that does not correlate with findings typical of organic pathology. Abnormal pain distributions, such as glove or stocking patterns, and exact hemianesthesia are common in patients with psychogenic pain.

E. Musculoskeletal System Examination

Abnormalities of the musculoskeletal system are often evident on inspection of the patient's posture and muscular symmetry. Muscle atrophy usually indicates disuse. Flaccidity indicates extreme weakness, usually from paralysis, and abnormal movements indicate neurologic damage or impaired proprioception. Limited range of motion

TABLE 5.4 Common Painful Root Syndromes

Root	Sensory Loss	Motor Changes: Weakness	Motor Changes: Decreased Deep Tendon Reflexes
Upper extremity			
C5	Lateral aspect of the upper arm	Deltoid and biceps	None/biceps
C6	Thumb and index finger	Biceps and brachioradialis	Brachioradialis and biceps
C7	Middle finger	Triceps and pronator teres	Triceps
Lower extremity			
L4	Medial calf	Quadriceps	Knee
L5	Medial half of the foot and lateral calf	Peroneal, anterior, and posterior tibial and toe extension	Internal hamstring
S1	Lower posterior calf and lateral foot	Plantar flexion	Ankle

of a major joint can indicate pain, disk disease, or arthritis. Palpation of muscles will help in evaluating range of motion and in determining whether trigger points are present. Coordination and strength are also tested.

F. Assessment of Psychological Factors

Complete assessment of pain includes analysis of the psychological aspects of pain and the effects of pain on behavior and emotional stability. Such assessment is challenging because many patients are unaware of or are reluctant to present psychological issues. It is also more socially acceptable to seek medical than psychiatric care. Initially, the use of a descriptive pain questionnaire such as the MPQ may provide some evidence of a patient's affective responses to pain. For example, words such as "aching" and "tingling" refer to sensory aspects of pain, whereas words such as "agonizing" and "dreadful" suggest negative feelings and do not aid in characterizing the pain sensation. For a better description of psychological evaluation in pain management, see Chapter 15.

A patient's personality and mood greatly influence his or her response to pain and choice of the coping strategy. Some patients may benefit from the use of strategies of control such as distraction and relaxation. Patients who have an underlying anxiety disorder may be more likely to seek high doses of analgesics. Therefore, inquiry regarding a patient's history of coping with stress is often useful.

As part of the pain history, the clinician should include questions about some of the common symptoms in patients with chronic pain: depressed mood, sleep disturbance, preoccupation with somatic symptoms, reduced activity, reduced libido, and fatigue. Standardized questionnaires, such as the Beck Depression Inventory (BDI), the Beck Anxiety Inventory (BAI), and the Minnesota Multiphasic Personality Inventory (MMPI), may expand the assessment. On the MMPI, patients with chronic pain characteristically score very high on the depression, hysteria, and

TABLE 5.5 Painful Sensory Neuropathies

Endocrinologic
- Diabetes mellitus
- Hypothyroidism

Metabolic
- Uremia
- Thiamine deficiency
- Acute intermittent porphyria

Toxic
- Vincristine
- Acrylamide
- Heavy metals
- Organic solvents

Infectious/inflammatory
- HIV-related painful neuropathies
- Herpes zoster—acute and chronic postherpetic neuralgia
- Guillain-Barré syndrome
- Chronic inflammatory polyneuropathy

Immunologic
- Polyarteritis nodosa
- Cryoglobulinemia
- Systemic lupus erythematosus

Physical
- Brachial plexopathies
- Compressive (such as carpal, ulnar, or tarsal tunnel syndromes

Neoplastic
- Multiple myeloma
- Cancer (including nonmetastatic effects and carcinomatosis)

Genetic
- Fabry disease
- Tangier disease
- Familial dysautonomia (Riley-Day syndrome, inherited sensory neuropathy III)
- Amyloidosis
- Inherited erythromelalgia

- Thermal allodynia: warm/cold test tube or tuning fork
- Hyperalgesia: single pinprick; multiple pinpricks for summation/aftersensations

hypochondriasis scales. However, the MMPI may reflect functional limitation secondary to pain, as well as psychological abnormality associated with chronic pain, limiting its interpretation for some patients suspected of having psychogenic pain.

Several psychological processes and syndromes predispose patients to chronic pain. Predisposing disorders include major depression, somatization disorder, conversion disorder, hypochondriasis, and psychogenic pain disorder. The diagnosis of somatization disorder is quite specific, although many patients with chronic pain may "somatize" (focus on somatic complaints). Somatization disorder as such requires a history of physical symptoms of several years' duration, beginning before the age of 30 years and including complaints of at least 14 specific symptoms for women and 12 for men. These symptoms are not adequately explained by physical disorder, injury, or toxic reaction.

Psychogenic pain may occur in susceptible individuals. In some patients, pain may ameliorate more unpleasant feelings, such as depression, guilt, or anxiety, and distract the patient from environmental stress factors. Historic features that suggest a psychogenic component to chronic pain include the following:

- Multiple locations of pain at different times
- Pain problems dating since adolescence
- Pain without obvious somatic cause (especially in the facial or perineal area)
- Multiple, elective surgical procedures
- Substance abuse (patient and/or significant other)
- Social or work failure

Psychogenic pain is clearly distinct from malingering. Malingerers have an obvious, identifiable environmental goal in producing symptoms, such as evading law enforcement, avoiding work, or obtaining financial compensation. Patients with psychogenic pain may make illness and hospitalization their primary goals. Being a patient is their primary way of life. Such patients are unable to stop symptom production when it is no longer obviously beneficial. Specific diagnoses include somatic symptom disorder and factitious disorder (previously Munchausen syndrome)

The physical examination in patients with psychological factors exacerbating pain may be perplexing or inconsistent. Some findings may not correspond to known anatomic or physiologic information. Examples of such findings include the following:

- Manual testing inconsistent with patient observation during sitting, turning, and dressing
  - Grasping with three fingers
    - Antagonist muscle contraction on attempted movement
    - Decreased tremor during mental arithmetic exercises
    - A positive Romberg sign with one eye closed
    - Vibration sense absent on one side of midline (eg, right side of the skull or sternum)
    - Inconsistency of timed vibration when the affected side is tested first
    - Patterned miscount of touches
    - Difficulty touching the good limb with the bad
    - A slight difference in sensation on one side of the body

Useful neurologic signs are deep tendon reflexes, motor tone and bulk, and the plantar response (Babinski).

III. DIAGNOSTIC STUDIES

The diagnosis and understanding of a patient's pain complaint can usually be obtained after a thorough history and physical examination. Diagnostic and physiologic studies are used to support a clinician's suspicion, as well as to assist in the diagnosis. Some of the more common studies used for pain assessment are described in following text.

A. **Conventional radiography** is used to diagnose bony abnormalities such as pathologic fractures seen in bony metastases; spine pathology, including spondylolisthesis, stenosis, and osteophyte formation; and bone tumors. Some soft tissue tumors and bowel abnormalities can also be seen. X-rays of the painful area have usually been obtained by the referring physician.

B. A **computerized tomography** scan is most often used to define bony abnormalities, and **magnetic resonance imaging** best shows soft tissue pathology. Spinal stenosis, disk herniation or bulge, nerve root compression, and tumors in all tissues can be diagnosed, as well as some causes of central pain, such as CNS infarcts or plaques of demyelination.

C. **Diagnostic blocks** may differentiate somatic pain from visceral pain and confirm the anatomic location of peripheral nerve pain. These blocks may help localize painful pathology or contribute to the diagnosis of complex regional pain syndrome (CRPS). They are also necessary precedents to neurolytic blocks for malignant pain or radiofrequency lesions. The various diagnostic blocks are described in detail in Chapter 12.

D. **Drug challenges** are used to predict drug treatment utility and help in the assessment of pain etiology. For example, brief intravenous infusions of lidocaine and ketamine may be used to assess sensitivity to sodium channel and NMDA blockade in neuropathic pain.

   1. Various **neurophysiologic tests** are used to help in the diagnosis of pain syndromes and related neurologic diseases. These tests are described in Chapter 7. EMG and NCS primarily assess large nerve fiber dysfunction suggested by findings of weakness and sensory loss on the physical examination. For small fiber neuralgia and neuropathy, quantitative sensory testing (QST) evaluates patients' responses to carefully quantify physical stimuli.
   2. **Mechanical nonpainful sensation**: Large myelinated Aβ fiber function, most decreased after peripheral nerve injury and sensitive to ischemia; tuning fork and von Frey hairs.
   3. **Mechanical painful sensation**: Single stimulus tests, Aδ and C fibers; repetitive tests, C fibers; and pinch algometer.
   4. **Thermal sensation**: Cool sensation, Aδ; warm sensation, C; cold pain sensation, Aδ + C; and heat pain sensation, C fiber.
   5. **Cool sensation** is first to decrease after peripheral nerve injury and cold allodynia is prominent in CRPS.
   6. Pediatric patients (<14 years) with diabetes may have subclinical neuropathy per QST.

E. **Quantitative sudomotor axon reflex test (QSART)** is a **test** that measures the autonomic nerves that control sweating. The **test** is useful in assessing autonomic nervous system disorders, peripheral neuropathies, and some types of pain disorders. The **test** requires a mild electrical stimulation on the skin, which allows to stimulate the sweat glands.

F. **Thermography** is a noninvasive way of displaying the body's thermal patterns. A normal thermal pattern is relatively symmetric. Tissue pathology is associated with chemical and metabolic changes that may cause abnormal thermal patterns by altering vascularity, such as in CRPS. The patterns of color difference seen are not specific for the underlying central or peripheral pathology.

G. **Myelography** is the injection of radiopaque dye into the subarachnoid space to visualize spinal cord/column abnormalities radiographically, such as disk herniation, nerve root impingement, arachnoiditis, and spinal stenosis. Major disadvantages of this procedure are postdural puncture headache and meningeal irritation.

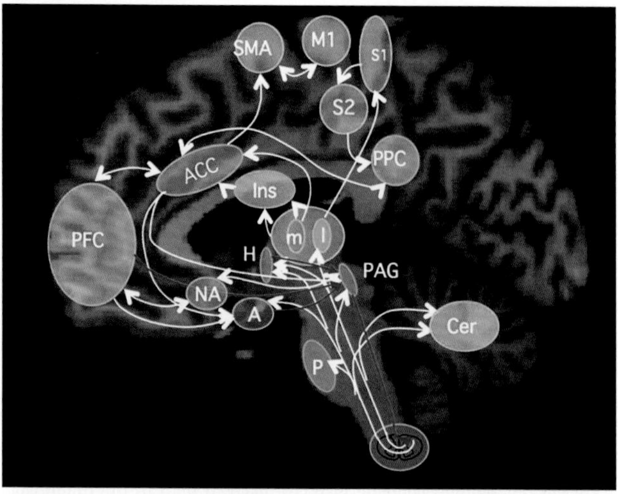

FIGURE 5.4 Overview of pain pathways and altered neural systems in chronic pain. *White arrows*, ascending and intracerebral pain pathways; *blue arrows*, modulatory descending pathways. A, amygdala; ACC, anterior cingulate cortex; Cer, cerebellum; H, hypothalamus; Ins, insula; I, m, lateral and medial thalamus; M1, primary motor cortex; NA, nucleus accumbens; PAG, periaqueductal gray; PFC, prefrontal cortex; PPC, posterior parietal cortex; S1, S2, primary and secondary somatosensory cortices; SMA, supplementary motor area.

H. **Bone scanning** is the use of a radioactive compound to detect a number of bone lesions, including neoplastic, infectious, arthritic, and traumatic, Paget disease, and the osteodystrophy of reflex sympathetic dystrophy. The radioactive compound accumulates in the areas of increased bone growth or turnover. It is a very sensitive test for subtle bone abnormalities that may not appear on conventional radiographs.
I. The removal of small punch **skin biopsies** (immunolabeled to show the cutaneous sensory nerve endings) has provided a new tool with which to directly visualize the cutaneous endings of pain neurons. Although currently available at only a few centers, this technique is replacing sural nerve biopsy for the diagnosis of sensory neuropathies. The technique appears to be helpful for diagnosing small fiber neuropathy, in which there is loss of nociceptive terminals, and potentially focal painful nerve injuries. Skin biopsies are only minimally invasive, can be repeated, and can be performed in areas other than those innervated by the sural nerve. Corneal fiber density per confocal microscopy may also be a less invasive measure of small fiber neuralgia.
J. **Functional brain imaging**, such as positron emission tomography and functional magnetic resonance imaging (fMRI), is an investigative tool, at present, with provocative findings about the cortical and subcortical processing of pain information. The fMRI shows pain to be remarkably distributed at the cortical level. Figures 5.4-5.6 detail select advances in the understanding of pain pathways and pain processing elucidated through fMRI.

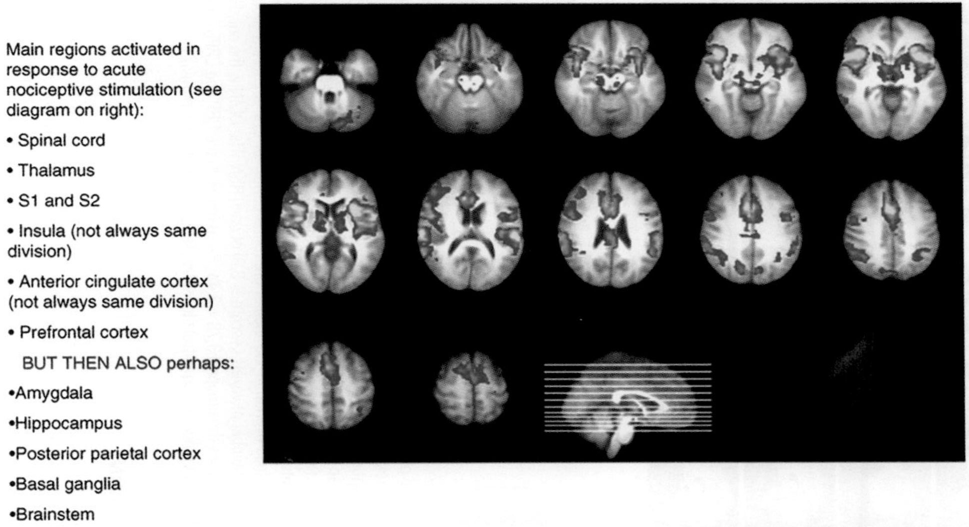
Main regions activated in response to acute nociceptive stimulation (see diagram on right):
• Spinal cord
• Thalamus
• S1 and S2
• Insula (not always same division)
• Anterior cingulate cortex (not always same division)
• Prefrontal cortex
BUT THEN ALSO perhaps:
•Amygdala
•Hippocampus
•Posterior parietal cortex
•Basal ganglia
•Brainstem

FIGURE 5.5 Neuroanatomy of pain processing. The main brain regions that activate during a painful experience are highlighted as bilaterally active but with more dominant activation on the contralateral hemisphere (*red*).

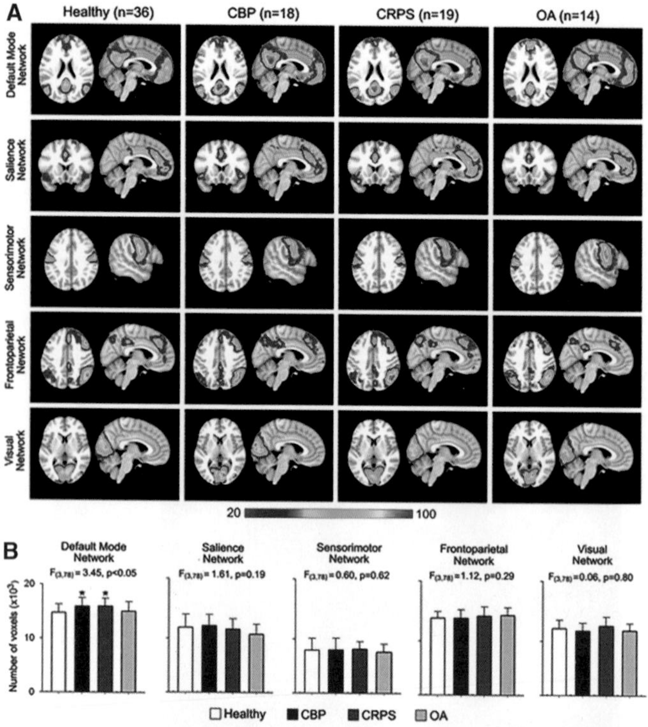

FIGURE 5.6 Spatial properties of resting state networks in three chronic pain patient groups and in healthy controls. **A.** Percent spatial overlap of five resting state networks (RSNs) for healthy and pain patient groups. Colors represent the percentage of subjects whose best fit component overlap at each voxel. *Red* denotes much overlap, while *purple* denotes little overlap. Overall, All RSNs show similar spatial representation across all groups except for the default mode network (DMN), which exhibits larger overlap in the precuneus and posterior cingulate and less overlap in the medial prefrontal cortex for CBP and CRPS groups. **B.** Mean ± S.E.M. of number of voxels (*z*-score > 3.0) of each RSN. The DMN is the only RSN that differs in size across the groups ($F3,78 = 3.45$, $P < 0.05$), with the CBP and CRPS groups having a larger DMN compared to controls (post hoc test, $^{*}P < 0.05$ vs controls).

IV. CONCLUSION

The assessment of pain can be challenging and intensive but is an essential component of pain management and allows the pain physician to devise optimal treatment of some of the most complex pain issues of patients. It is important to treat the patient as a complete person and not just the painful location. Believing the patient and establishing rapport with the patient are of the utmost importance. A systematic approach, grounded in knowledge of anatomy and physiology, will assist the clinician in determining the pathophysiology of the patient's pain complaint. With this essential knowledge, the therapy can be formulated, promptly initiated, and easily reassessed.

Selected Readings

Beecher HK. *Measurement of Subjective Responses.* New York, NY: Oxford University Press; 1959.

Borsook D, Sava S, Becerra, L. The pain imaging revolution: advancing pain into the 21st century. *Neuroscientist.* 2010;16:171-185.

Bovie J, Hansson P, Lindblom U, eds. *Touch, Temperature and Pain in Health and Disease: Mechanisms and Assessments,* Vol. 3. Seattle, WA: IASP Press; 1994.

Carlsson AM. Assessment of chronic pain I: aspects of the reliability and validity of the visual analogue scale. *Pain.* 1983;16:87-101.

Galer BS, Dworkin RH. *A Clinical Guide to Neuropathic Pain.* Minneapolis, MN: McGraw-Hill; 2000.

Gracely RH. Evaluation of multidimensional pain scales. *Pain.* 1992;48:297-300.

Harris CA, Joyce LD. Psychometric properties of the Beck Depression Inventory-(BDI-II) in individuals with chronic pain. *Pain.* 2008;137:609-622.

Katz J. Psychophysical correlates of phantom limb experience. *J Neurol Neurosurg Psychiatry.* 1992;55:811-821.

Lowe NK, Walder SM, McCallum RC. Confirming the theoretic structure of the McGill pain questionnaire in acute clinical pain. *Pain.* 1991;46:53-60.

McGrath PA. *Pain in Children: Nature, Assessment and Treatment.* New York, NY: Guildford Press; 1990.

Melzack R, Katz J. Pain measurement in persons in pain. In: Wall PD, Melzack R, eds. *Textbook of Pain.* 4th ed. New York, NY: Churchill Livingstone; 1999.

Melzack R. The McGill questionnaire: major properties and scoring methods. *Pain.* 1975;1:277-299.

Price DD, Bush FM, Long S, et al. A comparison of pain measurement characteristics of mechanical visual analogue and simple numerical rating scales. *Pain.* 1994;56:217-226.

Woolf CJ. What is this thing called pain? *J of Clin Invest.* 2010;120(11):3742-3744.

6 Psychological Assessment of Pain and Headache

Ellen S. Patterson, María F. Hernández-Nuño de la Rosa, Kelly M. Wawrzyniak, and Ronald J. Kulich

I. THE BIOPSYCHOSOCIAL MODEL OF PAIN ASSESSMENT

In clinical practice, the biopsychosocial model of pain represents a widely accepted approach to understanding the complex and dynamic interaction of biological, psychological, and social factors relevant to the assessment and care of acute and chronic pain conditions. This model assumes four dimensions associated with pain: nociception, pain, suffering, and pain behavior. While *nociception* (sensory input) and *pain* (subjective perception) represent methods of communication to the central nervous system, *suffering* represents the affective response to pain that may occur concurrently with other psychological comorbidities, such as depression and anxiety. Suffering also includes a social component, as significant distress may be associated with isolation, impaired interpersonal relationships, and loss of role or identity that frequently accompanies the experience of physical pain. *Pain behaviors*, or the individual's actions while experiencing pain, are reactions to these inputs and are influenced by a myriad of factors including environmental context, prior pain and health care experiences, and anticipation of potential consequences. The interplay and expression of these four dimensions of pain are unique to each individual and impact the clinical presentation, progression of the condition, and response to treatment. Evaluating the patient using the biopsychosocial model, the clinician must recognize that expressions of these dimensions occur concurrently and are interactive and closely intertwined. Chronic pain cannot be viewed from a cartesian dualist perspective, that is, pain is neither purely "psychological" nor purely "physical."

The biopsychosocial model directs the clinician to comprehensively assess all aspects of the *illness*, rather than to focus solely on the underlying *disease* process. Kleinman explains this distinction as follows: "Illness refers to how the sick person and the members of the family or wider social network perceive, live with, and respond to symptoms and disability. Illness is the lived experience of monitoring bodily processes such as respiratory wheezes, abdominal cramps, stuffed sinuses, or painful joints. Illness involves the appraisal of those processes as expectable, serious, or requiring treatment."

Applying a biopsychosocial approach, the clinician acknowledges and responds therapeutically to the individual's unique overall pain experience by comprehensively assessing multiple dimensions. Important variables for the clinician to consider in the comprehensive psychological assessment of pain include prior experiences with pain, experiences with medical/surgical interventions or events related to treatment of the pain condition, history of past and current psychiatric disorders, and contextual social and work-related factors. Each of these factors may have a significant impact on the presentation, course, and response to treatment of the pain condition. It is also prudent for the clinician to explore any adversarial relationships (such as involvement in a legal case related to an injury or a worker's compensation claim) as well as rewarding or solicitous relationships, as these may be relevant to the assessment and will likely impact, consciously or unconsciously, self-reported symptoms and functional impact of the pain condition. Contextual factors also contribute to the emergence of depression, disability, and substance abuse, comorbidities that are significantly more common in pain populations.

Poor adherence to recommended treatments is common across clinical settings; in the context of acute medical problems, only 50% of patients will completely follow the clinician's treatment recommendations, and analysis of CDC data revealed that for every 100 prescriptions written, 50%-70% were filled and only 20%-30% were taken as directed. Adherence tends to be even lower when psychiatric comorbidities or chronic medical conditions are present; therefore, assessment of potential barriers to adherence should be included as part of the psychological assessment. To improve adherence in the context of pain, a template of assessment steps has been proposed that addresses numerous relevant factors including (but not limited to) beliefs about the underlying cause of the pain, biases about the proposed treatments, and past personal experiences with pain interventions.

II. PSYCHOLOGICAL RISK SCREENING VS COMPREHENSIVE PSYCHOSOCIAL ASSESSMENT

The term **psychological risk screening** denotes a brief assessment process that typically includes one or more validated screening instruments. The goal of risk screening is to stratify the likelihood that an individual suffers from a relevant mental health or substance use disorder; screening may assist with diagnosis, but it should be stressed that this screening is only an initial step to help identify the need for further evaluation. In contrast, *comprehensive psychosocial assessment* is a more intensive process in which detailed information is gathered to establish relevant diagnoses and identify other risk factors. Comprehensive psychosocial assessments are more time-consuming, typically synthesize data from multiple primary and secondary sources, and are critical for individualized treatment planning. The use of *risk screening measures* is becoming the standard of care for initial or preintervention pain assessments, including prior to surgery, neuromodulation, and prescription of opioid analgesics.

Given the multiple complex and intersecting variables that may impact outcomes of chronic pain management, psychological assessment should be considered an ongoing process and not limited to a onetime, preintervention screening. Periodic follow-up assessments are important as they provide opportunities to (1) monitor changes in risk factors that affect treatment options and prognosis allowing for earlier effective intervention; (2) promote rapport building with the patient and family; (3) collect valuable information regarding the impact of social, family, and functional/vocational issues; (4) encourage periodic review of health records and data collection from cotreating clinicians; and (5) longitudinally document relevant data, including data from other sources such as a state prescription monitoring program. All of these are valuable contributions to comprehensive pain assessment and care planning. The initial psychological evaluation should address preliminary goal setting and clarify patient expectations of care, and subsequent follow-up assessments will provide information about progress toward functional goals, address barriers to adherence, and help to engage the patient in targeted psychosocial interventions as well as acceptance of any recommended referrals.

III. THE PROGRESSION FROM ACUTE TO CHRONIC PAIN CONDITIONS

The progression from acute injury or tissue damage to the development of a chronic pain condition typically follows a predictable course (Fig. 6.1) and usually occurs in the context of multiple premorbid risk factors. For example, after a musculoskeletal injury, an individual may engage in self-directed treatments, use over-the-counter medications, and/or seek care from a physician or other primary health care provider. Most mild to moderate injuries are self-limited and recovery occurs without complications. However, when there is prolonged or residual pain (with or without

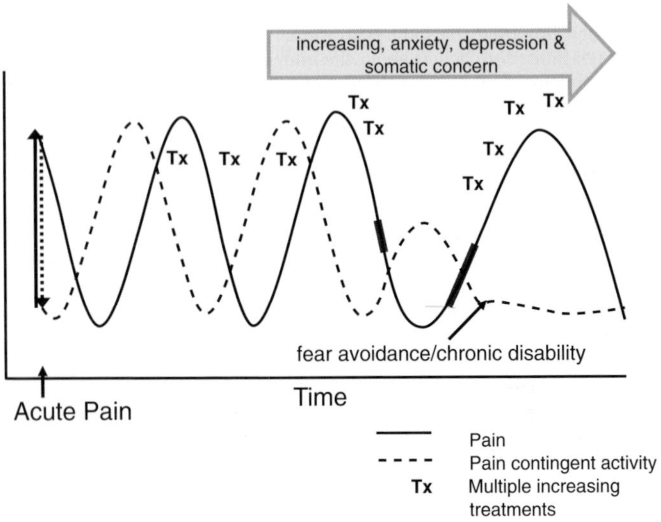

FIGURE 6.1 Development of chronic pain (graphic).

objective evidence of persistent tissue damage), the individual typically seeks specialist care, diagnostic studies, and more intensive treatments. Multiple clinicians may be consulted with varying levels of coordination or communication between providers. If the pain persists, the patient typically experiences increasing frustration and psychological distress; repeated unsuccessful interventions may stretch into weeks, months, or years, and reduction in normal activities typically ensues. This pattern can lead to a negative spiral of progressively invasive interventions and concomitant reductions in social, occupational, physical, and psychological functioning.

As this pattern progresses, a well-meaning but potentially countertherapeutic alliance may develop between the treating clinician, the patient, and the patient's support system, each struggling to "fix" the underlying problem with additional interventions at the first sign of a pain exacerbation or "flare." New conditions may be diagnosed, prompting additional consultations. Passive treatment approaches (such as massage, various braces, or ultrasound) may be recommended in an effort to reduce pain. Although there may be a role for such interventions, care must be taken to avoid promoting the sick role and pain contingent behavior, and efforts should be taken by the clinician to minimize the reinforcement of behaviors that promote chronic disability. For example, temporary pain relief attributed to a passive treatment may in fact represent the waxing and waning pattern typical of many chronic pain conditions, potentially confusing the clinical picture. New pain complaints and other secondary problems may emerge due to iatrogenic consequences of multiple interventions, deconditioning from extended periods of bed rest, or the emergence of undertreated psychiatric concomitants. Ensuing emergence of multiple psychosocial challenges such as chronic depression, anxiety, disability, substance misuse, family disruption, financial stress, and work loss may also occur, and an ingrained lifestyle pattern of help seeking (the "professional patient") can compromise the individual's chances for a successful pain treatment outcome (Fig. 6.1).

To ameliorate this pattern, the clinician will ideally identify and address salient psychosocial variables early in care. Although research on psychological assessment has focused primarily on individuals with chronic pain, an increasingly robust scientific literature is emerging on the role of psychosocial factors in acute pain, particularly preemptive strategies to identify factors that predict the progression to chronic pain syndromes. **Primary psychosocial risk factors** that have been associated with worse outcomes in surgical patients include the presence of anxiety, depression, maladaptive coping strategies (such as pain catastrophizing), and substance misuse or abuse. Relevant **situational or environmental factors** include stressors related to finances, employment, or dysfunctional family dynamics.

Typically, individuals will present for specialized pain care somewhere in the midst of the process described in Figure 6.1. The treating clinician, understandably frustrated by the psychosocial complexity of the patient's presentation, may require the patient to submit to a psychological assessment by a mental health provider as a prerequisite for further intervention, but this step may be interpreted as punitive and dismissive, with patients sometimes voicing the fear that "The doctors think it's all in my head." Positively framing of the value of early psychosocial assessment and stressing the value of interdisciplinary care for improved treatment outcomes will help to normalize the behavioral dimensions of pain and support recommended psychological interventions. Ideally, the pain psychologist or psychiatrist will be an integral part of a team-based treatment approach, ensuring that communication and education are patient centered, positive, and consistent. This integrative approach is becoming more common in primary care and other settings and can reduce the risk that the patient and family perceive any recommended behavioral interventions as "punishment" for "failing" prior treatments.

IV. COMMON PSYCHOLOGICAL COMORBIDITIES WITH CHRONIC PAIN

Individuals with chronic pain conditions commonly experience worry associated with fear of pain exacerbations, fear of inability to perform important tasks, and fear of being deprived of access to treatments or medications perceived as critical to his or her well-being. The normal and biologically adaptive responses to acute pain may secondarily evolve, especially in the context of chronic pain, into a strong (but typically mistaken) belief that "hurt" always equals "harm." The individual concludes that any atypical pain or any exacerbation following a triggering activity necessarily indicates that additional tissue damage or irreversible worsening of the underlying pain condition has occurred. This may lead to **fear-avoidance** of activities and certain irrational thinking patterns (**catastrophizing**). Catastrophic thinking leads the patient to believe that his or her condition is much worse than it is, as illustrated by comments such as "I will never be able to cope with this pain," "This pain must mean I have a new herniated disc," "The degenerative disc disease is getting worse," "I need someone else to look at/take another MRI," "I will never be able to work again," or "I know I can't live without these pain medications."

Posttraumatic stress disorder (PTSD) is prevalent in chronic pain populations, although it is frequently underdiagnosed. Multiple investigations have demonstrated an association between PTSD linked to early trauma or victimization and the development of chronic pain conditions. It is important to note that in the context of a comorbid pain condition, individuals with PTSD (as well as other psychiatric conditions) frequently experience exacerbations of their mental health symptoms. Effectively treating comorbid PTSD will not necessarily resolve the coexisting chronic pain syndrome; however, aggressive concomitant treatment of PTSD will likely improve adherence, enhance the patient's capacity for self-management and emotional regulation, reduce autonomic arousal and hypervigilance, and optimize pain treatment outcomes.

Major depressive disorder is common in individuals suffering from chronic pain conditions, with more than half developing a major depressive disorder within several years of pain onset. Most pain patients experience some symptoms of depression. In one study of individuals with a disabling occupational spine disorder, prior history of depression was associated with the emergence of treatment-resistant pain, although no clear cause-and-effect relationship was established. Several classes of antidepressants are commonly prescribed as adjuvant pharmacotherapy for pain, particularly for management of neuropathic pain conditions and for pain-associated sleep disturbance, although adjuvant antidepressant doses are typically subtherapeutic for treatment of major depression. Given the high prevalence of major depression in pain populations, clinicians must take care to recognize and aggressively treat comorbid mood disorder to avoid potentially dangerous undertreatment. Periodic assessment of suicidal thoughts is always warranted for individuals living with chronic pain; a depressed patient with unused tricyclic antidepressants or opioid analgesics (especially in combination with benzodiazepines, alcohol, or other CNS depressants) may be at significant risk for death by intentional or accidental overdose. Individuals experiencing depression need to be informed that effective behavioral and pharmacologic treatments are available and that there are overlapping benefits for treating both pain and depression concomitantly. To maximize the reciprocal efficacy of interventions for both conditions, patients with depression should be referred for comprehensive psychological assessment by a psychologist or psychiatrist with experience treating pain populations to integrate depression treatment into the patient's individualized pain management plan.

Although many individuals with persistent pain *report disordered sleep*, the association of sleep and pain varies across chronic pain disorders, and sleep problems should be evaluated and addressed at the earliest phases of pain care. In addition to the direct impact of the pain condition, sleep disturbance may be related to adverse effects of medications, poor sleep hygiene, secondary effects of drugs or alcohol, reduced activity and exercise, and comorbid depression and/or anxiety disorders. Sleep disruption can also function as symptom trigger for certain chronic pain conditions, such as migraine headaches, and central and obstructive sleep apneas are more prevalent in chronic pain populations compared to the general population. Numerous diverse studies have investigated the complex associations between sleep and pain; a review concluded that there is convincing evidence that disrupted sleep patterns increase the risk of future chronic pain disorders in individuals previously pain free but that existing pain is not a strong predictor of a new-onset sleep disturbance. Optimizing management of depression, anxiety, and pain may lead to improved sleep quality, but persistent sleep disorders are common and should be assessed and monitored as part of the overall care plan. Since patients typically do not consider sleep disturbance to be stigmatizing, they are typically quite willing to discuss details about their sleep, making a thorough sleep history a helpful jumping-off point to inquire about other mental health–related symptoms. Discussions about managing sleep problems also present an opportunity to normalize the range of psychological factors typically associated with pain conditions.

The presence of **substance abuse or prescription medication misuse** is associated with poorer surgical outcomes, poorer rehabilitation outcomes, and greater psychiatric symptomatology. Referral to a psychologist, psychiatrist, or other qualified mental health provider is indicated whenever there is suspicion of a substance use disorder. Selected validated substance use screening tools are included in Table 6.1. The practice of routine, serial substance use screening is highly recommended in all pain patients, with documentation and consistent follow-up intervention when elevated risk is identified. Screening tools may be administered by trained staff and integrated for easy access into electronic health records. The four-item NIDA Quick Screen includes questions about prescription medication misuse, alcohol use, tobacco use, and illicit drug use and is easily administered by using a short form, an online interface, or smartphone application. The longer NIDA-Modified ASSIST V2.0 provides prompts for a brief intervention, including standardized scripts that guide the clinician to appropriate follow-up assessment and options for intervention.

Although it is quite common for individuals with pain to experience anxiety and significant subjective distress, *excessive somatic concern* is a common psychological concomitant in chronic pain conditions. When an extreme focus on physical symptoms develops, **somatization** and the related distorted thinking pattern of **catastrophizing** may emerge. When

TABLE 6.1 Brief Screening and Outcomes Measures

Psychological/ Behavioral Domain	Measure	Notes
Anxiety	GAD-7 (Generalized Anxiety Disorder-7)	7-item generalized anxiety screener, extensively studied with multiple acute and chronic pain populations (Bener et al., 2013)
Depression	PHQ-9 (Patient Health Questionnaire-9)	9-item depression screener, extensively studied with multiple acute and chronic pain population; addresses suicidal ideation (Bener et al., 2013; Choi, Mayer, Williams, & Gatchel, 2014)
Sleep	**SDQ (Sleep Disturbance Questionnaire)**	12-item scale evaluates subjective experiences of insomnia including mental anxiety and physical tension (Cheatle et al., 2016)
Fear avoidance/ pain catastrophizing	**TSK (Tampa Scale of Kinesiophobia)**	17-item scale addressing fear-avoidance of activity, predicting other disability measures; has been studied with multiple chronic pain populations (Cleland, Fritz, & Childs, 2008; Gregg et al., 2015)
	PCS (Pain Catastrophizing Scale)	13-item scale, one of several available to address this construct and frequently used for assessment with pain conditions; addresses rumination, magnification, and helplessness (Sullivan, 2009; Wertli et al., 2014a; Wertli, Rasmussen-Barr, Weiser, Bachmann, & Brunner, 2014b)
Somatization	PHQ-15 (Patient Health Questionnaire-15)	Widely used 15-item self-report measure for somatization syndromes; normative data available for pain populations; not sensitive to when patient only endorsed pain-related symptoms (Bener et al., 2013)
Disease specific: fibromyalgia	FIQ-R (Fibromyalgia Impact Questionnaire-R)	21-item, covers ADLs, recreational and work functional limitations common to FM and other chronic pain conditions; face valid items encourage goal setting discussion (Collado-Mateo et al., 2017)
Disease specific: headache	HIT (Headache Impact Test)	6-item test validated with migraine and other headache diagnoses; can be used as repeated measures scale to assess outcomes (Rendas-Baum et al., 2014)

TABLE 6.1 Brief Screening and Outcomes Measures (*Continued*)

Psychological/ Behavioral Domain	Measure	Notes
Disability and function	WHODAS 2.0 (WHO Disability Assessment Schedule 2.0)	36-item self-report questionnaire that addresses six domains of functioning: cognition, mobility, self-care, interacting with others, life activities, and participation; used across diseases, including pain conditions, useful for goal setting (Garin et al., 2010; Silva et al., 2013; Williams et al., 2015)
Combined scale: emotional status + disability and function	PROMIS (Patient-Reported Outcomes Measurement Information System)	PROMIS is a flexible set measures of physical, mental, and social health; available in multiple languages and formats, including short form and computer adaptive tests, which adapt questions offered based on respondent's previous answers; validated in multiple pain populations (Deyo et al., 2016). Guide to PROMIS measures: http://www.healthmeasures.net/explore-measurement-systems/promis/intro-to-promis
Substance use/ misuse	NIDA (National Institute on Drug Abuse) Quick Screen	4-item clinician-administered screening instrument for substance use, including prescription medication use; available by Web application; NIDA-Modified ASSIST guides clinician through brief intervention (SBIRT, National institute on drug abuse, 2018)
	SOAPP-R (Screener and Opioid Assessment for Patients with Pain-Revised)	24-item risk screener for patients being considered for chronic opioid therapy; also used in populations already using opioids. Validated short form available, as well as computer-based applications (Butler, Fernandez, Benoit, Budman, & Jamison, 2008; Finkelman et al., 2017b)
	COMM (Current Opioid Misuse Measure)	17-item screener for patients using chronic opioids, addresses risk for current/future aberrancy; intended for as one component of comprehensive opioid risk assessment. Validated short form available, as well as computer-based applications (Butler, Budman, Fanciullo, & Jamison, 2010; Butler et al., 2007)
Cognitive functioning	MoCA (Montreal Cognitive Assessment)	8-item, clinician-administered cognitive impairment screening tool commonly employed in health care settings (Nasreddine et al., 2005)

somatization is present, the clinician must take particular care to avoid further medicalizing or overtreating somatic complaints. The individual with excessive somatic concern experiences intense distress and/or significant disruption in functioning as well as excessive thoughts, feelings, and behaviors related to their pain symptoms. Rumination often leads to lost sleep, feelings of hopelessness, and expressions of excessive worry. A downward cycle of repeated requests for evaluation, anxiety symptoms, and heightened reactivity to any perceived worsening or change in the pain condition may emerge, leading the patient to make frequent requests for office visits, prescription medications, diagnostic tests, and interventions. If efforts to reassure the patient are unsuccessful, conflicts in the clinician-patient relationship may emerge and may lead to the clinician erroneously labeling the patient a "symptom magnifier," "hypochondriac," or "malingerer." Labeling, blaming, or accusing the patient of conscious manipulation of the pain condition for financial or other secondary gain is typically misguided and countertherapeutic, as the excessive or disproportionate thoughts, feelings, and behaviors more likely indicate a psychological condition. Individuals exhibiting these behavior patterns benefit from a combination of behavioral approaches and a coordinated, interdisciplinary care model that directs the patient toward functional, rather than symptom-driven, treatment goals.

Patients may present for specialized pain care having had multiple prior surgeries or concurrent providers, and family members may unintentionally reinforce excessive somatic concern by encouraging online searches for new or experimental treatments or by endorsing self-imposed functional restrictions or disability behavior. Recognizing and responding therapeutically to the individual with excessive somatic concern is essential to preventing excessive, unnecessary, and potentially harmful interventions. Consolidation and coordination of care is the most important management strategy, typically by centralization of care referrals through a single primary care provider who takes the role of health care team leader. This approach can effectively limit excessive subspecialist assessments, facilitate communication, and prevent costly and unnecessary interventions.

V. PAIN BEHAVIORS

According to operant learning theory, behavior is a function of its consequences; behaviors are exhibited more frequently when followed by a pleasant stimulus (positive reinforcement) or removal of an unpleasant stimulus (negative reinforcement); behaviors become less frequent when negative outcomes follow (positive punishment) or when positive outcomes are removed (negative punishment). The operant model of pain focuses on **pain behaviors** as a central component of the pain problem and emphasizes the role that **learning** plays in maintaining or diminishing these behaviors. Although operant approaches to pain management are relevant to any chronic pain condition, these approaches are particularly relevant to the individual with somatic overconcern or excessive pain behaviors. As illustrated in Figure 6.1, the individual exhibits an increase in a behavior after negative reinforcement (eg, rest or a short-acting analgesic is followed by a transient reduction in pain.) Pain complaints may also evoke increased care and attention from a spouse or caregiver (positive reinforcement), who then offers to take over aversive responsibilities (negative reinforcement). In this way, social reinforcements can become a major factor in maintaining or increasing pain behaviors, even without intentional manipulation or "malingering" on the part of the patient or the family. Behaviors that reduce pain are typically reinforced intermittently, further strengthening their association, and over time the disability or pain-contingent behaviors can become ingrained within the individual's environment and social support relationships.

Assessment of the unique factors relevant to the complex reinforcement of pain behaviors by an experienced behavioral specialist can help the treatment team to effectively apply operant principles to the overall care plan. Behavioral clinicians can also engage with willing family members and caregivers to help them recognize the most helpful strategies to provide caring support for the patient while reducing their responses that will reinforce pain behaviors. Best practices for behavioral management include implementation of high-frequency, regularly scheduled visits with the primary care provider for noninvasive assessment and reassurance, supportive reinforcement of pain self-management strategies, regular physical activity, and individualized treatment goals that focus on functional outcomes (rather than pain measures).

VI. STANDARDIZED MEASURES

Efforts over the past 20 years to improve pain management by promoting routine systematic pain assessment, termed the "fifth vital sign," have been linked to unintended consequences, including overmedicalization and overuse of opioid analgesics. Efforts are under way to promote implementation of clinical guidelines to assess and manage pain, including guidelines for the prescription of opioids for chronic pain and the use of defined criteria to screen, assess, and reassess pain in various treatment contexts. Standardized measures can be used effectively to aid clinical assessment, monitor treatment progress, and compare efficacy of treatment interventions. Commonly used self-report measures and observational measures of pain, relevant comorbidities, and functional status are included in Table 6.1. Some measures are simple **screening tools** to help the clinician identify when more comprehensive assessment is warranted. Other measures are **assessment instruments** designed to evaluate the severity of a condition and predict risk and/or prognosis. Some measures may be administered as a self-report form and others are clinician administered (through interview or observation). Although not an exhaustive list, Table 6.1 describes measures commonly used in pain care settings and that have validation and normative data available for pain populations.

To promote development of generalizable, well-constructed, and clinically relevant patient-reported measures, the National Institutes of Health created the Patient-Reported Outcomes Measurement Information System (PROMIS) to evaluate instruments targeting pain-related domains across multiple chronic conditions. PROMIS domains include pain intensity (pain rating), pain quality, perceived life interference, emotional functioning, pain behavior, and disability. PROMIS measures can be administered electronically and readily integrated into electronic health records. Although there is increasing use and integration of PROMIS measures, their clinical utility has been challenged and many clinicians still opt to use the various disease-specific scales that are currently available.

VII. SELF-REPORT MEASURES

Despite concerns regarding validity and bias associated with self-report measures, their availability and cost-effectiveness make them an important component of clinical assessment. Self-reported domains include **pain**

perception (such as pain intensity and degree of pain relief), **mood and affect** (depression and anxiety), **pain beliefs** and/or **coping strategies** (somatization, fear-avoidance, catastrophizing), **pain-related suffering** (pain acceptance), and pain-related **functional assessment and quality of life.**

The GAD-7 and PHQ-9 are self-report questionnaires that address anxiety and pain, respectively. The PHQ-9 has been extensively studied in multiple acute and chronic pain populations and grades the severity of depression symptoms and addresses suicidal ideation and global impairment. Sleep problems are common in chronic pain, and the Sleep Disturbance Questionnaire addresses subjective experiences of insomnia including restlessness, mental overactivity, consequences of insomnia, sleep readiness concerns, sleep hygiene, anxiety-related sleep issues, and symptoms of obstructive sleep apnea. As with other screeners, this measure is not intended to replace a clinical interview and sleep history.

A brief screening instrument to address problematic pain beliefs and somatization is the Pain Catastrophizing Scale (PCS), which is widely used to assess rumination, "symptom magnification," and helplessness with respect to pain; higher scores predict poor outcomes with many pain treatment interventions. The self-report Patient Health Questionnaire-15 (PHQ-15) measures the level of concern about 15 somatic symptoms. It may be less relevant for assessing the patient who only presents with marked concern about particular pain issues, a place where the PCS may be more appropriate. The Tampa Scale of Kinesiophobia addresses fear-avoidance of activity, has demonstrated adequate psychometric properties, and correlates with objective and other subjective measures of disability.

The World Health Organization Disability Assessment Scale (WHODAS-R) is a longer, 36-item measure with specific disability domains that can help to establish goals for treatment and define a baseline as well as a pre-post measure for clinically relevant areas of functioning. The six domains of functioning included are cognition (understanding and communication), mobility (ability to move and get around), self-care (ability to attend to personal hygiene, dressing, and eating and to live alone), getting along (ability to interact with other people), life activities (ability to carry out responsibilities at home, work, and school), and participation in society (ability to engage in community, civil, and recreational activities). A shorter form of this measure (WHODAS 2.0) may reduce respondent burden but with a risk of missing critically important areas of disability important for the assessment and management of the patient suffering from persistent pain.

Although measures that cut across persistent pain conditions are typically preferred, disease-specific measures also have a role. Measures have been developed for almost every pain-related condition. Other chapters address some of these measures specifically for spine pain, and other multiple measures are also available for fibromyalgia and headache. The Fibromyalgia Impact Questionnaire-R (FIQ-R) includes 21 items that address specific complaints and functional limitations typically associated with that disorder. It is often important to document a diagnostic picture suggestive of fibromyalgia, as the presence of this diagnosis often predicts a problematic course with treatments for other pain conditions. Similarly, the Headache Impact Questionnaire-6 (HIT-6) offers another brief screening measure that has been validated with migraine and other headache conditions, addressing the full range of symptoms and their impact.

VIII. OBSERVATIONAL MEASURES

Observational measures have long been used in the pain field in an effort to standardize the assessment of physical functioning or **physical capacity**. Standardized **work capacity** assessments typically address the individual's ability to engage in specific tasks that simulate the work environment by observing effort in various lifting, bending, standing, or walking activities. Studies of these measures, however, have not supported their efficacy in assessing malingering, and critics have noted that their generalizability to actual work settings may be limited. The clinician-administered Waddell's signs test has been used extensively to identify "nonorganic" pain, but the validity of conclusions drawn from Waddell's signs has been questioned by clinicians and in court cases, leading to decreased reliance on this observational tool.

Certain chronic pain populations have increased prevalence of cognitive impairment. An interview-based mental status examination administered by mental health providers may include observational screening tools and can provide important screening data with particular relevance in settings where impaired psychiatric and/or cognitive functioning occurs more frequently than in the general chronic pain population, for example, nursing home settings. Cognitive impairment is a potential adverse effect of commonly prescribed pharmacologic agents, and psychiatric comorbidities including depression, disordered sleep, and anxiety may also contribute. A review of instruments to assess cognitive function revealed limited normative data for chronic pain populations, although several clinician-administered instruments have been studied with chronic pain populations. Many are long, several are not sensitive to mild levels of impairment, and some require specialized training by the clinician. The Montreal Cognitive Assessment (MoCA) is a short, validated, clinician-administered screener available in multiple languages that addresses attention and concentration, executive function and memory, conceptual thinking, orientation, and ability to perform calculations. It can be valuable with respect to cognitive function, but it does not address anxiety, depression, or personality disorder features.

In the content of chronic pain, the most clinically relevant observational approach is the provider's careful observation of the patient's appearance, display of pain behaviors, attentiveness to interview questions, and recall of recent specific events. Interview questions about specific recent and past events may be used to assess memory if the accuracy of the patient's responses can be confirmed by a significant other or medical record. The clinician should always note the presence of depressed affect, statements about suicidal intent or plans, or slurred speech, and patient beliefs and attitudes are best documented by quoting specific statements in the record. Simply documenting broad, nonspecific descriptors such as "the patient presents as hostile" or "cooperative" is of little value in the absence of specific details, examples, or thorough descriptions of the relevant behaviors. Health literacy, language, or other communication barriers should also be assessed and noted, as these are important potential barriers to effective assessment, adherence, and patient engagement. Any vision or hearing deficits should be documented so that adaptive strategies may be consistently applied by all care team members.

There has traditionally been an overreliance on self-report measures in pain medicine because standardized observational measures have been limited and complex assessments are time-intensive and difficult to execute consistently. For example, a review of over 2700 studies of mindfulness interventions for chronic pain found only one study that used an observational performance-based outcome measure. Data from digital monitoring devices are emerging as promising, cost-effective strategies for objective measurement, and data from wearable activity tracking devices can be transferred electronically and integrated into the patient's ongoing pain and disability assessment and goal setting. Useful activity tracker data may include step counts, sleep time and quality, and intensity of activity, and trackers have been used to study outcomes in a wide range of pain conditions and interventions, including fibromyalgia, postlaminectomy, and total knee arthroplasty (Mobbs, Phan, Maharaj & Rao, 2016; Phan & Mobbs, 2016; Rao et al., 2016; Roe, Salmon & Twiggs, 2016; Scheer et al., 2017). It has also been suggested that activity trackers may potentially encourage increased activity and reduce self-report bias by consistently cuing the patient when planned activity goals are reached.

IX. BEHAVIORAL ASSESSMENT FOR EFFECTIVE GOAL SETTING

While the goals of care for acute pain or injury are to return the patient to baseline health status, it can be much more difficult to identify appropriate goals for chronic pain management, as the complete resolution of pain or return to full functioning may not be realistic. In order to establish realistic and measurable short- and long-term treatment goals, it is essential to assess and openly discuss the patient's expectations. If a patient with a chronic pain condition reports a potentially unrealistic goal such as "I just want the pain fixed" or "I just need to find the right dose/kind of pain reliever," clinician intervention to redefine appropriate goals will head off later misunderstandings and frustrations for both patient and clinician. Goals should ideally reflect measurable functional targets such as improved mood (evidenced by increased interest in pleasurable activities), increased activity (evidenced by returning to regular participation in a specific activity), improved sleep (evidenced by data from a fitness tracker or other record-keeping), or improved energy (evidenced by activity intensity or duration). The patient should be informed that preliminary goals that are established in the assessment phase will be periodically reviewed and revised over the course of treatment, but the primary focus will remain on identifying clear, specific, time-based goals that can be objectively assessed and systematically reinforced. When appropriate treatment goals are addressed early and prior to an intervention or surgery, postprocedure frustrations and disappointment may be reduced and outcomes optimized. Similarly, prior to initiating chronic opioid therapy, clear expectations for objective goals should be in place and documented in a written treatment agreement. Sharing proposed treatment goals with important stakeholders, including family and other treating clinicians, and soliciting their feedback is also a key strategy to encourage consistency and motivation toward measurable functional goals.

X. BARRIERS AND STIGMA ASSOCIATED WITH PSYCHOLOGICAL ASSESSMENT

When a pain condition becomes chronic, some degree of anxiety and somatic concern is common. If marked anxiety, depression, or irrational beliefs about the underlying condition and interventions are present, behavioral intervention may improve treatment satisfaction and effectiveness. Barriers to behavioral assessment and interventions, including patient resistance or refusal to participate, may be related to societal and cultural stigma associated with mental health diagnoses and treatments.

Depending on the setting or the patient's financial resources, access to care may be another barrier.

The following steps maximize the likelihood of a successful mental health referral:

- **Explain that mental health assessment is a normal component of a comprehensive pain assessment,** and reassure the patient that referral does not imply that the pain complaints are being minimized or dismissed as "psychosomatic." Preface the referral by acknowledging the profound impact of serious pain conditions on a wide range of functions, including emotional functioning, for example, "We're addressing mental health concerns because it's so common for individuals with significant or prolonged pain to have consequences such as sleep loss, anxiety, and frustration. We want to make sure we address you as a whole person in order to best manage your pain."
- **Initiate the psychological assessment and referral early in treatment.** Do not wait until a crisis or major setback emerges, as this can lead to resistance and anger from the patient, who may perceive the referral as distancing or a negative clinician response to an unsuccessful treatment.
- **Identify and engage key stakeholders** (such as a spouse or a trusted cotreating clinician), and encourage them to support behavioral referrals and interventions. Whenever possible, educate family members and other stakeholders, and provide evidence for the success of behavioral interventions.
- **Recognize and address potential financial, access, and insurance barriers.** Despite mental health insurance parity laws, coverage limits and shortages of qualified providers remain a serious problem for many patients. Increasingly, tertiary pain care centers and primary care practices directly contract for behavioral services; when available, these greatly facilitate access to on-site, integrated mental health consultations and treatment.
- **Despite absence of conflict or difficulty during your clinical encounters, significant psychosocial barriers to successful treatment may still be present.** For example, patients with certain personality disorders will report immediate benefit from your treatment interventions, comply with clinical recommendations, and report satisfaction with care, only to deny any measurable improvements in symptoms or function, becoming high utilizers of escalating levels of medical care. Alternatively, many individuals with significant depression can "put on a happy face" during interactions with others, but privately suffer with serious untreated symptoms.

Psychologists or psychiatrists who provide comprehensive chronic pain assessments should, at a minimum, have basic training and experience with this complex patient population. Although specialty fellowships are available, currently there is no board certification for mental health providers in the specialty area of pain management. It is prudent for the pain clinician to refer to mental health professionals who follow subspecialty ethical standards that require the behavioral clinician to practice within the scope of their training and skills. Some state guidelines require increased levels of training for clinicians practicing in the fields of pain psychology or psychiatry.

XI. SPECIAL CONSIDERATIONS FOR INDIVIDUALS RECEIVING CHRONIC OPIOID THERAPY

As the risks associated with chronic opioid therapy have become widely recognized, specific assessment for chronic opioid therapy (sometimes termed **opioid risk stratification**) is becoming increasingly common. This assessment, however, should never be considered a onetime evaluation, as risk factors and patient goals and expectations change over time. Unfortunately, this risk assessment may be perceived by the patient as adversarial, further complicating the clinician's ability to gather accurate clinical information. As noted above, patient education and efforts to normalize the assessment as a component of routine care and patient safety can help overcome this barrier.

Controlled substance assessments are typically applied to **assess risk of medication misuse or abuse**, either before initiating chronic opioid therapy or to guide ongoing treatment. As many variables may be considered within the realm of "risk," it is helpful to define the subset of risks that are most relevant to the individual, for example, overdose risk, risk for aberrant behaviors such as dose escalation or diversion, or likelihood of poor response to the intervention. Risk-related variables associated with chronic opioid therapy are well established, although many of these factors are also associated with poorer medical, psychological, and social outcomes. The Opioid Risk Tool offers a useful template for classifying the patient risk into low, medium, and high categories, but robust data are lacking to support this classification system. Validated self-report instruments such as the COMM or SOAPP-R (Screener and Opioid Assessment for Patients with Pain-Revised) can add valuable data to the clinical assessment. Abbreviated and computer-based versions of these tools have been studied, although all of these measures should be considered adjuncts to a comprehensive interview-based assessment. Especially when assessing risks of chronic opioid therapy, obtaining data from multiple information sources is strongly recommended. These include (but are not limited to)

- Thorough review of the patient's medical and mental health records, particularly those that predate beginning opioid therapy
- Urine toxicology screening
- Routine, serial reviews of state databases for prescription monitoring of controlled substances
- Permission to engage the patient's significant others/caregivers in care planning

Clinicians should engage in ongoing conversations with the patient that include empathy for their difficult situation as well as frank and open conversations about the serious potential risks of chronic opioid treatment. Informed consent should always include efficacy and safety of alternative, nonopioid options. Plain-language reviews of the scientific literature on chronic opioid therapy are available online to help the clinician effectively communicate to patients and families potential medical complications, including hyperalgesia, dangerous drug interactions, and other risks. Written and verbal instructions for safe storage and disposal of controlled substances should be provided to all patients, and benefits of providing the patient and family access to naloxone should also be routinely discussed.

XII. SPECIAL CONSIDERATIONS FOR WORK-INJURED POPULATIONS

Chronic pain associated with occupational injury is typically complex and measurable outcomes tend to be poorer. The compensation and legal processes associated with work-related injuries are often adversarial, and challenges to the validity of the patient's self-reported symptoms may complicate assessment and treatment. To maintain an effective therapeutic alliance, it is important for the clinician to avoid blaming the patient for their injury. Clinicians may at times support delayed return to work, although it is important to underscore to patients and their families that in most cases, rapid return to work-related activities predicts better long-term outcomes for pain and overall disability. As outlined previously, fear-avoidance and multiple other psychological comorbidities typically develop with extended periods of disability, further complicated by the stressors associated with financial losses and legal proceedings. At times, the clinician may be called upon to communicate directly with the patient's employer, occupational physician, or the patient's attorney. In Chapter 9, a template for communication with the complex array of stakeholders involved in an occupational injury is supplied.

As with all complex pain conditions, an interdisciplinary and collaborative care approach is ideally applied in cases of pain-related work injury; single modality treatments often lead to failed outcomes, and knowledge of disability and work-related treatment guidelines as well as consultation with specialists in occupational medicine can help the clinician set appropriate treatment expectations. Caring for patients with chronic pain associated with work injury can be especially complex and challenging—engaging the appropriate care team, including psychological expertise, can contribute to improved outcomes, enhanced coordination of care, and effective return-to-work transition strategies.

XIII. KEY POINTS

- Multidimensional psychosocial assessment is a necessary and integral component of comprehensive evaluation of pain conditions. The psychological and social contexts of pain, as well as past health care experiences and consequences of the pain condition (current and anticipated), will have a profound impact on pain symptom expression, patient and family engagement in recommended care, and clinical outcomes.
- Psychological assessment is ideally integrated into the initial phase of care planning. For individuals with chronic pain conditions, follow-up assessments benefit both the patient and the treatment team, as behavioral clinicians can help monitor the effectiveness of interventions, individualize and update treatment goals, and promote collaboration and communication between care providers and other important stakeholders.
- Depression, anxiety, posttraumatic stress, and substance use disorders are common psychological comorbidities and should be assessed in all patients with chronic pain conditions.
- Screening and assessment measures (self-report, clinician-administered, or observational) are useful adjuncts to the comprehensive psychological assessment and help clinicians identify individuals who will benefit from referral for more in-depth psychosocial evaluation. Table 6.1 includes a selected list of useful screeners and assessment tools that address substance abuse and misuse and risk associated with opioid therapy; severity of anxiety, depression, and sleep symptoms; fear avoidance, pain catastrophizing, and somatization; and cognitive functioning. Questionnaires that assess functional limitations/disability can be particularly useful for goal setting and evaluation of the effectiveness of interventions.
- Individuals with chronic pain typically have complex treatment histories and multiple care providers. Communication and coordination among care providers and other important stakeholders is a key management strategy, and integration of psychological assessment and treatment services within a team-based approach to pain care will enhance opportunities for individualized patient education, appropriate goal setting, and avoidance of unnecessary interventions.

Selected Readings

American Psychiatric Association. *Diagnostic and Statistical Manual of Mental Disorders (DSM-5®).* Washington, DC: American Psychiatric Publishing; 2013.

Bener A, Verjee M, Dafeeah EE, et al. Psychological factors: anxiety, depression, and somatization symptoms in low back pain patients. *J Pain Res.* 2013;6:95-101.

Block AR. Spine surgery. In: Block AR, Sarwer DB, eds. *Presurgical Psychological Screening: Understanding Patients, Improving Outcomes.* Washington, DC: American Psychological Association; 2013:43-60.

Burress E, Burress J, Kulich RJ. Assessment and management of disability in the chronic pain patient. In: Ballantyne J, ed. *The Massachusetts General Hospital Handbook of Pain Management.* 4th ed. Philadelphia, PA: Lippincott Williams & Wilkins; 2018.

Butler SF, Budman SH, Fanciullo GJ, Jamison RN. Cross validation of the current opioid misuse measure to monitor chronic pain patients on opioid therapy. *Clin J Pain.* 2010;26(9):770-776.

Butler SF, Budman SH, Fernandez KC, et al. Development and validation of the current opioid misuse measure. *Pain.* 2007;130(1-2):144-156.

Butler SF, Fernandez K, Benoit C, Budman SH, Jamison RN. Validation of the revised screener and opioid assessment for patients with pain (SOAPP-R). *J Pain.* 2008;9(4):360-372.

Centers for Disease Control and Prevention, National Center for Injury Prevention and Control, Division of Unintentional Injury Prevention. Guideline for prescribing opioids for chronic pain. 2017. Retrieved from https://www.cdc.gov/drugoverdose/pdf/Guidelines_Factsheet-a.pdf

Cheatle M, Fine PG. *Facilitating Treatment Adherence in Pain Medicine.* 1st ed. New York, NY: Oxford University Press; 2017.

Cheatle MD, Foster S, Pinkett A, Lesneski M, Qu D, Dhingra L. Assessing and managing sleep disturbance in patients with chronic pain. *Anesthesiol Clin.* 2016;34(2):379-393.

Choi Y, Mayer TG, Williams MJ, Gatchel RJ. What is the best screening test for depression in chronic spinal pain patients? *Spine J.* 2014;14(7):1175-1182.

Chou R, Turner JA, Devine EB, et al. The effectiveness and risks of long-term opioid therapy for chronic pain: a systematic review for a national institutes of health pathways to prevention workshop. *Ann Intern Med.* 2015;162(4):276-286.

Cleland JA, Fritz JM, Childs JD. Psychometric properties of the fear-avoidance beliefs questionnaire and tampa scale of kinesiophobia in patients with neck pain. *Am J Phys Med Rehabil.* 2008;87(2):109-117.

Collado-Mateo D, Chen G, Garcia-Gordillo MA, et al. Fibromyalgia and quality of life: mapping the revised fibromyalgia impact questionnaire to the preference-based instruments. *Health Qual Life Outcomes.* 2017;15(1):114.

Dersh J, Gatchel RJ, Mayer T, Polatin P, Temple OR. Prevalence of psychiatric disorders in patients with chronic disabling occupational spinal disorders. *Spine.* 2006;31(10):1156-1162.

Dersh J, Mayer T, Theodore BR, Polatin P, Gatchel RJ. Do psychiatric disorders first appear preinjury or postinjury in chronic disabling occupational spinal disorders? *Spine.* 2007;32(9):1045-1051.

Deshpande A, Furlan A, Mailis-Gagnon A, Atlas S, Turk D. Opioids for chronic low-back pain. *Cochrane Database Syst Rev.* 2007;(3):CD004959.

Deyo RA, Ramsey K, Buckley DI, et al. Performance of a patient reported outcomes measurement information system (PROMIS) short form in older adults with chronic musculoskeletal pain. *Pain Med.* 2016;17(2):314-324.

Fernández-de-Las-Peñas C, Fernández-Muñoz JJ, Palacios-Ceña M, Parás-Bravo P, Cigarán-Méndez M, Navarro-Pardo E. Sleep disturbances in tension-type headache and migraine. *Ther Adv Neurol Disord.* 2018;11:1756285617745444.

Finan PH, Goodin BR, Smith MT. The association of sleep and pain: an update and a path forward. *J Pain.* 2013;14(12):1539-1552.

Finkelman MD, Jamison RN, Kulich RJ, et al. Cross-validation of short forms of the screener and opioid assessment for patients with pain-revised (SOAPP-R). *Drug Alcohol Depend.* 2017a;178:94-100.

Finkelman MD, Smits N, Kulich RJ, et al. Development of short-form versions of the screener and opioid assessment for patients with pain-revised (SOAPP-R): a proof-of-principle study. *Pain Med.* 2017b;18(7):1292-1302.

Garin O, Ayuso-Mateos JL, Almansa J, et al. Validation of the "world health organization disability assessment schedule, WHODAS-2" in patients with chronic diseases. *Health Qual Life Outcomes.* 2010;8:51.

Gatchel RJ, Peng YB, Peters ML, Fuchs PN, Turk DC. The biopsychosocial approach to chronic pain: scientific advances and future directions. *Psychol Bull.* 2007;133(4):581-624.

Geriatrics and Extended Care Strategic Healthcare Group, National Pain Management Coordinating Committee, Veterans Health Administration. Pain as the 5th vital sign toolkit. 2000. Retrieved from https://www.va.gov/PAINMANAGEMENT/docs/Pain_As_the_5th_Vital_Sign_Toolkit.pdf

Green SM, Krauss BS. The numeric scoring of pain: this practice rates a zero out of ten. *Ann Emerg Med.* 2016;67(5):573-575.

Gregg CD, McIntosh G, Hall H, Watson H, Williams D, Hoffman CW. The relationship between the tampa scale of kinesiophobia and low back pain rehabilitation outcomes. *Spine J.* 2015;15(12):2466-2471.

Humeniuk R, Henry-Edwards S, Ali R, Poznyak V, Monteiro MG. *The ASSIST-linked Brief Intervention for Hazardous and Harmful Substance Use: A Manual for Use in Primary Care.* 1st ed. Geneva: World Health Organization; 2010.

Jackson W, Kulich R, Malacarne A, Lapidow A, Vranceanu A. Physical functioning and mindfulness based interventions in chronic pain: a systematic review. *J Pain.* 2016;17(4):S99.

Kaye AD, Jones MR, Kaye AM, et al. Prescription opioid abuse in chronic pain: an updated review of opioid abuse predictors and strategies to curb opioid abuse (part 2). *Pain Physician.* 2017;20(2S):S133.

Kleiman V, Clarke H, Katz J. Sensitivity to pain traumatization: a higher-order factor underlying pain-related anxiety, pain catastrophizing and anxiety sensitivity among patients scheduled for major surgery. *Pain Res Manage.* 2011;16(3):169-177.

Kleinman A. *The Illness Narratives: Suffering, Healing, and the Human Condition.* 1st ed. New York, NY: Basic books; 1988.

Kroenke K, Spitzer RL, Williams JB. The PHQ-15: validity of a new measure for evaluating the severity of somatic symptoms. *Psychosom Med.* 2002;64(2):258-266.

Kulich RJ, Backstrom J, Healey E. Chronic pain: a template for biopsychosocial assessment. In: Bonakdar RA, Sukiennik AW, eds. *Integrative Pain Management.* 1st ed. New York, NY: Oxford University Press; 2016:141-152.

Kulich RJ, Driscoll J, Prescott JC, et al. The Daubert standard, a primer for pain specialists. *Pain Med.* 2003;4(1):75-80.

Kulich RJ, Gottlieb B. The management of chronic pain: a cognitive-functioning approach. In: Upper D, Ross SM, eds. *Handbook of Behavioral Group Therapy.* 1st ed. New York, NY: Plenum; 1985:489-507.

Kulich RJ, Walsh EA, Vranceanu A. Psychological assessment and management of pain after surgery in adults: relevance to chronic post-surgical pain. In: Carr DB, Morlion B, eds. *Pain After Surgery.* 1st ed. Washington, DC: International Association for the Study of Pain; 2018.

López-Martínez AE, Ramírez-Maestre C, Esteve R. An examination of the structural link between post-traumatic stress symptoms and chronic pain in the framework of fear-avoidance models. *Eur J Pain.* 2014;18(8):1129-1138.

Mobbs RJ, Phan K, Maharaj M, Rao PJ. Physical activity measured with accelerometer and self-rated disability in lumbar spine surgery: a prospective study. *Global Spine J.* 2016;6(5):459-464.

Moeller-Bertram T, Keltner J, Strigo IA. Pain and post traumatic stress disorder–review of clinical and experimental evidence. *Neuropharmacology.* 2012;62(2):586-597.

Murray AM, Toussaint A, Althaus A, Löwe B. The challenge of diagnosing non-specific, functional, and somatoform disorders: a systematic review of barriers to diagnosis in primary care. *J Psychosom Res.* 2016;80:1-10.

Nasreddine ZS, Phillips NA, Bédirian V, et al. The montreal cognitive assessment, MoCA: a brief screening tool for mild cognitive impairment. *J Am Geriatr Soc.* 2005;53(4):695-699.

Ojeda B, Failde I, Dueñas M, Salazar A, Eccleston C. Methods and instruments to evaluate cognitive function in chronic pain patients: a systematic review. *Pain Med.* 2016;17(8):1465-1489.

Pampati S, Manchikanti L. What is the prevalence of symptomatic obstructive sleep apnea syndrome in chronic spinal pain patients? An assessment of the correlation of OSAS with chronic opioid therapy, obesity, and smoking. *Pain Physician.* 2016;19(4):E579.

Phan K, Mobbs RJ. Long-term objective physical activity measurements using a wireless accelerometer following minimally invasive transforaminal interbody fusion surgery. *Asian Spine J.* 2016;10(2):366-369.

Rao PJ, Phan K, Maharaj MM, Pelletier MH, Walsh WR, Mobbs RJ. Accelerometers for objective evaluation of physical activity following spine surgery. *J Clin Neurosci.* 2016;26:14-18.

Rendas-Baum R, Yang M, Varon SF, Bloudek LM, DeGryse RE, Kosinski M. Validation of the headache impact test (HIT-6) in patients with chronic migraine. *Health Qual Life Outcomes.* 2014;12(1):117.

Roe J, Salmon L, Twiggs J. Objective measure of activity level after total knee arthroplasty with the use of the 'Fitbit' Device. *Orthopaedic J Sports Med.* 2016;4(2):2325967116S00012.

SBIRT, National institute on drug abuse. NIDA drug screening tool. 2018. Retrieved from https://www.drugabuse.gov/nmassist/

Scheer JK, Bakhsheshian J, Keefe MK, et al. Initial experience with real-time continuous physical activity monitoring in patients undergoing spine surgery. *Clin Spine Surg.* 2017;30(10):E1443.

Schneider F, Karoly P. Conceptions of the pain experience: the emergence of multidimensional models and their implications for contemporary clinical practice. *Clin Psychol Rev.* 1983;3(1):61-86.

Silva C, Coleta I, Silva AG, et al. Adaptation and validation of WHODAS 2.0 in patients with musculoskeletal pain. *Revista De Saude Publica.* 2013;47(4):752-758.

Sitnikova K, Dijkstra-Kersten S, Mokkink LB, et al. Systematic review of measurement properties of questionnaires measuring somatization in primary care patients. *J Psychosom Res* 2017;103:42-62.

Sullivan M. *The Pain Catastrophizing Scale: User Manual.* Montreal, Quebec: McGill University; 2009.

The Commonwealth of Massachusetts, Department of Industrial Accidents. Guideline 27 - chronic pain. 2012. Retrieved from https://www.mass.gov/files/documents/2016/08/tp/cl-340.pdf

The Joint Commission. New and revised pain assessment and management standards for accredited hospitals. 2018. Retrieved from https://www.jointcommission.org/topics/pain_management.aspx

Turner JA, Shortreed SM, Saunders KW, LeResche L, Berlin JA, Von Korff M. Optimizing prediction of back pain outcomes. *Pain.* 2013;154(8):1391-1401.

Wawrzyniak KM, Backstrom J, Kulich RJ. Integrating behavioral care into interdisciplinary pain settings: unique ethical dilemmas. *Psychol Inj Law.* 2015;8(4):323-333.

Webster LR. Opioid risk tool. 2005. Retrieved from https://www.drugabuse.gov/sites/default/files/files/OpioidRiskTool.pdf

Wertli MM, Eugster R, Held U, Steurer J, Kofmehl R, Weiser S. Catastrophizing—a prognostic factor for outcome in patients with low back pain: a systematic review. *Spine J.* 2014a;14(11):2639-2657.

Wertli MM, Rasmussen-Barr E, Weiser S, Bachmann LM, Brunner F. The role of fear avoidance beliefs as a prognostic factor for outcome in patients with nonspecific low back pain: a systematic review. *Spine J.* 2014b;14(5):816-836.

Williams JS, Ng N, Peltzer K, et al. Risk factors and disability associated with low back pain in older adults in low- and middle-income countries. Results from the WHO study on global AGEing and adult health (SAGE). *PLoS One.* 2015;10(6):e0127880.

Zanocchi M, Maero B, Nicola E, et al. Chronic pain in a sample of nursing home residents: prevalence, characteristics, influence on quality of life (QoL). *Arch Gerontol Geriatr.* 2008;47(1):121-128.

7 Diagnostic Imaging and Pain Management

James P. Rathmell

I. OVERVIEW

Diagnostic imaging techniques have rapidly advanced in sophistication in recent years at the same time that our understanding of how and when to use these techniques most effectively has grown. Diagnostic imaging is an essential tool for the pain physician, aiding in the accurate diagnosis and treatment of painful conditions. Although plain x-rays remain in common use, advanced modalities including computed tomography (CT), magnetic resonance imaging (MRI), and nuclear medicine studies have proved to be valuable diagnostic tools for patients with pain. Functional imaging modalities, including positron emission tomography (PET) scanning and functional magnetic resonance imaging (fMRI), have added to our understanding of the mechanisms that underlie pain and pain-related behavior. The frequent and indiscriminate use of imaging has contributed to the rapid rise in health care costs. It is important to have a clear understanding of how and when imaging studies should be used. When in doubt, direct consultation with a radiologist can help select the most cost-effective approach to using imaging studies. This chapter will provide a brief introduction to diagnostic imaging modalities and some of their primary uses in caring for patients with painful disorders.

II. IMAGING TECHNIQUES AND STUDIES

A. Plain Films

Plain x-rays generate two-dimensional images that are most effective at identifying abnormalities in skeletal structures—soft tissue abnormalities are often subtle or inferred from changes in bony anatomy. Contemporary x-ray technology generally produces high-quality images with minimal radiation exposure. The x-ray beam is differentially absorbed as it passes through a section of the patient and then goes on to expose the film or electronic image intensifier. Radiopaque contrast materials given orally, locally, intravenously, and intrathecally may be used to aid the study by outlining a specific compartment with a radiopaque material. Most contrast agents used with plain x-rays are iodine based. Plain x-rays are the first-line examination for fewer and fewer conditions but remain invaluable in assessing for fractures and abnormal alignment of bony structures.

B. Fluoroscopy

The principles of fluoroscopy are the same as those of plain x-rays; they are two-dimensional x-ray images. The transmitted radiation is viewed on a fluorescent screen rather than on a static film. Fluoroscopy also allows for repeated images to be taken in sequence providing a motion picture-like recording of moving structures (often called "real-time" fluoroscopy or cineangiography when used to show blood flow through vascular structures). Digital subtraction angiography is a variant of cineangiography in which the baseline static image is digitally subtracted from subsequent images to produce a combined image that more clearly reveals the pattern of contrast spread without the shadows of the overlying structures interfering. Fluoroscopy has become a mainstay in assisting with safe and accurate needle placement in the pain clinic, and digital subtraction techniques have also come into common use for detecting intravascular needle placement during techniques like transforaminal injection.

C. Computed Tomography

The first CT scanners were developed in the 1960s and revolutionized diagnosis of many conditions by providing a cross-sectional reconstruction of the imaged anatomy. For the first time, the exact location and contours of many structures, like the brain, could be directly visualized. Today's CT scanners quickly provide high-resolution diagnostic images, and three-dimensional reconstruction of these images is now commonplace. In CT imaging, the x-ray tube produces a beam of energy that passes through and is detected by a circular array of detectors on the opposite side. Both the detector and the x-ray source rotate around the axis of the patient and produce exposures at various angles and at numerous, closely spaced intervals from top to bottom of the area being imaged. Computer algorithms are then used to reconstruct the data in the desired anatomic plane. CT studies now routinely include axial, sagittal, and frontal planar reconstructions. Intravenous contrast can be used to enhance the imaging of vascular structures and normal tissues.

Quantitative CT is particularly useful in measuring bone density for the assessment of osteoporosis. Newer CT techniques have greatly improved the ability to distinguish subtle differences in soft tissue structures and can be used when MRI (which provides superior soft tissue contrast) is not available, if the patient cannot tolerate MRI because of claustrophobia, or when time is of the essence (eg, rapid diagnosis of epidural hematoma in the emergency department).

D. Magnetic Resonance Imaging

Nuclear magnetic resonance (NMR) was developed in the 1940s to characterize chemical structures by exposing them to strong magnetic fields. In the 1980s, clinical application of NMR became feasible, and the name was changed to MRI to allay public anxiety engendered by the word *nuclear*. MRI has revolutionized diagnostic imaging and our understanding of many diseases without the use of ionizing radiation. MRI signals are obtained by subjecting the tissues to strong magnetic fields, which induce hydrogen ions in tissues to align. Tiny radiofrequency signals are emitted as the hydrogen ions "relax" to their native conformation when the magnetic field is removed. The image represents the intensities of the electromagnetic signals emitted from the hydrogen nuclei at various discrete points at a depth within the tissues being imaged. A tissue such as fat, which is rich in hydrogen ions, gives a bright signal, whereas bone gives a void or essentially no signal. Abnormal tissue generally has more free water and displays different magnetic resonance characteristics. The MR signal is a complex function of the concentration of deflected normal hydrogen ions, buildup and relaxation times (T1 and T2) of the magnetic field, flow or motion within the sample, and the MR sequence protocol (Table 7.1).

There are numerous protocols for both MR data acquisition and image reconstruction that have been developed to aid in diagnosis of specific disorders. Most MR studies provide images that are weighted to emphasize T1 and T2 relaxation times. T1-weighted images are used to discern soft tissue structures: fat remains bright (white/light gray) and water is dark (dark gray/black). T2-weighted images are useful to pain clinicians because they highlight soft tissue/water interfaces: fat and water are bright (white/light gray) and soft tissues remain dark (dark gray/black). T2-weighted images are helpful in evaluating patients with spine-related pain, because many of the problems that cause spinal nerve compression occur where the bony and soft tissue structures of the spine interface with the CSF-containing dural sac. MRI is easily able to provide multiplanar images. Its advantage over CT scan is its superior resolution of subtle differences in soft tissues, especially neural tissues. The addition of gadolinium as an intravenous contrast material aids in defining vascular tumors and inflammatory processes.

E. Myelography

Injection of a radiocontrast material into the intrathecal space, followed by imaging using conventional x-ray techniques or CT, provides diagnostic information about potential structural abnormalities affecting the spinal nerves. When noninvasive imaging with either MRI or CT does not provide adequate information, myelography remains an option for diagnosing a structural spine disease. It is also useful for imaging patients who have had spinal instrumentation, which tends to produce extensive artifact on both CT and MR. Post-myelogram CT imaging can be useful for detecting subtle spinal nerve impingement caused by posterior/lateral intervertebral disc herniation that can be been missed by MRI. However, myelography is invasive and uses ionizing radiation, so it is reserved for unusual scenarios where conventional imaging is inadequate.

F. Bone Scans and Nuclear Medicine

Nuclear medicine studies rely on three types of radioactive emissions: positive particles (α-particles), negative particles (β-particles), and high-penetration radiation (γ-radiation). Nuclear medicine uses the tracer principle, "radiolabeling-" specific physiologic substances with radioactive

TABLE 7.1 MRI Sequences and Appearances of Various Structures

MRI Sequences	Lipid	CSF/Edema	Bone	Spinal Cord/Nerve	White Matter	Gray Matter
T1-weighted	Hyperintense	Hypointense	Hypointense	Intermediate	Brighter	Darker
T2-weighted	Less hyperintense	Hyperintense	Hypointense	Intermediate	Darker	Brighter
Short tau inversion recovery (STIR)	Hypointense	Hyperintense	Hypointense	Intermediate	Darker	Brighter
T1-postcontrast	Normal enhancement of vascular structures, abnormal enhancement at sites of blood-brain barrier disruption, and hypervascularity (tumor, infection, inflammation, demyelination)					

moieties that produce more of these emissions. A radiopharmaceutical agent is injected into the patient, and the radioactive decay is detected by a detection device (eg, a γ-counter). Emissions are detected by a scintillation camera and are mapped in 2D space, demonstrating distribution of the radiolabeled agent in specific target tissues, revealing information about both the structure and function of various tissues.

Bone scans are one common nuclear medicine study that can be helpful in evaluating complaints of skeletal pain. Technetium-99m (99mTc) is a metastable nuclear isomer of technetium-99 that emits γ-rays about the same wavelength as emitted by conventional x-rays. This radiolabel localizes to areas of increased bone turnover that represent increased rates of osteoblastic activity. Bone scans are more sensitive than x-rays in detecting subtle skeletal pathology. Bone scans are particularly helpful in detecting bony metastases and subtle stress fractures: while the sensitivity for detection is high, the low specificity of abnormal findings can be problematic.

G. Discography

Degeneration of the intervertebral discs including loss of disc height and hydration of the nucleus pulposus and the development of radial tears within the annulus fibrosis are common. It is difficult to discern patients who have pain related to these anatomic abnormalities from those with pain unrelated to disc degeneration. Discography was developed to assist in identifying pain arising from the intervertebral discs. Using fluoroscopic guidance, a needle is placed under into the central nucleus pulposus, and a radiographic contrast is injected under low to moderate pressure (high-pressure injection can further damage the disc and is almost universally painful). The level of pain produced in the anatomically abnormal disc is compared with the level of pain produced in an adjacent normal "control" disc. This process can provide objective structural and anatomic information about the intervertebral disc. In addition, it can provide subjective information on whether a specific disc is the source of a patient's axial lumbar pain. Discography has fallen out of favor in recent years after the publication of studies that demonstrated accelerated degeneration of the adjacent normal intervertebral disc that was used as a control during the diagnostic procedure.

H. Positron Emission Tomography

PET is a nuclear medicine technique used to observe metabolic processes to aid diagnosis. A radioactive tracer, most commonly fluorine-18 combined with a biologically active molecule, is injected and emits gamma rays. PET is a sensitive and specific technique for early detection of metastases in many types of cancer, often combined with CT as PET-CT for a precise localization. PET is being used to characterize the physiologic processes that are associated with acute and chronic pain, and the literature on PET and functional neuroimaging of pain is growing.

I. Functional Magnetic Resonance Imaging

MRI has evolved as a powerful research tool for functional imaging of the human brain. Functional imaging, including fMRI, has helped identify mechanisms and anatomic targets that may help to develop more effective and specific treatments for pain. Functional activation of brain regions is reflected by increases in the blood-oxygen-level-dependent (BOLD) signal on fMRI. This modality has been used to examine the contribution of thalamic and cortical areas to the human pain experience. The cortical areas identified include the primary and secondary somatosensory cortices (S1 and S2), the anterior insula, and the anterior cingulate cortex. Abnormal pain evoked by innocuous stimuli (allodynia) has been associated with the specific patterns of activation that differ from those activated by an acute pain stimulus.

III. HEADACHE

Headache is a common complaint among patients presenting to both the primary care physician and the pain clinic. The pain physician must be familiar with indications for imaging in the assessment of patients with headache. Most patients who complain of headache and whose neurologic examinations are normal findings have normal CT studies. Thus, taking a detailed history and performing a neurologic examination are crucial before deciding whether to order a diagnostic test.

A. Primary Headache

In patients who present with a history characteristic of primary headache (new-onset headache without an identifiable underlying cause) without additional neurologic symptoms and with normal findings on neurologic examination, it is rare to find imaging abnormalities, and imaging is not indicated.

B. Secondary Headache

Subarachnoid hemorrhage should be considered in patients without chronic headache but with an initial presentation of the "worst headache of my life." Emergent CT without contrast is the evaluation of choice because it is sensitive to the presence of acute blood. When there is new headache plus fever, lumbar puncture may be indicated. Before proceeding to lumbar puncture, CT is used to exclude any space-occupying lesion—a contraindication to lumbar puncture. CT is also indicated in acute trauma because it best identifies acute hemorrhage and bone fractures. CT with contrast is indicated when there is clinical suspicion of vascular lesions, neoplastic lesions, or inflammatory conditions. Plain x-rays are rarely helpful in evaluating the patient with chronic headache. MRI is preferred as it is highly sensitive for detecting intracranial pathology. Diagnostic criteria and imaging for secondary headache are discussed in more detail in Chapter 38.

IV. CRANIOFACIAL PAIN SYNDROMES

A. Trigeminal Neuralgia

Severe unilateral paroxysmal lancinating pain in the distribution of the trigeminal nerve is a characteristic of trigeminal neuralgia. Trigeminal neuralgia is idiopathic and imaging studies generally show no abnormalities. In patients with trigeminal neuropathy and trigeminal neuropathic pain in which atypical features exist, it is important to evaluate for other diagnostic possibilities. MRI is the imaging modality of choice. Occasionally, vascular malformations, aneurysms, and tumors cause trigeminal neuralgia. Multiple sclerosis is sometimes associated with neuropathic facial pain, and lesions of increased T2-weighted signal intensity on MRI may be seen in the trigeminal brain stem dorsal root entry zones.

B. Glossopharyngeal Neuralgia

The characteristic pain of glossopharyngeal neuralgia is similar to that of trigeminal neuralgia but is located unilaterally in the posterior tongue throughout the tonsillar area and sometimes in the auricular area. It is frequently idiopathic, and, in isolated glossopharyngeal neuralgia, imaging studies rarely show abnormalities. In patients with evidence of associated pathology, particularly at the brain stem, MRI with contrast is the imaging study of choice.

V. CENTRAL PAIN SYNDROMES

Central neuropathic pain can result after an injury to the primary somatosensory nervous system. Constant burning neuropathic pain is typically seen. Infarction, trauma, and radiation are frequent causes. Thalamic pain syndromes and pain following spinal cord injury are two common central pain syndromes, and there are no universally effective treatments for these devastating conditions.

VI. THALAMIC PAIN SYNDROMES

Injury to the thalamus, specifically to the ventral posterolateral nucleus, typically results in constant burning pain on the contralateral side of the body, including the face, arm, trunk, and leg. This pain frequently results from thalamic infarction but can also result from hemorrhage, trauma, or space-occupying lesions including tumor, infection, and abscess. Imaging reveals signal abnormalities in the thalamus contralateral to the site of pain. A "pseudothalamic pain syndrome" can result after injury to the thalamocortical white matter tract. Clinical presentation is similar, but MRI reveals abnormalities in the thalamocortical radiations.

VII. SPINAL CORD INJURY

Injury to the spinal cord at any level can result in a central pain syndrome. Damage to the spinothalamic tract frequently results in central neuropathic pain. Considerable central neuropathic pain accompanies spinal cord injury in 25% of patients. Causes include trauma, space-occupying lesions including neoplasms, demyelinating processes including multiple sclerosis, and syringomyelia. MRI is the imaging modality of choice. In multiple sclerosis, lesions of increased T2-weighted signal intensity are seen in the white matter tracts of the spinal cord. In syringomyelia, MRI reveals a central cavity that shows high signal intensity on T2-weighted images and diminished signal on T1-weighted images.

A. Axial Low Back Pain

Low back pain is a common complaint in patients presenting to both primary care physicians and pain clinics. Pathologic processes affecting the lumbar spine include disc degeneration, intervertebral disc herniation, facet joint arthropathy, vertebral fracture, vertebral dislocation, spondylolisthesis, and osteoporosis. Degenerative causes of low back pain may be difficult to distinguish from other common causes such as simple lumbar sprain-strain. Less common causes include intradural and extradural neoplasms, infections, and congenital abnormalities of the spine. The history and physical examination are the basis for deciding when imaging studies may be helpful in establishing a definitive diagnosis.

The primary rationale for radiographic imaging of low back pain is to exclude or define a serious pathology. Most low back pain originates from the soft tissues, and imaging studies are not helpful. In older patients, imaging studies frequently reveal abnormalities that may or may not be responsible for the pain. Plain x-rays can help diagnose spondylolysis (pars interarticularis defects, usually at the L5 or sometimes L4), ankylosing spondylitis, and fractures but have little utility in routine diagnosis. When neurologic signs or symptoms are present, including those of sciatica, MRI is the imaging modality of choice. MRI without contrast can detect herniation of lumbar discs with compression of nerve roots causing radicular symptoms. In patients with a previous history of lumbar surgery, contrast-enhanced MRI helps differentiate recurrence of disc herniation from epidural scar tissue; the latter is detected by T1-weighted signal enhancement after administration of contrast. In patients with a clinical complaint of lumbar claudication and suspected spinal stenosis, both CT scan and MRI are appropriate. CT scan offers the advantage of superior imaging of bony hypertrophic changes of the lumbar spine.

B. Plain X-ray Evaluation of Low Back Pain

Plain x-ray provides an assessment of the configuration and alignment of the lumbar vertebral spine with a high degree of accuracy. There have been a number of natural history and comparative studies evaluating the usefulness of plain x-rays in evaluating low back pain. In a large retrospective study reviewing 1000 lumbar spine radiographs of patients with low back pain, more than one-half of the radiographs were normal. In another study of 780 patients, only 2.4% had unique diagnostic findings on plain radiographs.

Most episodes of low back pain resolve within 6 weeks. Evidence-based guidelines state that radiographs are not indicated for a first presentation of low back pain (see Chapter 36). General recommendations for radiographs in patients with low back pain are as follows:

- For a first episode of low back pain for fewer than 6 weeks, with improvement with or without active treatment, no radiographs are indicated unless an atypical clinical finding or special psychological or social circumstances exist. Atypical history ("red flags") includes age of more than 65 years, history suggesting a high risk for osteoporosis, symptoms of persistent sensory deficit, pain worsening despite treatment, intense pain at rest, fever, chills, unexplained weight loss, and recurrent back pain with no radiographs within the last 2 years. Atypical physical findings include considerable motor deficit and unexplained deformity.
- For recurrent low back pain, radiographs are not indicated if a previous radiographic study had been done within 2 years.

In general, anteroposterior and lateral views are the only views needed initially. In patients with chronic pain or additional history and physical findings suggesting stenosis or instability, flexion and extension films may be helpful.

C. MRI and Low Back Pain

MRI has a high sensitivity for detecting pathology of the lumbar spine. A poor correlation exists between the severity of pain symptoms and the extent of morphologic changes seen on MRI: a statistically significant percentage of healthy individuals without lumbar pain have degenerative changes on MRI (as many as 50%-60%) and even disc herniation (as many as 20%). Careful attention must be paid to correlate clinical symptoms with radiographic findings; otherwise, imaging findings may be used inappropriately to justify unneeded intervention or treatment.

Age-related morphologic changes occur in the spine throughout life. There is a decrease in concentration of water and glycosaminoglycans in the intervertebral disc, and there is an increase in concentration of collagen. On the MRI, these changes show up as a loss of signal intensity on T2-weighted images, a reduction in the height of vertebral bodies, a reduction in the height of the intervertebral discs, and a reduction in the diameter of the central spinal canal. The onset of degenerative processes of the lumbosacral spine seems to be consistently marked by tears of the annulus fibrosis and by MRI and histologic changes of the vertebral bone marrow adjacent to the intervertebral spaces. Facet degeneration rarely occurs in the absence of disc degeneration, and it seems likely that facet osteoarthropathy results from the added stress of increased loading after disc space narrowing has occurred. Multiple studies have found an association between disc degeneration and facet osteoarthritis using imaging criteria. In patients with radicular symptoms, clinical evaluation can usually predict the spinal nerve involved. The actual spinal pathology cannot be predicted with clinical evaluation alone, and MRI examination can be of assistance. A spinal nerve can be compressed by a disc either at the traversing segment by central disc herniation or at the exiting segment by a lateral disc herniation. Imaging is beneficial for defining the site of pathology. Symptomatic patients may have neuroimaging abnormalities at more than one spinal level.

The MRI appearance of progressive degeneration of the vertebral endplates (the bone facing the intervertebral discs) was classified by Modic (Fig. 7.1).

Type I Modic changes are T1 hypointense and T2 hyperintense and correlate with the formation of granulation tissue subjacent to the endplates. Type II changes are T1 and T2 hyperintense and correlate with replacement of bone marrow by fat. Suppression of the T2 hyperintensity on STIR sequence further confirms the presence of fat. Type III changes appear T1 and T2 hypointense and correlate with long-standing and chronic degeneration of the endplates. Other common degenerative changes seen on both CT and MRI are the formation of osteophytes and/or disc-osteophyte complexes. These bony overgrowths occur most commonly along the margins of the vertebral endplates and at the margins of the articular surfaces of the facet joints. As they enlarge, these bony deposits can narrow the dimensions of the spinal foramina and the central spinal canal and impinge on adjacent neural structures, causing pain and other characteristic neurologic symptoms of spinal and foraminal stenosis.

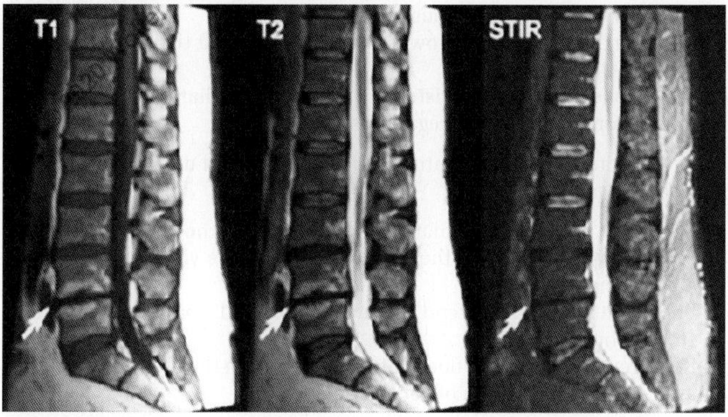

FIGURE 7.1 Type 2 Modic changes (*arrows*) in the vertebral bodies adjacent to the L4/5 intervertebral disc. Type II changes are T1 and T2 hyperintense and correlate with replacement of bone marrow by fat. Suppression of the T2 hyperintensity on STIR sequence further confirms the presence of fat.

D. Pain After Lumbar Surgery

When evaluating patients who have had prior lumbar surgery, it is important to identify those who have recurrent pain that has appeared after a pain-free interval after surgery. The appearance of new pain in this group of patients should signal the need for careful evaluation. New onset of axial low back pain after prior instrumented lumbar surgery can signal hardware failure. This group of patients often describe sudden onset of pain in the area of prior surgery; the pain is often localized, and the pain may resolve completely when they stop moving. Plain x-rays are often invaluable in assessing the integrity of prior spinal instrumentation. In patients who have had previous back surgery and now complain of recurrent radicular pain, the differential diagnosis includes the following:

- Incorrect original diagnosis or residual disease
- Spinal nerve or dorsal root ganglion injury
- Retained or recurrent intervertebral disc fragment
- Epidural fibrosis

Fibrosis is a natural consequence of surgical procedures. Numerous reports suggest that fibrosis and adhesions cause compression or tethering of the spinal nerves and their roots, which in turn can lead to recurrent radicular pain and physical impairment. The literature repeatedly suggests that fibrosis is a major cause of recurrent symptoms when no alternative bone or disc pathology can be found, but definitive proof of this causality is lacking. It has also been suggested that fibrosis may be causal in as many as 25% of patients with failed back surgery syndrome.

Recurrent radicular pain is radicular pain occurring 6 months or later after primary surgery after a successful initial result (eg, at 1 month postoperatively). A considerable association between the size of the peridural scar and the incidence of pain has been demonstrated. MRI with and without contrast helps differentiate recurrent or retained disc fragment from epidural scarring. The criteria used to identify epidural fibrosis by MRI include the following:

- Epidural scar is isointense or hypointense relative to the intervertebral disc on T1-weighted images on an MRI scan.
- Peridural scar tends to form in a curvilinear pattern surrounding the dural tube, with homogenous intensity.
- Traction of the dural tube toward the side of the soft tissue is more characteristic of scar.
- Scar tissue is seen to consistently enhance immediately after the injection of contrast material, regardless of its location.

The criteria used to identify recurrent herniated disc by MRI include the following:

- Recurrent herniated disc material is isointense to the intervertebral disc on T1-weighted images. There tends to be a more variable appearance on T2-weighted images.
- Recurrent herniations tend to have a polypoid configuration with a smooth outer margin.
- Recurrent disc material does not enhance within the first 10-20 minutes after the administration of contrast material.

E. Arachnoiditis

Arachnoiditis, which is distinct from epidural scar formation, involves inflammation within the dura surrounding the spinal nerves. Arachnoiditis is largely a diagnosis made by excluding other causes of pain. Patients present with pain in the lower extremities that involves multiple dermatomes and does not follow the distribution of a single peripheral nerve. The pain often has neuropathic characteristics and is described as tingling, burning, or lancinating; weakness, bowel and bladder dysfunction, and sexual dysfunction are variable. The MRI characteristics of arachnoiditis have been described in three possible patterns. The first is centrally clumped spinal nerve roots in the thecal sac seen on T1-weighted images, the second is peripheral adhesions of roots to the thecal sac, and the third is an increased soft tissue signal within the thecal sac below the conus. These MRI findings are often seen in patients without pain; thus, establishing an unequivocal diagnosis even in the presence of MRI findings can be difficult.

VIII. METASTATIC DISEASE OF THE SPINE

Severe back pain is a common presentation of cancer metastasis to the lumbar spine. The most common tumors that metastasize to bone and therefore to the lumbar spine are lung, prostate, and breast. Multiple myeloma and breast cancer typically are osteolytic, whereas prostate cancer tends to cause osteosclerotic changes. Bone scans are sensitive for detecting metastatic involvement of the lumbar spine. The correlation between the severity of bone scan and the intensity of pain is poor.

When spinal cord compression resulting from epidural metastatic disease is suspected, MRI is the imaging modality of choice and contrast enhancement is recommended. Severe back pain is a\the most common presentation of spinal cord compression. When considerable reduction of vertebral body height is seen, concomitant epidural involvement is common. Disruption of the pedicle on imaging suggests metastatic disease and, when seen on a plain radiograph, warrants further investigation.

IX. INFECTIOUS PROCESSES OF THE VERTEBRAL SPINE

Plain x-rays can be used to assess osteomyelitis. Characteristic changes include loss of endplate definition, associated soft tissue swelling, destruction of vertebral bodies, and loss of intervertebral disc height. MRI detects involvement of the disc space. Occasionally, tMRI is negative and radionucleotide imaging studies can help establish the diagnosis. The characteristics of osteomyelitis on MRI include decreased signal intensity, a loss of delineation and demarcation of the vertebral endplate on T1-weighted images, and increased signal intensity in the intervertebral disc on T2-weighted images.

X. CONCLUSION

Diagnostic imaging studies and image-guided intervention are indispensable tools for the pain physician. Gaining a basic understanding of how and when to use different imaging modalities is a critical part of being an effective clinician. Inappropriate use of these expensive tests not only raises health care costs, it also subjects patients to the unnecessary risks involved in chasing incidental findings irrelevant to the presenting symptoms. While we have given a broad overview of these modalities, consultation with a radiologist is invaluable in choosing the best approach whenever uncertainties arise.

ACKNOWLEDGMENT

This chapter was updated By James P. Rathmell from an earlier version first written by Onassis A. Caneris for the previous edition of this text.

Selected Readings

Chou R, Fu R, Carrino JA, Deyo RA. Imaging strategies for low-back pain: systematic review and meta-analysis. *Lancet.* 2009;373:463-472.

Klein JP. A practical approach to spine imaging. *Continuum (Minneap Minn).* 2015;21:36-51.

Lurie JD. What diagnostic tests are useful for low back pain? *Best Pract Res Clin Rheumatol.* 2005;19:557-575.

Modic MT, Ross JS. Lumbar degenerative disk disease. *Radiology.* 2007;245:43-61.

8 Neurophysiologic Testing in Pain Management

Kenneth S. Tseng

I. INTRODUCTION

Neurophysiologic testing can be a useful adjunct in the clinical evaluation of patients who present with pain and not just those with neuropathic pain. However, because the subspecialty of clinical neurophysiology and electrodiagnostic medicine intersects several different specialties, encompasses tests that may evaluate both painful and nonpainful disease, and is often compartmentalized in large hospitals or academic centers, it may be difficult for pain specialists to fully realize the scope of testing that is available to them.

Nociceptive signals can be transmitted along many different pathways in the peripheral and central nervous systems, before being interpreted in the cerebral cortex. Neurophysiologic testing attempts to delineate the portions of the nervous system that may be responsible for that pain. Electrodiagnostic studies can be helpful in differentiating radiculopathy from peripheral nerve entrapment or axonal injury from demyelinating disease. Quantitative sensory testing (QST) can evaluate the function of small-diameter nerve fibers (nociceptive fibers), isolating conduction through Aδ, C, or Aβ fibers. Somatosensory evoked potential (SEP) can be useful for identifying more centrally located lesions in cases where tests of peripheral nerve function are normal. Parts of the nervous system that are not normally involved in pain messaging, such as the sympathetic and parasympathetic systems, can become involved in certain disease states, after injury, or following sensitization; abnormalities of these systems can also be evaluated using various neurophysiologic tests. Since neuronal activity in various afferent systems can overlap or change functionally (both anatomically and at a cellular and molecular level), the diagnosis and treatment of some pain problems can be complex, and being able to utilize neurophysiologic testing can help provide clarity to the mechanisms underlying the pain and direct targeted treatment. In addition to the tests mentioned above, there are several other tests that may also be performed by neurophysiologists—such as microneurography, contact heat evoked potentials, or nociceptive flexion reflex testing—but are beyond the scope of this review. Figure 8.1 summarizes the utility of various tests for different parts of the nervous system.

II. ELECTRODIAGNOSTIC TESTING

Electrodiagnostic testing can be a useful aid in the diagnosis of nervous system disorders. These studies can help to localize lesions to the central or peripheral nervous system and, within the latter group, can further narrow the diagnosis to radiculopathies, plexopathies, mononeuropathies, neuromuscular junction disorders, or myopathies. Certain patterns on testing results can also suggest specific diagnoses. Once an abnormality is identified, results of electrodiagnostic testing can also be used to monitor the progression of disease.

Routine electrodiagnostic evaluations include both nerve conduction studies and needle examination of muscles or electromyography (EMG). The term "nerve conduction study" is commonly abbreviated as NCV, where the "V" stands for velocity, although nerve conduction studies also measure amplitude, latency, duration, temporal dispersion, conduction block, and other measurements, in addition to velocity. The combination of the two tests—EMG and NCV—is commonly referred to as simply "EMG." An electrodiagnostic study must include both components to provide a complete assessment of peripheral nervous system function.

A. Nerve Conduction Studies

Nerve conduction studies are performed by electrically stimulating a peripheral nerve with supramaximal intensity and then measuring the response from either the nerve itself or a muscle it innervates. The nerves being studied can be motor nerves, sensory nerves, or mixed.

Stimulation of a motor nerve produces a compound muscle action potential (CMAP) measured in the muscle belly of the muscle being stimulated. For example, one of the more commonly performed tests for the diagnosis of carpal tunnel syndrome is the stimulation of the median nerve at the wrist and the measurement of a CMAP from the abductor pollicis brevis (APB) muscle, as pictured in Figure 8.2. The amplitude of the CMAP is measured from baseline to negative peak in millivolt units. The onset and peak latencies of the stimulation are the times between the onset of the stimulation and the onset and peak of the CMAP, respectively, measured in millisecond units. The conduction velocity of the nerve is calculated by measuring the latency from different points—proximal and distal—along the nerve and dividing the distance by the difference between the latencies of the distal and proximal points.

Stimulation of a sensory nerve produces a sensory nerve action potential (SNAP), measured at a distal point along the same nerve. For example, the median sensory study is performed by stimulating the median nerve at the wrist and by recording a SNAP from the digital nerves of the second finger. Because they are nerve-generated potentials rather than muscle-generated potentials, the amplitude of SNAPs are smaller than CMAPs and are measured in microvolt units (compared to millivolt units for CMAPs).

A characteristic feature of demyelinating neuropathy, conduction block can be seen when the amplitude or area under the CMAP is significantly reduced from distal stimulation compared to proximal stimulation. If the amplitude is decreased, but the duration of the CMAP generated by the proximal stimulation is increased, this may be a sign of temporal

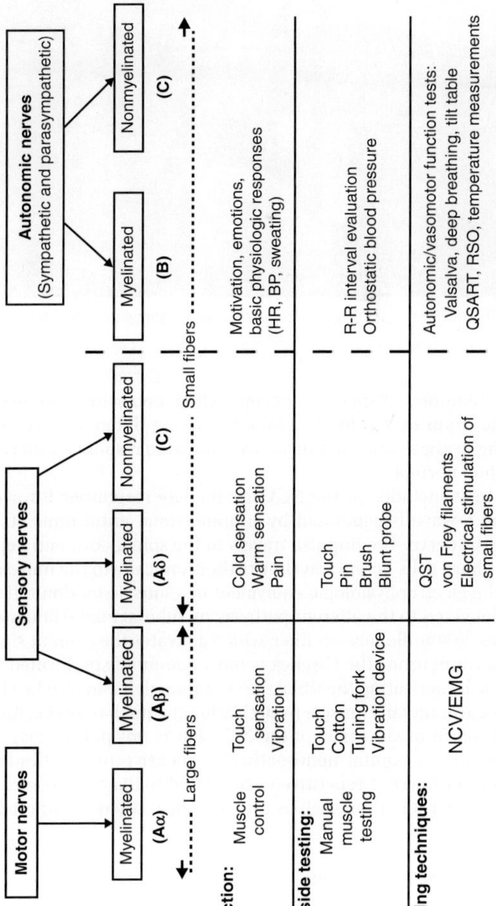

FIGURE 8.1 The peripheral nerve fibers. NCV, nerve conduction velocity; EMG, electromyography; QST, quantitative sensory testing; QSART, quantitative sudomotor axon reflex testing; RSO, resting sweat output.

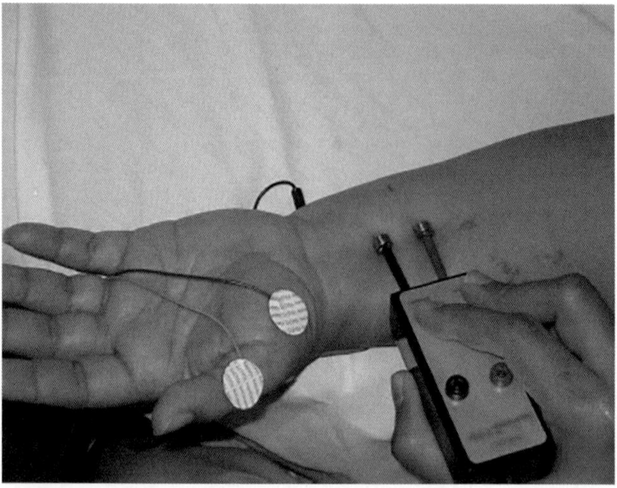

FIGURE 8.2 The median motor study being performed by stimulating the median nerve at the wrist.

dispersion. Temporal dispersion occurs when demyelination leads to increased variation in conduction velocity among different nerve fibers, thus resulting in phase cancellation and a summated response with smaller amplitude than normal.

Other tests included in the NCV are the late responses: F-wave and H-reflex. The F-wave is generated by supramaximal antidromic stimulation of a motor nerve. The impulse travels to the spinal cord and depolarizes anterior horn cells before traveling orthodromically to the muscle. The H-reflex is the electrophysiologic equivalent of a muscle tendon reflex. An impulse is delivered to the afferent pathway by submaximal stimulation of a type 1a muscle spindle sensory fiber, which activates the efferent signal in the alpha motor neuron. The H-reflex is most commonly performed in the soleus muscle by activating the tibial nerve, although it can also be elicited in the flexor carpi radialis muscle by activating the median nerve. Another study that is performed as part of the NCV, but is not particularly useful in the evaluation of painful neuropathy, is repetitive nerve stimulation, in which a motor nerve is repetitively stimulated to diagnose disorders of the neuromuscular junction, such as myasthenia gravis or Lambert-Eaton syndrome.

B. Needle Electrode Examination

The electromyogram or needle electrode examination of muscles is used to evaluate for denervation changes and myopathic disorders. A disposable needle electrode is inserted into the muscle belly. Insertion activity is caused by mechanical damage to the muscle fibers from the needle insertion, and abnormal activity can be manifested as fibrillation potentials or positive sharp waves. Once the needle is resting in place, the examiner evaluates any spontaneous activity in the relaxed muscle. Normal resting muscle should not exhibit any electrical activity, and pathologic findings can include signs of abnormal muscle fiber potentials (fibrillation potentials, positive sharp waves, complex repetitive discharges, myotonic discharges) and abnormal motor unit potentials (fasciculations, myokymic discharges, cramp discharges, neuromyotonic discharges).

Contraction activity is measured as a motor unit action potential (MUAP) during voluntary contraction of the muscle fibers. A motor unit is defined as the alpha motoneuron, its axon, the skeletal muscle fibers it innervates, and the neuromuscular junctions. Normally, individual motor units contain muscle fibers of the same type; for example, motor units containing slow-twitch, fatigue-resistant muscle fibers are the first to be activated when a low load is placed on the muscle. If the load on the muscle increases, the central nervous system can either increase the rate at which the motor unit fires (also known as temporal recruitment) or recruit more motor units to fire at the same time (also known as spatial recruitment). Generally, larger motor units containing fast-twitch, fatigable muscle fibers are reserved for larger loads. One way to measure the recruitment pattern in a given muscle is to measure the recruitment frequency, which is the frequency of the first motor unit at which a second motor unit is recruited. In myopathic disorders, early recruitment occurs because many motor units fire at a normal rate despite minimal force production. After a denervation injury and subsequent reinnervation, the motor units are reduced in number but fire excessively fast, producing reduced or neurogenic recruitment. Chronic neuropathic disorders cause motor units to become larger than normal. In myopathic disorders, the motor units are smaller than normal.

C. Localizing a Nerve Injury

One reason to order an EMG/NCV as a pain physician is to attempt to localize a painful process, such as differentiating between a radiculopathy, plexopathy, or mononeuropathy. EMG/NCV can be used in two ways to localize an injury: by "intersection" or by direct localization of an abnormality across a segment of nerve. In the intersection method, abnormalities in two or more nerve overlapping pathways indicate that the lesion is likely at the overlap or intersection of the two pathways. In the direct localization method, a focal nerve abnormality, such as a conduction block, decreased conduction velocity, or increased temporal dispersion is demonstrated on nerve conduction study.

D. Aiding in Diagnosis

Certain characteristics EMG findings of nerve injury may help to differentiate axonal injury from demyelinating injury. After an axonal injury, axonal degeneration occurs over several weeks. The nerve conduction study generally shows a normal latency, but may show decreased motor and sensory amplitudes on CMAP and SNAP, respectively. The NCV may be slightly slower than normal. On needle electrode examination, fibrillation potentials and positive sharp waves can be present after axonal nerve lesions. After prolonged axonal injury, uninjured motor units may reinnervate denervated muscle fibers, producing larger MUAPs. In contrast to axonal injury, demyelination injury generally causes a prolonged latency and a more profound decrease in conduction velocity. A conduction block or increased temporal dispersion may be more prominent if individual myelinated nerve fibers are affected, such as in acquired (segmental demyelination) neuropathy, as opposed to hereditary (uniform demyelination) neuropathies, in which diffuse demyelination leads to a more pronounced latency prolongation or decrease in conduction velocity. Unlike with axonal injury, the needle electrode examination findings in demyelinating injury show no abnormal spontaneous activity and normal insertional activity. There can be evidence of reduced recruitment and rapidly firing motor units in both types of injury.

Because NCV measures both CMAPs and SNAPs, it can be used to differentiate motor and sensory fiber abnormalities. When a mixed nerve, such as the median nerve, is involved, sensory fibers are usually involved to a greater extent than motor fibers. In the special case of radiculopathy, SNAPs are normal—even when there is clinical hypoesthesia over a dermatome—because the dorsal root ganglia is distal to the lesion and therefore unaffected.

The timing of an EMG/NCV after axonal injury will also affect the findings. After the initial injury, Wallerian degeneration occurs in the segment distal to the lesion. This process often takes several weeks, and CMAP and SNAP amplitudes may be normal at first. CMAP amplitudes recorded distal to the lesion begin to decline at 3 days and reach their nadir at 7 days; SNAP amplitudes begin to drop at 6 days and reach their nadir at 11 days. Needle electrode studies may be normal for up to 3 weeks after axonal injury before fibrillation potentials and positive sharp waves are present. Therefore, the EMG study should not be performed sooner than 3 weeks postinjury to avoid underdiagnosing the severity of an axonal or demyelinating injury.

E. Clinical Applications

The American Association of Neuromuscular and Electrodiagnostic Medicine (AANEM), in conjunction with the American Academy of Neurology and the American Academy of Physical Medicine and Rehabilitation, has provided several guidelines for the use of electrodiagnostic testing in certain clinical situations. They recommend use of EMG/NCS for suspected cases of carpal tunnel syndrome. NCS can be useful to confirm diagnosis and localize injury in suspected cases of peroneal mononeuropathy or tarsal tunnel syndrome; the use of EMG is unclear in these cases. Guidelines for the electrodiagnostic evaluation of ulnar neuropathy at the elbow have been published, but the authors stopped short of recommending that EMG/NCS be performed for all suspected cases, since there were no outcome studies evaluating the risks and benefits of performing electrodiagnostic evaluation for suspected cases.

The utility of electrodiagnostic testing has also been evaluated in cervical and lumbar radiculopathy. In some cases, NCS can differentiate radiculopathies from entrapment neuropathies that present with similar symptoms. Needle EMG of cervical paraspinal muscles can be used to pinpoint the involved nerve root. Median and/or ulnar nerve F-wave tests are an option for suspected C8 or T1 radiculopathy and the flexor carpi radialis H-reflex test is an option for suspected C6 or C7 radiculopathy. For lumbar radiculopathy, electrodiagnostic testing can be particularly helpful in cases with negative or discordant imaging findings or when clinical examination is limited by patient effort or discomfort. Suggested studies that may aid in the diagnosis of lumbosacral radiculopathy include peripheral limb EMG, needle EMG of paraspinal muscles, and possibly H-reflex test in S1 radiculopathy.

III. QUANTITATIVE SENSORY TESTING

QST evaluates high-threshold pain and temperature-sensing mechanisms and provides information on the function of the entire afferent pain pathway (from receptor to brain). Patients are asked to respond to thermal (warm, cool, hot, and cold), mechanical (light touch and pinprick), vibratory, and electrical stimuli at varying intensity to detect hypoesthesia, allodynia, hypoalgesia, or hyperalgesia that can be associated with abnormal pain states. These are considered psychophysical tests because they lack the objectivity seen in electrodiagnostic testing and are dependent on patient cooperation, examiner proficiency, and maintenance of equipment. QST relies on subjective responses to calibrated sensory stimuli. Different testing centers vary in the methods that they use, and it is difficult to amass a body of normative data that allows for comparison of results. However, QST may still be able to detect subtle abnormalities in patients who have normal NCV/EMG studies.

Evidence of hypoesthesia can be elicited using mechanical, vibratory, or electrical stimuli. The "sensory detection threshold" is the lowest intensity at which the stimulus can be felt half of the time. Thermal or electrical stimuli can be used to elicit pain responses. Abnormalities of specific modalities can indicate pathology in certain central nervous system tracts: vibratory and thermal sensations are specific to the dorsal columns and spinothalamic tracts, respectively. Peripheral nerve function—particularly nociceptive transmission in the Aδ fibers, C fibers, and Aβ fibers—can also be elucidated based on responses to different stimuli. The Aδ and C fibers are activated by cold and warm stimuli, respectively, and their function can be measured by heat pain and cold pain thresholds. The Aβ fibers can be evaluated by vibration sense. Common test findings and their association with various pain processes are listed in Table 8.1. The American Academy of Neurology has recommended that while QST can be useful for demonstrating altered pain thresholds in several pain syndromes, the sensitivity of QST is unclear, and it should not be used as the sole criteria in a diagnostic evaluation.

A. Thermal Stimuli

Pain and temperature sensation are both transmitted to higher brain centers by small, high-threshold fibers (C and Aδ) via the lateral spinothalamic tracts. Thermal thresholds are most commonly tested using devices

TABLE 8.1 Pain Processes and Their Association With Test Findings

Pain Processes	Test Findings
Painful neuropathies (including *CRPS II*)	Thermal hypoesthesia, hyperesthesia, *hypoalgesia, or hyperalgesia*
Peripheral sensitization and inflammation (including erythromelalgia or angry backfiring C [ABC] nociceptor syndrome)	Heat hyperalgesia
CRPS I	Cold or heat hyperalgesia without *hypoesthesia* or hyperesthesia
Central sensitization	Tactile allodynia, mechanical hyperalgesia
Postherpetic neuralgia	Thermal hypoesthesia and hyperalgesia (anesthesia dolorosa)
Triple cold syndrome	Cold hyperalgesia, cold hypoesthesia, and cold skin
Sympathetically mediated pain (CRPS I and II)	Changes in sudomotor reflexes (QSART), sweat output (RSO), and vasomotor function

CRPS, complex regional pain syndrome; QSART, quantitative sudomotor axon reflex testing; RSO, resting sweat output.

that rely on the Peltier effect to generate or remove heat from a small-surface thermode that is placed flat against the skin. Most systems utilize a computer to regulate the rate and degree of thermal changes within prespecified limits. Different testing systems have different size thermodes, sometimes depending on the site chosen for testing. Patients are initially asked to identify cold and warm detection thresholds, followed by cold and hot pain thresholds. The threshold for detection of temperature change is usually within 1°C-2°C above or below baseline. Hot pain is typically felt at ~45°C. The cold pain threshold is quite variable but can occur starting at ~10°C or less. Attempts have been made to collect age- and gender-adjusted normative data as a reference.

B. Vibration Stimuli

The vibration test measures the sensitivity of the larger Aβ fibers. Several different devices are in use, including the Rydel-Seiffer graduated tuning fork and the electromagnetic biothesiometer, which produce vibrations at a single frequency at varying amplitudes and are commonly used in clinical practice as screening devices for neuropathy. Newer devices can produce vibration in a range of frequencies. To avoid variability in the amount of pressure transmitted by the tester when using handheld devices, some newer devices are mounted on supports.

C. Mechanical Stimuli

One of the most common ways to quantify sensitivity to mechanical stimuli is through the use of von Frey hairs, which were initially made of horsehair when they were first developed in 1896. The Semmes-Weinstein series is a standardized set of von Frey monofilaments with graduated diameters that produce a repeatable, calibrated force when pressed down on the skin hard enough to cause them to bend. In addition to screening for early changes in peripheral neuropathy, the monofilaments can be used to detect allodynia and areas of primary and secondary hyperalgesia.

Mechanical pain threshold can also be measured using pinprick stimuli applied with varying degrees of force. Enhanced temporal summation (windup) is the phenomenon where rhythmic application of a pinprick to the same site on the skin over a period of at least eight repetitions, each being delivered within 2-3 seconds of the previous one, causes escalation of discomfort in a person with hyperalgesia. It is typically present in neuropathic pain states (eg, spinal cord injury and postherpetic neuralgia).

D. Electrical Stimuli

Responses to electrical stimuli are occasionally included as part of QST, although its use is mostly limited to research studies. Previously described machines generate frequencies of 5 Hz, 250 Hz, and 2000 Hz at varying intensities. Abnormally elevated current perception thresholds (CPT) may reflect a hypoesthetic state and indicate a loss of nerve function. The utility of CPT measurements has been questioned, since electrical stimuli are not naturally occurring.

IV. EVOKED POTENTIALS

A. Somatosensory Evoked Potentials

SEPs can be used to evaluate the entire somatosensory pathways, from the distal peripheral nerve, through the dorsal root ganglion, dorsal columns, thalamocortical projections, to the sensory cortex. In the clinical setting, repeated electrical stimuli are applied at a peripheral mixed nerve, such as the median nerve at the wrist, the common peroneal nerve at the knee, or the posterior tibial nerve at the ankle. The evoked potential responses are then measured at certain points along the sensory pathway: on the scalp, over the cervical or lumbar spine, and over peripheral nerves proximal to the stimuli. Measurements at each component include peak latencies, polarity, and amplitude. Peak latencies exhibit less intersubject variability than amplitude and are used to calculate interpeak intervals. Prolonged interpeak intervals or absent obligate waves are generally considered to be abnormal. Individual laboratories may also use other variables to determine abnormal tests based on their own normative data.

SEPs can be useful in situations when the clinical diagnosis is uncertain based on conventional EMG or NCS, particularly if those latter studies are normal or if no peripheral sensory response can be obtained. They may also be useful for identifying central sensory pathway lesions. Some authors have suggested that SEPs may be useful to delineate the spinal levels involved in lumbar spinal stenosis. However, it is generally agreed that SEPs are not superior to EMG/NCS for acute lumbar radiculopathy, chronic thoracic root disease, chronic cervical root disease, or entrapment neuropathies.

B. Laser Evoked Potentials

Measuring laser evoked potentials is another method that has been used to evaluate the spinothalamic tract. Infrared laser pulses are applied to the skin, causing rapid heating and activation of C and Aδ fibers. The stimuli normally produce one early and one late cerebral response as measured by EEG, which could correspond to the difference in conduction velocity between the thin myelinated and unmyelinated fibers. Clinically, laser evoked potentials can be used to distinguish a neuropathy in the small pain fibers from a neuropathy affecting the larger nerve fibers responsible for touch or vibration. However, there are studies suggesting that the cerebral activity may not be nociceptive-specific and could be affected by other stimuli such as attentional reorientation.

V. AUTONOMIC TESTING

Small fiber sensory neuropathy causing severe neuropathic pain can often be associated with changes to autonomic and somatic C fibers, as well. Routine EMG/NCV testing, which does not include autonomic tests, can be normal in patients with a purely small fiber neuropathy because motor and sensory nerve conduction studies measure conduction along large-diameter myelinated nerve fibers only. Therefore, in patients with symptoms suggesting neuropathic pain who have normal NCSs, autonomic testing can be used along with QST or skin biopsy to diagnose small fiber neuropathy. Autonomic testing should also be considered in patients with other symptoms suggesting dysautonomia, such as syncope, orthostatic hypotension, gastrointestinal or urologic disturbances, and sweating disorders.

Sudomotor function refers to the autonomic pathways that activate sweat gland production via cholinergic innervation. Sweating can occur as a response to pain, stress, fear, or anxiety. This occurs most frequently in the sweat glands of the palms, soles, and axilla. The sympathetic skin response, now also known as electrodermal activity, is a test that measures a change in skin conductance, thought to be due to secretion of electrolytes in sweat. This test can be performed using standard EMG equipment, placing the recording electrode on either the palmar surface of the hand or the plantar surface of the foot and stimulating at the contralateral median or tibial nerve, respectively. Accumulation of normative data is difficult due to large intersubject variability, habituation of the response with repeated stimuli, and attenuation from medications (such as anticholinergics), age, and low skin temperature; thus, the test is generally only considered abnormal in cases when the sudomotor response is absent.

The quantitative sudomotor axon reflex test (QSART) is a sensitive, reproducible test that produces quantifiable results. A special sweat capsule with two compartments is attached to the skin. Acetylcholine is iontophoresed through the skin under the outer compartment to produce a sweat response that is measured by a change in humidity in the inner compartment. In addition to binding the muscarinic receptors on the sweat glands, the iontophoresed acetylcholine also binds to nicotinic receptors on the nerve terminals, activating an antidromic impulse along the postganglionic sympathetic nerve back to branch points where the impulse then travels orthodromically to neighboring sweat glands. QSART is thus a measure of the fidelity of postganglionic neurons, but does not assess preganglionic pathology.

An older method of assessing sudomotor function which tests both pre- and postganglionic function is the thermoregulatory sweat test (TST). The TST is performed in a temperature- and humidity-controlled room or sweat chamber. An activator dye that changes color when exposed to sweating is applied to the skin over the entire body, allowing areas of anhidrosis to be mapped. TST sweat patterns can show loss of sweat response in a stocking and glove distribution, such as in length-dependent neuropathy, focal defects corresponding to individual nerves, dermatomal defects corresponding to nerve root defects, or complete autonomic failure. Abnormal TST results combined with normal QSART results could indicate a preganglionic autonomic lesion.

AANEM has made several recommendations with regard to the use of autonomic testing in distal symmetric polyneuropathy. In cases of polyneuropathy, they recommended consideration of autonomic testing to document autonomic involvement. For patients with suspected small fiber sensory polyneuropathy, which can present as a burning sensation and allodynia in both feet, autonomic testing can be considered as part of the evaluation. In addition to the tests of sudomotor function listed above, tests of cardiovagal and adrenal function (eg, orthostatic blood pressure, heart rate response to tilt, heart rate response to deep breathing, the Valsalva ratio, etc.) should also be considered in the battery of autonomic function tests to provide the greatest diagnostic accuracy.

VI. CONCLUSION

This chapter describes some of the neurophysiologic tests available in pain management. Used together with a careful physical exam and appropriate imaging, in certain situations, these tests can help localize pathology to the central or peripheral nervous system, confirm peripheral entrapment neuropathies, pinpoint abnormalities in certain nerve fiber types, or document autonomic involvement. They are reliant on the accumulation of normative data, and in many cases, different labs have their own reference ranges for normal values.

Selected Readings

American Association of Electrodiagnostic Medicine. Guidelines in electrodiagnostic medicine. Somatosensory evoked potentials: clinical uses. *Muscle Nerve Suppl.* 1999;8:S111-S118.

Campbell WW. Guidelines in electrodiagnostic medicine. Practice parameter for electrodiagnostic studies in ulnar neuropathy at the elbow. *Muscle Nerve Suppl.* 1999;8:S171-S205.

Cho SC, Ferrante MA, Levin KH, et al. Utility of electrodiagnostic testing in evaluating patients with lumbosacral radiculopathy: an evidence-based review. *Muscle Nerve.* 2010;42(2):276-282.

England JD, Gronseth GS, Franklin G, et al. Practice parameter: evaluation of distal symmetric polyneuropathy: role of autonomic testing, nerve biopsy, and skin biopsy (an evidence-based review). Report of the American Academy of Neurology, American Association of Neuromuscular and Electrodiagnostic Medicine, and American Academy of Physical Medicine and Rehabilitation. *Neurology.* 2009;72(2):177-184.

Illigens BM, Gibbons CH. Sweat testing to evaluate autonomic function. *Clin Auton Res.* 2009;19(2):79-87.

Jablecki CK, Andary MT, Floeter MK, et al. Practice parameter: electrodiagnostic studies in carpal tunnel syndrome. Report of the American Association of Electrodiagnostic Medicine, American Academy of Neurology, and the American Academy of Physical Medicine and Rehabilitation. *Neurology.* 2002;58(11):1589-1592.

Katims JJ, Naviasky EH, Rendell MS, et al. Constant current sine wave transcutaneous nerve stimulation for the evaluation of peripheral neuropathy. *Arch Phys Med Rehabil.* 1987;68(4):210-213.

Legrain V, Bruyer R, Guerit JM, et al. Involuntary orientation of attention to unattended deviant nociceptive stimuli is modulated by concomitant visual task difficulty. Evidence from laser evoked potentials. *Clin Neurophysiol.* 2005;116(9):2165-2174.

Marciniak C, Armon C, Wilson J, et al. Practice parameter: utility of electrodiagnostic techniques in evaluating patients with suspected peroneal neuropathy: an evidence-based review. *Muscle Nerve.* 2005;31(4):520-527.

Mouraux A, Iannetti GD. Nociceptive laser-evoked brain potentials do not reflect nociceptive-specific neural activity. *J Neurophysiol.* 2009;101(6):3258-3269.

Namer B, Bickel A, Kramer H, et al. Chemically and electrically induced sweating and flare reaction. *Auton Neurosci.* 2004;114(1-2):72-82.

Rolke R, Magerl W, Campbell KA, et al. Quantitative sensory testing: a comprehensive protocol for clinical trials. *Eur J Pain.* 2006;10(1):77-88.

Shy ME, Frohman EM, So YT, et al. Quantitative sensory testing: report of the Therapeutics and Technology Assessment Subcommittee of the American Academy of Neurology. *Neurology.* 2003;60(6):898-904.

Singer W, Spies JM, McArthur J, et al. Prospective evaluation of somatic and autonomic small fibers in selected autonomic neuropathies. *Neurology.* 2004;62(4):612-618.

Snowden ML, Haselkorn JK, Kraft GH, et al. Dermatomal somatosensory evoked potentials in the diagnosis of lumbosacral spinal stenosis: comparison with imaging studies. *Muscle Nerve.* 1992;15(9):1036-1044.

So YT. Guidelines in electrodiagnostic medicine. Practice parameter for needle electromyographic evaluation of patients with suspected cervical radiculopathy. *Muscle Nerve Suppl.* 1999;8:S209-S221.

Wilke K, Martin A, Terstegen L, et al. A short history of sweat gland biology. *Int J Cosmet Sci.* 2007;29(3):169-179.

9 Disability Assessment

John W. Burress, Emily J. Burress, and Ronald J. Kulich

Disability, as a term used by society, refers to a status where an individual is unable to carry out necessary tasks in any important domain of life because of a medical or psychosocial condition. Pain remains as one of the greatest contributors to this problem. Society asks health care providers to assist in the determination of disability. Why? This chapter strives to answer that question and improve disability assessment skills with special focus on the person with persistent pain.

In contrast to disability, the term ***impairment*** has a more narrowed focus to connote a loss or abnormality of body structure or of a physiologic or psychosocial function. Impairment can be more objectively defined and reliably measured than disability. Impairment, according to the American Medical Association (AMA), provides the underpinnings of assessing disability. The AMA Guide defines disability as "an alteration of an individual's capacity to meet personal, social, or occupational demands or statutory or regulatory requirements because of an impairment."

Patients and other stakeholders (eg, school, workplace, coach, family) often want the health care provider to opine on the individual's ability to perform in a specific setting. For example, a patient being treated for a chronic pain condition may ask the provider to complete a return-to-work (RTW) note. A pragmatic approach that the health care provider can deploy to address this challenge includes breaking the question down into three distinct components: **limitations, restrictions, and tolerance.** Limitation refers to what the person cannot do, for example, raise the arm. Limitations coincide with impairment (can be measured). Restriction refers to what he should not do, for example, climb a ladder. Restriction implies consideration of risk, for example, if the patient is sedated or has vertigo, then it is best not to climb a ladder or operate a vehicle. Of the three components, tolerance is the most difficult to assess. Some would argue for ignoring tolerance altogether when assessing ability because it cannot be measured and depends on the individual. However, to ignore what often represents the deciding influence in a person's disability represents an abdication of role. Further, understanding the determinates of tolerance allows insight into the human condition. That insight can reveal clinical opportunities to achieve tertiary prevention (reduce impact of existing disease by restoring function and reducing disease-related complications) and thus manage the degree of disability. Whether the original insult or injury stemmed from work or not, chronic pain represents a common pathway toward disruption of purposeful/fulfilling activity, including employment. Regardless of niche or specialty within medicine, this chapter provides the background necessary for the clinician to unlock the process of disability assessment. Importantly, once done, a credible disability assessment pivots the focus of care toward improving that person's human condition.

I. BURDEN OF DISABILITY ASSOCIATED WITH PAIN

The economic and personal costs associated with disability continue to escalate despite advances in medical care and some improvements in the accessing of health care services. Overall estimates of the cost of disability in the United States typically exceed $300 billion per year. Much of this loss is directly due to pain conditions, with an estimated 13% of the workforce having a loss of productive time over a 2-week period due to headache, back pain, musculoskeletal pain, and pain associated with arthritis. Back pain employer costs are $7.4 billion per year for workers over 40, with 71.6% of the cost due to repeat exacerbations of pain. Putting this into perspective with other illnesses impacting society, the annual cost of pain remains greater than that of heart disease and 30% higher than the combined costs of diabetes and cancer.

The burden of disability associated with pain, in addition to the financial costs, includes often devastating impacts on the patient and family. Disabling pain conditions can be intermittent or constant, and common consequences include psychological concomitants such as anxiety, depression, sleep disorder, and family and marital disruptions. Exacerbation of psychiatric conditions also is particularly common. Many patients develop substance use disorders as a result of long-term treatment with controlled substances. Persistent use of opioids after surgery also may lead to surgical complications. For example, Cron et al. (2017) found that 21% of patients were using opioids preoperatively and those users had 9.2% higher costs, a 12.4% longer length of stay, more complications, and more readmissions.

In contrast to disability from major trauma with immediate and often permanent deficits, creeping catastrophic disability begins with a minor injury that balloons over-time often leading to high dollar costs and loss of livelihood. Creeping catastrophic disability claims stem from influences both internal to the worker (eg, pre-incident coping ability; reaction to injury) and/or external to the worker (eg, glitches in how claim is administrated or care provided). Importantly, targeted interventions that begin with careful assessment can halt the evolution of creeping catastrophic cases and prevent unnecessary disability burden and pain.

II. WHY PROVIDERS ARE ASKED TO ASSESS DISABILITY

Why does society ask health care providers to assess disability? One explanation stems from early military aviation and underscores that to assess disability, the provider's understanding of the individual together with a sense of the job or life domain in question allows the provider to formulate an opinion. Early in World War I, officers were reassigned into aviation when they became physically unfit for infantry or cavalry. British studies showed that most plane crashes (90%) were due to physical or mental deficiencies. A medical board established to vet prospective pilots and assess injured pilots produced such striking statistical evidence of success that the United States quickly adopted a similar model, thus beginning the "formal authority" role for the health care provider. Since then, health care providers in the United States and other countries have been asked to assess the abilities of individuals in a variety of settings including those with statutory mandate. Examples include Americans with Disability Act (ADA), Social Security Disability Insurance (SSDI), short-term disability (STD) policies or long-term disability (LTD) policies, return to work (RTW), fitness for duty (FFD), driving a commercial motor vehicle (DOT, Department of Transportation), and flying a plane (FAA, Federal Aviation Administration). To fulfill the role of evaluator designated by society, the clinician must combine an understanding of the individual with a sense of the ergonomics, defined as matching people to their machines or work settings, of the job in question and then formulate an opinion.

III. KEY INSIGHTS ON ASSESSING DISABILITY

Critical to formulating your opinion regarding disability is to **appreciate the function of your patient.** From the preceding paragraph on "why," we see that the provider's insights on the physical and psychological makeup of a person lead to our being picked as society's best choice for assessing disability. Medical training generally focuses on diagnosing the patient and managing disease processes. For many, identifying a person's functional deficits seems foreign. **However, to assess disability, the clinician must overcome the impulse to defer this assessment to others.**

There are courses and certifying exams to formally assess permanent impairment ratings, for example, the use of a goniometer to measure range of motion for a specific joint and then apply tables to ascertain whole body impairment. Techniques are recommended within relevant chapters of the AMA Guide. Further, there are courses and reference books on performing a formal independent medical evaluation (IME). However, the majority of disability assessment questions that arise do not entail the assessment of impairment rating and are within the scope of practice of most clinicians. Stakeholders give deference to the treating provider's input. Many retirement systems by statute or law explicitly request the opinions of the treating providers. Not providing an accurate, well-reasoned assessment of functional status represents a disservice to patients.

Understanding the role of observation and psychometrics should boost your confidence in assessing disability. The psychologist-turned-ergonomist that developed the NIOSH Safe Lifting Guides, Stover Snook, PhD, observed and measured repetitive lifts of sequential weights by hundreds of individuals. During the evaluation of a specific individual, the clinician can deploy the same psychometric principles by having that person lift, pull, push, transfer, and/or perform a cognitive task designed to bring sharp focus on potential rate-limiting ergonomic challenges. What the patient is asked to do during the evaluation is important, but your observations are critical and inform what you document. You should be aware that medical professionals address disease, but those that adjudicate disability rewards want practical information on how disease impacts function. Assessing disability of the patient with pain represents an exercise in writing to your audience. Requested forms to be completed vary, but the common theme remains the communication of the functional impact of disease.

Pain diagrams (visual representation of anatomical location and character or distribution of pain) and questionnaires can be utilized to augment and facilitate assessment. Still, questionnaires and other tools should always be an adjunct to the evaluation, with the clinician obtaining a comprehensive activity tolerance history as an integral aspect of the assessment.

Patients may be reluctant to discuss any actual or perceived functional limitations in an interview setting, preferring to focus on evaluation and "fixing" their particular pain condition. Refocusing the patient on the importance of function can be facilitated by a frank discussion about the impact of pain on their life. Further, addressing those areas of function may prove more successful vs efforts that target underlying initial tissue damage or nociception. Most importantly, this focus should not stop with the patient's initial assessment. Standardized measures can be administered on a repeated basis as a means of assessing success with the treatment, as well as engaging the patient in the process of self-directed care aimed at improving function.

Self-report measures of disability measure various domains, for example, the inability to engage in specific tasks or fear-avoidance of activities. Some are brief, pain-specific measures such as the Pain Disability Questionnaire or the Tampa Kinesiophobia Scale, measures that are intended for use across a range of pain conditions. Others are disease specific and include pain content, for example, disability associated with spine conditions has been assessed with the Quebec Back Pain Disability Score, the Roland-Morris Disability Scale, the Oswestry Disability Index, or the Neck Disability Index. Other common disabling pain conditions also have been assessed with measures such as the Headache Impact Test and the Fibromyalgia Impact Questionnaire-R. Finally, there are well-studied global measures of disability that have normative data on multiple pain conditions. In an effort to facilitate the use of standardized assessment that could be used across conditions, the PROMIS group initiated a series of extensive studies through the National Institute of Health, producing a series of disability measures ranging from 4 to 20 items. The PROMIS questionnaire is meant to easily integrate into an e-record and place a low burden on the patient.

The World Health Organization Disability Scale 2.0 provides another alternative that may have the benefit of better clinical utility as it covers very specific domains of disability. It can be particularly helpful with respect to treatment planning and goal setting for the patient. Specific domains include (1) understanding and communication; (2) getting around (eg, standing, walking); (3) self-care (eg, dressing, eating); (4) getting along with people; (5) household activities; (6) school/work activities; and (7) participation in society (eg, participating in community activities, sexual activity, time focused on health concerns). Chronic pain is a condition that commonly leads to disability, regardless of the location of pain or the initial disease-specific entity. When the pain has persisted for months or years, the disabling features of the illness tend to be similar. Hence, global self-report measures of disability (Table 9.1) may be the best measures to consider in clinical practice.

Fortunately, newer technological advances have started to provide better and more cost-effective options for assessing disability. Digital monitoring devices are increasingly being studied with chronic pain conditions that include chronic low back pain, fibromyalgia, and mixed musculoskeletal disorders. Normative data for specific pain populations is becoming available, and devices can be readily integrated into the patient's care. Devices such as the Fitbit provide ongoing reinforcement for increase in activity. These measures fail to be unobtrusive, so there are issues of bias when used in a research setting. In a clinical setting, this generally is less of a concern. Indeed, the clinician can integrate the device into the initial evaluation and over time to measure progress. In subsequent visits, the patient can be engaged in discussions about functional goals during review of the results of the digital monitoring.

TABLE 9.1 Self-report Disability Measures

Measures	General Disability
World Health Organization Disability Assessment Scale (WHODAS-2)	36-item scale, covering six domains of functioning: (1) cognition (understanding and communication); (2) mobility (ability to move and get around); (3) self-care (ability to attend to personal hygiene, dressing, and eating and to live alone); (4) getting along (ability to interact with other people); (5) life activities (ability to carry out responsibilities at home, work, and school); and (6) participation in society (ability to engage in community, civil, and recreational activities). Not intended as a brief screening of disability, but well-established validity and reliability with normative data and utility for assisting the patient with goal setting.
PROMIS Scales	Through an extensive NIH-funded effort, a set of validated self-report outcome measures were produced to monitor physical, mental, and social health in the general population and in patients with chronic medical conditions. Depending upon their intended use, there are short and longer forms with some as short as 4-12 items. There also are innovative Computerized Adaptive Technology (CAT) versions where the burden on the respondent may be reduced. With respect to disability, physical functioning and psychological PROMIS scales have been used with multiple types of pain.
Pain Disability Questionnaire (PDQ)	14-item, addressing physical functioning as well as psychological domains related to disability. Widely used in clinical settings and referenced in the AMA Guide to Permanent Impairment, 6th addition. More recent data are limited with respect to psychometric properties including predictive validity.
	Back Pain Scales
Oswestry Disability Index (OSI)	10-item index, listing degrees of severity for each domain, extensively studied with low back pain, addressing mostly functional variables such as sitting, standing, walking, but also social and sexual activity impacted by disability.
Acute Low Back Pain Screening Questionnaire	20-item questionnaire, with primary focus on screening of psychosocial variables; additional data available for neck pain. Cutoff scores may predict disability and sick leave.[a]
Roland-Morris Disability Questionnaire (RMDQ)	24-item questionnaire, primarily studied on low back pain, and there is a modified version for general pain. Covers similar disability domains as ODI, including psychosocial areas, but less sensitive as a measure of severe disability.

TABLE 9.1 Self-report Disability Measures (*Continued*)

Measures	**General Disability**
	Other Pain Conditions
Orebro Musculoskeletal Pain Screening Questionnaire	25-item questionnaire, screens for six common factors impacting disability including perceived function, pain, fear avoidance, distress, return to work expectancy, and pain coping. General wording permits use with multiple-location pain conditions.
Fibromyalgia Impact Questionnaire (FIQ-R)	21-item questionnaire, covers ADL, recreational, and work functional limitations common to FM and other chronic pain conditions, longer than most screeners. Transparent question domains facilitate discussion with patient about goals and can be used repeatedly to measure outcome.
Neck Disability Index (NDI)	10-item widely used measure that correlates with quality of life and other emotional functioning measures. Also shows predictive validity with other self-report and objective measures of function.
Headache Impact Test (HIT)	6-item test validated on migraine and other headache diagnoses, most common brief self-report assessment in headache, can be used as repeated measures scale to assess outcomes.
	Disability Related Psychological Constructs
Tampa Scale of Kinesiophobia	17-item scale, covers fear-avoidance of activity, and scores predict to other disability measures. Most studies are in low back and neck pain, but relevant across all pain conditions.[b]
Pain Catastrophizing Scale (PCS)	13-item scale, one of several scales available to address the catastrophizing construct, with the PCS frequently used with spine conditions. Constructs include rumination, somatization, and helplessness.[c,d]

[a]Sattelmayer M, Lorenz T, Röder C, Hilfiker R. Predictive value of the Acute Low Back Pain Screening Questionnaire and the Örebro Musculoskeletal Pain Screening Questionnaire for persisting problems. *Eur Spine J.* 2012;21(suppl 6):773-784. doi: 10.1007/s00586-011-1910-7.

[b]Cleland J, Fritz J, Childs J. Psychometric properties of the Fear-Avoidance Beliefs Questionnaire and Tampa Scale of Kinesiophobia in patients with neck pain. *Am J Phys Med Rehabil.* 2008;87(2):109-117. doi: 10.1097/phm.0b013e31815b61f1 7.

[c]Wertli M, Eugster R, Held U, Steurer J, Kofmehl R, Weiser S. Catastrophizing—a prognostic factor for outcome in patients with low back pain: a systematic review. *Spine J.* 2014;14(11):2639-2657. doi: 10.1016/j.spinee.2014.03.003.

[d]Wertli M, Rasmussen-Barr E, Weiser S, Bachmann L, Brunner F. The role of fear avoidance beliefs as a prognostic factor for outcome in patients with nonspecific low back pain: a systematic review. *Spine J.* 2014;14(5):816-836.e4. doi: 10.1016/j.spinee.2013.09.036.

IV. HOW TO ASSESS DISABILITY

The following steps comprise a pragmatic approach that any provider can utilize.

A. Preparation

Before the assessment visit, you will review records. Based on your record review, you should consider which if any self-report instruments to administer. The clinician can choose the instrument(s) that best fit the patient's circumstances (see Table 9.2).

Pain diagrams give a visual illustration that can stimulate useful discussion during the interview; however, they should be interpreted with caution. Certain questionnaires assess activity tolerance across key domains (eg, WHODAS-2 scale, PROMIS) and may provide information more useful for assessing function compared to questionnaires that focus on impacts of pain (eg, PDQ, Oswestry). In short, responses to self-report instruments can help focus the discussion during your interview, substantiate conclusions, and enhance stakeholder acceptance of evaluation process.

B. Face-to-Face Interview

In addition to obtaining the usual medical history which should include mechanism of injury, presenting complaints, treatment to date, occupational history, and psychosocial history (see also MGH Handbook of Pain chapters on History and Clinical Examination as well as Pain Assessment), a careful activity tolerance history should be taken. Questions should start with an open-ended approach. For example, an initial question or statement might be "Describe a typical day." Then ask the patient to describe activities that provoke pain with attention to what is being avoided in their daily life or work setting. Interview may then proceed to more directed questions as needed. For example: "Can you sit through a 30 minute TV show? A movie?" As mentioned in the above section on preparation, self-report measures such as a pain diagram and questionnaire(s) should be incorporated into the discussion.[29] These instruments address specific areas of functional limitation and can augment, especially when the clinician has a conversation with the patient about the specific limitations and abilities that are endorsed in the questionnaire. Further, the scores of the WHODAS-2 scale may be helpful in documenting overall functional level and provide a basis for comparison over time. Specific items may be more helpful to shape the assessment process, for example, "You checked that you have problems walking long distances and have trouble with household tasks. How far do you typically walk every day? What specific household tasks are a problem completing because of the pain?"

TABLE 9.2 How to Assess Disability

Prepare	Record review, choose self-report instruments to be administered including pain diagram and questionnaire(s) that ask about activity tolerance across key life domains
Interview and examine	Obtain HPI, mechanism of injury, current symptoms, etc. Go beyond standard history to include questions on activities tolerated that inform functional assessment. Incorporate pain diagram and questionnaire responses in your discussion. Digital monitoring data, if available, may corroborate.
Hands-on functional assessment	Components created based on tolerance history, pain diagram, and questionnaire data. Document observations include gradation of lifts or other exertions plus any subsequent level of discomfort or lack thereof.
Conclude	Complete requested forms and/or generate report. Summarize what was done and how patient reacted/responded. Communicate appraised function when answering specific questions and offering opinions.

Have the person you are evaluating commit to a narrative that includes their self-perceived tolerance to activities of daily living (ADLs) and instrumental activities of daily living (IADLs) such as cooking, household chores, yardwork, shopping, exercise, as well as avocational and vocational pursuits. From an activity tolerance history, the clinician can customize or target the hands-on portion of a functional assessment where you observe various activity tasks.

C. Functional Assessment

Observe the patient engaging in movement and activities. Create components of your hands-on functional assessment based on your interview, interpretation of self-report information, and discussion with the patient. Focus your functional assessment on body parts known to be limiting the patient's activity. Start with low weight and easy height to allow patient to succeed with movement and acknowledge minimal, if any, discomfort. Then sequentially increase weight, resistance, and/or height until patient's mechanics falter or patient relays discomfort. Observe for lifting mechanics and body language. Ask the patient how this or that feels while performing the task or motion. Before starting, inform the person you're evaluating that he/she should speak up and stop if anything causes undue pain but that the objective is to identify what is and is not comfortable or tolerated. Inquire afterward as to the presence and character of any increased soreness and document the patient's responses. These techniques help convey empathy while underscoring that the evaluation process is careful and comprehensive. To facilitate functional evaluation, consider having available basic materials. Examples include a crate with pavers (each 5 lb, total 50 no.), a bucket or bag weighing 25 lb (for asymmetric or one hand lifts/carries), and an axe handle. If these are unavailable, then improvise. For example, use the ubiquitous provider's stool (often about 15 lb depending on make) to assess lifting tolerance, for example, hold close, then arms out, then to sides, then have the person bend knees, and hold close while you push down on stool to simulate greater weight. Assess hand grip tolerance by having your patient perform power grip (all fingers) of the edge of the provider stool's padded seat. Tolerance to push/pull can be assessed either with using provider's hand or arms (set your feet apart; warn patient to pull or push easy not yank), while both you and the person being evaluated, grasp the stool. Pinch grips can be assessed using metal paper clasp of varying sizes if a hand grip manometer is not readily available. Lack of specific equipment should not limit your efforts to assess function. Importantly, observe patient walk and traverse stairs. The 6-minute walk test has been standardized and well studied for pain conditions. Lastly, many jobs or tasks require endurance. Your activity history should include markers of endurance (eg, distance/time walked, back-to-back errands, time raking leaves). During the hands-on component of your assessment, you should also be attentive to signs of early fatigue, for example, patient slows movement, limbs shake, and patient hesitates.

D. Document Observations, Answer Specific Questions, and Develop Report

Record/describe what you had the patient complete and how he/she responded. Document the gradation (often extremely useful in answering specific disability questions) of lifts and how the patient responded. Comment on whether activity tolerance by history matches your observations. Depending on the setting, consider asking patient for permission to photograph key lifts or movements, and include those pictures in your report. Your findings regarding function will inform and increase the credibility of your disability determination.

V. PITFALLS OF FORMAL FUNCTIONAL CAPACITY EVALUATIONS

Lengthy and elaborate physical and functional capacity evaluations (FCEs) may be requested by stakeholders. Often conducted by the physical or occupational therapist, typically they involve a series of lifting, bending, and related movement tasks to assess the patient's capacity. Some FCEs will attempt to simulate job tasks specific to that patient's occupation. An FCE may last 4 hours or be conducted over more than 1 day. FCEs are generally designed to test several physical parameters including strength and endurance, positional or postural tolerance, coordination, body mechanics, ability to perform repeated activities, and work-simulation activities. FCEs are associated with a risk of new or repeat injury and may be contraindicated or unwise in certain settings, especially when the patient being evaluated is hesitant and feels forced to participate. Standardized measures of lifting and movement have a long history of receiving attention by insurance companies attempting to assess disability, often for purposes of financial compensation or judging whether an individual is "safe" to RTW. Lengthy and elaborate physical and FCEs may be requested by stakeholders. Recent Cochrane reviews report mixed results from multiple studies that employed structured pre-employment screening assessments to predict work-related musculoskeletal injuries. The studies that address predictive validity of structured observational measures for successful RTW with individuals who sustained a work injury are equally disappointing. Some observational measures such as the 6-minute walk test have been shown to have sufficient reliability and predictive validity and have been used with chronic pain. However, standardized tests of this sort may not be practical in general clinical practice. In short, FCEs are best for motivated patients wherein the benefit of greater quantification of capacity outweighs the risks of potential injury and the cost.

VI. MALINGERING AND NONMEDICAL INFORMATION

Disability and the use of standardized measures cannot be discussed without addressing the issue of malingering or feigning. There is no question that patients may seek to deceive the clinician for purposes of financial compensation, acquisition of controlled substances, or other rewards. Conscious deception does not always imply the absence of a legitimate medical or psychiatric condition or the absence of disability related to that condition. A patient may have a severe disabling disorder but seek to embellish or to minimize symptoms for gain. With respect to the latter, a patient may deceive the clinician about a health condition in order to continue their work status due to financial or job security pressures. Performing work tasks when ill-advised may place the patient at risk of further injury or delayed recovery and present undue liability for other stakeholders, for example, the employer. Standardized physical examinations and psychological tests aimed at assessing maligning of pain tend to perform poorly in controlled studies. In fact, some examinations such as the "Waddell signs" have been debunked by US courts when they purport to measure deception. When the veracity of the patient is in question, workers' compensation or disability policy carriers may resort to surveillance and other strategies to obtain nonmedical information. As the treating provider or evaluator of the patient disabled from pain, you may be asked to review such nonmedical information and comment. Your assessment of function as depicted/performed by the patient during your care or evaluation would then be compared to presented footage, providing a basis for an opinion on any disparity. If a clear discrepancy appears to exist that brings into question the veracity of the patient's history, then the strength of opinions based on that history should be adjusted. A critical eye regarding content and quality of any image is prudent as others may have been overly quick in drawing conclusions. The goal is to represent the patient's functional abilities or limitations as accurately as possible based on available information, both medical and nonmedical.

VII. CONCLUSION

The clinician assessing the patient with persistent pain should be confident to undertake a hands-on assessment of function/tolerance, incorporate standardized questionnaires, access a pain diagram, and utilize real-time digital monitoring where feasible. The process of how you assess disability impacts the quality and credibility of the output. Assessment of disability for those in pain fulfills an important service for the patient, as well as a critical role designated by society. This chapter aspires to build your confidence and ability to fulfill that role. Disability assessment allows an opportunity to learn more about your patient. This chapter emphasizes the functional impact of the overall condition, inclusive of pain. The central goal is to provide the groundwork for you to create a well-substantiated report that details your findings and opinions. This chapter also outlines opportunities to exceed expectations by identifying ways to reduce disease-related complications, restore the patient's function, and improve quality of life.

Selected Readings

Alhowimel A, AlOtaibi M, Radford K, Coulson N. Psychosocial factors associated with change in pain and disability outcomes in chronic low back pain patients treated by physiotherapist: a systematic review. *SAGE Open Med.* 2018;6:2050312118757387. doi: 10.1177/2050312118757387.

Anagnostis C, Gatchel RJ, Mayer TG. The pain disability questionnaire: a new psychometrically sound measure for chronic musculoskeletal disorders. *Spine* 2004;29(20):2290-2302.

Anderson HG. The medical aspects of aeroplane accidents. *Br Med J.* 1918;1(2977):73-76.

ATS Committee on Proficiency Standards for Clinical Pulmonary Function Laboratories. ATS Statement: guidelines for the six-minute walk test. *Am J Respir Crit Care Med.* 2002;166:111-117.

Bennett RM, Friend R, Jones KD, Ward R, Han BK, Ross RL. The Revised Fibromyalgia Impact Questionnaire (FIQR): validation and psychometric properties. *Arthritis Res Ther.* 2009;11(4):R120. doi: 10.1186/ar2783.

Cella D, Riley W, Stone A, et al. The Patient-Reported Outcomes Measurement Information System (PROMIS) developed and tested its first wave of adult self-reported health outcome item banks: 2005-2008. *J Clin Epidemiol.* 2010;63(11):1179-1194.

Chiarotto A, Maxwell L, Terwee C, Wells G, Tugwell P, Ostelo R. Roland-Morris disability questionnaire and oswestry disability index: which has better measurement properties for measuring physical functioning in nonspecific low back pain? Systematic review and meta-analysis. *Phys Ther.* 2016;96(10):1620-1637. doi: 10.2522/ptj.20150420.

Chiarotto A, Ostelo R, Boers M, Terwee C. A systematic review highlights the need to investigate the content validity of patient-reported outcome measures for physical functioning in patients with low back pain. *J Clin Epidemiol.* 2018;95:73-93. doi: 10.1016/j.jclinepi.2017.11.005.

Clement R, Welander A, Stowell C, et al. A proposed set of metrics for standardized outcome reporting in the management of low back pain. *Acta Orthop.* 2015;86(5):523-533. doi: 10.3109/17453674.2015.1036696.

Collado-Mateo D, Domínguez-Muñoz FJ, Olivares PR, Adsuar JC, Gusi N. Stair negotiation in women with fibromyalgia: a descriptive correlational study. Tarantino G, ed. *Medicine.* 2017;96(43):e8364. doi: 10.1097/MD.0000000000008364.

Cron DC, Englesbe MJ, Bolton CJ, et al. Preoperative opioid use is independently associated with increased costs and worse outcomes after major abdominal surgery. *Ann Surg.* 2017;265(4):695-701. doi: 10.1097/SLA.0000000000001901.

Dersh J, Mayer T, Theodore BR, Polatin P, Gatchel RJ. Do psychiatric disorders first appear preinjury or postinjury in chronic disabling occupational spinal disorders? *Spine*. 2007;32(9):1045-1051. doi: 10.1097/01.brs.0000261027.28779.52.

Froud R, Patel S, Rajendran D, et al. A systematic review of outcome measures use, analytical approaches, reporting methods, and publication volume by year in low back pain trials published between 1980 and 2012: respice, adspice, et prospice. *PLoS One*. 2016;11(10):e0164573. doi: 10.1371/journal.pone.0164573.

Garin O, Ayuso-Mateos JL, Almansa J, et al. Validation of the "World Health Organization Disability Assessment Schedule, WHODAS-2" in patients with chronic diseases. *Health Qual Life Outcomes*. 2010;8:51.

Gaskin DJ, Richard P. The economic costs of pain in the United States. In: Institute of Medicine (US) Committee on Advancing Pain Research, Care, and Education, ed. *Relieving Pain in America: A Blueprint for Transforming Prevention, Care, Education, and Research*. Washington, DC: National Academies Press (US); 2011.

Gibson TM, Harrison M. Aviation medicine in the UK: early years, 1911-1918. *Aviat Space Environ Med*. 2005;76:599-600.

Gregg C, McIntosh G, Hall H, Watson H, Williams D, Hoffman C. The relationship between the Tampa Scale of Kinesiophobia and low back pain rehabilitation outcomes. *Spine J*. 2015;15(12):2466-2471. doi: 10.1016/j.spinee.2015.08.018.

MacDermid JC, Walton DM, Avery S, et al. Measurement properties of the neck disability index: a systematic review. *J Orthop Sports Phys Ther*. 2009;39:400–417.

Martin DW. *Independent Medical Evaluation: A Practical Guide*. Cham, Switzerland: Springer International Publishing AG; 2018. doi: 10.1007/978-3-319-71906-1.

Mitchell SJ. Health assessment in aviation medicine. *Occup Med*. 2003;53:3-4.

Rendas-Baum R, Yang M, Varon SF, Bloudek LM, DeGryse RE, Kosinski M. Validation of the Headache Impact Test (HIT-6) in patients with chronic migraine. *Health Qual Life Outcomes*. 2014;12:117. doi: 10.1186/s12955-014-0117-0.

Revicki DA, Cook KF, Amtmann D, Harnam N, Chen WH, Keefe FJ. Exploratory and confirmatory factor analysis of the PROMIS Pain Quality item bank. *Qual Life Res*. 2014;23(1):245-255.

Rondinelli RD, Eskay-Auerbach M; American Medical Association. *Transition to the AMA Guides Sixth: Guides to the Evaluation of Permanent Impairment*. 6th ed. Chicago, IL: American Medical Association; 2010.

Silva C, Coleta I, Silva AG, et al. Adaptation and validation of WHODAS 2.0 in patients with musculoskeletal pain. *Rev Saude Publica*. 2013;47(4):752-758.

Southerst D, Côté P, Stupar M, Stern P, Mior S. The reliability of body pain diagrams in the quantitative measurement of pain distribution and location in patients with musculoskeletal pain: a systematic review. *J Manipulative Physiol Ther*. 2013;36(7):450-459. doi: 10.1016/j.jmpt.2013.05.021.

Steenstra IA, Munhall C, Irvin E, et al. Systematic review of prognostic factors for return to work in workers with sub acute and chronic low back pain. *J Occup Rehabil*. 2017;27(3):369-381. doi: 10.1007/s10926-016-9666-x.

Talmage JB, Melhorn JM, Hyman MH; American Medical Association. *AMA Guides to the Evaluation of Work Ability and Return to Work*. 2nd ed. Chicago, IL: American Medical Association; 2011.

Waljee J, Cron D, Steiger R, Zhong L, Englesbe M, Brummett C. The effect of preoperative opioid exposure on healthcare utilization and expenditures following elective abdominal surgery. *Ann Surg*. 2017;265(4):715-721. doi: 10.1097/SLA.0000000000002117.

Williams JS, Ng N, Peltzer K, Yawson A, Biritwum R, Maximova T, et al. Risk factors and disability associated with low back pain in older adults in low- and middle-income countries. Results from the WHO Study on Global AGEing and Adult Health (SAGE). *PLoS One*. 2015;10(6):e0127880.

Yang M, Rendas-Baum R, Varon SF, Kosinski M. Validation of the Headache Impact Test (HIT-6™) across episodic and chronic migraine. *Cephalalgia*. 2011;31(3):357-367. doi: 10.1177/0333102410379890.

SECTION III

Therapeutic Options: Pharmacologic Approaches

10 Neuropathic Pain Medications

Dermot P. Maher and Lucy Chen

Neuropathic pain may develop as a result of traumatic insult or inflammation involving the central or peripheral nerve tissue. The nature of neuropathic pain often affords it the qualities of being both difficult to fully clinically characterize and refractory to complete resolution with currently available therapies. Effective management of neuropathic pain is often considered to be the reduction, but not complete resolution, of symptoms. In order to achieve an optimal treatment regimen, therapy with several different medications at various doses should be sequentially attempted and balanced against side effects. Often, combinations of neuropathic pain medications must also be evaluated for possible therapeutic benefit. This uncertainty is partially due to the heterogeneous nature of neuropathic pain diagnoses and the interpatient and intrapatient variability in symptomatology and the response to pharmacological agents.

Many pain physicians are trained to evaluate disease based on anatomical location and symptomatology in order to arrive at pathology and potential treatment. However, among neuropathic pain patients with similar clinical presentations and even those with the same diagnoses, the pathology may be variable, and therefore responsiveness to equivalent treatments is frustratingly difficult to predict. Further complicating the situation is the relatively incomplete current understanding of the molecular processes leading to the development and maintenance of chronic neuropathic pain. Without a full understanding of discreet neuropathic pathologies, determination of optimal pharmacologic targets must be accomplished by trial and, frequently, error. Physicians must also take care to rule out similar appearing nonneuropathic sources of pain, such as musculoskeletal or other organic medical causes, which are often refractory to neuropathic pain agents.

Many neuropathic pain agents were initially developed for use in nonpain diagnoses and were later found to be effective in neuropathic pain management. Efficacy of medications is often seen gradually with initial onset in 2-4 weeks and full clinical effect often taking up 8 weeks in some cases.

I. ANTIDEPRESSANTS

In many chronic pain patients, antidepressant therapy has a dual function: treating a depressive disorder, which are frequently concurrent with chronic pain, and addressing the chronic pain. The first reports of analgesic properties of antidepressants were attributed solely to treatment of the depression component of pain. Although treatment of depression may result in better coping and decreased reports of chronic pain complaints, some antidepressants were noted to have independent effects on pain via modulation of the noradrenergic, serotonergic, cholinergic, and possibly other neurotransmitter systems. However, simple monoamine neurotransmitter modulation incompletely explains the observed effects of these medications. Monoamine neurotransmitter levels are increased almost instantaneously, but therapeutic benefit is often only seen after several weeks of use.

By having a plurality of therapeutic mechanisms, many of the medications are subject to dose-limiting side effects. A reasonable goal for the use of such medications is to reduce, but not completely eliminate, a patient's pain with tolerable, but not completely absent, side effects. Antidepressant medication is classified by chemical structure and/or a medication specific pattern of monoamine neurotransmitter inhibition.

II. TRICYCLIC ANTIDEPRESSANTS

Tricyclic antidepressants (TCAs) are one of the oldest classes of antidepressant medications. While the initial analgesic studies were conducted using amitriptyline and desipramine, it is thought that all TCAs have approximately equal analgesic properties at therapeutic doses. It should be noted that the effective analgesic dose of these medications is often lower than the effective antidepressant dose. The choice of individual medications is largely determined by an optimal side effect profile.

A. Mechanism of Action

All TCAs inhibit the reuptake of serotonin and norepinephrine into presynaptic neurons to varying degrees as outlined in Table 10.1. Increased levels of synaptic serotonin and norepinephrine cause analgesia through augmentation of outflow from the descending inhibitory spinal tracts. The tertiary amines, including imipramine, amitriptyline, and doxepin, tend to have a broader spectrum of action than the secondary amines, including nortriptyline and desipramine. Additional therapeutic benefit is thought to be conferred through sodium channel blockade, NMDA antagonist,

TABLE 10.1 Summary of TCA Properties

Medication	Trade Names	Dosage Range (mg/d)	Effective Serum Concentration	Maximum Dose (mg/d)	Elimination Half-Life	Anticholinergic Activity	Serotonin-Norepinephrine Selectivity Ratio	Sedation
Tertiary Amines								
Imipramine	Tofranil	10-300 mg	200-300 ng/mL	300 mg	5-30 h	Moderate	27	Moderate
Amitriptyline	Elavil, Levate	10-150 mg	80-200 ng/mL	300 mg	9-27 h	Strong	8	Strong
Clomipramine	Anafranil	25-250 mg	230-450 ng/mL	250 mg	15-60 h	Moderate	130	Mild
Doxepin	Sinequan, Deptran	10-150 mg	150-250 ng/mL	300 mg	15 h *N*-desmethyldoxepin 31 h	Moderate	2	Mild
Secondary Amines								
Desipramine	Norpramin, Pertofrane	10-150 mg	100-300 ng/mL	300 mg	10-30 h	Minimal	0.05	Minimal
Nortriptyline	Pamelor, Allegron, Sensoval	10-150 mg	50-150 ng/mL	200 mg	20-55 h	Mild	0.24	Mild

α_1-adrenergic inhibition, TRPV1, and mu-opioid receptor modulation. The mechanism of action tramadol and cyclobenzaprine may be partially attributed to TCA-like activity.

B. Pharmacology

TCAs as a class have nearly complete bioavailability. In general, they undergo about 50% first-pass hepatic metabolism and are over 80%-90% protein bound. Tertiary amines are metabolized to secondary amines. Amitriptyline is demethylated to nortriptyline. Imipramine is demethylated to desipramine. Terminal metabolism is through inactivation by CYP 2D6, 1A2, 3A4, and 1C19 and eventual urinary clearance.

C. Dosing and Monitoring

Serum level monitoring of TCAs can be used to establish dosing, especially in slow or rapid metabolizers. The serum concentration seems to be best correlated to the analgesic benefit for desipramine, nortriptyline, amitriptyline, clomipramine, and imipramine. Discontinuation should be done over 4 weeks to prevent cholinergic rebound and the recrudescence of depressive symptoms.

D. Adverse Side Effects

Side effects of these medications are largely determined by anticholinergic and antihistaminic properties of individual medications. TCAs are contraindicated in patients with cardiac arrhythmias, QTc prolongation, recent heart attacks, epilepsy, narrow angle glaucoma, heart block, hyperthyroidism, urinary outflow obstruction due to benign prostatic hyperplasia, and current use of monoamine oxidase inhibitors. Due to the risk of decreased cardiac conduction, an EKG should be obtained prior to initiating therapy but does not need to be rechecked unless the patient is symptomatic. TCAs lower the seizure threshold. Major side effects include orthostatic hypotension, cardiac conduction anomalies due to quinidinelike properties, weight gain, sedation, sexual dysfunction, alcohol abuse, and restlessness. Patients should be monitored for worsening depression and risk of suicidal ideations. Unlike newer selective serotonin reuptake inhibitors (SSRIs), overdoses can be lethal at three to five times the therapeutic dose. TCAs are generally considered safe to use during pregnancy.

E. Indications and Evidence

Prior to the development of SSRIs, TCAs were the most commonly used medication to treat depression. There are now numerous subsequent well-conducted studies and meta-analyses to support their use for central and neuropathic pain states including diabetic peripheral neuropathy, postherpetic neuralgia, CRPS, poststroke pain, radiculopathy, migraines, and fibromyalgia. TCAs have also been demonstrated to be effective preemptive analgesia with an opioid sparing effect observed in the postoperative phase of care. Despite a prolonged history of safe and effective use, TCA therapy for neuropathic pain is considered "off-label." The number needed to treat (NNT) is ~2-3, and the number needed to harm (NNH) for minor adverse events is 6, and NNH for major adverse events is 28. The generic availability and low NNT makes TCA therapy a very cost-effective modality to treat chronic pain.

III. SELECTIVE SEROTONIN-NOREPINEPHRINE REUPTAKE INHIBITORS

Serotonin-norepinephrine reuptake inhibitors (SNRIs) are a nontricyclic class of antidepressants. Although they have a similar mechanism of action to TCAs, fewer side effects are observed due to less interaction with cholinergic and histaminic receptors. The NNT also appears to be higher compared to TCAs possibly due to the TCA's antagonism of multiple pain pathways.

A. Mechanism of Action

SNRIs inhibit the central reuptake of both serotonin and norepinephrine into presynaptic neurons. At doses <150 mg/day, venlafaxine primarily inhibits the reuptake of serotonin. However, at doses >150 mg/day, venlafaxine inhibits both serotonin and norepinephrine reuptake. Venlafaxine may also have naloxone reversible agonist activity at the opioid receptors due to its structural similarity to tramadol. SNRIs differ from TCAs in that they produce no or very little anticholinergic, dopaminergic, α_1-adrenergic, and antihistaminic effects. They do not inhibit monoamine oxidase.

B. Pharmacology

The pharmacokinetic profiles are described in Table 10.2. Available SNRIs are structurally unrelated compounds. They have a widely variable bioavailability and time to peak plasma concentration. Their absorption is not affected by food, but consumption with food may decrease the incidence of nausea. Venlafaxine is hepatically metabolized to an active metabolite, *O*-desmethylvenlafaxine. Regular and extended-release venlafaxine seem to produce similar plasma levels for equivalent total daily doses. Duloxetine moderately inhibits the function of CYP2D6. Renally excreted and dose adjustments are needed in the setting of renal insufficiency for all SNRIs.

C. Dosing and Monitoring

No laboratory studies are needed prior to initiating therapy. Duloxetine's optimal dosage for pain control is 60 mg/day. 120 mg/day has not been shown to be more effective than 60 mg/day. 20 mg/day has not been effective in the treatment of pain. Venlafaxine at doses between 150 and 225 mg/day are effective pain treatment. 75 mg/day has not been demonstrated to be effective in the treatment of pain possibly due to a lack of significant norepinephrine reuptake antagonism. Milnacipran is generally started at 12.5 mg twice a day (bid) and then increased to 50 mg bid.

D. Adverse Side Effects

Adverse side effects are seen in ~21% of patient utilizing duloxetine therapy including nausea, headaches, insomnia, dizziness, constipation, and dry mouth. Duloxetine has been associated with rare, but sometimes fatal, cases of hepatic failure. Venlafaxine at high doses has significant norepinephrine reuptake inhibition and may be associated with an increase in systolic blood pressure and should be used with caution in patients with pre-existing hypertension. Venlafaxine may also be associated with an increased risk of upper gastrointestinal (GI) bleeds. Other common side effects of SNRIs include nausea, dry mouth, dizziness, nervousness, constipation, anorexia, and sexual dysfunction. SNRIs have a class C rating if taken during pregnancy (eg, risk cannot be ruled out).

E. Indications and Evidence

Duloxetine is FDA approved for the treatment of depression, chronic musculoskeletal pain, painful diabetic neuropathy, fibromyalgia, and generalized anxiety. There is also evidence for a synergistic effect when combined with a gabapentinoid medication. It should be noted that comparative effectiveness trails of duloxetine against vastly less expensive TCAs did

TABLE 10.2 Pharmacokinetics of SSRIs and SNRIs

Medication	Typical Starting Dose	Normal Daily Dose	Maximum Daily Dose	Bioavailability (%)	Time to Peak Plasma Concentration	Primary Elimination	Elimination Half-Life	Serotonin-Norepinephrine Selectivity Ratio
SSRI								
Citalopram	20 mg/d	20-40 mg/d	40 mg/d	80%	4 h	CYP3A4 CYP2C19	35 h	3500-3900
Escitalopram	10 mg/d	10-20 mg/d	20 mg/d	80%	5 h	CYP3A4 CYP2C19	27-32 h	7100
Fluoxetine	20 mg/d	20-50 mg/d	80 mg/d	100%	1-2 h	CYP2C19 CYP2D6	96-144 h (chronic use), norfluoxetine 96-384 h	300-545
Fluvoxamine	50 mg/d	100-300 mg/d	300 mg/d	53%	3-8 h	CYP1A2 CYP2D6	16 h	580-620
Paroxetine HCl	20 mg	20-50 mg/d	50 mg/d	100%	3-8 h	CYP2D6	21 h	300-450
Sertraline	50 mg/d	50-200 mg/d	200 mg/d		4.5-8.4 h	CYP2C19 CYP2D6	62-104 h	1400-2750
SNRI								
Venlafaxine	37.5 mg bid	150-225 mg/d	225 mg/d	13%	1-2 h	CYP2D6 CYP3A4	3-7 h, ODV 9-13 h	115-120
Duloxetine	30 mg (20 mg in elderly)	60 mg/d	120 mg/d	50%	6 h	CYP1A2 CYP2D6	8-17 h	9
Milnacipran	12.5 mg/d	50 mg bid	100 mg bid	85%-90%	2-4 h	Glucuronidation	8-10 h	0.5

ODV, *O*-desmethylvenlafaxine.

not demonstrate statistical differences in observed pain control but did produce more insomnia. Milnacipran is FDA approved for the treatment of fibromyalgia. Its use is supported by seven prospective randomized controlled trials. Venlafaxine is used for neuropathic pain diagnoses but may be less efficacious than other SNRIs due to dose-dependent variation in serotonin reuptake inhibition.

IV. SELECTIVE SEROTONIN REUPTAKE INHIBITORS

Fluoxetine (Prozac) is the prototypical SSRI. It was first introduced in 1987 and, due to a much lower side effect profile compared to TCA, quickly became first-line treatment for the treatment of depression. Several other SSRI medications have been approved for the treatment of depression including citalopram, fluvoxamine, paroxetine, and sertraline. However, analysis of published material has failed to find an independent analgesic effect of SSRI. As such, these medications are rarely prescribed purely for the treatment of chronic pain. They can be extremely useful for the management of coexisting depression, but care must be taken to ensure that there will not be a potentially serious pharmacological interaction, such as serotonin syndrome.

A. Mechanism of Action

All SSRIs inhibit the reuptake of serotonin into presynaptic neurons in the CNS. SSRIs differ from TCAs in that they produce no or very little anticholinergic, dopaminergic, α_1-adrenergic, and antihistaminic effects. They are different from SNRIs in that they do not produce clinically relevant norepinephrine reuptake inhibition.

B. Pharmacology

The pharmacokinetic profiles are described in Table 10.2. In general, SSRIs are rapidly and completely absorbed from the GI tract and reach peak plasma concentrations in 1-8 hours. Absorption is generally not affected by concurrent food consumption. Fluoxetine is metabolized to norfluoxetine which is pharmacologically active as a serotonin reuptake inhibitor.

C. Dosing and Monitoring

Among the SSRIs, fluoxetine is the most potent inhibitor of CYP 2D6. However, paroxetine, fluvoxamine, and sertraline at doses >100 mg also inhibit the metabolic action of CYP 2D6. This may cause decreased metabolism and increased side effects from other medications metabolized by the same enzyme. Abrupt discontinuation of an SSRI may be associated with dizziness, paresthesias, myalgias, irritability, insomnia, and visual disturbances.

D. Adverse Side Effects

SSRIs have minimal anticholinergic properties compared to TCAs and produce less sedation, and orthostatic hypotension and no delayed conduction of cardiac impulses are reported. They do not lower the seizure threshold. Common side effects can include headaches, stimulation or sedation, fine tremor, neuromuscular restlessness which can mimic akathisia, increased bruising and bleeding, predisposition to osteoporosis, nausea, vomiting, anorexia, bloating, and diarrhea. 10%-15% of patients will experience sexual side effects resulting in medication noncompliance such as decreased libido, impotence, ejaculatory disturbances, and anorgasmia. Concurrent use of other serotonergic drugs should be avoided to minimize the risk of precipitating serotonin syndrome. The FDA has a "Black Box" warning due to a possible increase risk of suicidal tendencies in adolescent and teenage patients. Overdoses are rarely lethal. SSRIs have a class C rating if taken during pregnancy (eg, risk cannot be ruled out).

E. Indications and Evidence

FDA approved for the treatment of depression, anxiety disorders, bulimia nervosa, and obsessive compulsive disorders. The does needed to treat anxiety is typically higher than the dose needed to treat depression. Also frequently used for premenstrual syndrome, posttraumatic stress disorder, social phobia, chronic fatigue syndrome, and intermittent explosive disorder.

V. OTHER MEDICATIONS

A. Trazodone

1. Mechanism of Action

Trazodone primarily acts through the inhibition of both the serotonin-2 receptor and presynaptic serotonin reuptake pump. Additionally, trazodone inhibits histamine-1 receptors and α_1-adrenergic receptors. Trazodone does not have anticholinergic activity at clinically relevant doses.

2. Pharmacology

The bioavailability of trazodone is 86% and can be increased with concurrent consumption of food. The time to peak serum concentration is 0.5-2.5 hours but can be increased to 2.5 hours with food. Trazodone is 85%-95% protein bound. It is extensively metabolized by CYP3A4 and primarily renally excreted and secondarily fecally excreted. The elimination halftime of trazodone is 3-9 hours. Trazodone can decrease the hepatic metabolism of other medications that are metabolized by CYP3A4 including astemizole, terfenadine, triazolam, and alprazolam.

3. Dosing and Monitoring

No laboratory studies are needed prior to initiating therapy. Initial dosing should start at 50-100 mg at night and then increased weekly. Doses of up to 600 mg daily have been studied. However, the most effective treatment for insomnia usually occurs between 50 and 300 mg.

4. Adverse Side Effects

Major reported side effects include sedation, orthostatic hypotension, nausea, dizziness, headache, nausea, dry mouth, and GI upset. Rarely, cardiac arrhythmias have been reported. A rare but serious side effect is priapism, which can occur in 1/100/ to 1/10 000 patients. Similar to SSRI therapy, the FDA has a "black box" warning due to a possible increase risk of suicidal tendencies in adolescent and teenage patients. Trazodone has a class C rating if taken during pregnancy (eg, risk cannot be ruled out).

5. Indications and Evidence

Trazodone has not been reported to be efficacious for the treatment of chronic pain. However, it can be useful as a sedative to address insomnia often present in depression, anxiety, and chronic pain states. It is rarely used as an antidepressant as few patients are able to tolerate the significant sedative side effects.

B. Mirtazapine

1. Mechanism of Action

Mirtazapine acts through inhibition of serotonin receptors and presynaptic α_2 adrenergic receptor in the CNS. Inhibition of presynaptic α_2 receptors stimulates serotonin and norepinephrine release. At doses between 15 and 30 mg/day, it is thought to primarily stimulate serotonin release. At higher doses of 45-60 mg/day, it augments primarily noradrenergic release.

2. Pharmacology

The bioavailability of mirtazapine is ~50% with a time to peak plasma concentration of 2 hours. It is ~85% protein bound. Mirtazapine is extensively hepatically metabolized by CYP1A2, 2D6, and 3A4 and has an elimination halftime of 20-40 hours. It is ultimately excreted primarily in the urine and, to a less extent, in the feces.

3. Dosing and Monitoring

Starting dose is usually 15 mg QHs which can then be increased gradually to a maximum of 45 mg daily.

4. Adverse Side Effects

At lower doses, which preferentially facilitate serotonin transmission, it is more sedating and has an antianxiety effect. At higher doses, which preferentially facilitate norepinephrine transmission, it is more activating and can provoke anxiety symptoms. 0.3% of patients on this medication can develop agranulocytosis and neutropenia. There are also reports of patients developing new arthralgias following initiation of therapy. Mirtazapine has a class C rating if taken during pregnancy (eg, risk cannot be ruled out).

5. Indications and Evidence

Mirtazapine is currently indicated for the treatment of major depressive disorders. It does not have activity as an analgesic medication.

C. Bupropion

1. Mechanism of Action

Bupropion is a centrally acting stimulant and that inhibits the presynaptic reuptake of both norepinephrine and dopamine in the CNS. At higher doses, presynaptic serotonin reuptake is also inhibited. It is structurally related to amphetamine.

2. Pharmacology

Bupropion has a high bioavailability allowing for a rapid time to peak plasma concentration of 2 hours. It is 84% protein bound. It is extensively metabolized by CYP2B6 to hydroxybupropion, which has about 20%-50% of the norepinephrine and dopamine reuptake inhibition of bupropion. Bupropion is primarily eliminated through the urine and, secondarily, through the feces.

3. Dosing and Monitoring

The starting dose of bupropion is 75-100 mg in order to avoid insomnia at the time of initiation. After 5 days, the dose is advanced to a therapeutic dose, which is usually 300 mg daily. Different formulations allow for dosing to be once a day, twice a day, or three times a day.

4. Adverse Side Effects

The most commonly observed side effects are headaches, insomnia, upper respiratory tract complications, nausea, restlessness, agitation, and irritability. An observed dose-dependent decrease in the seizure threshold is observed with 0.4% of patients on <450 mg/day experienced seizures and 4% of those using between 450 and 600 mg/day experienced seizures. Patients with known seizure disorders, those that are using other seizure threshold lowering medications, or those with eating disorders should avoid this medication. It is not associated with sexual side effects. Bupropion has a class C rating if taken during pregnancy (eg, risk cannot be ruled out).

5. Indications and Evidence

Bupropion is FDA approved for attention deficit disorder, Parkinson disease, and narcolepsy. The medication has been used for smoking cessation with very encouraging results. Studies have produced mixed results as to whether this medication is useful for the treatment of a variety of neuropathic pain syndromes and chronic low back pain. However, it is often utilized as a stimulant in order to minimize or counteract the sedating effects of certain sedating pain medications such as opioid therapy.

D. Ketamine

1. Mechanism of Action

Noncompetitively inhibits NMDA receptors at the level of both the CNS and the dorsal root ganglia. Subanesthetic doses will produce analgesia, reduce hyperesthesia, allodynia, and opioid tolerance.

2. Pharmacology

Numerous routes have been described for administration including oral, IV, and intranasal. The oral bioavailability of ketamine is 17% and the intranasal bioavailability is 45%. IV infusions are also commonly employed in the outpatient setting for the treatment of neuropathic pain. The onset of action is <10 minutes and maintains analgesic properties for 1 hour with the intranasal preparation. Ketamine undergoes hepatic *N*-dealkylation to form norketamine, which is ~33% as potent as the parent compound.

3. Dosing and Monitoring

Numerous IV infusion protocols have been described for the treatment of discreet neuropathic pain pathologies. In general, a starting concentration on 0.15 mg/kg in a monitored outpatient setting is the starting dose with gradual increases as tolerated. Intranasal use starts at 10 mg every 90 seconds until analgesia is achieved for a maximum of 50 mg. The oral preparation may start at 0.5 mg/kg and increase 0.5 mg/kg as appropriate 3-4 times daily.

4. Adverse Side Effects

Numerous unpleasant side effects have been described which have historically limited the role of ketamine in the widespread treatment of neuropathic pain. Described side effects may include cardiac arrhythmias, hyper- or hypotension, bradycardia, confusion, delirium, dreamlike state, vivid imagery, increases in cerebrospinal fluid (CSF) pressure, central diabetes insipidus, nausea, sialorrhea, cystitis, diplopia, nystagmus, increased intraocular pressure, and respiratory depression. Ketamine has a class C rating if taken during pregnancy (eg, risk cannot be ruled out).

5. Indications and Evidence

Ketamine has been demonstrated to be effective for the treatment of numerous chronic neuropathic pain states including fibromyalgia, CRPS, postherpetic trigeminal neuralgia, painful diabetic neuropathy, spinal cord injury, and other pain diagnoses. Other NMDA antagonists that are being investigated as potentially therapeutic NMDA antagonists are dextromethorphan, memantine, magnesium, nitrous oxide, and dizocilpine (MK-801).

VI. CALCIUM CHANNEL BLOCKERS

A. Gabapentin

1. Mechanism of Action

Gabapentin has an incompletely understood mechanism of action. It has a cyclohexane amino acid chemical structure that is related to the neurotransmitter GABA. However, it does not bind to or augment the function of the GABA receptor. The primary binding site has been localized to the α-2-δ subunit of the L-type presynaptic voltage-gated calcium channel. Binding and inhibition by gabapentin subsequently prevents excessive presynaptic glutamate, substance P, and norepinephrine release.

2. Pharmacology

The bioavailability of gabapentin is inversely related to the dose. L-Amino acid transporter is saturable. At low doses of 300 mg tid, the average bioavailability is 60%, which is not altered by food. Absorption from the GI tract decreases after 900 mg tid with excessive gabapentin eliminated in the stool. Less than 3% of gabapentin is protein bound in the plasma. It is eliminated unchanged via urinary excretion. Elimination kinetics are not altered by dose or chronicity but are directly related to creatinine clearance and should be adjusted in the setting of decreased renal function. The bioavailability of the prodrug gabapentin enacarbil, which received FDA approval in 2012, is substantially increased. It is not certain if this change results in better pain control at a higher cost.

3. Dosing and Monitoring

Numerous reasonable dosing and titration schedules have been described. A reasonable starting dose is 300 mg at bedtime and then increases to 300 mg tid after 1-2 days in a patient with normal renal function. Thereafter, if no side effects are observed, the dose should be increased by 300 mg every 3-5 days as tolerated to a maximal dose of 1200 mg tid. A next step may be to increase the dose to 1200 mg qid in certain patients. Dose adjustments are required for patients with renal impairment or who are on dialysis. No adjustment for hepatic impairment is required. Therapy should only be considered a failure if a dose of >1800 mg/d for several weeks was achieved.

4. Adverse Side Effects

Somnolence, weight gain, fatigue, ataxia, dizziness, inability to concentrate, GI disturbances, and nystagmus are the most commonly observed side effects at 2-4 weeks. Pedal edema can occur in 1.7% of patients. Abrupt discontinuation can precipitate seizures. Discontinuation of the medication requires a taper over at least 1 week. Gabapentin has a class C rating if taken during pregnancy (eg, risk cannot be ruled out).

5. Indications and Evidence

Initially approved for epilepsy in 1993, the drug was later FDA approved for treatment of postherpetic neuralgia in 2002. Generic availability makes gabapentin a cost-effective method of treating many neuropathic pain diagnoses. Other indications include painful diabetic neuropathy, multiple sclerosis, migraine headaches, HIV neuropathy, trigeminal neuralgia, malignant pain, and phantom limb pain. The NNT of gabapentin depends on the exact diagnosis that is being addressed but ranges from 5.9 to 8.0. Evidence suggests that the combination of gabapentin with TCA has a synergistic effect for the treatment of pain. It is not known how this can be extrapolated to the combination of other medications such as pregabalin and SNRIs.

B. Pregabalin

1. Mechanism of Action

Pregabalin is the *S*-3-isobutyl isomer of GABA. As with gabapentin, the exact mechanism is not fully delineated at this point. It has been demonstrated to bind to the α-2-δ subunit of presynaptic voltage-gated calcium channel with approximately five to six times the affinity of gabapentin. There is also suggestion that it additionally augments the activity of glutamic acid decarboxylase in the presynaptic neuron.

2. Pharmacology

The bioavailability is ~90% in healthy subjects. The average time to peak plasma concentrations is 1.5 hours. Unlike gabapentin, absorption is not saturable or affected by food, which results in a more linear pharmacokinetic profile. The plasma half-life is ~5.8 hours and the time to steady state is 24-48 hours. It is 99% is excreted in the urine unchanged. The clearance of pregabalin is directly related to creatinine clearance and should be adjusted in the setting of decreased renal function.

3. Dosing and Monitoring

A reasonable starting dose is 75 mg bid for 1 week and then increased to 150 mg bid. The usual effective dose range is 150-600 mg divided into bid or tid dosing. If pregabalin is to be discontinued, it should be done slowly over the course of a week. It is available as an oral solution.

4. Adverse Side Effects

The most common side effects are peripheral edema, ataxia, weight gain, xerostomia, blurred vision, diplopia, dizziness, somnolence, and headaches. Pregabalin has a class C rating if taken during pregnancy (eg, risk cannot be ruled out).

5. Indications and Evidence

It currently has FDA approval for painful diabetic neuropathy, postherpetic neuralgia, spinal cord injury–associated pain, and fibromyalgia. Therapeutic benefit for the treatment of pain is usually seen within a week. The differences between gabapentin and pregabalin are given in Table 10.3.

TABLE 10.3 Differences Between Gabapentin and Pregabalin

	Gabapentin	Pregabalin
Bioavailability	27%-60% (dose dependent)	90%
T max (hours)	2-3	1
Plasma protein binding	<3%	0
Plasma half-life	5-7 h	5.5-6.7 h
Elimination	100% renal unchanged	92%-99% renal unchanged
Average neuropathic pain dose	1800-3600 mg/d	150-600 mg/d
Time to effective dose	6-9 d	1-3 d
Number needed to treat	6.3	7.7

C. Ziconotide

1. Mechanism of Action

ω-Conopeptide previously known as SNX-111. Ziconotide inhibits calcium flux through N-type calcium channels that are present in the dorsal horn lamina and preventing conduction of aberrant signals in the ascending neural tracts.

2. Pharmacology

Ziconotide has a peptide structure that necessitates intrathecal administration for therapeutic benefit. It is currently administered through an implanted intrathecal infusion pump. Approximately 50% becomes protein bound when it enters the blood stream. Half-life elimination is 2.9-6.5 hours in the CSF and 1-1.6 hours in blood. It is metabolized to inactive produced by endopeptidases and exopeptidases found in various organs.

3. Dosing and Monitoring

Initial intrathecal dosing should be started at a low dose of 2.4 μg/d. The medication has a prolonged time to effect and should be only increased slowly at intervals of 2-3 times per week. The maximum recommended dose is 19.2 μg/d. It can be used as monotherapy or combined with other intrathecal medications.

4. Adverse Side Effects

Dizziness, ataxia, confusion, and headaches have been reported. The medication is not reported to cause respiratory depression, tolerance, or dependence. Hallucinations have been reported, and therapy is not recommended in patients who have a history of psychosis. Ziconotide has a class C rating if taken during pregnancy (eg, risk cannot be ruled out).

5. Indications and Evidence

Some evidence suggests efficacy for the treatment of trigeminal neuralgia, CRPS, diabetic neuropathy, radicular extremity pain, postherpetic neuralgia, and chemotherapy-induced peripheral neuropathy.

D. Zonisamide

1. Mechanism of Action

Zonisamide is a sulfonamide-derived medication. It has diffuse mechanisms of action including inhibition of voltage-gated sodium channels, voltage-dependent T-type calcium channels, potassium-evoked glutamate responses, and augmenting serotonergic, dopaminergic, and GABAnergic transmission. This diffuse mechanism of action serves to stabilize membranes and prevent neuronal hypersynchronization.

2. Pharmacology

Approximately 100% bioavailability with food causing a delay of time to maximal plasma concentration but not overall bioavailability. Time to peak plasma concentration in normal individuals is 2-6 hours and can be delayed up to 2 hours if taken with food. The mean half-life is 60 hours and takes ~2 weeks to reach steady state. It is hepatically metabolized by CYP3A4 to a glucuronic acid conjugate and is excreted mostly in the urine. About one-third of the drug is excreted unchanged in the urine. The plasma half-life can be decreased by up to 50% by concurrent use of other cytochrome-inducing antiepileptic drugs (AEDs).

3. Dosing and Monitoring

The initial starting dose is 100 mg daily. Every 2 weeks, the dosage may be increased by 100 mg to a maximal dose of 400 mg daily. The usual effective dose is between 200 and 400 mg daily with little benefit seen at higher doses. Higher doses are associated with increased side effects such as weight loss.

4. Adverse Side Effects

The most common side effects are somnolence, ataxia, anorexia, difficulty in concentrating, agitation, and headaches. Patients who are allergic to sulfonamides should not be prescribed zonisamide. Pediatric patients are at an increased risk of developing oligohidrosis and susceptibility to hyperthermia. Serious complications such as Stevens-Johnson syndrome have occurred. Zonisamide has a class C rating if taken during pregnancy (eg, risk cannot be ruled out).

5. Indications and Evidence

FDA approved for seizure management. Several RCTs and reviews have demonstrated evidence for the treatment of different types of neuropathic pain and headaches.

VII. ANTICONVULSANTS

Anticonvulsants, also known as AEDs have been utilized for the management of pain since the 1960s, soon after they were initially introduced for the management of epilepsy. These medications were initially thought to have utility only in the treatment of burning neuropathic pain. However, recent evidence suggests a therapeutic benefit for numerous pain conditions.

Similar to other neuropathic pain agents, treatment of pain with an AED often requires serial trials of different medications, which can often take months or even years. In general each medication should be initiated a relatively low dose and then increased according to a predefined slow titration schedule until therapeutic effects or limiting side effects are observed. The early observation of side effects may indicate the need to revert to a lower dose and continue to up-titrate the medication at a slower rate. An adequate trial length should be at least 4-6 weeks. Serum levels do not appear to correlate well to pain response. The medications should be gradually tapered down, rather than abruptly discontinued, in order to avoid potentially serious withdrawal effects.

A. Carbamazepine

1. Mechanism of Action

Although structurally similar to TCAs, carbamazepine has a unique mechanism of action. It has its therapeutic effect through inhibition of voltage-gated sodium channel currents in the inactive state, thus prolonging the refractive and suppressing high-frequency conduction. It preferentially binds to highly active fibers, having very little effect on normally functioning C and Aδ nociceptive fibers. Additionally, carbamazepine centrally inhibits the reuptake of norepinephrine.

2. Pharmacology

The bioavailability of carbamazepine is 85%-95%. Peak concentrations are seen after 2-8 hours. Serum half-life is 10-20 hours with an average of 14 hours and 75%-90% protein binding. It is metabolized by CPY3A4, has biologically active metabolites, and is ultimately renally excreted and, secondarily, through the feces. As carbamazepine causes hepatic enzyme autoinduction of CYP3A4, increased metabolism and decreased side effects are seen with continued treatment.

3. Dosing and Monitoring

The starting dose is 100-200 mg/d and increased by 200 mg every 1-3 days to a maximum recommended dose of 2500 mg in divided doses. Therapeutic benefit is usually observed at 800-1200 mg/d. As carbamazepine is a gastric irritant, it should be taken with food.

4. Adverse Side Effects

Sedation, nausea, diplopia, ataxia, and vertigo are the most frequently observed side effects. Potentially serious hematologic side effects that have been reported include aplastic anemia, agranulocytosis, and pancytopenia thrombocytopenia. Monitoring of serial CBCs is recommended for patients taking carbamazepine starting with baseline values, then every 2 weeks for the first month, then monthly for the next 3 months, then every 6 months for the next year, and then yearly thereafter. Hematologic problems may be exacerbated if the patient is concurrently receiving bone marrow suppressing chemotherapy agents. Additionally, hepatocellular and cholestatic jaundice may occur necessitating monitoring of liver function. Oliguria, hypertension, and acute left ventricular heart failure have also been reported. Analysis has determined that the NNH of 24 for major adverse side effects and 3 for minor side effects. Carbamazepine has a black box warning for Stevens-Johnson syndrome in the setting of HLA B*1502 allele. The HLA B*1502 allele is almost universally found in persons of Asian descent. Carbamazepine has a class D rating if taken during pregnancy (eg, fetal harm will occur if taken during pregnancy).

5. Indications and Evidence

Carbamazepine is most frequently utilized to treat generalized and partial seizures. Strong evidence exists for the treatment of trigeminal neuralgia, painful diabetic neuropathy, and other neuropathic pain diagnoses with lancinating qualities. It is FDA approved and most widely studied for treatment of trigeminal neuralgia with a NNT < 2. Less well-established evidence suggests efficacy in the treatment of postherpetic neuralgia, central pain, and restless leg syndrome.

B. Oxcarbazepine

1. Mechanism of Action

Oxcarbazepine is a structural derivative of carbamazepine. Alterations in the metabolic profile of oxcarbazepine are derived from oxcarbazepine being the 10-keto analog of carbamazepine. It has a similar mechanism to carbamazepine. Additionally, oxcarbazepine has a pharmacologically active monohydroxy metabolite (10-MHD) with a longer elimination half-life. It may additionally increase potassium channel conductance and modulate high-voltage–activated calcium channels.

2. Pharmacology

The bioavailability of oxcarbazepine is >95% reaching peak plasma concentrations in 1-3 hours. The rate and extent of absorption are not modulated by consumption of food. It is extensively metabolized to 10-MHD. Parent drug half-life is 1-5 hours and 10-MHD half-life is 9 hours. Steady-state concentrations are reached following 2-3 days of use at a certain dose.

3. Dosing and Monitoring

A reasonable starting dose of 150 mg daily and then increased by 150-300 mg weekly. The dose recommended for seizure prophylaxis is 1200 mg daily. 600-1200 mg daily is the typical dose for pain treatment.

4. Adverse Side Effects

Hyponatremia (Na < 125 mmol/L) can rarely occur and monitoring of serum sodium levels is recommended. This usually develops after an average of 3 months of therapy and rapidly corrects with discontinuation of the medication. The most common side effects include dizziness, somnolence, diplopia, fatigue, ataxia, nausea, and abnormal vision. Oxcarbazepine has a class C rating if taken during pregnancy (eg, risk cannot be ruled out).

5. Indications and Evidence

The equal analgesic effectiveness and decreased incidence of serious side effects has resulted in oxcarbazepine usurping carbamazepine as the treatment of choice for trigeminal neuralgia. It is also used off label for several additional neuropathic pain indications.

C. Lamotrigine

1. Mechanism of Action

Lamotrigine is a phenyltriazine derivative that inhibits voltage-gated sodium channels and inhibits the release of glutamate from presynaptic neurons. Additionally, it may augment potassium and calcium currents. It has a weak inhibitory effect on serotonin-3 receptor.

2. Pharmacology

Lamotrigine has 98% bioavailability, which is not altered by concurrent food intake. The plasma concentration reaches peak levels after 1.4-5 hours, and the plasma half-life is ~24 hours. It is about 55% protein bound. Lamotrigine has limited first-pass metabolism but is extensively metabolized via hepatic glucuronic acid conjugation. Its pharmacokinetic profile is significantly altered by hepatic enzyme inhibition and induction. This typically occurs through concurrent use other AEDs. It is eliminated in the urine as a glucuronide conjugate. Dose adjustment is required with hepatic and renal insufficiency or dialysis.

3. Dosing and Monitoring

The exact starting dose depends on concurrent medication use. A starting dose may be 25 mg daily increased by 25 mg/week to 100 mg bid. Subsequently, the dose may increase by 50 mg/week to a maximum dose of 250 mg bid. Discontinuation requires a minimum of 2 weeks taper in order to avoid withdrawal side effects.

4. Adverse Side Effects

Nine to ten percent of patients will develop a benign and self-limiting rash. However, 1% of adolescent patients and 0.3% of adult patients may develop potentially life-threatening Stevens-Johnson syndrome also known as toxic epidermal necrolysis. The incidence of Stevens-Johnson syndrome appears related to the starting dose of lamotrigine and rate of increase. Therapy should be discontinued if a rash develops as there is no reliable way to discriminate between early-stage serious Stevens-Johnson rashes and benign self-limited rashes. Patients should be cautioned to be mindful of dizziness, nausea, headaches, ataxia, diplopia, blurred vision, and somnolence. Some patients can also develop back pain arthralgias and myalgias in response to therapy. Lamotrigine has a class C rating if taken during pregnancy (eg, risk cannot be ruled out).

5. Indications and Evidence

Mixed evidence suggests that lamotrigine is effective for the treatment of CRPS, oxcarbazepine-resistant trigeminal neuralgia, HIV-induced distal sensory polyneuropathy, and antiretroviral toxic neuropathy, spinal cord injury, multiple sclerosis, and central poststroke pain. It is most commonly utilized for the treatment of seizure control, mood stabilization, and the treatment of depressive components of bipolar disorder.

D. Topiramate

1. Mechanism of Action

Topiramate is a sulfamate-substituted monosaccharide. It has numerous mechanisms of actions including inhibition of voltage-gated sodium channels, voltage-activated L-type calcium channels, AMPA, and kainite receptors. Additionally, it has activity as an allosteric GABA-A agonist.

2. Pharmacology

The bioavailability of topiramate is 80% reaching peak serum concentration in 2 hours. The time to peak serum concentration is not affected by food. It is 15%-40% protein bound. Plasma half-life is 21 hours, and steady state is reached in ~4 days in patients with normal renal function. It undergoes minor hepatic metabolism. Approximately 70% is excreted unchanged in the urine.

3. Dosing and Monitoring

A reasonable starting dose is 25 mg, which is then increased by 25-50 mg/week. Therapeutic benefit is usually observed at a dose between 200 and 300 mg bid.

4. Adverse Side Effects

Weight loss occurs in a dose-dependent manner peaking after 15-18 months of therapy. Weight will usually return to pretreatment weight thereafter. Typical weight loss is reported to be 1.7%-7.2% of the pretreatment weight. 1.5% of patients develop renal calculi due to its inhibition of carbonic anhydrase. Stone formation may be limited with maintenance of hydration. Somnolence, dizziness, ataxia, paresthesias, nervousness, abnormal vision, and cognitive difficulties manifesting as problems with memory and concentration have also been reported with topiramate use. Topiramate has a class D rating if taken during pregnancy (eg, fetal harm will occur if taken during pregnancy).

5. Indications and Evidence

It is indicated as a prophylactic treatment for migraine headaches. Additional benefits suggest benefit for treatment of spinal cord injuries and diabetic neuropathy.

E. Lithium

Lithium is extensively utilized for the treatment of migraines and cluster headaches. However, there is no strong evidence for any other type of chronic pain. It has been prescribed for the treatment of bipolar disorder, but a low therapeutic index and the development of safer and equally efficacious medications has caused a decline in its overall utilization. Lethal overdoses have been observed at four to five times the therapeutic dose. Lithium can produce euthyroid goiter and hypothyroidism, and thyroid function should be monitored during therapy. Additionally, renal function should be monitored as chronic use can lead to the development of nephrogenic diabetes insipidus. Hypercalcemia with and without hyperparathyroidism has been reported.

F. Phenytoin

1. Mechanism of Action

Phenytoin inhibits the function of voltage-gated sodium channels, thereby inhibiting the development and propagation of ectopic discharges on excitatory neurons. Antiepileptic effect of phenytoin is derived from stabilization of membranes in the motor cortex.

2. Pharmacology

The bioavailability is formulation dependent and requires 1-3 hours until peak plasma levels are observed. Protein binding is 90%-95% in adults and 80% in small children. Halftime elimination is 7-14 hours. It is hepatically metabolized by CPY2C9 and CYP2C19. Metabolism is highly altered depending on cytochrome phenotypic expression, which has significant interpatient variability. It is ultimately excreted in the urine.

3. Dosing and Monitoring

100 mg bid to tid is considered an effective dose. The optimal dose for the treatment of neuropathic pain has not been clearly established.

4. Adverse Side Effects

Common side effects include the development of somnolence, motor disturbances, and slowing of mentation which may be related to the rate of administration. Unique side effects include the development of gingival hyperplasia and coarsening of facial features. The blockade of sodium channels on ventricular pacemaker cells can result in cardiac dysrhythmias and is usually seen in pediatric patients after rapid IV administration. Phenytoin has a class D rating if taken during pregnancy (eg, fetal harm will occur if taken during pregnancy).

5. Indications and Evidence

It is previously used for the treatment of diabetic neuropathy. However, the development of newer medications with fewer side effects has caused it to be supplanted as a first-line agent.

VIII. LOCAL ANESTHETICS

A. Lidocaine

1. Mechanism of Action

All local anesthetics, including lidocaine, exhibit therapeutic benefit from inhibition of sodium channels in the inactive state at an intraneural binding site. This prevents the initiation and propagation of nerve cell depolarization in both abnormally and normally functioning neural fibers.

2. Pharmacology

In general, it is administered as an IV infusion. However, numerous effective infusion protocols have been described over time. It is 60%-80% protein bound. The elimination half-life in adults is 1.5-2 hours. It is 90% metabolized by CYP3A4 to inactive metabolites that are excreted in the urine.

3. Dosing and Monitoring

Multiple infusion protocols have been described as effective for the treatment of various discreet pain disorders. However, in general a starting doe of 1-5 mg/kg IV lidocaine is given over 15 minutes in a monitored setting. A decrease in pain by 50% warrants continuation of therapy with mexiletine or possibly an anticonvulsant with sodium channel inhibitory properties.

Prior to infusion, a baseline EKG and hepatic function tests are recommended.

Topical lidocaine is available as a gel solution or a transdermal patch, which produce analgesia without causing local anesthesia. The patches are designed to be used for 12 hours and then to leave the skin exposed for 12 hours. Up to three patches per day may be used for certain pain indications.

4. Adverse Side Effects

The most commonly reported side effects with lidocaine infusions are tinnitus, perioral numbness, a metallic taste in the mouth, and dizziness during the trial. There is also the possibility of arrhythmia, syncope, hypotension, ataxia, tremors, nervousness, upper GI distress, dizziness, hepatotoxicity, skin rashes, visual changes, fevers, and chills. Cardiac arrhythmias occur with doses >20-25 mg/mL and must be done with extreme caution and with close cardiac monitoring. Lidocaine has a class B rating if taken during pregnancy (animal models do not demonstrate harm but no adequate human studies have been done).

5. Indications and Evidence

Evidence for infusion lidocaine therapy for the treatment of continuous and lancinating dysesthesias including pain due to herpes zoster, phantom limb pain, and diabetic neuropathy. Superficial causes of neuropathic pain, such as postherpetic neuralgias, are ideally suited to treatment with topical lidocaine. Lidocaine patches are also effective for trigeminal neuralgia and CRPS where the patches also protect against mechanical dermal irritation. Additional indications include myofascial pain, postthoracotomy pain, postmastectomy pain, postamputation pain, neuroma-induced pain, diabetic peripheral neuropathy, meralgia paresthetica, intercostal neuralgia, and ilioinguinal neuralgia.

B. Mexiletine

1. Mechanism of Action

Similar to lidocaine and other local anesthetics, mexiletine blocks sodium channels in the inactive state at an intraneural binding site. This prevents the initiation and propagation of nerve cell depolarization. Mexiletine is an amide local anesthetic that is structurally related to lidocaine.

2. Pharmacology

The bioavailability of mexiletine is 90% with time to peak serum concentration of 2-3 hours. It is 50%-60% protein bound and has an elimination halftime of 10-12 hours. Mexiletine is metabolized by CYP2D6 to inactive metabolites, which are ultimately excreted in the urine.

3. Dosing and Monitoring

The recommended starting dose is 150 mg at bedtime for 1 week, which is then increased to 300-450 mg tid over 3 weeks. If additional pain relief is required, then a maximal safe dose of 1200 mg daily is recommended with close monitoring of cardiac conduction.

4. Adverse Side Effects

Commonly reported side effects include somnolence, irritability, blurred vision, nausea, and vomiting. There is also a risk of developing blood dyscrasias in certain patients. The FDA has a black box warning for acute liver injury, which is usually seen in patients taking mexiletine who have congestive heart failure or cardiac ischemia. The exact link to mexiletine has not been established.

5. Indications and Evidence

Mexiletine has been found to be effective in the treatment of painful diabetic neuropathy, thalamic stroke pain, spasticity-related pain, and myotonia. Its therapeutic effect on the latter has been reported to be minimal.

IX. NEUROLEPTICS

Antipsychotics are medications that are primarily used in the treatment of schizophrenia. They have also found utility in the treatment of psychotic symptoms associated with mood disorders and delirium. Other uses include anxiety, insomnia, and agitation associated with dementia and personality disorders. They are referred to as neuroleptics due to the often irreversible seen with older typical agents. Although not often used as first-line agents in the treatment of neuropathic pain, in some cases, they do offer benefit for symptomatic management. There are broadly subdivided into typical and atypical neuroleptics based on an individual medications antagonism of the postsynaptic D2 receptor.

A. Typical

Included in the typical neuroleptic class of medications are fluphenazine, haloperidol, perphenazine, thiothixene, trifluoperazine, loxapine, chlorpromazine, and thioridazine.

1. Mechanism of Action

As a class, the primarily mechanism of action is antagonism at postsynaptic D2 receptors in neural tracts originating in the midbrain and ramifying in the limbic system. Other receptors which may contribute to these medication's analgesic properties include cholinergic, α_1-adrenergic, and histaminic receptors. However, these later systems may also contribute to the side effect profile of these medications. It is felt that the sedating and anxiolytic effects of these atypical neuroleptics do not adequately account for their therapeutic properties in the treatment of multiple pain conditions.

2. Pharmacology

Haloperidol is the only typical antipsychotic that is available for IV use in the United States. The efficacy and potency of typical neuroleptics is directly proportional to the degree of antagonist at the D2 receptor. Most first-generation neuroleptics have a high bioavailability and rapidly reach therapeutic concentrations in the brain. α_1-Adrenergic antagonism may contribute to orthostatic hypotension, and histaminic stimulation may result in sedation. These medications are usually metabolized by CYP2D6 and excreted in the urine.

3. Adverse Side Effects

All typical antipsychotics carry a risk of extrapyramidal symptoms including tardive dyskinesia, akathisia, acute dystonia, and pseudoparkinsonism. The risk seems to be inversely proportional to the degree of anticholinergic effects. Prolactin levels have been reported to be elevated in response to neuroleptics causing amenorrhea, galactorrhea, false-positive pregnancy tests in women, and gynecomastia in men. Other neurohumoral alterations include hypothalamic dysfunction and syndrome of inappropriate antidiuretic hormone, temperature dysregulation, and serum glucose level disruption.

Anticholinergic activity may cause xerostomia, blurry vision, constipation, urinary retention, and confusion and delirium. Histaminic side effects that may be observed include sedation, cognitive impairment, and weight gain. Additional side effects may include sexual dysfunction, hypotension, fainting, nonspecific changes on EKG, and rarely, arrhythmias including torsades de pointes and, rarely, cardiac death. The seizure threshold is lowered in a manner inverse to the potency of the medication with the highest seizure risk with chlorpromazine and lowest seizure risk with haloperidol. The risk if taken during pregnancy is variable for each medication.

4. Indications and Evidence

Phenothiazines, such as chlorpromazine and prochlorperazine, have evidence as being effective as adjuvants for the treatment of migraines and nonmigraine headaches. Evidence suggests that haloperidol and fluphenazine have analgesic properties for the treatment of neuropathic pain and can be useful in the treatment of pain-related suffering and distress.

B. Atypical

1. Mechanism of Action

The primary therapeutic target of atypical neuroleptics continues to be the postsynaptic D2 receptors, similar to the typical neuroleptics, albeit to a reduced degree. These medications preferentially inhibit serotonin 2 receptors and dopaminergic 4 receptors to a greater degree than typical neuroleptics. They are possibly more effective at treating the negative symptoms associated with psychotic symptoms. However, their use in chronic pain has not been thoroughly studied.

2. Pharmacology

The bioavailability and metabolic profile varies widely from one drug to another.

3. Adverse Side Effects

The significant advantage of atypical antipsychotic agents over typical agents is the lower incidence of extrapyramidal side effects. Quetiapine is thought to have the lowest incidence of extrapyramidal side effects. The side effect profile is variable among medications within the class. However, patients should be monitored for sedation, weight gain, dizziness, and insulin resistance. No laboratory tests are required when initiating or maintaining therapy in healthy adults. The risk if taken during pregnancy is variable for each medication.

4. Indications and Evidence

Small RCTs have demonstrated that olanzapine may decrease pain in cancer pain patients with coexisting anxiety and mild cognitive impairment. They are possibly effective as second- or third-line agents in prophylaxis of migraines or chronic daily headaches. The dosage range for analgesic benefit of atypical neuroleptics has not been firmly established.

C. Capsaicin

1. Mechanism of Action

The mechanism of capsaicin is the subject of much ongoing research. The primary mechanism of action is the depletion of substance P and neuropeptides from nociceptive fibers, causing analgesia. Capsaicin binds the vanilloid receptor-1 (TRPV1).

2. Pharmacology

It depolarizes the neural membrane via TRPV1. Initially upon application, it stimulates skin nerve fiber conduction and then subsequently blocks skin nerve fiber conduction. Absorption from 8% patch at 60 minutes is <5 ng/mL and undetectable at 6 hours. The half-life of capsaicin is 1.6 hours.

3. Dosing and Monitoring

The topical cream usually dosed as a 0.025% or 0.075% lotion or cream applied 3-5 times daily is available over the counter. Therapeutic benefit is usually seen after 4-6 weeks of topical therapy. An 8% patch is also available as a prescription that is designed to be worn every day for 60 minutes for the treatment of PHN and 30 minutes for HIV-associated neuropathy. Therapeutic benefit with a patch can be seen with 1 week of therapy. Studies demonstrated durable benefit lasting over 12 weeks of treatment.

4. Adverse Side Effects

The most commonly reported side effect is localized burning or stinging upon application of either the patch or the cream. Erythema may develop at the site of application. Due to the very minimal systemic absorption, capsaicin is not associated with systemic adverse effects.

5. Indications and Evidence

Useful for postherpetic neuralgia, HIV-associated neuropathy, and osteoarthritis treatment.

There are a number of other medications that have been demonstrated in high-quality evidence to be effective for the treatment of certain neuropathic pain conditions. These medications may find utility in clinical use in the coming years and be valuable tools in the treatment of neuropathic agents. Such medications may include low-dose naltrexone, bisphosphonates, intranasal calcitonin, alpha-lipoic acid, acetyl-L-carnitine, medical marijuana, cannabinoid derivatives, and B vitamins. Numerous other medications are also at various stages of testing.

In conclusion, the effective treatment of neuropathic pain can be a prolonged and difficult process. However, the currently available library of neuropathic pain medications can be sequentially offered alone or in combination with each other. The therapeutic benefit of each medication must be balanced against a unique side effect profile. As the pathology and molecular biology allows our understanding of these diseases to evolve, new medications will continue to be developed allowing for improved management of patient's suffering with neuropathic pain.

Selected Readings

Attal N, Bouhassira D. Pharmacotherapy of neuropathic pain: which drugs, which treatment algorithms? *Pain.* 2015;156(suppl 1):S104-S114.

Boyle J, Eriksson ME, Gribble L, et al. Randomized, placebo-controlled comparison of amitriptyline, duloxetine, and pregabalin in patients with chronic diabetic peripheral neuropathic pain: impact on pain, polysomnographic sleep, daytime functioning, and quality of life. *Diabetes Care.* 2012;35(12):2451-2458.

Challapalli V, Tremont-Lukats IW, McNicol ED, Lau J, Carr DB. Systemic administration of local anesthetic agents to relieve neuropathic pain. *Cochrane Database Syst Rev.* 2005;(4):CD003345.

Chaparro LE, Wiffen PJ, Moore RA, Gilron I. Combination pharmacotherapy for the treatment of neuropathic pain in adults. *Cochrane Database Syst Rev.* 2012;7:CD008943.

Chappell AS, Littlejohn G, Kajdasz DK, Scheinberg M, D'Souza DN, Moldofsky H. A 1-year safety and efficacy study of duloxetine in patients with fibromyalgia. *Clin J Pain.* 2009;25(5):365-375.

Chung H. Dosing of selective serotonin reuptake inhibitors. *Prim Care Companion J Clin Psychiatry.* 2001;3(5):224-225.

Cohen SP, Mao J. Neuropathic pain: mechanisms and their clinical implications. *BMJ.* 2014;348:f7656.

Derry S, Phillips T, Moore RA, Wiffen PJ. Milnacipran for neuropathic pain in adults. *Cochrane Database Syst Rev.* 2015;7:CD011789.

Derry S, Wiffen PJ, Aldington D, Moore RA. Nortriptyline for neuropathic pain in adults. *Cochrane Database Syst Rev.* 2015;1:CD011209.

Finnerup NB, Attal N, Haroutounian S, et al. Pharmacotherapy for neuropathic pain in adults: a systematic review and meta-analysis. *Lancet Neurol.* 2015;14(2):162-173.

Fishbain DA, Cutler R, Rosomoff HL, Rosomoff RS. Evidence-based data from animal and human experimental studies on pain relief with antidepressants: a structured review. *Pain Med.* 2000;1(4):310-316.

Gallagher HC, Gallagher RM, Butler M, Buggy DJ, Henman MC. Venlafaxine for neuropathic pain in adults. *Cochrane Database Syst Rev.* 2015;8:CD011091.

Ghio L, Puppo S, Presta A. Venlafaxine and risk of upper gastrointestinal bleeding in elderly depression. *Curr Drug Saf.* 2012;7(5):389-390.

Gilron I, Bailey JM, Tu D, Holden RR, Jackson AC, Houlden RL. Nortriptyline and gabapentin, alone and in combination for neuropathic pain: a double-blind, randomised controlled crossover trial. *Lancet.* 2009;374(9697):1252-1261.

Gilron I, Baron R, Jensen T. Neuropathic pain: principles of diagnosis and treatment. *Mayo Clin Proc.* 2015;90(4):532-545.

Grundmann M, Kacirova I, Urinovska R. Therapeutic drug monitoring of atypical antipsychotic drugs. *Acta Pharm.* 2014;64(4):387-401.

Hauser W, Urrutia G, Tort S, Uceyler N, Walitt B. Serotonin and noradrenaline reuptake inhibitors (SNRIs) for fibromyalgia syndrome. *Cochrane Database Syst Rev.* 2013;1:CD010292.

Hearn L, Derry S, Phillips T, Moore RA, Wiffen PJ. Imipramine for neuropathic pain in adults. *Cochrane Database Syst Rev.* 2014;5:CD010769.

Hearn L, Moore RA, Derry S, Wiffen PJ, Phillips T. Desipramine for neuropathic pain in adults. *Cochrane Database Syst Rev.* 2014;9:CD011003.

Jensen TS. Anticonvulsants in neuropathic pain: rationale and clinical evidence. *Eur J Pain.* 2002;6(suppl A):61-68.

Johannessen Landmark C, Henning O, Johannessen SI. Proconvulsant effects of antidepressants—what is the current evidence? *Epilepsy Behav.* 2016;61:287-291.

Lunn MP, Hughes RA, Wiffen PJ. Duloxetine for treating painful neuropathy, chronic pain or fibromyalgia. *Cochrane Database Syst Rev.* 2014;1:CD007115.

Max MB, Culnane M, Schafer SC, et al. Amitriptyline relieves diabetic neuropathy pain in patients with normal or depressed mood. *Neurology.* 1987;37(4):589-596.

McDowell GC II, Pope JE. Intrathecal ziconotide: dosing and administration strategies in patients with refractory chronic pain. *Neuromodulation.* 2016;19(5):522-532.

Mease PJ, Clauw DJ, Gendreau RM, et al. The efficacy and safety of milnacipran for treatment of fibromyalgia. a randomized, double-blind, placebo-controlled trial. *J Rheumatol.* 2009;36(2):398-409.

Mico JA, Ardid D, Berrocoso E, Eschalier A. Antidepressants and pain. *Trends Pharmacol Sci.* 2006;27(7):348-354.

Mittur A. Trazodone: properties and utility in multiple disorders. *Expert Rev Clin Pharmacol.* 2011;4(2):181-196.

Moore RA, Derry S, Aldington D, Cole P, Wiffen PJ. Amitriptyline for neuropathic pain in adults. *Cochrane Database Syst Rev.* 2015;7:CD008242.

Moore RA, Wiffen PJ, Derry S, Lunn MP. Zonisamide for neuropathic pain in adults. *Cochrane Database Syst Rev.* 2015;1:CD011241.

Moore RA, Wiffen PJ, Derry S, Toelle T, Rice AS. Gabapentin for chronic neuropathic pain and fibromyalgia in adults. *Cochrane Database Syst Rev.* 2014;4:CD007938.

Morillas-Arques P, Rodriguez-Lopez CM, Molina-Barea R, Rico-Villademoros F, Calandre EP. Trazodone for the treatment of fibromyalgia: an open-label, 12-week study. *BMC Musculoskelet Disord.* 2010;11:204.

Niesters M, Martini C, Dahan A. Ketamine for chronic pain: risks and benefits. *Br J Clin Pharmacol.* 2014;77(2):357-367.

O'Connor AB, Dworkin RH. Treatment of neuropathic pain: an overview of recent guidelines. *Am J Med.* 2009;122(10 suppl):S22-S32.

Passier A, van Puijenbroek E. Mirtazapine-induced arthralgia. *Br J Clin Pharmacol.* 2005;60(5):570-572.

Saarto T, Wiffen PJ. Antidepressants for neuropathic pain. *Cochrane Database Syst Rev.* 2007;(4):CD005454.

Scadding JW. Treatment of neuropathic pain: historical aspects. *Pain Med.* 2004; 5(suppl 1):S3-S8.

Seidel S, Aigner M, Ossege M, Pernicka E, Wildner B, Sycha T. Antipsychotics for acute and chronic pain in adults. *Cochrane Database Syst Rev.* 2013;8:CD004844.

Shah TH, Moradimehr A. Bupropion for the treatment of neuropathic pain. *Am J Hosp Palliat Care.* 2010;27(5):333-336.

Sindrup SH, Bach FW, Madsen C, Gram LF, Jensen TS. Venlafaxine versus imipramine in painful polyneuropathy: a randomized, controlled trial. *Neurology.* 2003;60(8):1284-1289.

Smith EM, Pang H, Cirrincione C, et al. Effect of duloxetine on pain, function, and quality of life among patients with chemotherapy-induced painful peripheral neuropathy: a randomized clinical trial. *JAMA.* 2013;309(13):1359-1367.

Tasmuth T, von Smitten K, Hietanen P, Kataja M, Kalso E. Pain and other symptoms after different treatment modalities of breast cancer. *Ann Oncol.* 1995;6(5):453-459.

Tesfaye S, Wilhelm S, Lledo A, et al. Duloxetine and pregabalin: high-dose monotherapy or their combination? The "COMBO-DN study"—a multinational, randomized, double-blind, parallel-group study in patients with diabetic peripheral neuropathic pain. *Pain.* 2013;154(12):2616-2625.

Thase ME. Effects of venlafaxine on blood pressure: a meta-analysis of original data from 3744 depressed patients. *J Clin Psychiatry.* 1998;59(10):502-508.

VanderWeide LA, Smith SM, Trinkley KE. A systematic review of the efficacy of venlafaxine for the treatment of fibromyalgia. *J Clin Pharm Ther.* 2015;40(1):1-6.

Verdu B, Decosterd I, Buclin T, Stiefel F, Berney A. Antidepressants for the treatment of chronic pain. *Drugs.* 2008;68(18):2611-2632.

Vorobeychik Y, Gordin V, Mao J, Chen L. Combination therapy for neuropathic pain: a review of current evidence. *CNS Drugs.* 2011;25(12):1023-1034.

Walitt B, Urrutia G, Nishishinya MB, Cantrell SE, Hauser W. Selective serotonin reuptake inhibitors for fibromyalgia syndrome. *Cochrane Database Syst Rev.* 2015;6:CD011735.

Zakrzewska JM, Linskey ME. Trigeminal neuralgia. *BMJ.* 2014;348:g474.

Zhang L, Rainka M, Freeman R, et al. A randomized, double-blind, placebo-controlled trial to assess the efficacy and safety of gabapentin enacarbil in subjects with neuropathic pain associated with postherpetic neuralgia (PXN110748). *J Pain.* 2013;14(6):590-603.

11 Opioids

Mark A. Hoeft

I. DEFINITIONS

A. Addiction

A primary, chronic, neurobiological disease, with genetic, psychosocial, and environmental factors influencing its development and manifestations. It is characterized by behaviors that include one or more of the following: impaired control over drug use, compulsive use, continued use despite harm, and craving.

B. Physical Dependence

A state of adaptation that is manifested by a drug class–specific withdrawal syndrome that can be produced by abrupt cessation, rapid dose reduction, decreasing blood level of the drug, and/or administration of an antagonist.

C. Tolerance

A state of adaptation in which exposure to a drug induces changes that result in a diminution of one or more of the drug's effects over time.

D. Opium

A bitter brownish addictive narcotic drug that consists of the dried latex obtained from immature seed capsules of the opium poppy.

E. Opioid

All substances, both natural and synthetic, that bind to opioid receptors (including antagonists).

F. Opiate

Opium or a drug derived from opium-possessing morphinelike effects.

G. Narcotic

A drug that in moderate doses dulls the senses, relieves pain, and induces profound sleep but in excessive doses causes stupor, coma, or convulsions.

H. Opioid-Induced Hyperalgesia

A state of nociceptive sensitization caused by exposure to opioids. The condition is characterized by a paradoxical response whereby a patient receiving opioids for the treatment of pain could become more sensitive to certain painful stimuli. The type of pain experienced might be the same as the underlying pain or might be different from the original underlying pain.

II. HISTORY

The first utilization of opioids was noted in 3400 BC in Mesopotamia (current regions of Syria, Kuwait, Turkey, Iraq, and Iran). The opium poppy was called the "Joy Plant." Hippocrates (460-357 BC), the Greek "father of medicine," describes "meconium" (the opium poppy) as sleep producing in his writings on *The Diseases of Women*.

III. OPIOID CRISIS

In 2015, the CDC quotes 33 000 opioid (prescription opioid and heroin)-related deaths of which half were from prescription pain medications. One out of every 550 patients started on opioid therapy died from opioid-related complications within 2.6 years. In the primary care setting, the prevalence of opioid addiction for patient with chronic, noncancer pain may be as high as 26%. Risk of opioid overdose increases twofold in patients taking 50-99 morphine milligram equivalents (MME)/d. This increases up to ninefold for those taking over 100 MME/d. The quoted rate of overdose for patients taking over 200 MME/d is 1 in 32.

IV. MECHANISM OF ACTION

Opioids act on multiple receptors including the μ (mu), κ (kappa), δ (delta), opioid receptor–like-1 (OLR-1) (Table 11.1). Receptors are located centrally in the dorsal horn of the spinal cord and dorsal root ganglia and peripheral nerves. The opioid receptors act at pre- and postsynaptic G (guanine)-coupled receptor proteins in the central and peripheral nervous system.

Activation of opioid receptors in the locus coeruleus, medulla, and periaqueductal gray area modulate descending pain pathways by directly inhibiting neurons in these locations which inhibit pain transmission from the spinal cord.

V. DURATION OF TREATMENT

Opioid prescriptions for acute and chronic pain and the risk of addiction potential are currently undergoing a paradigm shift. Data are currently inconclusive for the efficacy of opioids for the treatment of chronic pain. Recent CDC studies demonstrated that those patients with a first time course of opioids for ≥8 days have a 13.9% chance of being prescribed opioids at 1 year. This increased to 29.9% when patients were prescribed opioids for ≥31 days. This study found factors for the continued use of opioids >1 year included older age, female, pain diagnosis prior to initiation of opioids, initiation of higher doses of opioids, and publically or self-insured. The highest probability of continued opioid use at 1 and 3 years was

TABLE 11.1 Putative Opioid Receptor Location, Function/Effect and Specific Opioid Ligands

Pharmacological Subtype	Location	Function/Effect	Subtype-Specific Opioid Ligands	Subtype Nonspecific Opioid Ligands
μ1	Brain, spinal cord, periphery	Analgesia	Morphine (agonist), naloxone (antagonist), codeine (agonist), oxycodone (agonist)	Codeine (+), fentanyl (+++), hydromorphone (+++), Methadone (+++), morphine (+++), oxycodone (+), tramadol (+), tapentadol (+++)
μ2	Brain, spinal cord, periphery	Analgesia, GI transit, respiratory depression, itching	Morphine (lower affinity agonist), naloxone (lower affinity antagonist), M6G (agonist), heroin (agonist)	
μ3	Immune cells, amygdala, peripheral neural, cardiovascular endothelial cells	NO release	Morphine (lower affinity agonist), naloxone (lower affinity antagonist), M6G (lower affinity agonist), heroin (agonist)	
δ1	Brain, periphery	Analgesia, cardioprotection	Naltrexone (antagonist), enkephalin (agonist), deltorphin-D (agonist)	
δ2	Brain and spinal	Analgesia, cardioprotection, thermoregulation	Naltrexone (antagonist), enkephalin (agonist), deltorphin-D (agonist), deltorphin-II (agonist)	
κ 1a, κ 1b	Brain (nucleus accumbens, neocortex, cerebellum)	Analgesia, feeding		Morphine (+), oxycodone (++)
κ 2a, κ 2b	Brain (hippocampus, thalamus, brainstem)	Analgesia, diuresis, neuroendocrine		
κ 3	Brain	Spinal analgesia, peripheral effects		

Adapted from Dietis N, Rowbotham DJ, Lambert DG. Opioid receptor subtypes: fact or artifact? *Br J Anaesth.* 2011;107(1):8-18, Table 1 and Drewes AM, Jensen RD, Nielsen LM, et al. Differences between opioids: pharmacological, experimental, clinical and economical perspectives. *Br J Clin Pharmacol.* 2013;75(1):60-78.

observed in patients initially prescribed long-acting opioids, tramadol, or a short-acting opioid other than hydrocodone or oxycodone. See Table 11.2 for the CDC's current recommendations regarding the prescribing of opioids for chronic noncancer pain.

TABLE 11.2 CDC Recommendations for Prescribing Opioids for Chronic Pain Outside of Active Cancer, Palliative, and End-of-Life Care

Determining When to Initiate or Continue Opioids for Chronic Pain	**1.** Nonpharmacologic therapy and nonopioid pharmacologic therapy are preferred for chronic pain. Clinicians should consider opioid therapy only if expected benefits for both pain and function are anticipated to outweigh risks to the patient. If opioids are used, they should be combined with nonpharmacologic therapy and nonopioid pharmacologic therapy, as appropriate **2.** Before starting opioid therapy for chronic pain, clinicians should establish treatment goals with all patients, including realistic goals for pain and function, and should consider how therapy will be discontinued if benefits do not outweigh risks. Clinicians should continue opioid therapy only if there is clinically meaningful improvement in pain and function that outweighs risks to patient safety **3.** Before starting and periodically during opioid therapy, clinicians should discuss with patients known risks and realistic benefits of opioid therapy and patient and clinician responsibilities for managing therapy
Opioid Selection, Dosage, Duration, Follow-up, and Discontinuation	**1.** When starting opioid therapy for chronic pain, clinicians should prescribe immediate-release opioids instead of extended-release/long-acting (ER/LA) opioids **2.** When opioids are started, clinicians should prescribe the lowest effective dosage. Clinicians should use caution when prescribing opioids at any dosage, should carefully reassess evidence of individual benefits and risks when increasing dosage to ≥50 morphine milligram equivalents (MME)/d, and should avoid increasing dosage to ≥90 MME/d or carefully justify a decision to titrate dosage to ≥90 MME/d **3.** Long-term opioid use often begins with treatment of acute pain. When opioids are used for acute pain, clinicians should prescribe the lowest effective dose of immediate-release opioids and should prescribe no greater quantity than needed for the expected duration of pain severe enough to require opioids. Three days or less will often be sufficient; more than seven days will rarely be needed **4.** Clinicians should evaluate benefits and harms with patients within 1-4 wk of starting opioid therapy for chronic pain or of dose escalation. Clinicians should evaluate benefits and harms of continued therapy with patients every 3 mo or more frequently. If benefits do not outweigh harms of continued opioid therapy, clinicians should optimize other therapies and work with patients to taper opioids to lower dosages or to taper and discontinue opioids

TABLE 11.2 CDC Recommendations for Prescribing Opioids for Chronic Pain Outside of Active Cancer, Palliative, and End-of-Life Care (*Continued*)

Assessing Risk and Addressing Harms of Opioid Use	**1.** Before starting and periodically during continuation of opioid therapy, clinicians should evaluate risk factors for opioid-related harms. Clinicians should incorporate into the management plan strategies to mitigate risk, including considering offering naloxone when factors that increase risk for opioid overdose, such as history of overdose, history of substance use disorder, higher opioid dosages (≥50 MME/d), or concurrent benzodiazepine use, are present **2.** Clinicians should review the patient's history of controlled substance prescriptions using state prescription drug monitoring program (PDMP) data to determine whether the patient is receiving opioid dosages or dangerous combinations that put him or her at high risk for overdose. Clinicians should review PDMP data when starting opioid therapy for chronic pain and periodically during opioid therapy for chronic pain, ranging from every prescription to every 3 mo. **3.** When prescribing opioids for chronic pain, clinicians should use urine drug testing before starting opioid therapy and consider urine drug testing at least annually to assess for prescribed medications as well as other controlled prescription drugs and illicit drugs **4.** Clinicians should avoid prescribing opioid pain medication and benzodiazepines concurrently whenever possible **5.** Clinicians should offer or arrange evidence-based treatment (usually medication-assisted treatment with buprenorphine or methadone in combination with behavioral therapies) for patients with opioid use disorder

Taken from CDC Guideline for Prescribing Opioids for Chronic Pain — United States. *MMWR.* 2016;65(1);1-49.

VI. OPIOID RISK STRATIFICATION

Opioid risk stratification should be utilized prior to prescribing opioids to a patient for the first time. Tools such as the Opioid Risk Tool (ORT) consider age, sex, personal and family substance abuse history, and mental health history to stratify a patient into low, medium, and high risk for opioid abuse.

VII. COMMON OUTPATIENT OPIOIDS

A. Buprenorphine

1. **Routes of administration:** Sublingual, buccal, intramuscular, oral, transdermal.
2. **Peak effect:** Intravenous 0.25-3 hours, sublingual 3-7 hours. Transdermal patch steady state is reached within 3 days after the application of the patch.

3. **Mechanism of action:** Partial agonist at the μ-opioid receptor and an antagonist at the κ-opioid receptor, an agonist at the δ-opioid receptors, and a partial agonist at ORL-1 receptor.
4. **Metabolism:** Metabolized primary in the liver via cytochrome P-450.
5. **Excretion:** Majority excreted via the feces. Less than 30% is excreted in the urine. The mean elimination half-life is ~37 hours.
6. **Dosing (adult):** Please consult trained buprenorphine prescriber for initiation and maintenance of therapy.
7. **Special considerations:** Cases of hepatotoxicity (cytolytic hepatitis and hepatitis with jaundice) have been observed with buprenorphine administration. For patients at risk for hepatotoxicity (eg, excessive alcohol intake, intravenous drug abuse, or liver disease), baseline liver function tests should be obtained prior to starting buprenorphine. Monitor patients who are taking cytochrome P-450 inducers or inhibitors when the mediation is initiated.
8. Data are sparse regarding the continuation or discontinuation of buprenorphine in the perioperative setting. For mildly painful surgeries, buprenorphine maybe continued perioperatively and used as the primary analgesic postoperatively. For elective moderate to severely painful surgeries, some have recommended discontinuing buprenorphine 3-7 days preoperatively. Others have recommended reducing the dose to 8 mg or less, but maintaining the patient on some buprenorphine to reduce the risk of relapse and prevent the need for reinduction onto buprenorphine. In either case, the patient may be given a minimal prescription for a full opioid agonist for withdrawal symptoms. Consider multimodal analgesia in those patients taking buprenorphine chronically including neuraxial or regional anesthesia. Postoperatively, high-dose opioids may be necessary given the opioid antagonist action of the buprenorphine.

B. Codeine

1. **Formulations:** Oral.
2. **Peak effect:** 1-1.5 hours.
3. **Metabolism:** Codeine is metabolized to codeine-6-glucuronide (C6G) (70%-80%) and via *O*-demethylation to morphine (about 5%-10%) and *N*-demethylation to norcodeine (about 10%).
4. **Excretion:** Approximately 90% of codeine is excreted through the kidneys. Approximately 10% of this is unchanged codeine. Plasma half-lives of codeine and its metabolites have been reported to be ~3 hours.
5. **Dosing (adult):** 15-60 mg po q4h prn, not to exceed 360 mg/d.
6. **Special considerations:** Patients metabolize codeine at varying rates secondary to a specific CYP2D6 genotype. Ultrarapid metabolizers breakdown the codeine to morphine at extremely high rates which may cause toxicity and potential for life-threatening respiratory depression and death. This is seen in ~2% of the population but has a prevalence of 0.5%-1% in Chinese and Japanese, 0.5%-1% in Hispanics, 1%-10% in Caucasians, 3% in African Americans, and 16%-28% in North Africans, Ethiopians, and Arabs. Poor metabolizers are seen in 5%-10% of the population resulting in poor pain control. It is recommended to use morphine in this patient population as tramadol, and to a lesser extent, hydrocodone and oxycodone are metabolized by CYP2D6.

C. Fentanyl

1. **Formulations:** Intravenous, transdermal, buccal, sublingual, transnasal, epidural, intrathecal.
2. **Peak effect:** Intravenous, 3-5 minutes. Fentanyl transdermal patch: Peak serum levels are reached within 20-72 hours following application of the

patch. Steady-state levels are reached within 6 days (the end of 72 hours following the application of the second patch).

3. **Metabolism:** Metabolized primarily via human cytochrome P-450 3A4.
4. **Excretion:** Approximately 75% of the dose is excreted in urine within 72 hours of intravenous fentanyl administration, mostly as metabolites with <10% representing unchanged drug. Approximately 9% of the dose is excreted in the feces, primarily as metabolites.
5. **Dosing:** For chronic pain use in patients already on chronic opioids. Please consult a pain specialist for fentanyl patient controlled analgesia, transdermal, or mucosal use.
6. **Special considerations:** As elderly, cachectic, or debilitated patients may have altered pharmacokinetics due to poor fat stores, muscle wasting, or altered clearance; the fentanyl patch is often a poor choice given the unpredictability of the medication.

D. Hydrocodone

1. **Routes of administration:** Oral, rectal.
2. **Peak effect:** 30-60 minutes.
3. **Metabolism:** CYP3A4-mediated *N*-demethylation to norhydrocodone. Watch use with CYP inducers and inhibitors.
4. **Excretion:** Hydrocodone and its metabolites are primarily excreted via the kidneys.
5. **Dosing (adult):** 5-10 mg po q4-6h prn.
6. **Special considerations:** Do not exceed 3000 mg/d of acetaminophen in formulations containing acetaminophen.

E. Hydromorphone

1. **Formulations:** Oral, intravenous, intramuscular, subcutaneous, intranasal, rectal, sublingual, transmucosal, buccal, epidural.
2. **Onset of analgesia:** Intravenous, 5 minutes.
3. **Maximum analgesia effect:**
4. **Intravenous:** Maximum analgesia effect 10-20 minutes.
5. **Oral immediate-release:** 1.5 hours.
6. **Oral long-acting:** 9 hours.
7. **Metabolism:** Hydromorphone is metabolized via glucuronidation in the liver, with >95% of the dose metabolized to hydromorphone-3-glucuronide along with minor amounts of 6-hydroxy reduction metabolites.
8. **Excretion:** Most of the dose of hydromorphone is excreted as hydromorphone-3-glucuronide along with minor amounts of 6-hydroxy reduction metabolites.
9. **Dosing (adult):** Hydromorphone immediate-release 2 mg po q4h prn.
10. **Special considerations:** The mean exposure to hydromorphone (Cmax and AUC) is increased fourfold in patients with moderate (Child-Pugh Group B) hepatic impairment. Patients with moderate hepatic impairment should be started at lower doses and closely monitored. Severe hepatic failure has not been studied.
11. Mean exposure to hydromorphone (Cmax and AUC) is increased in patients with impaired renal function by twofold, in moderate (CLcr = 40-60 mL/min) renal impairment and threefold in severe (CLcr < 30 mL/min) renal impairment. During dose titration, patients with renal dysfunction should be started at lower doses and closely monitored.

F. Morphine

1. **Formulations:** Intravenous, buccal, oral, subcutaneous, intramuscular, rectal, epidural, intrathecal.

2. **Peak effect:** Intravenous, 3-5 minutes; oral, 80% of peak effect in 20 minutes but peak effect around 90 minutes.
3. **Metabolism:** Almost all morphine is converted by hepatic metabolism to the 3- and 6-glucuronide metabolites (M3G and M6G; 50% and 15%, respectively). M6G has analgesic activity but crosses the blood-brain barrier poorly. M3G has no significant analgesic activity.
4. **Excretion:** Almost all morphine is excreted in urine as M3G and M6G. A small amount is excreted in bile and the feces.
5. **Dosing (adult):** Oral: Morphine immediate-release 15-30 mg po q4h prn.

G. Oxycodone

1. **Formulations:** Oral, sublingual, transdermal.
2. **Analgesic onset (immediate-release):** 20-30 minutes.
3. **Peak effect (immediate-release):** 1-1.5 hours.
4. **Metabolism:** The primary metabolic pathway of oxycodone CYP3A-mediated *N*-demethylation to noroxycodone. Therefore, metabolism can be affected by CYP inducers and inhibitors.
5. **Excretion:** Oxycodone and its metabolites are excreted primarily via the kidney.
6. **Dosing (adult):** Oxycodone immediate-release 5 mg po q4-6h prn.
7. **Special considerations:** Rifampin, St. John's wort, and carbamazepine are inducers of cytochrome P-450. In combination with oxycodone, these mediations may lead to subtherapeutic doses of oxycodone and poor pain control as a result.

H. Methadone

1. **Formulations:** Oral, intravenous, sublingual, rectal.
2. **Analgesic onset (oral):** 0.5-1 hours.
3. **Peak effect (oral):** 1.5-7.5 hours.
4. **Receptors:** Beyond the μ receptor, methadone acts as an antagonist to the NMDA receptor.
5. **Metabolism:** Methadone is primarily metabolized through cytochrome P-450 enzymes.
6. **Excretion:** Methadone is eliminated by extensive biotransformation, followed by renal and fecal excretion.
7. **Dosing:** Consult pain specialist.
8. **Special considerations**
   a. The long half-life of methadone increases the risk of respiratory depression. Methadone therapy should only be initiated in consultation with a clinician with experience in chronic methadone therapy.
   b. Check a QTc prior to initiation of therapy and prior to dose increases. QTc values >460-480 ms have been used to define long QTc intervals, but this is also within the range of normal values. QTc > 500 ms are abnormal and is a known risk for development of torsade de pointe. Female sex, methadone dosage, concomitant use of cytochrome P-450 3A4 inhibitors, hypokalemia, and impaired liver function contribute to QT prolongation.

I. Tramadol

1. **Formulations:** Oral.
2. **Peak plasma concentration:** 1.6-1.9 hours.
3. **Receptors:** The μ opioid receptors account for 40% of the analgesia of tramadol, while serotonergic (20%) and noradrenergic (40%) account for the remainder.

4. **Metabolism:** Tramadol and its active metabolite (M1) have metabolic and renal elimination. The terminal half-life may be prolonged in hepatic or renal function disorders. The prolongation of the elimination half-life is relatively slight, as long as one of the two excretion organs is virtually intact. In patients with severe liver cirrhosis, the elimination half-life of tramadol was extended to a mean of about 13 hours; extreme values reached up to 22 hours.
5. **Excretion:** Mainly excreted via the kidneys (~90%) with the remainder excreted in the feces.
6. **Dosing (adult):** Tramadol immediate-release 25-50 mg po q4h prn. Not to exceed 400 mg/d. Do not exceed 200 mg/d if CrCl < 30.
7. **Special considerations:** The seizure risk with tramadol is <1%. The risk is highest among those aged 25-54 years, those with more than four tramadol prescriptions, and those with history of alcohol abuse, stroke, or head injury. Serotonin syndrome is another potential risk.

VIII. DIALYSIS-DEPENDENT PATIENTS

Pain management in dialysis-dependent patients can be a challenge given accumulation of metabolites between dialysis sessions and reduction in therapeutic levels during dialysis runs (Table 11.3).

IX. SIDE EFFECTS

Opioid side effects can be divided into peripheral and central effects. Peripheral effects include constipation, urinary retention, hives, and bronchospasm. Central effects include nausea, sedation, respiratory depression, hypotension, miosis, and cough suppression.

A. Endocrine Effects

The endocrine effects of opioids have demonstrated reduced release of gonadotropin-releasing hormone. As a result, testosterone levels have been demonstrated to be reduced in males. In males, reduced sex hormones may present with impotence and decreased muscle mass. Females may experience hot flashes and irregular menstrual cycles. Both sexes may experience infertility, decreased sexual function, loss of muscle mass, and anxiety and/or depression. In those taking chronic opioids, osteoporosis has been noted with increased risk of fractures.

B. Falls Risks

Opioids may increase the risk of falls which has been demonstrated in the elderly and the young. Fractures and falls appear to be more likely to occur immediately following the initial prescription of an opioid and decrease over time.

X. FUTURE OF OPIOIDS

The future of opioids include:

1. Determination of the efficacy of opioid therapy for acute and chronic, noncancer pain
2. Determination of the pain indications and optimal duration of opioid therapy
3. The creation of novel opioids that produce analgesia that minimize undesirable effects including euphoria (μ receptor), dysphoria (κ receptor), sedation, and respiratory depression

TABLE 11.3 Common Opioids and Dialysis

Drug	Dialysis	Metabolites	Comments
Morphine	Both morphine and metabolites can be removed by dialysis. Extra dosing may be needed during or after dialysis	Metabolites accumulate in between dialysis sessions	Morphine is best avoided in dialysis patients as better alternatives exist
Hydromorphone	Drug is partly removed by dialysis, but there are no data concerning dialysis of the metabolites	Metabolite accumulation is a risk	Used without adverse effects in dialysis patients. Careful use and monitor the patient
Oxycodone	Limited dialyzability of oxycodone and noroxycodone. Mean reduction in oxycodone and noroxycodone arterial concentrations was significant and higher with online hemodiafiltration than with standard hemodialysis	Limited dialyzability of noroxycodone. No oxymorphone or noroxymorphone metabolites detected at any time point	Insignificant postdialysis increase in pain. Use of oxycodone in dialysis patients is best avoided until there is further data
Codeine			Do not use. Metabolites accumulate in renal failure, and serious adverse effects have been reported in dialysis patients
Methadone	No dose adjustments are required in dialysis patients	The metabolites are inactive, and it is not dialyzed	The usual precautions taken when prescribing methadone should still be observed
Fentanyl	Fentanyl is not dialyzed, so in most cases, no dose adjustments have to be made for dialysis patients. Fentanyl may adsorb onto one filter type in which case changing the filter is recommended, but if that is not possible, changing to methadone is recommended	The metabolites are inactive	Appears safe over short periods. Fentanyl may accumulate in renal failure, but the clinical significance of this is not known

Tramadol	Dialysis appears not to have a significant effect on tramadol concentrations	Total amount of tramadol and M1 removed during a 4-hour dialysis period was <7% of the administered dose

Morphine Milligram Equivalent (MME) Conversion Factors[a]

Drug	Intravenous	Oral
Morphine[b]	3	1
Codeine	–	0.15
Hydrocodone	–	1
Hydromorphone[c]	20	4
Fentanyl (in mcg/hr)	2.4[a]	2.4
Methadone	Consult pain specialist	Consult pain specialist
Oxycodone[d]	–	1.5
Tapentadol	–	0.4
Tramadol[e]	–	0.25

[a]Caution: This conversion chart should not be used to determine doses when converting a patient from one opioid to another. This is especially important for fentanyl and methadone.
[b]Morphine 10 mg intravenous is equivalent to 30 mg oral MME. (Equation: morphine 10 mg IV × 3 conversion factor = 30 mg oral morphine mg equivalents.)
[c]Hydromorphone 8 mg oral is equivalent to 32 oral MME. (Equation: hydromorphone 8 mg oral × 4 conversion factor = 32 mg oral morphine mg equivalents.)
[d]Oxycodone 10 mg is equivalent to 15 oral MME. (Equation: oxycodone 10 mg oral × 1.5 conversion factor = 15 mg oral morphine mg equivalents.)
[e]Tramadol 50 mg oral is equivalent to 12.5 oral MME. (Equation: tramadol 50 mg oral × 0.25 conversion factor = 12.5 mg oral morphine mg equivalents.)
Data from Dean M. Opioids in renal failure and dialysis patients. *J Pain Symptom Manage.* 2004;28(5):497-504; and Samolsky Dekel BG, Donati G, et al. Dialyzability of oxycodone and its metabolites in chronic noncancer pain patients with end-stage renal disease. *Pain Pract.* 2017;17(5):604-615.

Selected Readings

Dowell D, Haegerich TM, Chou R. CDC guideline for prescribing opioids for chronic pain—United States, 2016. *MMWR Recomm Rep.* 2016;65(RR-1):1-49.

Frieden TR, Houry D. Reducing the risks of relief—the CDC opioid-prescribing guideline. *N Engl J Med.* 2016;374:1501-1504

Miller M, Stürmer T, Azrael D, Levin R, Solomon DH. Opioid analgesics and the risk of fractures among older adults with arthritis. *J Am Geriatr Soc.* 2011;59(3):430-438.

Roden DM. Predicting drug-induced QT prolongation and torsades de pointes. *J Physiol.* 2016;594(9):2459-2468.

Seyfried O, Hester J. Opioids and endocrine dysfunction. *Br J Pain.* 2012;6(1):17-24.

Shah A, Hayes CJ, Martin BC. Characteristics of initial prescription episodes and likelihood of long-term opioid use—United States, 2006–2015. *MMWR Morb Mortal Wkly Rep.* 2017;66(10):265-269.

Söderberg KC, Laflamme L, Möller J. Newly initiated opioid treatment and the risk of fall-related injuries. A nationwide, register-based, case-crossover study in Sweden. *CNS Drugs.* 2013;27(2):155-161.

12 Nonsteroidal Anti-inflammatory Medications

Dermot P. Maher

"Nonsteroidal anti-inflammatory drugs" (NSAIDs) is a general term representing a variety of chemically distinct medications that all possess analgesic, anti-inflammatory, and antipyretic properties. Additionally, acetaminophen, which is not a typical NSAID as it is centrally acting and has only weak anti-inflammatory properties, has analgesic and antipyretic properties that make it appropriate to discuss in this context. NSAIDs are the most widely used analgesics, both in the United States and worldwide, due to their diverse clinical applications, opioid-sparing effects, familiarity of use, and ease of access to most patients. NSAIDs differ from opioid analgesics in that (1) NSAIDs have an agent-specific maximal efficacious dose, sometimes called a "ceiling dose," beyond which no added analgesia is observed but adverse side effects continue, (2) there is a lack of either psychological or physical dependence, and (3) NSAIDs have potent antipyretic and anti-inflammatory effects. NSAIDs may be used for either acute or chronic pain and administered either locally (topical preparations) or systemically, either alone or as a coanalgesic to a centrally acting medication. NSAIDs have been demonstrated in numerous clinical trials to be effective for the treatment of a range of rheumatologic diseases, seronegative spondyloarthropathies, osteoarthritis, postoperative pain, low back and musculoskeletal pain, and also gout.

I. MECHANISM OF ACTION

NSAIDs exert pharmacological action through the inhibition of the cyclooxygenase (COX) enzyme through either reversible or irreversible binding. COX is a membrane-bound hemoprotein and glycoprotein homodimer that enzymatically cyclizes 20-carbon polyunsaturated fatty acids (arachidonic acid and eicosatrienoic acid) to produce prostaglandin E2 (PGE_2), thromboxane A2 (TXA_2), and prostacyclin (PGI_2) and other prostaglandins (PGs), which are then further processed (Fig. 12.1). Individual PGs produce varied physiological effects through paracrine signaling (Table 12.1). Receptors for individual PGs have been cloned.

COX exists as two isoforms encoded on separate chromosomes that share 60% sequence homology. However, COX-1 is constitutively expressed especially in the renal parenchyma, in the gastric mucosa, and on platelets and is only marginally up-regulated in response to inflammation. In contrast, COX-2

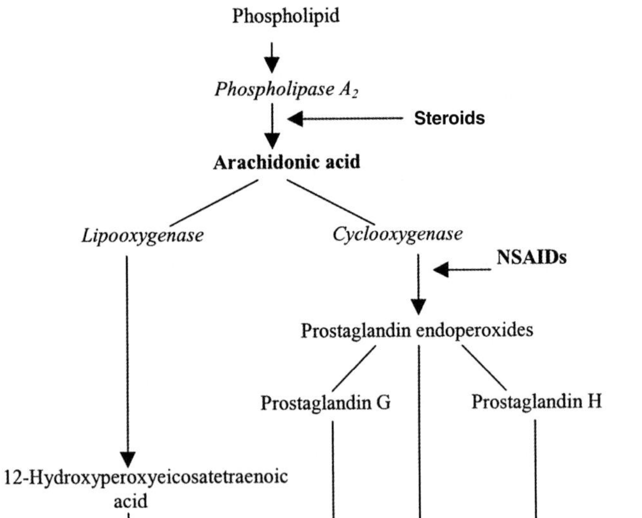

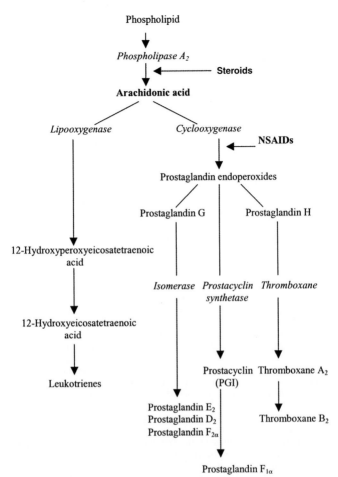

FIGURE 12.1 A schematic diagram showing the metabolism of phospholipid and arachidonic acid. Nonsteroidal anti-inflammatory drugs (NSAIDs) inhibit cyclooxygenase and thereby suppress the synthesis of prostaglandin E, prostacyclin, and thromboxane and alter the balance between these eicosanoids and the leukotrienes.

is inducible and expressed in tissue where local tissue trauma and inflammation have occurred and may be involved in oncogenic processes, such as cellular survival and angiogenesis. COX-2 is also constitutively expressed in some tissues, such as the kidney and CNS. PGs produced by COX-1 are generally responsible for a wide range of homeostatic processes. However, in response to increased levels of the inflammatory mediator IL-1β and NF-κB signaling, COX-2 is up-regulated and produces PGE_2, which sensitizes peripheral afferent nerve endings to the nociceptive actions of bradykinin, substance P, histamine, and other pain mediators inducing a state of hyperalgesia. In the CNS, IL-1β and NF-κB signaling also up-regulate COX-2 and PGE_2, but the response is not due to

TABLE 12.1 Prostaglandin and Thromboxane Actions

- Fever vascular smooth muscle relaxation (predominant action) (PGI_1 and PGE) and contraction (PGI_1 and TXA)
- Increased capillary permeability (LTB)
- Uterine smooth muscle contraction (PGE and PGI_2)
- Bronchial smooth muscle relaxation (PGE) and contraction (PGI_2 TXA, LTC, LTD)
- Increased GI contraction and motility (PGI_1 and PGI)
- Protection of GI tract by inhibiting gastric acid secretion and enhancing gastric mucous secretion (PGI_1 and PGI)
- Regulation of renal blood flow and sodium/potassium exchange (PGI_1 and PGI)
- Marked potentiation of the effects of other mediators of inflammation and pain (serotonin, bradykinin, and histamine) (PGI_1 and PGI)
- Sensitization of nociceptors (PGI_1 and PGI)
- Inhibition of platelet aggregation (PGI)
- Increased platelet aggregation (TXA)
- Constriction of vascular smooth muscle (TXA)

PGI, prostacyclin; PGE, prostaglandin E; PGF, prostaglandin F; TXA, thromboxane A; LTB, leukotriene B; LTC, leukotriene C; LTD, leukotriene D.

afferent neuron signaling or elevated systemic concentrations of IL-1β. Regional anesthesia will not block the CNS inflammatory effects. The result of CNS up-regulation of COX-2 is central hyperesthesia and sensitization.

II. PHARMACOKINETICS

As a class, NSAIDs are well-absorbed following oral administration and have a low first-pass hepatic extraction ratio. Peak plasma concentrations are generally reached within 2-3 hours. Analgesic efficacy is thought to be more dependent on the extent of absorption rather than the rate. Any factor that affects gastric emptying will greatly alter the time to peak plasma level. Topical absorption of NSAIDs has also resulted in the commercial development of three preparations; diclofenac gel (Voltaren, Pennsaid) and diclofenac epolamine patches 1.3% (Flector Patches) are available in the United States with other medications available in other countries. As NSAIDs are very weak acids with pK_a's usually between 3.5 and 5, these medications will preferentially concentrate in inflamed superficial tissue, such as inflamed and/or arthritic synovial joint capsules. Intravenous NSAID preparations are also currently available in the United States: ketorolac (Toradol), ibuprofen (Caldolor), and diclofenac (Dyloject).

The majority of NSAIDs are present in their ionized form and highly bound to plasma proteins, such as albumin. This results in volumes of distributions or between 0.1 and 0.3 L/kg, which approximates the plasma volume. The high degree of protein binding makes them susceptible to displacement and consequent alteration of the kinetics of other highly protein-bound medications, such as Coumadin. Decreased protein binding due to renal failure or hypoalbuminemia may increase the volume of distribution of the unbound fraction of the medication. More lipid-soluble members of the class may be able to exert more COX inhibition at the CNS due to their ability to traverse the blood-brain barrier.

NSAIDs undergo significant metabolism by oxidation, and glucuronidation catalyzed hepatic cytochromes with only minor excretion in the urine as unchanged drug. Renal failure will result in an increase in the unbound fraction of a medication resulting in increased renal clearance. NSAID medications that are metabolized to form acyl glucuronides (ketoprofen, naproxen, indoprofen) will accumulate rapidly in the setting of renal failure. Hemodialysis will not eliminate NSAIDs, and no dosage adjustment is required for patients undergoing hemodialysis although administration to such patients must be performed with caution. NSAID hepatic metabolism is not dependent on blood flow. ASA is rapidly metabolized in the liver to salicylic acid and then conjugated with glycine to form salicyluric acid, the urinary excretion of which is highly dependent on urinary pH, ranging from 85% with alkaline urine to <5% with highly acidic urine.

III. ADVERSE EFFECTS

Unfortunately, the NSAIDs are not free of bothersome, and sometimes serious, adverse effects (see Table 12.2). NSAIDs share adverse side effect profiles as a class though there are differences between agents.

A. Gastrointestinal Side Effects

Gastrointestinal toxicity associated with NSAID therapy, including gastritis, nausea, vomiting, diarrhea, and gastric ulceration, represents the most common adverse effects related to use of these medications. Approximately 50% of subjects chronically utilizing NSAIDs demonstrated some degree of gastric mucosal dysfunction. Symptomatic ulcers and ulcer complications associated with the use of standard NSAIDs may occur in 1% of patients treated for 3-6 months and in 2%-4% of patients treated for 1 year. Eighty percent of patients with GI toxicity have no preceding symptoms, and most have few or no risk factors. The incidence of upper GI ulcers is decreased by ~50% with the use of selective COX-2 inhibitors but remains above the background incidence of the non-NSAID using population. COX-1 is normally found in the gastric mucosa and maintains mucosal integrity through increased mucosal blood flow, epithelial cell growth, stimulation of the section of mucus, and bicarbonate. The use of nonselective NSAIDs is thought to cause gastric irritation through disruption of the protective mucosal barrier. NSAIDs do not directly cause lower esophageal dysfunction but may cause esophagitis due to a decrease in stomach pH. Risk factors for the development of NSAID-associated gastric adverse drug reactions include advanced age, prolonged use, use of high doses or multiple NSAIDs, alcohol use, smoking, concurrent steroid use, and a history of GI pathology such as ulcers of *Helicobacter pylori* infection.

Management of NSAID-induced gastritis may be achieved through the use of an H_2-antagonist such as ranitidine 150 mg twice daily, a synthetic

TABLE 12.2 Principal Adverse Effects of Long-term NSAID Therapy

- Dyspepsia, peptic ulcer disease
- Diarrhea, gastrointestinal hemorrhage
- Renal dysfunction and failure—acute papillary necrosis, chronic interstitial nephritis, decreased renal blood flow, decreased glomerular filtration rate, salt and water retention
- Inhibition of platelet aggregation; increased bleeding time
- Altered liver function tests, jaundice
- Drug interactions
- Impaired cartilage repair in osteoarthritis

PGE_1 analog such as misoprostol 200 mg four times daily, a proton pump inhibitor such as omeprazole 40 mg daily or sucralfate 1 g at night. The use of gastroprotective medications are not thought to decrease the analgesic efficacy of NSAID therapy. However, the choice of gastroprotective therapy should be individually tailored to the patient in order to prevent further drug-related adverse events. The use of enteric-coated NSAIDs does not consistently reduce the incidence of gastritis. NSAIDs should be used cautiously in patients with a history of ulcerative colitis or other inflammatory bowel diseases.

B. Cardiovascular Side Effects

The risk of experiencing a thrombotic episode or a myocardial infarction is elevated in individuals utilizing chronic NSID therapy. Although first described in COX-2-specific NSAIDs, the relative risk of NSAID-associated cardiovascular events appears to be highest with rofecoxib but is present for all NSAIDs compared to placebo. Subsequent studies demonstrated that celecoxib use is not associated with an increased risk of a cardiovascular event compared to other NSAIDs. The risk of hemorrhagic stroke, congestive heart failure, and cardiovascular death is also increased compared to placebo.

COX-2 in nucleated vascular endothelial cells catalyzes the production of prostacyclin (PGI_2), which functions as an anticoagulant preventing platelet activation under noninjured circumstances. COX-1 in nonnucleated platelets catalyzes the production of thromboxane (TXA_2), which is a potent vasoconstrictor, platelet stimulator and augments platelet aggregation. Platelets do not express COX-2. PGI_2 and TXA_2 work in concert to homeostatic anticoagulation state. The inhibition of COX-2 in nucleated cells will inhibit the production of PGI_2 while not affecting the production of TXA_2 in platelets causing a procoagulant state. This has been demonstrated to also lead to an increase in blood pressure, accelerate atherogenesis, and lead to an exaggerated response to rupture of an atherosclerotic plaque. This may explain the increase in severe cardiovascular events associated with diclofenac. Further, this has been exploited in the use of low-dose aspirin, which irreversibly binds to COX-1 and COX-2 in both platelets and endothelial cells. The platelets lack the capacity to synthesize new COX enzymes, while nucleated vascular endothelial cells can. The result is a relative increase in PGI_2 compared to TXA_2, which is thought to account for the cardioprotective effects of aspirin 81 mg. It should be noted that, as a class of medications, NSAIDs will cause fluid retention and modest hypertension (2-4 mm Hg), which potentially also contributes their increased risk of major cardiovascular events.

C. Hematologic Side Effects

Bleeding time is consistently prolonged in individuals undergoing long-term treatment with standard NSAIDs, but the consensus is that such prolongation is not excessive and that values remain below the upper limits of normal. The duration of elimination is related to the elimination half-life of the individual NSAID. Aspirin binds irreversibly to COX in platelets resulting in inhibition for the remaining lifespan of the platelet. Meta-analysis failed to demonstrate a meaningful increase in surgical bleeding in children using perioperative NSAID therapy undergoing tonsillectomies. However, intraoperative administration of NSAIDs, such as ketorolac, to subjects is not associated with an increase in surgical site bleeding but is associated with a small increase in GI ulcers. It is likely that the previously reported high incidence of GI hemorrhage associated with ketorolac was a function of the excessively high doses used before the manufacturers recommended a lower dose. COX-2 inhibitors do not appear to affect platelet aggregation, bleeding time, or postoperative blood loss.

D. Renal and Hepatic Side Effects

Nonselective COX inhibition by NSAIDs administration causes a decrease in the glomerular filtration rate and results in the release of renin from the juxtaglomerular cells, leading to further reduction in renal blood flow and a disturbance of renal function. Sodium and water retention, hyperkalemia, hypertension, papillary necrosis, and nephrotic syndrome are other possible consequences of the renal disturbance. Analgesic nephropathy caused by NSAIDs will usually resolve over several weeks with discontinuation. However, in certain cases, the renal side effects may result in fulminant renal failure, due to renal medullary ischemia. COX-2 inhibitors do not prevent the development of analgesic nephropathy. Elderly patients; patients with chronic renal dysfunction, dehydration, prolonged or high dose NSAID use, congestive heart failure, ascites, or hypovolemia; and patients treated with nephrotoxic drugs such as the aminoglycosides and vancomycin are at particular risk. The administration of preoperative ketorolac to otherwise healthy patients does not result in glomerular or tubular dysfunction.

The use of aspirin has been associated with transient and non–dose-dependent hepatic dysfunction.

E. Miscellaneous Side Effects

NSAIDs adversely affect the healing of bone in some studies using animal models while having no effect in other animal studies. While interesting, evidence from human studies has not substantiated this claim at this point.

NSAIDs may also cause a spontaneous degranulation of granulocytes in the skin and respiratory tract resulting in urticarial and bronchoconstriction. Although the etiology is thought to be due to a viral infection, Reye syndrome is often associated with the use of aspirin in pediatric populations.

Aspirin and other NSAIDs are not teratogenic at regular doses. However, NSAIDs are associated with a narrowing of the ductus arteriosus, possibly with gastroschisis and a decrease in fetal production of amniotic fluid. Additionally, the use of NSAIDs proximal to the time of delivery is associated with an increase in neonatal intracranial hemorrhage, and women are recommended against NSAID use during the third trimester. Aspirin and other NSAIDs are a class D medication in the third trimester and class C in the first two trimesters. Acetaminophen is class B throughout pregnancy. NSAIDs and acetaminophen are generally considered safe while nursing.

IV. SPECIFIC MEDICATIONS

A number of chemically and pharmacologically unique NSAIDs have been developed for a variety of clinical uses. The choice of a particular medication depends largely on the dosing schedule, cost, and history of NSAID use. It is well described that there is poorly understood variability across the population with regard to an individual's derived analgesic benefit. Often, in the setting of a patient who is not deriving acceptable analgesia from one NSAID, rotation to another may provide more adequate analgesia. Analgesia derived from NSAIDs for the treatment of arthritic joints is directly related to the amount of albumin and, consequently NSAID medication, in the joint. Table 12.3 describes the most widely clinically utilized NSAIDs.

TABLE 12.3 Survey of Commonly Utilized NSAIDs

Generic Medication Name	Half-Life (h)	Usual Adult Dose and Frequency	Comments
Aspirin	2-3	325-650 mg qid po	May cause severe GI side effects and platelet dysfunction Pharmacologic half-life is 7 d
Naproxen	14	250-500 mg bid po	
Ibuprofen	6 po or 2 IV	200-800 mg qid po or 400-800 mg IV qid	
Ketoprofen	2	50-75 mg tid	
Diclofenac	1 po or 12 h for 1% gel or 1.3% patch	50-75 mg bid-qid po or 2-4 g qid gel or 180 mg patch	Transdermal preparations have ~6% systemic absorption
Etodolac	7	200-300 mg bid-qid	
Indomethacin	4	25-75 mg bid po	Severe GI side effects
Sulindac	7 Parent drug 16 Active metabolite	150-200 mg bid po	Prodrug, excreted in bile, possibly reduced nephrotoxicity
Ketorolac	5	15-30 mg qid IV or IM	Bleeding time increased with spinal anesthesia but not general. May be used for 5 d
Nabumetone	20-24	500-750 mg bid	Prodrug
Meloxicam	15-20	7.5-15 mg daily	Lower dose is more selective for COX-2
Celecoxib	6-12	100-200 mg qd-bid	Increased risk of major cardiovascular event
Acetaminophen	2-3	325-1000 mg qid	

A. Acetaminophen

Acetaminophen or *N*-acetyl-*p*-aminophenol (APAP) is indicated for noninflammatory pain and for fever control. Despite very potent antipyretic and mild analgesic effects, it lacks significant peripheral anti-inflammatory properties. The mechanism of action of APAP is related to its ability to inhibit COX and decrease PGE_2 in the CNS but not in the periphery. Additionally, analgesic mechanism of action may involve the serotonergic system effects on the descending inhibitory pain pathways and possibly the cannabinoid system. Doses of 650 mg provide greater analgesia than doses of 325 mg, but no extra analgesia is observed with doses >1000 mg. This could indicate that 1000 mg is the maximal efficacious dose. APAP is frequently combined with opioids to exploit its opioid-sparing effect.

APAP has near complete gastric absorption and a peak serum concentration 30 minutes to 1 hour after oral consumption. IV and rectal formulations are also available and demonstrate similar kinetics. It is minimally protein bound, has a volume of distribution of 0.95 L/kg, and has a half-life of 2-3 hours. It is metabolized in the liver by glucuronidation and sulfation to mostly inert products with ~4% converted to the nephro- and hepatotoxic metabolite *N*-acetyl-*p*-benzoquinoneimine (NAPQI). Under normal circumstances, this is scavenged and neutralized by binding to glutathione. However, with cytochrome induction or glutathione depletion, both of which may be seen with chronic ethanol consumption, NAPQI serum concentrations may rise to toxic levels. Patients who consume more than three drinks per day are advised to avoid chronic APAP use. Liver function tests are mildly increased after 10 days of use in subjects who consume moderate amounts of alcohol and, to a lesser extent, in patients receiving <4 g/day.

APAP has not been demonstrated to affect platelet function or induce chronic analgesia nephropathy at clinically relevant doses. Hepatotoxiticity due to necrosis may occur after short-term administration of large doses (>10 g) or long-term use of APAP at lower doses (<4 g), especially in alcoholics. However, APAP may still be used in alcoholics at recommended doses and may be preferable to other NSAIDs due to a lack of platelet inhibitory effects, gastrointestinal irritation, and nephropathy. Despite a lack of platelet function alterations, APAP may cause severe rises in the INR of subjects who are concurrently taking Coumadin. APAP will not antagonize the effects of uricosuric medications. Dose adjustment is generally not required for renal dysfunction, but the half-life may be doubled in the setting of hepatic dysfunction.

Selected Readings

Curiel RV, Katz JD. Mitigating the cardiovascular and renal effects of NSAIDs. *Pain Med.* 2013;14(suppl 1):S23-S28.

Higuchi K, Umegaki E, Watanabe T, et al. Present status and strategy of NSAIDs-induced small bowel injury. *J Gastroenterol.* 2009;44(9):879-888.

Hooper L, Brown TJ, Elliott R, Payne K, Roberts C, Symmons D. The effectiveness of five strategies for the prevention of gastrointestinal toxicity induced by non-steroidal anti-inflammatory drugs: systematic review. *BMJ.* 2004;329(7472):948.

Kowalski ML, Woessner K, Sanak M. Approaches to the diagnosis and management of patients with a history of nonsteroidal anti-inflammatory drug-related urticaria and angioedema. *J Allergy Clin Immunol.* 2015;136(2):245-251.

Kurmis AP, Kurmis TP, O'Brien JX, Dalen T. The effect of nonsteroidal anti-inflammatory drug administration on acute phase fracture-healing: a review. *J Bone Joint Surg Am.* 2012;94(9):815-823.

Lewis SR, Nicholson A, Cardwell ME, Siviter G, Smith AF. Nonsteroidal anti-inflammatory drugs and perioperative bleeding in paediatric tonsillectomy. *Cochrane Database Syst Rev.* 2013(7);CD003591.

Moore RA, Derry S, Phillips CJ, McQuay HJ. Nonsteroidal anti-inflammatory drugs (NSAIDs), cyxlooxygenase-2 selective inhibitors (coxibs) and gastrointestinal harm: review of clinical trials and clinical practice. *BMC Musculoskelet Disord.* 2006;7:79.

Nasrallah R, Hassouneh R, Hebert RL. PGE2, kidney disease, and cardiovascular risk: beyond hypertension and diabetes. *J Am Soc Nephrol.* 2016;27(3):666-676.

National Clinical Guideline Centre. National Institute for Health and Clinical Excellence: Guidance. *Myocardial Infarction with ST-Segment Elevation: The Acute Management of Myocardial Infarction with ST-Segment Elevation.* London, England: Royal College of Physicians (UK), National Clinical Guideline Centre; 2013.

Nissen SE, Yeomans ND, Solomon DH, et al. Cardiovascular safety of celecoxib, naproxen, or ibuprofen for arthritis. *N Engl J Med.* 2016;375(26):2519-2529.

O'Connor N, Dargan PI, Jones AL. Hepatocellular damage from non-steroidal anti-inflammatory drugs. *QJM.* 2003;96(11):787-791.

Pope JE, Anderson JJ, Felson DT. A meta-analysis of the effects of nonsteroidal anti-inflammatory drugs on blood pressure. *Arch Intern Med.* 1993;153(4):477-484.

Schafer AI. Effects of nonsteroidal antiinflammatory drugs on platelet function and systemic hemostasis. *J Clin Pharmacol.* 1995;35(3):209-219.

Schjerning Olsen AM, Fosbol EL, Lindhardsen J, et al. Duration of treatment with nonsteroidal anti-inflammatory drugs and impact on risk of death and recurrent myocardial infarction in patients with prior myocardial infarction: a nationwide cohort study. *Circulation.* 2011;123(20):2226-2235.

Trelle S, Reichenbach S, Wandel S, et al. Cardiovascular safety of non-steroidal anti-inflammatory drugs: network meta-analysis. *BMJ.* 2011;342:c7086.

Ungprasert P, Matteson EL, Thongprayoon C. Nonaspirin nonsteroidal anti-inflammatory drugs and risk of hemorrhagic stroke: a systematic review and meta-analysis of observational studies. *Stroke.* 2016;47(2):356-364.

Ungprasert P, Srivali N, Thongprayoon C. Nonsteroidal anti-inflammatory drugs and risk of incident heart failure: a systematic review and meta-analysis of observational studies. *Clin Cardiol.* 2016;39(2):111-118.

Wallace JL. Prostaglandins, NSAIDs, and gastric mucosal protection: why doesn't the stomach digest itself? *Physiol Rev.* 2008;88(4):1547-1565.

13 Psychopharmacology for the Pain Specialist

Gregory Acampora

Pain serves a protective signaling function. Like the autonomic system (central and peripheral), coagulation pathways, and immune system, the pain system is complex and employs numerous feedforward and feedback mechanisms to achieve a physiologically functional, purposeful, and protective balance (ie, homeostasis). When this advantageous balance is disturbed, these systems can become disruptive and dangerous to the host organism.

Chronic pain patients deal with a fundamental biological dilemma—they are unable to escape from a signal that indicates something is to be changed or avoided; the signal has lost usual duration limits. Thus, one can imagine how a chronic pain patient is trapped—unable to change or avoid their circumstance and ameliorate their physical and now psychological discomfort. The dilemma resides in the duality of frontal-cortical and limbic processes. In a simple model, frontal is executive/proactive (judgment, foresight, and planning); limbic is fundamental/reactive. We need both systems in order to **operate securely** on a daily basis. Much of our day is spent unconsciously engaged in **security operations**: we look both ways before crossing, we avoid suspicious or threatening things, and we stop at stop lights—we even dress for security. The limbic system is effectively our early warning (sensitivity) of threat, and the frontal lobes provide executive oversight (specificity) for what to do with that hazard. **When we are threatened, it interferes with our security, self-esteem, and ambitions.** Thus, chronic pain moves well beyond an acute phase safety response and interferes with the homeostasis of the mind and body. For clinicians treating pain, understanding this all-encompassing duality with chronic pain will lead to a more sophisticated, comprehensive, and empathic treatment approach.

Good command of pharmacologic principals by a pain practitioner cannot be overemphasized. Understanding pharmacokinetic/pharmacodynamic (PK/PD), Ki, P450 subtypes, multicompartment models, context sensitivity, receptor heterogeneity, side effects, and the physiology of age will result in medication management mastery. An important clinical caveat in prescribing any medication is to **be careful** to avoid confounding what you want the medication to do and what the medication does in totality.

This chapter will address psychoactive medications that may be used concomitantly in those who present for pain management (opioids and nonopioid analgesics are addressed in other chapters). For the purposes of this chapter, think of psychoactive medications as falling into five main categories: (1) antidepressants, (2) mood stabilizers, (3) anxiolytics, (4) antipsychotics, and (5) psychostimulants. In broad terms, the first two categories are relied upon for their analgesic effect to expand the complement of nonopioid pharmacologic pain management. The others may be used with mood management as the goal with the expectation that a better mood will result in better response to pain. Put simply, pain affects mood and mood affects pain.

I. ANTIDEPRESSANTS

Absent opioid and nonsteroidal anti-inflammatory drugs (NSAID), the antidepressant class of psychoactive medications, are the medications most often utilized to treat chronic pain. The application of this medication group represents a confluence of separate but simultaneous actions. As mentioned in the introduction, mood affects pain, and pain affects mood. Through serendipitous observations in the 1950s of mood improvement when patients were treated with antituberculosis medications, attention was turned towards monoamine neurotransmitters (DA, NE 5-HT) as the putative mediators of mood. Unexpected reports of the analgesic effect of these monoamine-based agents were thought due to improvement in demeanor and improved general functions (appetite, sleep architecture, and motivation), but modern understanding of pain mechanisms reveals monoamines are implicated in descending spinal control pathways. Supraspinal circuits include the Central Autonomic Network (CAN) and strike system, which is composed of hypothalamic and parahypothalamic structures representing intracerebral circuits that influence afferent and efferent pathways to the periphery. Nociceptive pathways run parallel to this amine-mediated system and may well interact in visceral and autonomic responses. Thus, the amine active antidepressant class of drugs has been found directly and indirectly effective in the overall treatment of the chronic pain patient.

A. Tricyclic Antidepressants

1. Indications

Tricyclic antidepressants (TCAs) were developed in the 1950s and 1960s for the treatment of major depressive disorders as well as comorbid depression in other disorders. TCAs are considered to have independent analgesic effects in the treatment of chronic pain of a variety of etiologies including neuropathic and visceral. TCAs have a variety of side effects, some of which can be helpful (sedation as prohypnotic), while others (dry mouth and poor visual focus) must be evaluated as part of a risk/benefit decision for prescribing.

2. Mechanisms

TCAs inhibit both serotonin (5-HT, 5-hydroxytryptamine) and norepinephrine (NE) reuptake to varying degrees. Like all medications, they inhibit numerous receptors leading to their ultimate pharmacological profile. In pain management, the secondary-amine TCA nortriptyline and tertiary-amine TCA amitriptyline or imipramine have shown comparable analgesic efficacy. The time to onset of TCA analgesia varies between days and months supporting an old psychiatric adage of "wait, wait, wait" (if possible) for desired effect as well as for side effects to diminish.

Table 13.1 illustrates receptor $K_{d\ (dissociation)}$ activity complexity; it serves as a template demonstrating the complexity of any drug and its receptor interactions.

3. Adverse Effects

TCAs interact with many neuroreceptor types and subtypes (above) and, as a result, have wide side effect profiles that are dose dependent. Low $K_{d\ (dissociation)}$ at a specific receptor implies a low concentration of drug can sufficiently activate that receptor while insufficiently activating other receptors. Common TCA side effects include anticholinergic (constipation, dry mouth, altered visual accommodation), α_1 (orthostasis, weight gain), and histamine H_1 (sedation) side effects (Table 13.1). Caution is advised in patients with acute-angle glaucoma. TCAs tend to affect PR interval more than QT and thus can worsen some forms of heart block. TCAs have a low therapeutic index (amount beneficial vs lethal dose) and so should be used in caution with patients at risk of self-harm. The low therapeutic index of TCAs is the reason that selective serotonin reuptake inhibitor (SSRI) and serotonin norepinephrine reuptake inhibitor (SNRIs) are often chosen as first-line antidepressants over TCAs. Opportunely, the doses used for analgesia are typically lower than those used for major depression.

TCAs can lead to decreased intestinal motility; this should be considered in patients taking opioids. The combination of anticholinergic and opioid effects on the gastrointestinal tract can increase risk of constipation or ileus.

4. Dosages and Monitoring

As a general principle, "start low and go slow" is a common psychiatry adage. Realizing there is often a sense of urgency in pain patients, dosing should still start at the low end of the dosage range and then be titrated upward until a therapeutic level is reached. This schedule will minimize side effects and patients will be less likely to reject the therapy (Table 13.2).

B. Selective Serotonin Reuptake Inhibitors

1. Indications

SSRIs (see Table 13.3) revolutionized first-line therapy for depression because of a balance of good response in combination with muted side effects in comparison to TCAs. The safety profile of these agents promoted application to a variety of psychiatric presentations including anxiety, depressive disorders, anxiety disorders (GAD, OCD, panic), bulimia nervosa, premenstrual dysphoric disorder (PMDD), chronic fatigue syndrome, and PTSD. SSRIs are often prescribed for patients with chronic pain given the relatively high incidence of anxiety, depression and PTSD

TABLE 13.1 The Measured Affinities [K_d (Nm)] of Selected TCAs at Different Receptors or Transporter Binding Sites[a]

Compound	SERT	NET	DAT	5-HT_{1A}	5-HT_{2A}	5-HT_{2C}	5-HT_6	5-HT_7	α_1	α_2	D_2	H_1	mACh
Amitriptyline	**3.13**	**22.4**	**4430**	**320**	**24**	**6.15**	**103.1**	**114**	**26**	**815**	**1,230**	**1.03**	**13.8**
Butriptyline	1360	5100	3940	7000	380	?	?	?	570	4800	?	1.1	35
Clomipramine	0.21	45.85	2605	>10 000	35.5	64.6	53.8	127	3.2	525	119.8	31	37
Desipramine	179	0.63	3190	>10 000	315	?	?	?	115	6350	1561	45.4	232.6
Dosulepin	8.6	46	5310	4004	258	?	?	?	470	2400	?	4	63.6
Doxepin	68	29.5	12 100	276	27	8.8	136	?	24	1185	1380	0.21	81.4
Imipramine	**1.6**	**51.67**	**8500**	**>10 000**	**118.67**	**120**	**190.3**	**1000**	**61**	**3150**	**1310**	**24**	**68**
Iprindole	1620	1262	6530	2800	217	206	?	?	2300	8600	?	130	2100
Lofepramine	70	5.4	18 000	4600	200	?	?	?	100	2700	2000	360	67
Nortriptyline	**16.5**	**1.65**	**5000**	**302**	**43**	**8.5**	**148**	**?**	**58**	**2265**	**1885**	**8.2**	**94**
Protriptyline	19.6	1.41	2100	3800	70	?	?	?	130	6600	2300	60	25
Trimipramine	149	2450	3780	8000	32	?	?	?	24	680	180	0.27	58

Amitriptyline, imipramine, and nortriptyline have relatively potent affinity for 5-HT and NE transporter, as well as α_1 and *ACh* receptors. The bolded values are the TCA's most commonly used in clinical practice for pain management.

[a]The smaller the numerical value, the greater the affinity.

TABLE 13.2 Tricyclic Antidepressants

Medication	Proprietary Name	Dosage Range (mg)	Anticholinergic Activity	Central Action	Hypotension	Sedation
Tertiary Amines						
Imipramine	***Tofranil***	**10-300**	**Moderate**	**N/S**	**Moderate**	**Moderate**
Amitriptyline	***Elavil***	**10-300**	**Strong**	**S(N)**	**Strong**	**Strong**
Clomipramine	*Anafranil*	25-300	Moderate	S(N)	Strong	Mild
Doxepin	*Sinequan*	10-300	Moderate	S	Strong	Mild
Secondary Amines						
Desipramine	*Norpramin*	10-300	Minimal	N	Mild	Minimal
Nortriptyline	***Pamelor***	**10-200**	**Mild**	**N/S**	**Moderate**	**Mild**

S, serotonergic; N, norepinephrinergic; (N), weakly norepinephrinergic.
The bolded values are the TCA's most commonly used in clinical practice for pain management.

TABLE 13.3 Selective Serotonin Reuptake Inhibitors

Medication	Proprietary Name	Dosage Range (mg/d)
Fluoxetine	*Prozac*	10-60
Sertraline	*Zoloft*	25-200
Citalopram	*Celexa*	10-60
Escitalopram	*Lexapro*	10-30
Fluvoxamine	*Luvox*	50-300

found in this patient population. Although SSRIs have not historically been considered effective as analgesic agents, recent review of studies suggests a need for further investigation of these useful agents directly for pain.

2. Mechanisms

SSRIs act upon the serotonin transporter inhibiting the reuptake of the monoamine into the presynaptic cell, increasing the level of serotonin in the synaptic cleft. Review of the literature is lacking for a mechanism or evidence of a strong direct analgesic effect, but a number of studies found that SSRIs provided clinically important subjective pain relief. When SSRIs were compared to TCAs and SNRI, the latter two agents were shown to be statistically superior vs placebo.

3. Adverse Reactions

Despite a preferable side effect profile compared to SNRIS and TCAs, SSRIs still cause some undesirable symptoms. Gastrointestinal effects include GI upset, an interesting consequence of the GI tract being home to the greatest percentage of serotonin receptors in the body. Possible CNS effects include activation or slowing and occipital headaches (described as "tightness"). Some patients taking an SSRI will experience sexual side effects of decreased libido, ejaculatory changes, and anorgasmia, so it is important to ask about these in the first visit post initiation. These symptoms are often dose related. Although consideration should be taken when mixing with other serotonergic given the possibility of causing serotonergic syndrome, low doses can be used in combination with SNRIs for targeted effect (see additive risk in the Conclusions).

4. Dosages and Monitoring

No initial laboratory workup is required. Dosage titration is usually based on clinical response and side effects. These are psychoactive medications, and several fMRI studies suggest imaging changes correlating to patient's response to target stimuli within minutes to hours. Anecdotally patients have reported reduced anxiety, impulsivity, reactivity, and/or ruminations within days, whereas the antidepressant effect (feeling better about things) usually takes 2-4 weeks. When discontinuing SSRIs, taper dosages slowly to avoid withdrawal symptoms—the exceptions are citalopram and fluoxetine that have very long half-lives.

C. Serotonin-NE Reuptake Inhibitors

1. Indications

Duloxetine (Cymbalta) was the first serotonergic agent approved by the FDA for the treatment of pain (ie, in 2004 for painful diabetic neuropathy).

It was later approved for fibromyalgia pain in 2008 and for chronic musculoskeletal pain in 2010. There is ample medical evidence for analgesic efficacy of duloxetine. Duloxetine has also proven successful in treatment of depression and anxiety variants. Milnacipran (Savella) was approved in 2009 by the FDA for use in fibromyalgia. Venlafaxine (Effexor) has been used as an antidepressant since 1994; while it does not carry any FDA indications for pain treatment, there are limited data supporting its analgesic efficacy.

2. Mechanisms

SNRIs interfere with transporter systems to selectively inhibit the reuptake of 5-HT and NE from the synaptic clefts. SNRIs have differing selectivity for 5-HT and NE. Whereas milnacipran blocks 5HT and NE reuptake with equal affinity, duloxetine has a 10-fold greater selectivity for 5HT, and venlafaxine has a 30-fold greater selectivity for 5-HT.

3. Adverse Reactions

SNRIs all share qualities of which clinicians should be aware. These drugs tend to be "activating," which means they can result in tremors and a sense of anxiety via the NE effects. They should be "tapered up"—clinically start with regular formulations and "walk up" to effective dose then convert to long-acting formulations. They all can result in hypertension, so blood pressure should be monitored longitudinally. They all can result in "discontinuation syndrome," again via NE receptors requiring approximately a 2-week slow washout. This should not be confused with serotonin syndrome (SS), which is a hypermetabolic state caused by serotonin excess. The presentation resembles and should be included with a differential diagnosis including anticholinergic toxicity, heat stroke, meningitis, neuroleptic malignant syndrome (NMS), and malignant hyperthermia. For this reason, SNRIs should be used judiciously with other serotonin agents including SSRI, MAOI, TCA, buspirone, amphetamines, meperidine, tramadol, dextromethorphan, triptans, metoclopramide, or ondansetron.

4. Dosages and Monitoring

Dosage titration is usually based on clinical response and side effects with the caveat that up taper should not be accelerated and BP should be monitored. If activation is experienced, the medication should be held at the last "comfortable dose" to see if symptoms improve. Anecdotally patients have reported good pain response with duloxetine yet report dysphoria (worsening mood); equally some patients describe mood benefit without analgesic response. When discontinuing SNRIs, taper dosages slowly to avoid discontinuation syndrome. Some psychiatrists administer a very low dose of fluoxetine (10 mg) during the down taper as a serotonin "buffer" (Table 13.4).

TABLE 13.4 Serotonin Norepinephrine Reuptake Inhibitors (SNRI)

Medication	Proprietary Name	Dosage Range (mg/d)
Duloxetine	*Cymbalta*	40-120
Venlafaxine	*Effexor*	37.5-375
Milnacipran	*Savella*	12.5-200

D. Atypical Antidepressants

1. Indications

The atypical antidepressants include the medications bupropion, mirtazapine, and trazodone and recently vortioxetine. Bupropion received some attention for neuropathic pain showing superiority at a level similar to TCA over placebo using the 300 XL formulation but not for back pain. Mirtazapine and trazodone have been shown to help response to pain subjectively through mood enhancement. Vortioxetine is touted for cognition.

2. Mechanisms

Bupropion is referred to as a NE-DA reuptake inhibitor (NDRI), although it is significantly more potent as a DRI and has historically been described as such. Notably, it displays action at the $\alpha_3\beta_4$ nicotinic receptor giving it tobacco abatement qualities. Bupropion is typically used as an antidepressant which enhances mood. Historically it was given as the alternative antidepressant when patients complained of sexual side effects from TCAs, SSRIs, or SNRIs. There is a new evidence that it increases "dopaminergic tonic activity" (see Psychostimulants in the section that follows), lending to its proposed application in ADHD.

Mirtazapine is a noradrenergic and specific serotonergic antidepressant (NaSSA) typically viewed as a central α_2 adrenergic antagonist. It has high binding affinity for the H_1 histaminic receptor and as such promotes sleep induction. The increased appetite is believed to be due to its effect on noradrenergic transmission.

Trazodone is a serotonin antagonist and reuptake inhibitor (SARI) originally intended as an antidepressant used at higher doses. It too has high affinity for the H_1 histaminic receptor and represents a safe and commonly prescribed sleep induction agent at lower doses.

Vortioxetine, a serotonin modulator and activator, has drawn attention because it may affect sodium channels (see antiepileptic drugs [AEDs] below) and has demonstrated improvement in cognition for patients with severe MDD.

3. Adverse Reactions

Bupropion is considered "activating" and can result in feeling uncomfortably fidgety; hence, the dose is tapered up, like the SNRIs, by using regular formulations and converting to higher-dose LA preparations after tolerability has been established. At doses >450 mg/day, bupropion lowers seizure threshold (increases risk). The most common complaint by patients is "anxiety and jitteriness."

Mirtazapine's most dramatic deleterious side effect is weight gain, which often is the reason for discontinuation by those who are not seeking strong appetite promotion; the orexigenic (ie, appetite stimulating) effect is dose related but can occur at 7.5 mg/day. Trazodone can cause priapism, usually at higher doses. The beneficial sedating effect for sleep promotion must be balanced against sense of morning grogginess the following day.

Vortioxetine was associated with nausea and dizziness; although these were not dramatic, the very long $t_{1/2}$ of 66 hours should give any clinician pause before prescribing.

4. Dosages and Monitoring

Bupropion should be tapered up using regular formulations and then can be replaced with SR or XL formulations. Avoid higher doses in patients with vulnerability for seizure. Mirtazapine at low doses promotes hypnotic effects. Trazodone has hypnotic effects at doses as low as 25 mg, and some patients report tachyphylaxis; overall it is viewed as a safe "sleep medicine" (Table 13.5).

TABLE 13.5 Atypical Antidepressants

Medication	Proprietary Name	Dosage Range (mg/d)
Bupropion	*Wellbutrin*	75-450
Mirtazapine	*Remeron*	7.5-45
Trazodone	*Desyrel*	25-600[a]
Vortioxetine	*Trintellix*	5-20

[a]Antidepressant dose.

II. ANTIEPILEPTIC AGENTS (ANTICONVULSANTS)/ MOOD STABILIZERS

The second group of medications utilized to treat chronic pain not of the opioid or NSAIA category is the "mood stabilizer" class of psychoactive medications. Some drugs in this class are also called the anticonvulsants or, more accurately, AEDs or antiseizure drugs because they provide symptomatic treatment but may not alter the course of epilepsy. Herein they will be referred to as AEDs.

The first "mood stabilizer" was lithium, a salt that was marketed for the treatment of renal calculi in the early 1930s. Applied as a "cure-all," it was suggested as an anticonvulsant and hypnotic in 1870. After reports in 1890 that it was helpful in depression, little discussion was made of lithium until almost 1950 when reports of successful treatments for mania were reported. Not until the mid-1980s were valproate and carbamazepine (first-generation AEDs) introduced in specialty mood clinics. Eventually this led to the general realization that many of the AED class of drugs had mood effects leading to the study of this group of neurologic drugs in the field of psychiatry. In the last 50 years, under the Anticonvulsant Drug Development Program in the United States, there has been global licensing of numerous second-generation AEDs, in chronological order: vigabatrin, zonisamide, oxcarbazepine, lamotrigine, felbamate, gabapentin, topiramate, tiagabine, levetiracetam, pregabalin, and lacosamide. As was the case with mood clinics, nascent pain centers found putative pain benefit from AEDs and promulgated systematic study of this group. Today certain AEDs are considered valid agents for the treatment of neuropathic pain.

A. Indications

In concept, AEDs were developed to reduce the spread and generalization of an epileptic seizure focus, thereby preventing tonic-clonic or grand mal seizure. The gabapentinoids, gabapentin (Neurontin), and pregabalin (Lyrica) have a long history of application in chronic pain. A 2014 (updated 2017) Cochrane report indicated that gabapentin showed statistical improvement in diabetic neuropathy and postherpetic neuralgia. Pregabalin had evidence of efficacy in central neuropathic pain (typically pain after stroke) and in fibromyalgia. Unfortunately, there is limited or no evidence of validated effect with other AEDs for neuropathy. Topiramate is indicated in the treatment of headache.

From the psychiatric standpoint, certain AEDs are useful in the treatment of the elevated mood found in bipolar spectrum disorders (BPSD) type I and type II. Lamotrigine is effective in the treatment of combined mania and depression. Topiramate has found uses in treatment of mood variability associated with substance use disorders and has been shown to reduce craving in alcohol use disorder and cocaine use disorder.

B. Mechanisms

It has become clear that AEDs function through any number of mechanisms. These include (1) blocking voltage-sensitive sodium or calcium channels; (2) influencing γ-aminobutyric acid (GABA) levels through release and reuptake; (3) inhibition of *N*-methyl-D-aspartate (NMDA), alpha-amino-3-hydroxy-5-methylisoxazole-4-propionic acid (AMPA), or kainic acid receptors (KAR); and (4) by influencing neuronal glutamate. Gabapentinoids exerts their effect by binding to the alpha-2-delta 1 subunit of the voltage-gated calcium (Ca_V) channels (VGCC) that are required for many key functions in excitable cells, including transmitter release and muscle contraction. The exact molecular mechanism that results in analgesia remains to be determined.

C. Adverse Reactions

Unpleasant reactions (fatigue, dizziness, weight gain) were commonplace with AEDs resulting in very high noncompliance rates, especially with the first-generation AEDs. The gabapentinoids can produce significant weight gain and/or lower extremity edema. Lamotrigine must be increased slowly (to produce desensitization) to avoid a rare occurrence of Steven-Johnsons syndrome (SJS) that can lead to toxic epidermal necrolysis (TEN), a potentially fatal condition. Topiramate has earned the street-name "dopamax" because of speech dysfluency of sufficient density to result in significant rates of nonadherence. Recent functional MRI studies show this direct effect of topiramate on frontal lobe language management centers.

D. Dosages and Monitoring (Table 13.6)

III. ANXIOLYTICS

There are a broad number of drug classes that are utilized for reduction of anxiety including (alphabetically) antidepressants, antihistamines, barbiturates, benzodiazepines, opioids, and sympatholytics. There is often confusion about the terms anxiolytic, sedative, and hypnotic. Anxiolytics reduce anxiety and generate calm and quiet. Sedatives decrease activity, giving the appearance of calm and quiet. Hypnotics facilitate onset and maintenance of sleep by inducing drowsiness. Agents in this group often produce effects in all three of these domains opening the door to a not

TABLE 13.6 Antiepileptic Drugs (AEDs)

Medication	Proprietary Name	Dosage Range (mg/d)
Gabapentin	*Neurontin*	100-3200[a]
Pregabalin	*Lyrica*	50-300
Topiramate	*Topamax*	50-400
Lamotrigine	*Lamictal*	25-500[b]

[a]**Note**: An MGH Department of Psychiatry researcher studied the prescribing practice of Massachusetts MDs, which revealed gabapentin is one of the most prescribed medicines with the lowest specific indication for use. This implies gabapentin is prescribed often and in doses without solid rationale. A Canadian study similarly found gabapentin was among the medications with the highest proportion of off-label use, at 83% (Radley DC, Finkelstein SN, Stafford RS. Off-label prescribing among office-based physicians. *Intern Med.* 2006;166:1021-1026).

[b]FDA highly recommends slow taper up plans for initiation of lamotrigine to avoid TEN (toxic epidermal necrolysis).

infrequent behavior in prescribing; clinicians sometimes focus on achieving a target effect of a drug and inadvertently discount the full complement of actions (see additive risk at the Conclusions of this chapter).

Benzodiazepines (BzD) were discovered accidentally during a 1955 "lab cleanup"—a crystal residue yielded a six-ringed compound that produced muscle relaxation in mice and cats. Isolation techniques led to a very stable seven-ringed compound (diazepine) fused with a benzene ring that had sedating, hypnotic, and anxiolytic effects. This was chlordiazepoxide, later trademarked as Librium, which served as the springboard that allowed for the development of any number of compounds. These BzD compounds quickly replaced barbiturates, carbamates, and others because of superior safety profiles. These went on to become the most prescribed medication by 1970s because of their high therapeutic index and seductive efficacy at "calming"; unfortunately, they carried high tolerance and dependency risk. There are non-BzD agents that can result in "calming." The list of FDA-indicated and off-label application of drugs that have been used to induce anxiolytic, sedative, and hypnotic effects is manifold. Psychiatrists usually use SSRIs as first-line agents to address anxiety. Hydroxyzine can be considered as a safe anxiolytic adjunct with very high therapeutic index. Do not use quetiapine as an anxiolytic, hypnotic, or sedative (see Antipsychotic section next).

A. Indications

The benzodiazepines were understood early in the history of organized pain management to be ineffective as analgesics. On the other hand, they can serve in spasmodic conditions and can be of benefit for associated anxiety and panic. Nevertheless, the tolerance and dependency risk alone or concomitant when used with mu-receptor agonists (opioids) demands careful risk/benefit considerations before prescribing. Realizing risk can outweigh benefits particularly in a pain patient experiencing stress in several domains; it is preferable to rely on agents without misuse risk, such as an SSRI or hydroxyzine to address anxiety. On the other hand, if anxiety is obstructive to therapeutic progress, this class of agents can be advantageous. The "Z" class hypnotic agents (zolpidem, zaleplon, and eszopiclone) have found acceptance to address sleep issues, but there are risk concerns that are not trivial. With this group of agents, remember to reduce dose in the elderly given the association with increased fall risk.

B. Mechanisms

The BzD and Z classes of drugs increase the efficiency of the GABA-ligand/gated ion channel interaction that regulates the flow of chloride into the cell, causing neuron hyperpolarization that typically reduces interneuronal communications and thus sedative effects within the brain. The five protein hetero-complex has several binding sites, each of which generates different $GABA_A$ modulation results that roughly correlate to anxiolytic, sedative, hypnotic, and muscle relaxation qualities; BzDs bind at the interface of the α/γ subunits on the $GABA_A$ receptor (BZR), whereas Zs attach to sites between other protein pairs.

The BzD drugs differ in PK/PD parameters but, notably, active metabolites strongly define the observed clinical behavior. For example, alprazolam has an average terminal elimination half-life of 12 hours. Clonazepam shows a much slower elimination with a half-life of 20-80 hours. One of the active metabolites of diazepam, desmethyldiazepam, has an elimination half-life of between 30 and 200 hours leading to large interindividual variation.

TABLE 13.7 Bzds

Medication	Proprietary Name	Dosage Range (mg/d)
Lorazepam	*Ativan*	1-2
Clonazepam	*Klonopin*	0.5-1
Diazepam	*Valium*	5-15
Alprazolam	*Xanax*	0.25-0.50

C. Adverse Reactions

Both alprazolam and clonazepam are associated with agent-specific withdrawal; meaning, if detoxification is indicated, using an alternate agent in class (lorazepam or diazepam) will not provide full protection against acute withdrawal syndrome (AWS) and can leave a patient prone to dangerous autonomic or seizure risks. BzDs have been associated with post-acute withdrawal syndrome (PAWS), described as waves of symptoms occurring long after physiologic washout of the inciting drug; however, there is little scientific evidence to support this. BzDs are ranked seventh in dependence, physical harm, and social harm (in between alcohol and tobacco, each of which causes more mortality than all drugs combined). Alprazolam has both rapid onset and offset properties that are highly reinforcing qualities for addiction. The Z drugs have been associated with rapid tolerance, rebound with abrupt cessation and a significant incidence of complex "sleep-walking" behaviors, notably mysterious meal preparations, the results of which are discovered in the morning.

1. Dosages and Monitoring

A clinically prudent caveat with BzDs is to avoid any doses above 1-2 mg lorazepam equivalent (Table 13.7).

IV. ANTIPSYCHOTICS

The antipsychotic drugs have a particularly convoluted developmental history that eventually led to their primary application for disorders of thought, generally called psychosis. Methylene Blue, which had antimalarial qualities, led to further development of the phenothiazines that were used as antihistamines and anesthetics. Curiosity, newness, and serendipity led to the discovery that chlorpromazine had antipsychotic features and led to the first-generation antipsychotics (FGAs) whose hallmark was potent DA (D_2) inhibition. In the 1990s, the second-generation antipsychotics (SGAs) or "atypical antipsychotics" were discovered and found to have less extrapyramidal symptoms (EPS) that had proved deterring to wide use of FGAs.

A. Indications

There is no robust indication for the primary use of FGAs or SGAs in the treatment of pain. Cochrane reports of 2010 and 2013 note no robust studies but suggested further studies of SGAs for pain could be warranted. A 2016 review of quetiapine in fibromyalgia implied subjective superiority to placebo but no superiority to amitriptyline for fibromyalgia.

From the psychiatric standpoint, antipsychotics are intended to treat positive (hallucinations, delusions), negative (apathy, blunting, lack of social function), and cognitive (disorganized thought process) symptoms of schizophrenia as well as for psychosis associated with mood disorders.

The FGAs tend to treat positive symptoms, whereas the SGAs show added effect on negative and cognitive symptoms.

The practical result of SGAs is that they can result in beneficial mood and cognitive effects, which has led to their popularity and overuse. Aripiprazole, a D_2 partial agonist, has been proven beneficial as an antidepressant synergist.

B. Mechanisms

The hallmark of the antipsychotics is potent DA (D_2) inhibition. The major central DA paths originate in the ventral tegmental area (VTA), substantia nigra pars compacta (SNc), and hypothalamus, which then project to target frontal and central loci that govern emotions, executive function, learning, motivation, reward, and neuroendocrine control. Notable are striatal connections that are part of the cortico-basal ganglia-thalamo-cortical loop (CBGTC) pathways that are critical to initiation and reward discounting. The FGAs are D_2 antagonists with varying potencies at D_2, H_1, α_1, and muscarinic receptors. The SGAs have D_2 antagonistic activity but are unique for fast D_2 dissociation, 5-HT_{2A} antagonism, and 5-HT_{1A} agonism.

C. Adverse Reactions

The detriment of the antipsychotics is potent DA (D_2) inhibition. FGAs became associated with extrapyramidal side effects caused by nigrostriatal DA imbalance that could lead to tardive dyskinesia (TD), a troubling and potentially permanent side-effect with a treatment prevalence as high as 30%. SGAs have a greatly reduced risk of TD but carry risk of weight gain and/or metabolic syndrome (MetS). MetS occurs at up to 60% with certain SGAs—this in a treatment population that is already at risk for being overweight and having diabetes as well as against a U.S. general population prevalence of MetS of ~30%. The putative mechanism of MetS is that antipsychotics activate the TGFβ pathway effector SMAD3. One hypothalamic consequence of this group can be hyperprolactinemia manifested by galactorrhea. Both FGAs and SGAs have dose-related effects on cardiac Qtc (see Conclusions below). Rare, but necessary to remember is NMS, an emergency bradykinetic hyperthermia dysregulation event.

Given the weight gain, diabetes, endocrine, and MetS risks, the use of quetiapine (Seroquel) is contraindicated as an anxiolytic, hypnotic, or sedative. The partial agonist, aripiprazole, can be activating and lead to discomfort.

D. Dosages and Monitoring

Dosages of antipsychotics are outlined in reference manuals. Given their potent dopaminergic activity, prescribing this group of medicines is best left to skilled psychopharmacologists. Monitoring goes beyond behavioral observation; it is suggested that metabolic labs, blood pressure, and weight are closely followed. Quetiapine has unique sedating and hypnotic effects that have made it popular as a sleep medication, but the risk profile outweighs off-label use.

V. PSYCHOSTIMULANTS

Psychostimulants are the most used psychoactive compounds on earth. Caffeine and nicotine (tobacco), dated to 300 BC and 6000 BC, are consumed daily in great quantities. There are numerous illicit compounds like the cocaine analogues, *Catha edulis* (khat), MDMA, methadone, and methamphetamine. Appropriate to this chapter are the nootropics or cognitive enhancers, sometimes called "smart drugs." Pertinent examples include the amphetamines (AMPH) and methylphenidate (MPD) indicated for treatment of ADHD and the eugeroics (originally eugrégoiriques) like modafinil (MOD) and armodafinil used for sleep disorders and narcolepsy.

A. Indications

The stimulants do not have a primary indication in pain management. Literature review reveals entries suggesting adults with ADHD symptoms have higher odds for experiencing pain not explained by comorbid common mental disorders.

Stimulant medications have been the mainstay of treatment for ADHD since the late 1930s. Two sympathomimetics, atomoxetine and guanfacine, are nonstimulant medications that are FDA approved for the treatment of ADHD.

B. Mechanisms

MPD inhibits the neuronal DA transporter, increasing extracellular DA concentrations in the brain yielding a prolonged or intensified DA postsynaptic signal. AMPH also raises extracellular DA concentrations but through a more complex "triple mechanism." When comparing *in vitro* vs *in vivo* cellular stimulant response, it has become apparent that magnitude of **phasic DA** release relative to baseline DA levels (phasic/baseline), rather than general increases in overall DA levels (phasic + baseline) determines goal oriented behavior response. This can explain lower-dose functional behaviors vs higher-dose misuse behaviors.

MOD elevates extracellular DA, NE, 5HT, and glutamate levels suggesting the arousal and activity-promoting effects of MOD are largely a function of activity in catecholamine systems. Recent work suggests that activation of phasic DA signaling is also an important mechanism underlying the clinical efficacy for MOD arousal.

C. Adverse Reactions

The list of adverse effects from stimulants in general include symptoms consistent with amine excess. From the psychiatric standpoint, paranoia and psychosis can occur but need to be parsed from underlying comorbid common mental disorders, adulterants, or misuse of other agents. Cardiac events are usually limited to heart rate and blood pressure changes.

D. Dosages and Monitoring

Amphetamine and methylphenidate preparations exist in both regular release and extended release formulations. Clinical effectiveness is measured by functional status or formal testing and not patient reports of "focus and energy." Mental safety is assessed by behavioral successes and being attentive to subtle signs of thought disorder or paranoia.

VI. CONCLUSIONS

This chapter is meant to facilitate the interactive interface between disciplines that are offering relief for chronic pain, the potentially devastating condition that can result in a profound negative impact on the life and productivity, the center and circumference of individuals. Caregivers are exposed with high frequency to complex decision-making, which can lead to **underestimation of additive risk**. Additive risk assessment is the summation of active variables that can result in an observed negative outcome, which then may draw critical attention. To put in another way, a clinical presentation can arise within a busy case load that is either unfamiliar or very complex; this situation may result in an untoward outcome, which would then generate required review or scrutiny. Moreover, while seeking pragmatic solutions, a clinician can feel overwhelmed when met with the necessary mix of medical, pharmacological, procedural, and policy considerations. This combined burden could result in suboptimal inclusion of significant variables during the decision-making process.

A recent submission by the surgeon general placed landmark attention on the dangerous interaction of benzodiazepines and opioids on respiratory depression, an identified contributor in overdose death. In looking for this opioid/benzodiazepine burden, clinicians might overlook the additive effect of "other actors" that can add to respiratory depression, for example, gabapentin, clonidine, promethazine, and alcohol. In long QT syndrome, attention may turn to psychiatric medications (antipsychotics) that can prolong QT, while the dramatic problem event, torsades de pointes (TDP) leading to ventricular fibrillation (VF), is typically due to a confluence of factors: genetic loading, more than one drug that prolongs QT (including antiarrhythmic and or antibiotic medications); electrolytes; gender; fever; and even the time of day. Malignant hyperthermia, NMS, serotonin syndrome, stimulant-induced psychosis, and delirium all have complex causes, but the focus can trend towards a single causative influence, "a bad actor" if you will.

We can put an emphasis on **additive risk assessment** to expand our understanding of the cause and effect relationship to complex medical conditions that have high emotional associations. These emotional responses are amplified when there is potential significant bad outcome like death or significant morbidity. This emotive response can influence our thinking. Consideration of additive risk goes well beyond pharmacology. Clinicians incorporate this across many domains; medicine and surgery treatment options all require and involve consideration of additive risk. Please consider **"what is the additive risk?"** as a springboard question for expansive consideration for complex medical presentations.

Selected Readings

Bannister K, Dickenson AH. What do monoamines do in pain modulation? *Curr Opin Support Palliat Care.* 2016;10(2):143-148.

Bobak MJ, Weber MW, Doellman MA. Modafinil activates phasic dopamine signaling in dorsal and ventral striata. *J Pharmacol Exp Ther.* 2016;359(3):460-470.

Calipari ES, Ferris MJ. Amphetamine mechanisms and actions at the dopamine terminal revisited. *J Neurosci.* 2013;33(21):8923-8925.

Cates ME, Jackson CW, Feldman JM, Stimmel AE, Woolley TW. Metabolic consequences of using low-dose quetiapine for insomnia in psychiatric patients. *Community Ment Health J.* 2009;45:251-254.

Walitt B, Klose P, Üçeyler N, Phillips T, Häuser W. Antipsychotics for fibromyalgia in adults. *Cochrane Database Syst Rev.* 2016;(6). doi: 10.1002/14651858.CD011804.pub2.

Cohen T, Sundaresh S, Levine F. Antipsychotics activate the TGFβ pathway effector SMAD3. *Mol Psychiatry.* 2013;18:347-357.

Cunningham JL, Craner JR, Evans MM, Hooten WM. Benzodiazepine use in patients with chronic pain in an interdisciplinary pain rehabilitation program. *J Pain Res.* 2017;10:311-317.

DeVane CL, Ware MR, Lydiard RB. Pharmacokinetics, pharmacodynamics, and treatment issues of benzodiazepines: alprazolam, adinazolam, and clonazepam. *Psychopharmacol Bull.* 1991;27(4):463-473.

Dworkin RH, et al. Pharmacologic management of neuropathic pain: evidence-based recommendations. *Pain.* 2007;132:237-251.

http://neuroscience.uth.tmc.edu/s4/chapter03.html.

https://www.fda.gov/NewsEvents/Newsroom/PressAnnouncements/ucm232708.htm

http://profiles.nlm.nih. gov/ps/access/NNBBJB.pdf.

McIntyre RS, Harrison J, Loft H, Jacobson W, Olsen CK. The effects of vortioxetine on cognitive function in patients with major depressive disorder: A meta-analysis of three randomized controlled trials. *Int J Neuropsychopharmacol.* 2016;19(10): pyw055.

Katz J, Pennella-Vaughan J, Hetzel RD, Kanazi GE, Dworkin RH. A randomized, placebo-controlled trial of bupropion sustained release in chronic low back pain. *J Pain.* 2005;6(10):656-661.doi:10.1016/j.jpain.2005.05.002.

Llorca PM, Chereau I, Bayle FJ, Lancon C. Tardive dyskinesias and antipsychotics: a review. *Eur Psychiatry.* 17(3):129-138.

Nutt D, King LA, Saulsbury W, Blakemore C. Development of a rational scale to assess the harm of drugs of potential misuse. *Lancet.* 369(9566):1047-1053.

Papanastasiou E. The prevalence and mechanisms of metabolic syndrome in schizophrenia: a review. *Ther Adv Psychopharmacol.* 2013;3(1):33-51.

Patetsos E, Horjales-Araujo E. Treating chronic pain with SSRIs: what do we know? *Pain Res Manag.* 2016;2016:2020915.

Reddy S, Patt RB. The benzodiazepines as adjuvant analgesics. *J Pain Symptom Manage.* 1994;9(8):510-514.

Richelson E, Nelson A. Antagonism by antidepressants of neurotransmitter receptors of normal human brain in vitro. *J Pharmacol Exp Ther.* 1984;230(1):94-102.

Rossat A, Fantino B, Bongue B, et al. Association between benzodiazepines and recurrent falls: a cross-sectional elderly population-based study. *J Nutr Health Aging.* 2011;15(1):72-77.

Salerian AJ. Addictive potential: A = E/T(max)xt(1/2). *Med Hypotheses.* 2010;74(6): 1081-1083.

Saper CB. The central autonomic nervous system: conscious visceral perception and autonomic pattern generation. *Annu Rev Neurosci.* 2002;25:433-469.

Sinha A, Lewis O, Kumar R, Yeruva SL, Curry BH. Adult ADHD medications and their cardiovascular implications. *Case Rep Cardiol.* 2016. Article ID 2343691.

Skreta M. *Benzodiazepines Today and Tomorrow.* Lancaster, England: MTP Press Limited; 1980.

Stahl, et al. 2005. Stahl's essential psychopharmacology: the prescriber's guide / Stephen M. Stahl ; editorial assistant, Meghan M. Grady ; with illustrations by Nancy Muntner. – Fifth edition.

Stickley A, Koyanagi A, Takahashi H, Kamio Y. ADHD symptoms and pain among adults in England. *Psychiatry Res.* 2016;246:326-331.

Suliman NA, Taib M, Moklas M, et al. Establishing natural nootropics: recent molecular enhancement influenced by natural nootropic. *Evid Based Complement Alternat Med.* 2016;2016:4391375.

Wiffen PJ, Derry S, Bell RF, Rice ASC, Tölle TR, Phillips T, Moore RA. Gabapentin for chronic neuropathic pain in adults. *Cochrane Database Syst Rev.* 2017;6(6): CD007938. doi: 10.1002/14651858.CD007938.pub4.

Viswambharan V, Manepalli JN, Grossberg GT. Orexigenic agents in geriatric clinical practice. *Aging Health.* 2013;9(1):49-65. http://www.medscape.com/viewarticle/780506_6

Young LT. What exactly is a mood stabilizer? *J Psychiatry Neurosci.* 2004;29(2):87-88.

SECTION IV

Therapeutic Options: Interventional Approaches

14 Epidural Steroid Injection

M. Alexander Kiefer and Gary J. Brenner

Epidural steroid injection (ESI) is the most frequently utilized pain medicine intervention performed for the treatment of lower back and lower extremity pain (see Fig. 14.1), and, yet, a significant amount of controversy remains related to its efficacy and indications. Although many clinical trials and meta-analyses have been conducted, there is little expert consensus in the medical community, especially when assessed across specialties. This chapter outlines the periprocedural management and interventional approaches utilized at the Massachusetts General Hospital (MGH) Center for Pain Medicine in the performance of ESIs, as well as a brief discussion of the evidence supporting their use.

I. EFFICACY

A. Evidence of Efficacy

The use of ESIs to treat lower back pain is supported by >45 placebo-controlled studies and dozens of systematic reviews and meta-analyses; however, controversy surrounding their efficacy continues to persist with multiple studies and meta-analyses providing conflicting conclusions. The ESI literature is vast and complex. A full review is beyond the scope of this chapter, but a few recent meta-analyses and reviews will be briefly discussed.

In two systematic reviews sponsored by the National Health Service (NHS) and Health Technology Assessment Program, Lewis et al. strongly supported the use of ESI for the treatment of sciatica. In the more recent 2015 systematic review and meta-analysis of 122 studies and 21 treatment strategies, statistically significant improvements were demonstrated with ESIs. Additionally, this study showed that ESIs were superior to traction, percutaneous discectomy, and exercise therapy for the treatment of sciatica. This is in contrast to the recent technology assessment reviews for the Agency for Healthcare Research and Quality (AHRQ) published by Chou et al., which concluded a lack of effectiveness of ESIs in managing lumbar radiculopathy and spinal stenosis. These publications have been criticized as possessing a significant intellectual bias.

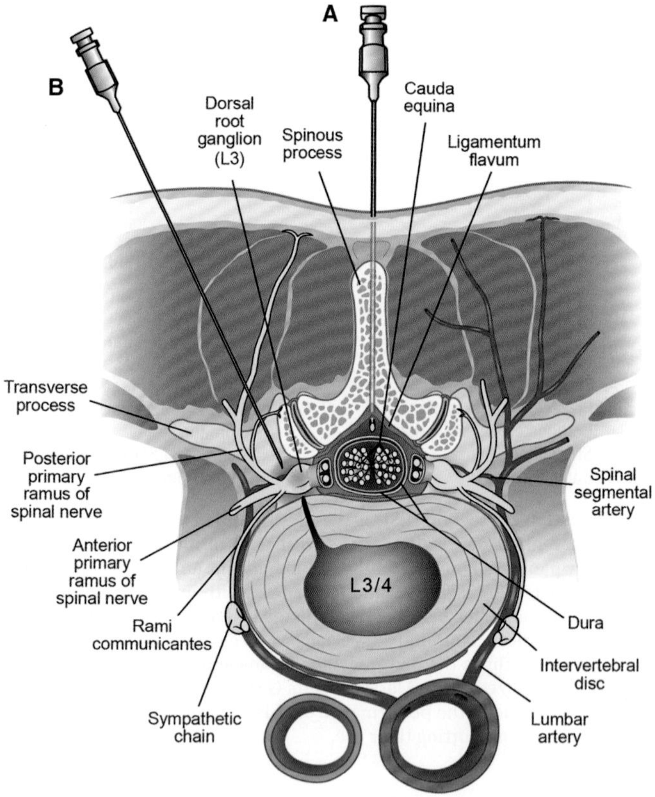

FIGURE 14.1 L3-L4 interlaminar **(A)** and transforaminal **(B)** epidural injections in a patient with an L3-L4 herniated disk. (Reprinted with permission from Rathmell J. *Atlas of Image-Guided Intervention in Regional Anesthesia and Pain Medicine.* 2nd ed. Philadelphia, PA: Lippincott Williams & Wilkins; 2012.)

Manchikanti et al., in a recent meta-analysis of seven studies, showed that epidural injection of lidocaine alone or in conjunction with steroid is significantly effective for analgesia and improvement of function at 3 months and 12 months in patients with spinal stenosis and radiculopathy. Interestingly, the authors concluded based on three randomized controlled trials with a total of 131 patients that there is no significant effect for ESI administered with saline (an ESI alone without local anesthetic).

In a systematic review of transforaminal (TFESI) vs interlaminar (ILESI) ESIs in the management of lumbosacral radicular pain, Chang-Chien et al. concluded that both TFESI and ILESI are effective in reducing pain and improving functional scores. However, TFESI demonstrated non–clinically significant superiority to ILESI only at the 2-week follow-up.

Despite the outcome data supporting clinically meaningful, albeit transient (weeks to months), benefit, the indications for ESIs continue to be controversial. ESI is commonly utilized for axial pain, postlaminectomy syndrome, central canal or neural foraminal stenosis, lumbar and cervical radiculopathy, degenerative disc disease, and neurogenic claudication.

B. Mechanisms of Efficacy

In lower back pain that is the consequence of a ruptured annulus fibrosus and resultant nucleus pulposus herniation, radicular pain is produced either by mechanical pressure or chemical irritation of the nerve root or both. The presumed effect of corticosteroid is to reduce the neuropathic pain, inflammation, edema, and scarring that can result from this pathology. The nucleus pulposus contains increased concentrations of phospholipase A_2, the enzyme responsible for the conversion of membrane phospholipids into arachidonic acid and lysophospholipids. Arachidonic acid is the principle substrate for the cyclooxygenase and lipooxygenase pathways, which result in the production of the inflammatory mediators (prostaglandins, prostacyclins, thromboxanes, and leukotrienes) responsible for the production and amplification of pain. Corticosteroids inhibit phospholipid A_2, thus producing an anti-inflammatory and analgesic effect. It has also been demonstrated that steroids may exert an analgesic effect by inhibiting ectopic discharges from injured nerve fibers and depressing conduction in normal C fibers. It also has been observed that steroids reduce the bulk of a scar by diminishing its hyaline portion while leaving the fibrous skeleton intact.

Recent research has revealed several potential mechanisms of action of ESIs that are not dependent on the pharmacologic action of corticosteroids. Injection of local anesthetics alone results in an increase of blood flow to ischemic nerve roots and is able to decrease conduction in injured nerves. Washout of inflammatory mediators and lysis of adhesions can also produce an analgesic effect following injection of saline, local anesthetic, or any nonsteroid injectate. Rabinovitch et al. found in a systematic review a significant correlation between epidural volume and degree of analgesia regardless of steroid dose.

II. GENERAL PRINCIPLES

A. Choice of Injectate

1. Corticosteroids

Glucocorticoids are the steroids most commonly used for ESIs and can be divided into particulate (triamcinolone, methylprednisolone, betamethasone, and prednisolone) and nonparticulate (dexamethasone) preparations based on the solubility of the steroid in water and their aggregation characteristics. Particulate steroids are thought to provide a longer duration of action at the injection site due to a continuous release of steroid over an extended time period. However, accidental intravascular injection of a particulate steroid into the artery of Adamkiewicz in the lumbar or thoracic spine or a radicular or vertebral artery in the cervical spine can result in serious adverse events. These unintended outcomes can include spinal cord ischemia and paralysis following a thoracic or lumbar ESI or stroke and even death for a cervical ESI. For this reason, many proceduralists will select a nonparticulate steroid (dexamethasone, 4-10 mg) when performing a transforaminal ESI (TFESI). Of note, no pharmacokinetic studies have been completed comparing the duration of action of particulate vs. nonparticulate preparations. For interlaminar ESIs (ILESIs), a dose ranging from 40 to 80 mg of triamcinolone is generally used. The steroids can be mixed with saline to increase volume or local anesthetics; however, we use small total volumes. Studies have shown that if adequately placed under fluoroscopic guidance, even small volumes will reach the site of pathology. Total volumes generally vary from 1 to 10 mL.

2. Local Anesthetic

The addition of a local anesthetic to the corticosteroid represents a clinical judgment based on such factors as fall risk, the vertebral levels targeted, and the degree of stenosis. Some proceduralists will omit local anesthetic in patients with a high degree of stenosis in order to conserve volume. Epinephrine is generally not added to the injectate. The presence of local anesthetic may have some diagnostic value, as a clear positive, albeit expectedly transient, decrease in symptoms may suggest that a major pain generator was targeted. Interestingly, clinical studies comparing epidural steroid to epidural local anesthetic alone have in some cases failed to demonstrate clear superiority of steroid over local anesthetic. This raises questions regarding the mechanisms of efficacy of ESI, though this needs to be considered in the context of the known immunomodulatory activities of lidocaine. Additionally, this equivocality supports the appropriateness of ESI with local anesthetic alone in patients who may not tolerate corticosteroids.

B. Physiologic Effects of Corticosteroids and Epidural Steroid Injections

According to a national survey, chronic pain patients undergo an average of five to seven ESIs per year. At our center, we limit this number to four per year in order to limit the risks caused by the physiologic effects of corticosteroids outlined below.

1. Immunosuppression

A prednisone equivalent of 2 mg/kg body weight is sufficient to produce clinically significant immunosuppression. ESIs performed on patients receiving systemic corticosteroids or repeat ESIs may exceed this recommended dosage limit. Immunosuppression and a resultant increase in infection risk is the result of the down regulation of inflammatory genes, up-regulation of anti-inflammatory genes, and suppression of B-cells, T-cells, and phagocytes. At particularly high risk are patients with preexisting immunosuppressive conditions, including cancer, diabetes, neutropenia, systemic steroid use, recent history of infections, renal failure, HIV infection, asplenia, and alcoholic cirrhosis.

2. Elevation of Blood Glucose

Injection of corticosteroid into the epidural space causes an elevation of blood glucose levels in patients with both insulin- and non–insulin-dependent diabetes mellitus. This elevation has a mean duration of 2 days; however, some studies have revealed a period of increased blood glucose of up to 6 days duration. Diabetic patients should be medically optimized prior to ESI and educated about postprocedural hyperglycemia and the potential need to change diet or medications following injection.

3. Suppression of the Hypothalamic-Pituitary-Adrenal Axis

Administration of exogenous corticosteroids can result in alterations of the hypothalamic-pituitary-adrenal (HPA) axis and cause adrenal suppression resulting in a decrease in endogenous cortisol and growth hormone levels. Additionally, Cushing syndrome secondary to iatrogenic hypercortisolism can result from a single ESI. HPA axis suppression is more likely to occur without Cushing syndrome and has been shown to persist from 3 weeks to 3 months following injection. However, suppression of the HPA axis can persist for up to 8 months in some extreme cases. Repeating injections within a 3-month window contributes to further axis suppression and potentiates the period of dysregulation.

Care should also be taken in patients with HIV infections undergoing active therapy with ritonavir, which, due to CYP3A4 inhibition, decreases the catabolic rate of corticosteroids, increases the risk of iatrogenic hypercortisolism and Cushing syndrome, and extends the duration of action of injected steroids. Coordination with the patient's primary care or infectious disease physician is recommended to ensure optimal care of an HIV-infected patient.

4. Bone Demineralization

Corticosteroids up-regulate the activity of osteoblasts while down-regulating the activity of osteoclasts, leading to decreased bone density and an increased risk of fractures. This effect is most pronounced in trabecular bone and thus commonly affects sites such as the vertebral body and the proximal femur. The dose at which bone demineralization begins to occur is controversial, but has been demonstrated to be as low as 2.5 mg/day of oral prednisone. A large retrospective cohort study, which compared 3000 patients who underwent ESI with 300 patients who did not, revealed that each ESI increases fracture risk by 21% (2). Special consideration of the risks and benefits of ESIs in populations at high risk for pathologic fracture (elderly women, osteoporosis, osteopenia) is recommended.

C. Complications

Major complications following ESI are rare, but can be catastrophic. The routine use of sedation should be avoided, especially for cervical procedures, to allow communication with the patient to assess inadvertent contact of the needle with the spinal cord, which could result in permanent spinal cord injury. Additionally, an alert patient can forewarn of potential neurologic damage during injection into a space with a high degree of stenosis, which can result in similar nerve damage. The American Society of Regional Anesthesia (ASRA) guidelines on anticoagulation management should be followed in order to reduce risk of epidural hematoma formation.

As an ESI is an elective procedure, it should not be performed in patients with active infections or who have not yet completed their antibiotic course for an infection. There is no consensus for how long an ESI should be postponed following resolution of an infection and completion of an antibiotic course. At our center, we will commonly wait 7 days. Meticulous attention to sterile technique should prevent most infectious complications including meningitis, epidural abscess formation, discitis, cutaneous infection, and osteomyelitis.

Inadvertent intravascular injection of a particulate corticosteroid into the artery of Adamkiewicz in the lumbar or thoracic spine or a radicular or vertebral artery in the cervical spine can result in serious adverse events including spinal cord ischemia and paralysis. For this reason, a nonparticulate steroid (dexamethasone, 4-10 mg) is recommended when performing a transforaminal ESI (TFESI). Additionally, the use of digital subtraction imaging (DSI) during injection of contrast increases the likelihood of diagnosing an intra-arterial injection if particulate steroid is used for a TFESI.

Use of fluoroscopy and injection of contrast media should greatly minimize the risk of intrathecal injection, arachnoiditis, seizure, or high spinal blockade. Likewise, the use of fluoroscopy with standardized technique should greatly reduce the risk of inadvertent puncture of viscera. Minor complications include dural puncture with associated post–dural puncture headache, vasovagal syncope, pneumocephalus, transient paresthesias, temporary increases in radicular pain, flushing due to an

IgE-mediated mechanism, and persistent hiccups. If available, the patient's MRI should always be reviewed prior to a procedure.

III. PROCEDURAL CONSIDERATIONS

A. Preprocedure Management

No restrictions to eating or drinking are required under routine circumstances. An IV is not required unless the patient has medical comorbidities, such as extreme anxiety, substantial cardiovascular disease, or a history of vasovagal syncope, that would indicate IV access. In general, medications that are either strongly analgesic or sedating are avoided so that baseline pain is not altered and patient cooperation is maintained. Antibiotics are not necessary. Baseline vital signs (including pain scale) are obtained upon arrival to the procedure suite. The level of monitoring is determined on a patient-to-patient basis using similar criteria to those for IV placement. The usual monitors are noninvasive blood pressure monitor, five-lead electrocardiogram (ECG), and pulse oximeter. The patient is placed prone with a pillow or cushion placed under the abdomen (between iliac crests and costal margin) to reduce lumbar lordosis. As the patient is generally not sedated, further cushioning and supports may be required to ensure patient comfort and cooperability. For the cervical approach, a small support (a stack of blue towels or a 1-L IV bag wrapped in towels) is placed under the patient's forehead or a specialized table is utilized. Arms should be relaxed over the sides of the table or placed at the patient's sides with the hands tucked under the patient's thighs.

B. Contrast Media

The use of fluoroscopy and contrast media is firmly supported during ESIs. Only nonionic contrast media (iopamidol) should be used when performing ESIs, as standard contrast media can result in neurotoxicity and should be avoided. In a case where standard contrast media are accidentally injected intrathecally, which can potentially result in anterior spinal artery syndrome, arachnoiditis, meningitis, urinary retention, and conus medullaris syndrome, the intrathecal space should be irrigated with large amounts of normal saline.

There is no consensus whether nonionic contrast should be used in patients allergic to IV contrast solutions. Traditionally, gadolinium has been used in patients with a perceived risk for allergic reaction. However, the safety of gadolinium-based contrast media is unclear and should be used with caution.

C. Postprocedure Management

Once the procedure is over, patients recover in the procedure suite or recovery room. The recovery time varies based on the choice of injectate, fall risk, and patient transportation arrangements following discharge. Once the patient meets standard recovery criteria, it is recommended he or she be discharged with an escort.

D. Lumbar and Cervical Interlaminar Approach

1. Achieve true anteroposterior (AP) fluoroscopic view ensuring the spinous process is midline between pedicles (Fig. 14.2).
2. Prepare skin with chlorhexidine and drape using meticulous sterile technique.
3. Mark needle insertion point ipsilateral to the side of pathology between the spinous process and pedicle or midline if the patient's symptoms

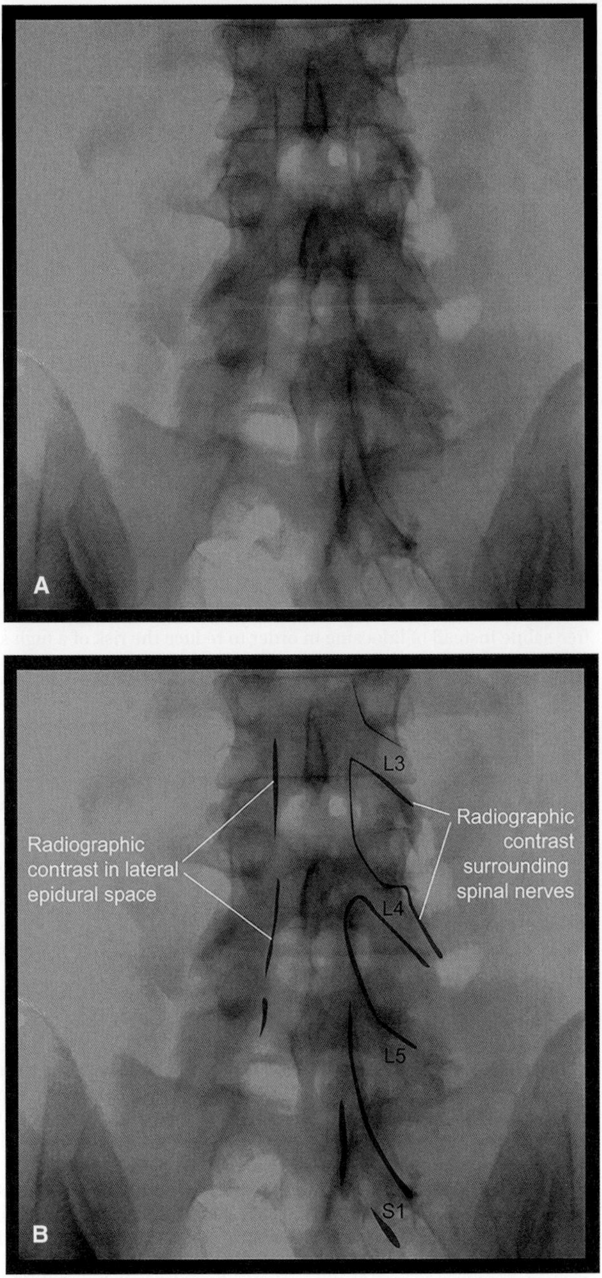

FIGURE 14.2 A. AP epidurogram of the lumbosacral spine demonstrating epidural contrast media spread following ILESI in a patient with right L4/L5 disc herniation. **B.** Labeled image. (Adapted from Rathmell JP, Torian D, Song T. Lumbar epidurography. *Reg Anesth Pain Med.* 2000;25:545.)

are bilateral. A radiopaque object, such as a Kelly clamp or needle, can be used to mark this location using fluoroscopy.

4. Infiltrate the insertion site with lidocaine (+/− sodium bicarbonate) using a 25-gauge 1.5-in needle. Skin wheals are painful and unnecessary.
5. Insert a 22-gauge Tuohy needle in a coaxial fashion (parallel to the x-rays), and advance until engaged in the ligamentum flavum. The approximate distance to engagement can be estimated from the patient's MRI.
6. Obtain a contralateral oblique view (45- to 55-degree oblique angle contralateral to the side of needle insertion). Without changing the orientation of the needle, advance the needle until the tip is at the anterior laminar line. Alternatively, the needle can be advanced in a lateral view (Fig. 14.3) until the tip is 2-3 mm shallow to the epidural space. Small adjustments are sometimes needed to navigate between lamina and osteophytes.
7. Remove the stylet from the Tuohy and proceed using a loss of resistance technique. It is recommended that the loss of resistance technique most familiar to the proceduralist should be utilized.
8. Once loss of resistance is achieved, inject 0.2-0.5 mL of nonionic contrast media and confirm its epidural spread.
9. Switching to an AP view, confirm medial/lateral spread of contrast to the side of patient's symptoms.
10. Slowly inject the injectate (commonly, 2 mL of 40 mg/mL triamcinolone and 1 mL 1% lidocaine). For cervical interlaminar injections, we recommend 2 mL of 40 mg/mL triamcinolone and 1 mL of sterile, preservative-free saline instead of lidocaine in order to reduce the risk of a high spinal. Pause if the patient feels severely uncomfortable.
11. Once injection is complete, immediately retract the needle from the epidural space.
12. Replace the stylet or flush the needle with local anesthetic to avoid tracking corticosteroid through the skin prior to withdrawal.
13. Slowly have the patient resume a sitting position. Do not leave him or her unattended. Take care when having the patient stand as he or she may have weakness in his or her legs.

E. Lumbar Transforaminal Approach

1. Obtain ipsilateral oblique ("Scottie dog", Fig. 14.4) fluoroscopic view (15-30 degrees) ensuring the superior endplate is "squared off."
2. Prepare skin with chlorhexidine and drape using meticulous sterile technique.
3. Using a radiopaque object, mark the needle insertion point at the 6 o'clock position on the projection of the pedicle at the skin.
4. Infiltrate the insertion site with lidocaine (+/− sodium bicarbonate) using a 25-gauge 1.5-in needle. Skin wheals are painful and unnecessary.
5. Using a 3.5-in 22- or 25-gauge needle with a tip slightly bent in the opposite direction to the bevel, enter the skin using a coaxial needle orientation. Advance the needle slowly. Longer needles may need to be used in patients with higher BMIs.
6. The radiographic target point is a "safe triangle" with sides: (a) the base is the inferior border of the pedicle; (b) the medial side is the exiting spinal nerve; and (c) the lateral side is the lateral border of the vertebral body.
7. Once the tip is on an appropriate coaxial trajectory toward the "safe triangle," utilize an AP view to ensure the needle is just below the midpoint of the pedicle.

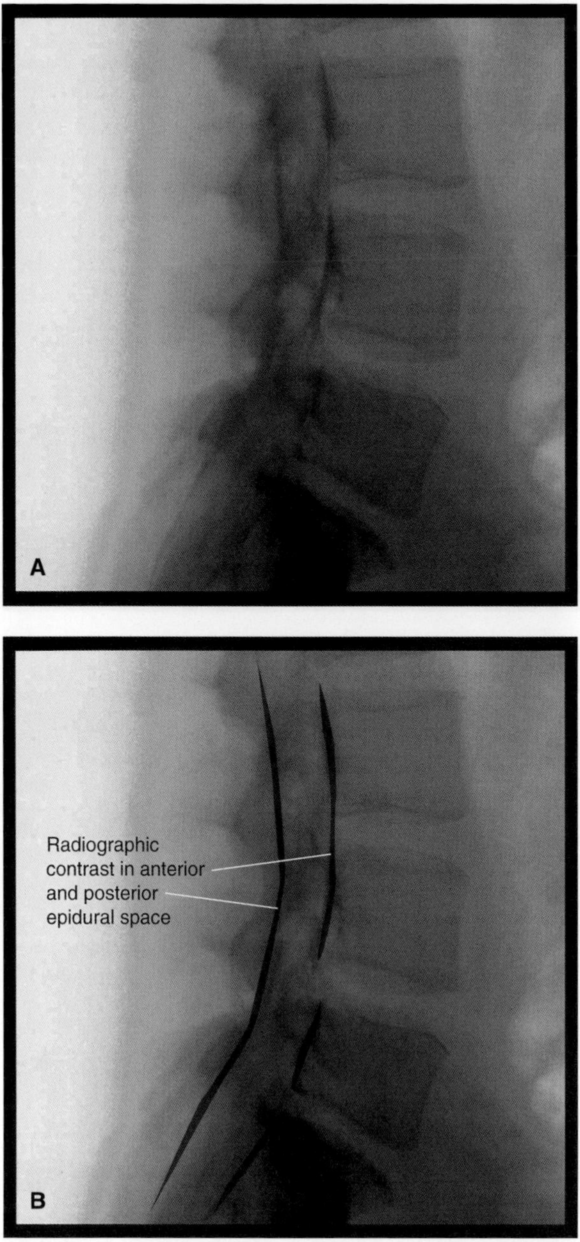

FIGURE 14.3 **A.** Lateral epidurogram of the lumbosacral spine demonstrating epidural contrast media spread following ILESI. **B.** Labeled image. (Adapted from Rathmell JP, Torian D, Song T. Lumbar epidurography. *Reg Anesth Pain Med.* 2000;25:545.)

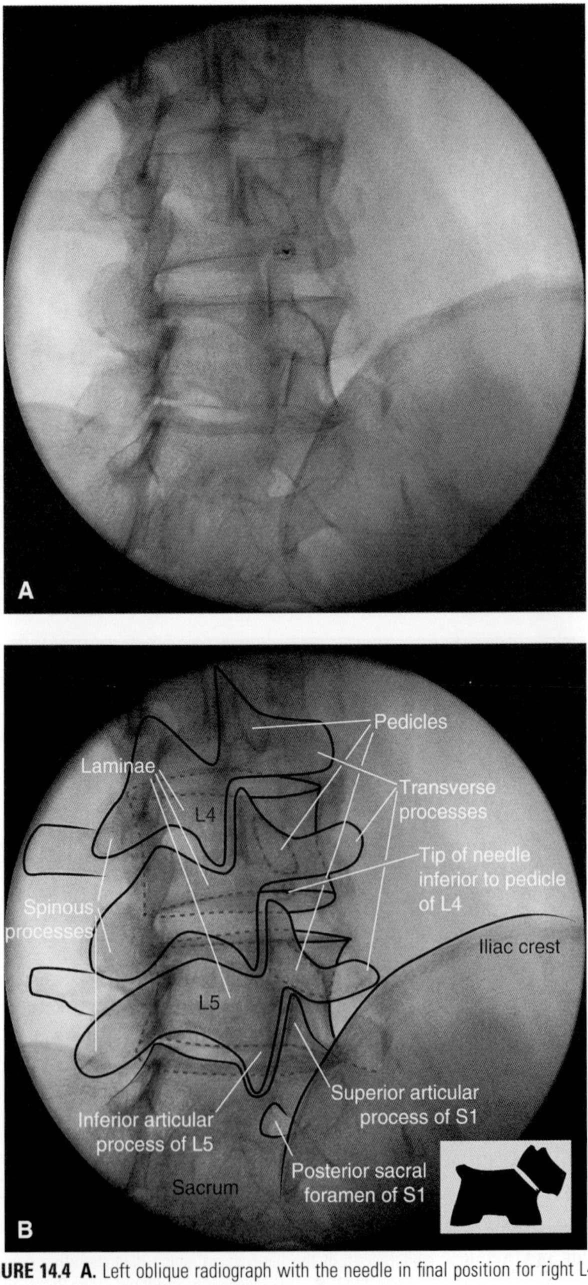

FIGURE 14.4 A. Left oblique radiograph with the needle in final position for right L4/L5 transforaminal injection. **B.** Labeled image.

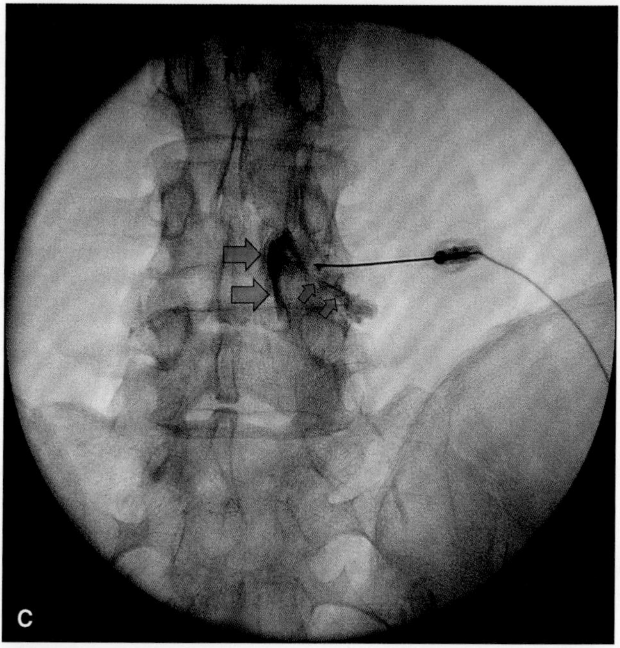

FIGURE 14.4 (*Continued*) **C.** AP radiograph with the needle in final position for right L4/L5 transforaminal injection after injection of 1 mL of radiographic contrast medium. Contrast outlines the spinal nerve (*small arrows*) and extends along the lateral aspect of the epidural space (*large arrows*). (Reprinted with permission from Rathmell J. *Atlas of Image-Guided Intervention in Regional Anesthesia and Pain Medicine.* 2nd ed. Philadelphia, PA: Lippincott Williams & Wilkins; 2012.)

8. Obtain a lateral view and guide the needle into the cephalad one-third of the intervertebral foramen.
9. Following negative aspiration of blood, inject 0.2-0.5 mL of nonionic contrast media under live fluoroscopy using DSI. Extension tubing can be flushed with contrast media and attached to the needle in order to avoid x-ray exposure to the proceduralist's hands.
10. After confirmation that the contrast medium was not inadvertently injected intravascularly, confirm appropriate epidural spread using AP and lateral views. Note that digital subtraction imaging (DSI) has been shown to reduce the risk of unrecognized intra-arterial injection.
11. Slowly inject 1-2 mL of nonparticulate corticosteroid (commonly 1 mL of 10-mg/mL dexamethasone). Keep in mind that injection of particulate matter in the artery of Adamkiewicz (T7-L4) can result in spinal cord infarction.
12. Replace stylet or flush needle with local anesthetic to avoid tracking corticosteroid through skin prior to withdrawal.
13. Slowly have the patient resume a sitting position. Do not leave him or her unattended. Take care when having the patient stand as he or she may have weakness in his or her legs.

F. Posterior S1 Foramen Approach

1. Remembering that the sacrum takes off posteriorly from the lumbar spine at about a 45-degree angle, scan the sacral area with the C-arm at different angles to see whether the posterior foramen can be made to overlie the anterior foramen (often only the anterior foramen can be visualized). The C-arm should have a slight caudad tilt.
2. Using a 25-gauge 3.5-in spinal needle, insert the needle 1 in caudad to the L5-S1 facet joint.
3. "Walk" the needle caudad until it falls through the posterior foramen. The posterior foramen is often found somewhat cephalad and lateral to the superomedial border of the elliptical image of the anterior foramen.
4. For epidural injections, the needle is advanced 1 cm into the foramen. For a selective nerve root block, the needle is advanced 2 cm until paresthesias are induced at the anterior foramen.
5. Needle position is confirmed in the lateral view with injection of 0.2-0.5 mL of nonionic contrast media.
6. Slowly inject the injectate.
7. Replace stylet or flush needle with local anesthetic to avoid tracking corticosteroid through skin prior to withdrawal.
8. Slowly have the patient resume a sitting position. Do not leave him or her unattended. Take care when having the patient stand as he or she may have weakness in his or her legs.

G. Caudal Approach

1. Achieve anteroposterior (AP) fluoroscopic view with a 20- to 30-degree caudal tilt, obtaining a good view of the sacrum, sacral hiatus, and coccyx.
2. Prepare skin with chlorhexidine and drape using meticulous sterile technique.
3. Mark needle insertion point with a radiopaque object over the sacral hiatus. If difficult to visualize, the approximate location can be found by palpating the paired sacral corneae in the midline.
4. Using a 22-gauge 3.5-in spinal needle, enter the skin and advance through the sacrococcygeal ligament.
5. Once the needle has transversed the ligament, decrease the angle of the needle to make it more acute with the skin and advance 1-2 cm into the caudal canal.
6. Inject 1-1.5 mL of nonionic contrast media and confirm epidural spread in the AP and lateral views.
7. Slowly inject the injectate (commonly 2 mL of 40 mg/mL triamcinolone, 1 mL 1% lidocaine, and saline to increase to the appropriate volume). A volume of 5 mL or more may be needed for the injectate to reach the lumbosacral junction.
8. Replace stylet or flush needle with local anesthetic to avoid tracking corticosteroid through skin prior to withdrawal.
9. Slowly have the patient resume a sitting position. Do not leave him or her unattended. Take care when having the patient stand as he or she may have weakness in his or her legs.

Selected Readings

Chang-Chien GC, Knezevic NN, McCormick Z, et al. Transforaminal versus interlaminar approaches to epidural steroid injections: a systematic review of comparative studies for lumbosacral radicular pain. *Pain Physician.* 2014;17(4):E509-E524.

Chou R, Hasimoto R, Friedly J, et al. Pain management injection therapies for low back pain. Technology Assessment Report ESIB0813. (Prepared by the Pacific Northwest Evidence-based Practice Center under Contract No. HHSA 290-2012-00014-I). Rockville, MD: Agency for Healthcare Research and Quality; March 20, 2015. https://www.cms.gov/medicare/coverage/determinationprocess/downloads/id98TA.pdf

Chou R, Huffman L. Epidural corticosteroid injections for radiculopathy and spinal stenosis: a systematic review and meta-analysis. *Ann Intern Med.* 2015;163:373-381.

Lewis RA, Williams NH, Matar HE, et al. The clinical effectiveness and cost-effectiveness of management strategies for sciatica. *Health Technol Assess.* 2011;15(39):1-578.

Lewis RA, Williams NH, Sutton AJ, et al. Comparative clinical effectiveness of management strategies for sciatica. *Spine J.* 2015;15(6):1461-1477.

Manchikanti L, Knezevic N, Boswell M, et al. Epidural Injections for lumbar radiculopathy and spinal stenosis: a comparative systematic review and meta-analysis. *Pain Physician.* 2016;19:E365-E410.

Mandel S, Schilling J, Peterson E, et al. A retrospective analysis of vertebral body fractures following epidural steroid injections. *J Bone Joint Surg Am.* 2013;95(11):961-964.

Rabinovitch DL, Peliowski A, Furlan AD. Influence of lumbar epidural injection volume on pain relief for radicular leg pain and/or low back pain. *Spine J.* 2009;9(6):509-517.

15 Radiofrequency Procedures for Chronic Pain

David E. Jamison and Steven P. Cohen

I. TYPES OF RFA
II. FACET JOINTS
III. SACROILIAC JOINT
IV. DORSAL ROOT GANGLIA
V. HIP
VI. KNEE
VII. OCCIPITAL NERVES
VIII. TRIGEMINAL NERVE
IX. SYMPATHETIC GANGLIA
X. CONCLUSIONS

In the field of pain management, radiofrequency ablation (RFA) refers to a range of procedures intended to interrupt afferent pain transmission by a specific nerve or ganglion. A radiofrequency generator is used to direct heat via a probe to thermally denature the target structure. The procedure is most typically performed after successful diagnostic or prognostic blockade with local anesthetic. Originally described for use in cordotomy (lesioning of ascending pain pathways in the spinal cord), the evolving use of radiofrequency allows its application to an increasing number of peripheral nerves, ganglia, and neural plexuses. The primary benefit of RFA over steroid-based injections is the potential for significantly longer-lasting relief. The supporting literature as a whole is mixed with more commonly performed RFA procedures being commensurately more studied and generally better supported by evidence.

I. TYPES OF RFA

Traditional, or continuous, RFA utilizes a high-frequency alternating current to achieve temperatures ranging from 60°C to 90°C and is typically performed for 90-180 seconds per site. The high temperatures associated with continuous RFA cause local tissue and neural destruction. Accordingly, continuous RFA is not generally suitable for use on neural structures that contain both sensory and motor function, and care must be taken during needle placement to avoid transmission of heat to nearby structures. Sensory and motor testing are considered by most experts to be necessary when performing continuous RFA given its high temperature, though some organizations claim that sensory and/or motor testing is not necessary if proper imaging is performed. Sensory testing suggests placement of the probe in proximity to the targeted structure, while motor testing confirms that the probe is not too close to nearby motor nerves. Local anesthetic is usually injected once appropriate probe placement is confirmed to lessen the pain associated with heating and enhance lesion size (known as "fluid amplification"). Some clinicians use a dilute steroid solution after heating to decrease postprocedure pain and neuritis. One study has shown that injecting steroid before heating can decrease lesion size.

Pulsed RF is primarily used for neuropathic pain. The rationale for pulsed RF is that by definition, neuropathic pain involves an injury or disease affecting the somatosensory system and cutting a nerve will inevitably lead to increased nerve damage, which may result in spontaneous pain from the ectopic discharge of neuromas, or deafferentation pain depending on the type of sensory nerve affected. Pulsed RF was first described in the mid-1990s and involves the use of a gated frequency to deliver bursts of energy. The pause between pulses of RF delivery allows for dissipation of heat; therefore, pulsed RF generates temperatures between 40°C and 42°C. Pulsed RF is usually performed for 120 seconds per site, and up to three cycles are utilized. The mechanism by which pulsed RF exerts a therapeutic effect is unclear, given that it operates at a temperature below the threshold for neural coagulation. It is thought to be related to the rapidly switching electrical field generated, alterations in gene expression, and enhancement of descending modulation systems. Pulsed RF preferentially affects the small nociceptive fibers in sensory nerves and is considered safe to use on nerves with a motor component or in close proximity to heat-sensitive structures.

Water-cooled RFA is one of the newer types of RFA. It is also used for tumor ablation. The probes used for cooled RFA have a hollow lumen through which water is circulated, thereby allowing constant cooling of the probe tip, which prevents local tissue charring and maintains low impedance in the area being treated. This allows improved transmission of heat, and studies have demonstrated creation of a larger lesion when compared to traditional RFA, although the clinical significance of this remains unclear. Water-cooled RFA probes achieve a temperature of 60°C at the site of the thermistor, but higher more distally from the electrode; heat is generally applied for at least 2½ minutes per site. Water-cooled RFA creates a circular lesion that extends beyond the probe tip, whereas continuous RFA creates a lesion along the side of the probe active tip that does not extend significantly beyond its tip. For this reason, a cooled electrode tip is located 2 mm proximal from where the stylet was located, which has implications for sensory and motor testing.

Introducer needles for all variants of RFA are similar in that they are composed of an insulated shaft and a noninsulated, or "active," tip. The active tip ranges from 3 mm to more than 10 mm and allows for the precise delivery of thermal energy to the distal end of the needle, not along its entire length. RF probe gauge and length must be matched to the introducer needle for proper functioning of the RF generator.

The potential complications of RFA include those of other pain interventions, such as infection, bleeding, and direct trauma to adjacent structures. The primary risks specific to RFA involve burns and the inadvertent ablation of nontargeted neural structures, such as a spinal nerve, which could lead to permanent neurological deficits. This latter risk is mitigated with adherence to proper probe placement, motor testing, and the avoidance of heavy sedation.

II. FACET JOINTS

The most common application of RFA is for the treatment of pain arising from the zygapophysial joints, also known as the facet joints, of the spine. The facet joints are innervated by the medial branch nerves, which arise from the posterior primary rami of their respective spinal nerves at each level. Pain is transmitted via the medial branch at the affected level, as well as that of the nerve arising at the level immediately superior, that is, the L4-L5 facet joint is innervated by the medial branches of L3 and L4. With the exception of L5, each medial branch innervates two consecutive facet joints, such that three consecutive medial branch nerves must be ablated to denervate two adjacent facet joints and two medial branch nerves must be ablated to completely block pain at a single level. RFA of the medial branches is typically performed after positive results are obtained from "diagnostic" blocks with local anesthetic. Medial branch blocks have been demonstrated to be more predictive of success with RFA than intra-articular facet joint injections. Sensory testing provides assurance that the probe is in close proximity to the medial branch, and motor testing assures that the probe is not too close to the exiting nerve root. Probe placement must be adjusted if muscle contractions are noted in an ipsilateral limb during motor stimulation or if the patient reports pain in the distal limb during RFA.

The anatomic locations of the posterior primary rami and medial branches vary with the region of the spine. The cervical medial branch nerves course posteriorly over the lateral masses of the C3-C7 vertebrae. The position of the medial branches is somewhat predictable and allows for placement of an RF probe in parallel with the nerve, which maximizes the amount of nerve susceptible to lesioning. At some levels, for example, C4 and C5, there are two medial branches innervating the facet joints. A posterior approach is typically used to direct a probe to the mediolateral border of the affected lateral mass, then the introducer is advanced slightly from a view lateral to the patient (see Figs. 15.1 and 15.2). The posterior primary rami of the C1, C2, and C3 spinal nerves give rise to the suboccipital (C1), greater and lesser occipital (C2 and C3) nerves. Ablation of these nerves is typically not performed for axial neck pain and is discussed in a separate section below. The third occipital nerve (TON) is the larger of the two medial branches arising from C3 and, unlike other spinal levels, provides the sole innervation to the C2-C3 facet joint.

The literature supporting cervical RFA is sparse. The 1996 randomized, sham-controlled trial (RCT) by Lord et al. showed significant improvement with RFA compared to sham RF but was conducted in only 24 patients with whiplash who underwent three diagnostic blocks. The 2004 RCT by Stovner et al. showed significant relief with RFA, but the

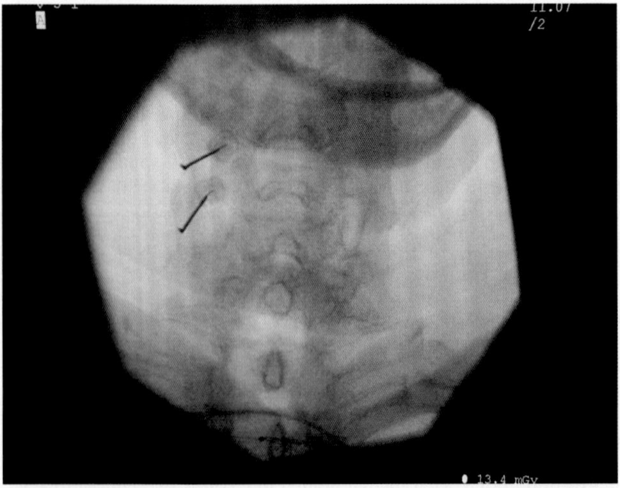

FIGURE 15.1 Anterior-posterior fluoroscopic view demonstrating probe placement for ablation of cervical medial branch nerves at C5 and C6.

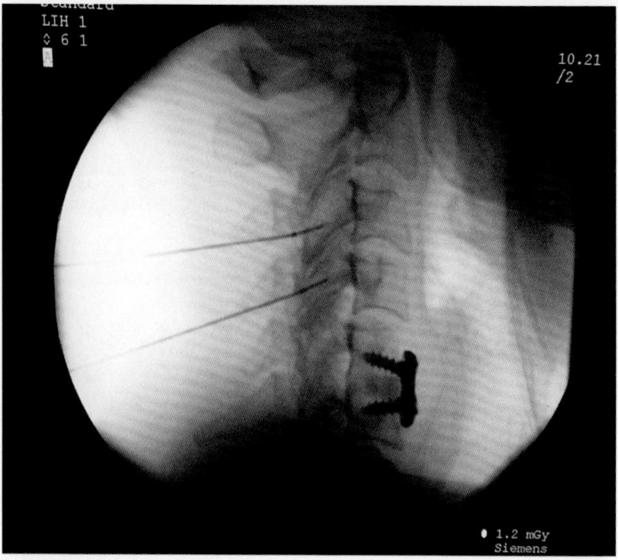

FIGURE 15.2 Lateral fluoroscopic view demonstrating probe placement for ablation of cervical medial branch nerves at C3 and C4.

study contained only 12 patients who underwent RFA regardless of their response to diagnostic blocks, and the primary outcome measure was improvement in cervicogenic headache. Aside from these trials, the bulk of evidence is in the form of positive, uncontrolled studies.

Thoracic medial branch anatomy is more variable than that of the cervical and lumbar regions. The upper thoracic (T1-T4) and low-mid-thoracic (T9-T10) medial branches are typically found at the superolateral corner of the transverse process (see Fig. 15.3). Mid-thoracic (T5-T8) medial branches may be suspended in the intertransverse space but then course over the medial transverse process. The lower thoracic medial branches cross the transverse process more medially in a fashion similar to that found in the lumbar region.

Mid-back pain occurs less frequently than neck or low-back pain, and accordingly, thoracic RFA has been less studied than its cervical and lumbar counterparts. High-quality randomized trials are lacking, and the evidence for performing thoracic RFA is mainly gleaned from prospective studies that have combined results of RFA done in all three regions of the spine.

The lumbar medial branches are uniform from L1 to L4 and can be ablated at the neck of the superior articulating process. An oblique, cephalad fluoroscopic view is typically used to direct an introducer needle to the superior portion of the lamina-transverse process junction parallel to the target nerve (see Fig. 15.4). The dorsal ramus of L5 is longer than those of higher lumbar levels and runs along the groove between the superior articulating process and the ala of the sacrum. For L5, the target nerve is the dorsal ramus itself, rather than the medial branch.

Most, but not all, RCTs have shown short- and long-term improvement with lumbar RFA when compared to sham treatment. In the past

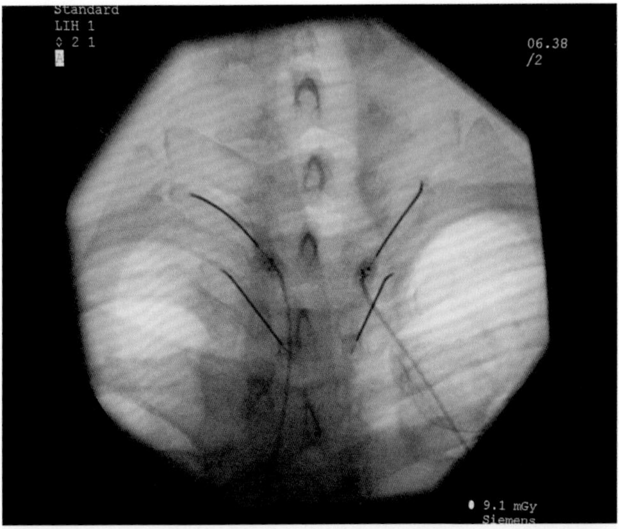

FIGURE 15.3 Anterior-posterior fluoroscopic view demonstrating probe placement for bilateral T1 and T2 medial branch denervation. Note that upper and mid-thoracic medial branches are located more laterally on the transverse process.

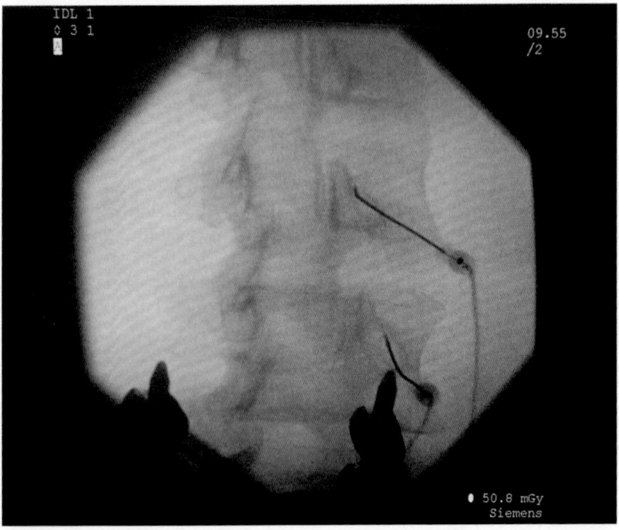

FIGURE 15.4 Oblique fluoroscopic view demonstrating probe placement for right-sided lumbar medial branch L3 and L4 denervation. Note the electrode placement parallel to the course of the nerves.

few years, several high-profile studies have arrived at conflicting conclusions. The 2017 MINT comparative-effectiveness trial by Juch et al. was a combination of three trials researching RFA of the lumbar facet joints, the sacroiliac joints, and a combination of the facet joints, sacroiliac joints, and intervertebral discs. In each group, an exercise program alone was compared to exercise plus RFA, with patients allowed to continue analgesics and receive psychotherapy as indicated. This study found nonstatistically significant benefits in favor of the RFA group for all three studies and was widely criticized on methodological (eg, they excluded patients over 70 years old who are more likely to suffer from facet arthropathy, over 70% of patients had positive diagnostic facet and sacroiliac joint blocks, and patients in all three studies had longer durations of pain), technical (the authors used small electrodes, which were placed perpendicular to the nerves), and statistical grounds. The 2018 FACTS trial by Cohen et al. was a double-blind, two-phase study in which intra-articular facet injections with local anesthetic and steroids were compared to medial branch blocks and saline control injections for therapeutic and prognostic value before RFA. The authors found no meaningful therapeutic benefit for intra-articular or medial branch blocks but reported that those who obtained positive diagnostic medial branch intra-articular facet blocks fared better after RFA than those who received a saline control injection. The authors concluded that these results showed that facet blocks have prognostic value and that the superior RFA results in the two treatment groups indirectly support the efficacy of lumbar medial branch RFA. In addition to the aforementioned RCTs, multiple observational studies have shown good therapeutic effect with lumbar RFA, with follow-up periods extending out several years with repeat procedures.

III. SACROILIAC JOINT

In addition to the medial branch nerves, the posterior primary rami also give rise to the intermediate and lateral branch nerves. In more cephalad portions of the spine, the lateral branches innervate the paraspinal muscles, but in the sacral region, they mainly transmit pain sensation from the sacroiliac joint and are thus a target for RFA. The position of the lateral branches is highly variable, to include differences between levels and even sides of the same patient. There is some discrepancy regarding the appropriate levels to target for RFA of the sacroiliac joint, but the prevailing method calls for ablation of the L5 medial branch in addition to the lateral branches from S1 to S3 and sometimes S4. There is significant variation in innervation patterns based on cadaveric studies, but the literature suggests that the L4 medial branch may infrequently innervate the upper portion of the sacroiliac joint in people with a sacralized L5. The S4 lateral branch supplies the lower joint in around 25% of people. Studies performed in volunteers have found that the lateral branches innervate the posterior sacroiliac joint ligaments rather than the capsule, suggesting it may be more effective in younger individuals with periarticular joint pain. The lateral branches are generally found lateral to the sacral foramina, and course to the sacroiliac joint, but their precise location in relation to the foramina varies. At each spinal level, there may multiple lateral branches, which typically range in number from 1 to 4. This suggests the need for a more aggressive lesioning strategy than for facetogenic pain. Water-cooled RFA (or other methods such as bipolar lesioning) to enhance lesion size has become the method of choice given its ability to create larger lesions that extend beyond the active tip of the probe and hence reduce the likelihood

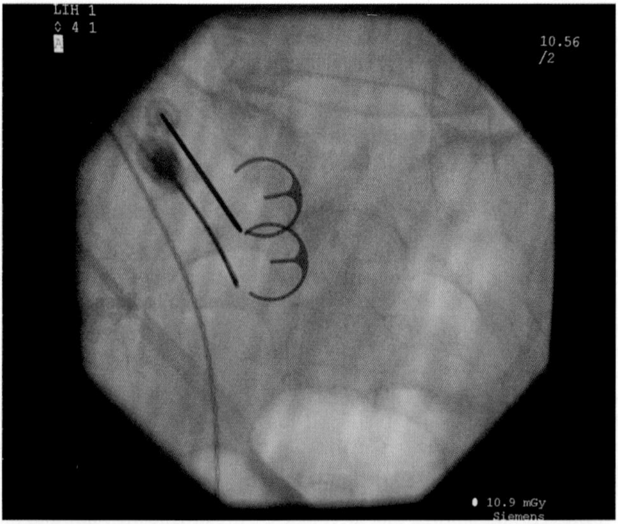

FIGURE 15.5 Anterior-posterior fluoroscopic view demonstrating probe placement for lateral branch water-cooled denervation. These lesions represent the most caudal of 3 lesions performed at the S1 and S2 levels.

of technical failure but require the creation of three lesions in an arc lateral to each foramen (see Fig. 15.5). Alternatively, a traditional RFA probe may be sequentially placed in a caudad-cephalad direction from a shallow angle to position the length of its active tip vertically along the sacrum lateral to each foramen, thereby creating a longitudinal strip lesion. A third method for lateral branch RFA involves placement of a proprietary curved RF wand that covers the distance between the S1 and S4 foramina and allows creation of a strip of monopolar and bipolar lesions along its length. Given the variable position of the lateral branches, similar to cooled and bipolar RF, this latter method theoretically increases the chance that the lesioned area will contain the targeted nerves, though a recent small, methodologically flawed, randomized study failed to demonstrate efficacy.

The evidence for traditional RFA of the lateral branches is limited. One randomized, comparative-effectiveness study performed in patients with ankylosing spondylitis showed that bipolar RFA was superior to celecoxib, and two retrospective studies comparing cooled to traditional RF were split as to whether cooled RF was superior. Cooled RFA for SIJ pain has been the subject of more extensive research, with two placebo-controlled trials demonstrating good, long-term (>6 months) outcomes.

IV. DORSAL ROOT GANGLIA

Dorsal root ganglia (DRG) contain the cell bodies of afferent sensory neurons and have emerged as a target for RF treatment of radicular limb pain. The DRG is located in the dorsal aspect of the neuroforamen and can be targeted with the aid of fluoroscopy in a manner akin to performing a selective nerve root block. Pulsed RF is usually performed after successful results are obtained from segmental selective nerve root blocks to accurately identify the spinal level associated with radicular pain. The most common treatment for radicular pain remains the epidural steroid injection (ESI), but pulsed RF of the DRG offers the possibility of longer-term pain relief.

The literature on pulsed RF of the DRG is modest. There is compelling evidence supporting the antinociceptive effects of pulsed RF in multiple animal models of neuropathic pain, and though a majority of clinical trials have yielded positive results, most tend to be small and methodologically flawed. Most available RCTs that compared pulsed RF to sham showed significant benefit in the RF group. Whereas some RCTs performed in individuals with radicular pain have shown results similar to control groups that received ESIs, others have shown better results with a combination of pulsed RF plus ESI or with combined continuous and pulsed RF. Preclinical studies and a clinical study examining pulsed RF outcomes in patients with postthoracotomy pain suggest that targeting the DRG may afford better results than treating a peripheral nerve. Given the generally good results shown with pulsed RF in neuropathic pain conditions, it is prudent to avoid conventional RFA in nerves that contain motor and nonpain sensory fibers.

V. HIP

Pain from the hip joint is transmitted via the articular branches of the obturator, femoral, sciatic, and gluteal nerves. The obturator and femoral branches innervate the anterior and superior portions of the joint, while the branches of the sciatic and gluteal nerves innervate its posterior portion. The articular branches of the obturator and femoral nerves contribute a majority of the pain sensation from the hip, and their position in the anterior joint space makes them more amenable to local anesthetic blockade and RF treatment. Accordingly, targeting these nerves with RF has emerged as a treatment for patients not deriving benefit from intra-articular corticosteroid injections or who are poor surgical candidates. Cadaveric studies have shown the number and position of the articular branches to be variable, with multiple branches per nerve coursing to the hip joint. The branches of the obturator nerve are found in a band across the anterior surface of the inferior pubic ramus lateral to the obturator foramen. The articular branches of the femoral nerve enter the joint at the anterosuperior portion of the acetabulum. Placement of probes along the inferior pubic ramus adjacent to the inferior acetabulum and at the anterosuperior border of the acetabulum allows for RF treatment of the branches of the obturator and femoral nerves, respectively (see Fig. 15.6). RF treatments are usually performed after positive results are obtained from nerve blocks with local anesthetic.

Evidence supporting the use of RF for treatment of hip pain is favorable, but RCTs are lacking. Multiple prospective studies have shown positive results in patients who failed traditional therapy to include intra-articular corticosteroid injections, but most were in small numbers of patients. One prospective study compared RF to conservative therapy and showed superior benefit in the RF group, but the study was not blinded and patients chose their treatment modality. Both continuous and pulsed RF have been utilized with similar reported benefit, though in general, both preclinical and clinical evidence are scant for treating nociceptive pain conditions with pulsed RF.

VI. KNEE

The most recent application of RFA is the lesioning of three genicular nerves for treatment of knee pain, first described in 2011. The innervation of the knee joint can be divided into anterior and posterior groups. The anterior compartment is innervated by branches from (1) the femoral

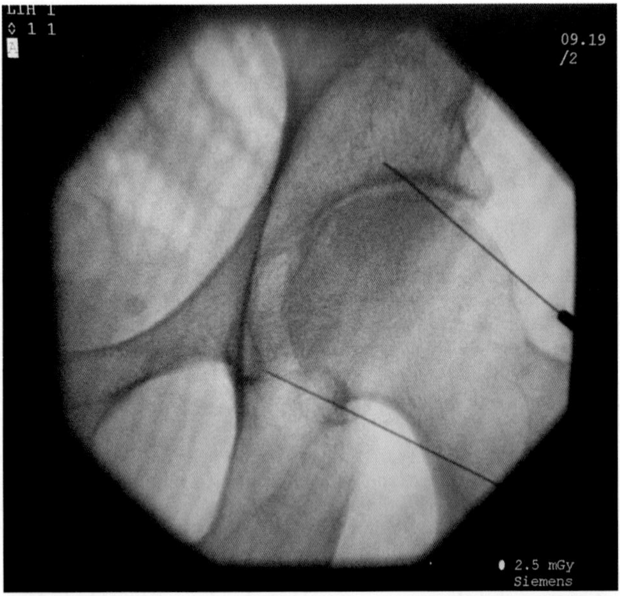

FIGURE 15.6 Anterior-posterior fluoroscopic view of the left hip demonstrating probe placement for denervation of the articular branches of the femoral and obturator nerves.

nerve, through branches to the vastus medialis, lateralis, and intermedius, as well as from the saphenous nerve branch, and (2) the common peroneal nerve, by its recurrent lateral retinacular branches. The posterior compartment is supplied by branches of the sciatic nerve, mainly its tibial branch, along with the posterior branch from the obturator nerve. According to the technique of Choi et al., the superior and inferior medial genicular nerves, which are branches of the tibial nerve, are ablated just proximal to the medial epicondyle of the femur and just distal to the medial epicondyle of the tibia, respectively. The superior lateral genicular nerve, a branch of the common peroneal nerve, is targeted in an area just proximal to the lateral epicondyle of the femur (see Figs. 15.7 and 15.8). RFA of these three genicular nerves allows blockade of some, but not all, of the afferent pain transmission from the knee joint. For example, several recent anatomical studies suggest that up to nine nerves should be targeted. In addition to the superior medial, superior lateral, and inferior medial genicular nerves, nerves to the vastus medialis, vastus lateralis, vastus intermedius (medial and lateral branches), infrapatellar branch of the saphenous nerve, recurrent fibular nerve, and the inferior lateral genicular nerves should be considered RFA targets in patients whose pain corresponds to these areas of innervation. For these reasons, some patients with true knee osteoarthritis who undergo successful ablation will fail to derive relief.

Support in the literature for a nonaggressive lesioning strategy is sparse given the recent advent of this RFA method. One small RCT ($N = 38$) by Choi et al. in which the superior medial, superior lateral, and inferior medial nerves were treated found significant improvement in pain, function, and patient satisfaction for up to 12 weeks with RFA vs sham. In addition to the small size, a significant flaw in this study is that the authors used

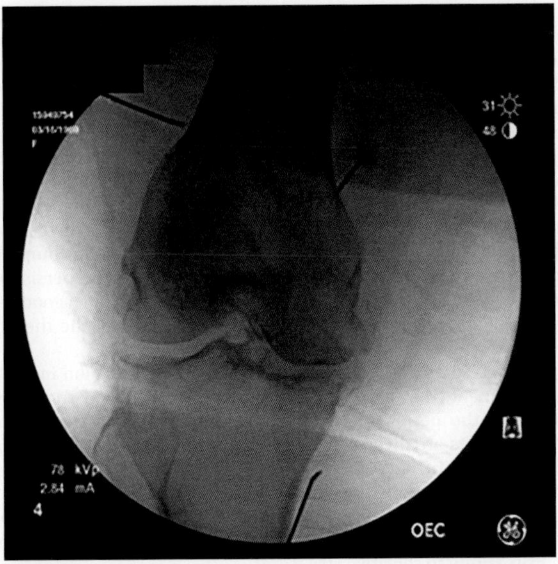

FIGURE 15.7 Anterior-posterior fluoroscopic view of the right knee demonstrating probe placement for genicular nerve denervation.

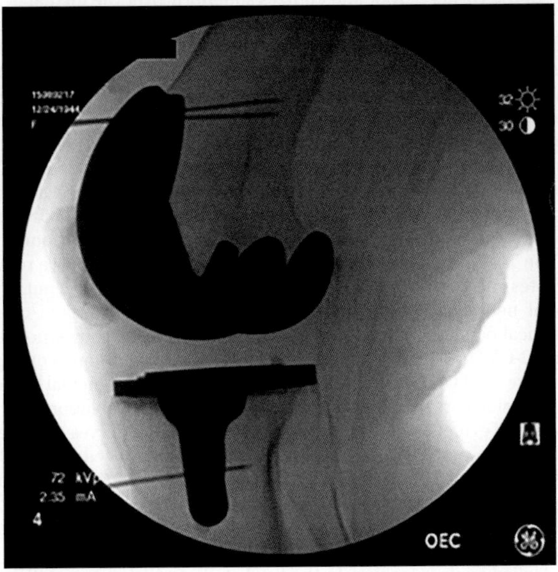

FIGURE 15.8 Lateral view of the knee demonstrating probe placement for genicular nerve denervation.

high volumes of local anesthetic (2 mL), relative to the size of the lesion they created with the small, 22-gauge electrodes and 70°C temperature utilized. However, two other RCTs targeted the same three nerves, one done in patients with persistent pain after knee arthroplasty and the other done preemptively in individuals scheduled to undergo knee arthroplasty, failed to demonstrate benefit. A nonrandomized, open-label controlled study performed in 35 patients compared RFA to local anesthetic nerve blocks of two nerves innervating the anterior segment of the knee joint: the intrapatellar branch of the saphenous nerve and the medial retinacular nerve, which is a terminal branch of the nerve supplying the vastus medialis muscle. This study found improvement in function in the RF group compared to the control group lasting 6 months and improvement in pain persisting for 3 months. Several case reports and case series have also shown good results with pulsed, conventional, and water-cooled RFA, though the theoretical basis for performing pulsed radiofrequency is unclear.

Although spine and knee pain remain the most common indications for RF treatment, thermal ablation has also been applied to numerous structures of the peripheral and sympathetic nervous systems. Peripheral nerve targets are diverse and include specific nerves or their sensory ganglia. Sympathetic nervous system targets include the stellate ganglion, lumbar sympathetic plexus, and splanchnic nerves. Pulsed RF is the preferred modality for many of these neural structures given their component of motor function, the presence of sensory nerves that could incur injury, or their proximity to sensitive structures.

VII. OCCIPITAL NERVES

The occipital nerve(s) can be a source of chronic neck pain and headaches. The greater occipital nerve (GON) is formed from the posterior primary ramus of the C2 nerve root and courses superiorly over the medial occiput from the base of the skull. The lesser occipital nerve (LON) is a terminal branch of the cervical plexus and usually is formed from contributions stemming from the C2 and C3 nerve roots. The LON innervates a cutaneous area of the head more lateral than that innervated by the GON. Since occipital neuralgia involves pain secondary to injury or entrapment of the occipital nerve(s), pulsed RF, which as noted above does not result in serious injury to neural architecture, is generally used to treat individuals who respond to diagnostic nerve blocks but fail to derive long-term benefit. Given the superficial and predictable courses of the GON and LON, pulsed RF may be performed using either sensory stimulation or ultrasound.

The TON is derived from the medial branch of the C3 nerve root and innervates the C2-C3 facet joint and an area of the lower occiput. Unlike occipital neuralgia that results from injury to the greater and/or LON, mechanical pain arising from C2-C3 is usually treated by conventional RFA at the C2-C3 facet joint interface, which is done using fluoroscopic guidance. Since the TON is much larger than the other cervical medial branches, multiple lesions are often performed to ensure adequate ablation.

Overall evidence for RF treatment of the occipital nerves is moderate. In addition to multiple case series, one large, randomized, double-blind study found pulsed RF to be superior to steroid injections for pain relief for up to 6 months in patients with occipital neuralgia with or without migraine. For third occipital headaches, although uncontrolled studies have demonstrated benefit with RF ablation, robust evidence in the form of controlled trials is lacking. In the Lord et al. study that found RFA to be superior to sham denervation in individuals with whiplash, patients with TON involvement were excluded from participation.

VIII. TRIGEMINAL NERVE

Facial pain presents a challenging clinical entity and can be difficult to treat. The trigeminal nerve transmits pain sensation from the face and is composed of three primary branches: the ophthalmic nerve (V1), the maxillary nerve (V2), and the mandibular nerve (V3). The three branches of the trigeminal nerve divide at the Gasserian ganglion within Meckel cave, and then each subdivides into multiple smaller branches. The mandibular nerve may be targeted with pulsed RF via a lateral, transcoronoid approach as it exits from the foramen ovale. The maxillary nerve can be targeted in the pterygopalatine fossa between the posterior border of the maxilla and the lateral pterygoid plate via a lateral, subzygomatic approach. The ophthalmic nerve's position within the skull precludes direct treatment with RF. Options for treatment of pain in a V1 distribution include targeting superficial tributaries of the ophthalmic nerve (eg, supraorbital or supratrochlear nerves) or treatment of the Gasserian ganglion itself by advancing an RF probed through the foramen ovale.

There are numerous, large case series, but no controlled studies supporting the use of RFA for either atypical facial pain or trigeminal neuralgia. Randomized studies have focused on the relative benefits of pulsed vs continuous RFA, and results are mixed with some studies showing equivalent improvement with each method but others showing better relief with continuous RFA. Conventional radiofrequency treatment for trigeminal neuralgia has become less common with the evolution of open neurosurgical decompression and external beam radiation treatments for many patients with this condition.

IX. SYMPATHETIC GANGLIA

As a group, the sympathetic ganglia are implicated in several chronic pain conditions, to include complex regional pain syndrome (CRPS), ischemic limb pain, and abdominal pain associated with malignancy. Blockade with local anesthetic can be therapeutic in some cases but can also be used to predict possible benefit with neurolysis. Some of the sympathetic ganglia, such as the celiac and superior hypogastric plexuses, have traditionally been chemically ablated with phenol or alcohol for abdominal and pelvic malignancies, but RFA of the lumbar sympathetic ganglia has also been employed to provide benefit for CRPS and other pain conditions in individuals with refractory, nonmalignant pain not associated with nerve injury. However, as noted above, the treatment of neuropathic pain conditions with neuroablative procedures may result in worsening pain after nerve regeneration and is considered controversial.

The stellate ganglion represents the fusion of the inferior cervical and upper thoracic sympathetic ganglia, which is present in 80% of individuals. It is located anterior to the transverse process of C7 and supplies sympathetic innervation to the head, neck, and arms. Both pulsed RF and RFA of the stellate ganglion have been performed for myriad neuropathic and nonneuropathic pain conditions, as well as posttraumatic stress disorder, with most studies reporting significant benefit. RF of the stellate ganglion can be performed by guiding an electrode to the anterior transverse process of C6 or C7 under fluoroscopic, computed tomography or ultrasound guidance. The vertebral artery lies within the transverse foramen at C6 but is usually unprotected at C7; hence, some experts consider the procedure safer to perform at C6 given the lower risk of intravascular injection of local anesthetic or arterial needle trauma. Although RF treatments of the stellate ganglion block are supported by favorable results in several prospective and retrospective reports, no RCTs have been performed. One randomized study that compared stellate ganglion block to RFA in patients with CRPS found significantly better pain relief in the RFA group lasting up to 2 years.

The splanchnic nerves converge in the celiac plexus and play a role in transmission of visceral pain from the upper abdomen. The celiac plexus's large area, and variable position surrounding the aorta at roughly the T11-T12 level, makes it a poor target for RF, but the splanchnic nerves originate in the retrocrural space, making them more amenable to RFA. Literature on this technique is exceedingly sparse, but one prospective study in patients with pain from chronic pancreatitis showed significant improvement in all 10 subjects.

The lumbar sympathetic chain may extend from L1 to L5, but the most common locations of the ganglia are between L2 and L4. The ganglia can be blocked with local anesthetic at one or more locations, which may provide diagnostic information (ie, is the pain sympathetically maintained?), alleviate pain and facilitate rehabilitation, and serve as a prognostic treatment before neurolysis, which has been shown to provide benefit in several uncontrolled studies. Two small, comparative-effectiveness studies compared phenol neurolysis to RF ablation in patients with CRPS, with one finding no difference between treatments and the other finding that phenol neurolysis was superior. Considering that the lumbar sympathetic ganglia vary significantly in number, spinal levels, and their location in relation to the vertebral bodies and that the lesions produced by RFA are much smaller in scope than the area affected by phenol injection, one might surmise that phenol neurolysis would provide better results.

X. CONCLUSIONS

Radiofrequency treatments represent a diverse array of interventions targeting pain in numerous anatomic locations. The most common application of RF remains the treatment of spine pain arising from the facet joints via ablation of the nociceptive afferent nerves, but the relative safety of pulsed RF has allowed the expansion of RF treatment to virtually any neural structure, particularly those associated with neuropathic pain. The quality of supporting evidence varies widely, mostly in proportion to the frequency with which a given RF treatment is performed. Among the RF applications herein discussed, only four (cooled RFA of the SIJ, pulsed RF of the DRG, pulsed RF of the GON, and RFA of the lumbar medial branches) are supported by high-quality RCTs. However, given their favorable side effect profile and potential for providing sustained pain relief, RF treatments should be entertained when positive results are obtained from prognostic blockade of neural structures with local anesthetic.

Selected Readings

Bhatia A, Peng P, Cohen S. Radiofrequency procedures to relieve chronic knee pain: an evidence-based narrative review. *Reg Anesth Pain Med.* 2016;41(4):501-510.

Choi J, Hwang J, Song G, et al. Radiofrequency treatment relieves chronic knee osteoarthritis pain: a double-blind randomized controlled trial. *Pain.* 2011;152(3): 481-487.

Chye C, Liang C, Lu K, Chen Y, Liliang P. Pulsed radiofrequency treatment of articular branches of femoral and obturator nerves for chronic hip pain. *Clin Interv Aging.* 2015;10:569-574.

Cohen S, Huang J, Brummett C. Facet joint pain—advances in patient selection and management. *Nat Rev Rheumatol.* 2013;9(2):101-116.

Cohen S, Hurley R, Buckenmaier C III, Kurihara C, Morlando B, Dragovich A. Randomized placebo-controlled study evaluating lateral branch radio frequency denervation for sacroiliac joint pain. *Anesthesiology.* 2008;109(2):279-288.

Cohen SP, Bhaskar A, Bhatia A, et al. Consensus practice guidelines on interventions for lumbar facet joint pain from an international, multispecialty working group. *Reg Anesth Pain Med.* 2020. pii: rapm-2019-101243. doi:10.1136/rapm-2019-101243. [Epub ahead of print].

Koh W, Choi S, Karm M, et al. Treatment of chronic lumbosacral radicular pain using adjuvant pulsed radio frequency: a randomized controlled study. *Pain Med.* 2015;16(3):432-441.

Lord S, Barnsley L, Wallis B, McDonald G, Bogduk N. Percutaneous radiofrequency neurotomy for chronic cervical zygapophyseal-joint pain. *N Engl J Med.* 1996;335(23):1721-1726.

Nath S, Nath CA, Pettersson K. Percutaneous lumbar zygapophysial (Facet) joint neurotomy using radiofrequency current, in the management of chronic low back pain: a randomized double-blind trial. *Spine (Phila Pa 1976).* 2008;33(12): 1291-1297.

Patel N, Gross A, Brown L, Gekht G. A randomized, placebo-controlled study to assess the efficacy of lateral branch neurotomy for chronic sacroiliac joint pain. *Pain Med.* 2012;13(3):383-398.

van Kleef M, Barendse G, Kessels A, Voets H, Weber W, de Lange S. Randomized trial of radiofrequency lumbar facet denervation for chronic low back pain. *Spine (Phila Pa 1976).* 1999;24(18):1937-1942.

Van Zundert J, Patijn J, Kessels A, Lamé I, van Suijlekom H, van Kleef M. Pulsed radiofrequency adjacent to the cervical dorsal root ganglion in chronic cervical radicular pain: a double blind sham controlled randomized clinical trial. *Pain.* 2007;127(1-2):173-182.

16 Sympathetic Blocks

Christopher Gilligan
and Divya Chirumamilla

I. LUMBAR SYMPATHETIC BLOCK

The sympathetic nervous system is involved in the pathophysiology of several different chronic pain conditions, including complex regional pain syndrome (CRPS) and ischemic limb pain. In some patients, these chronic pain states represent sympathetically mediated pain. Lumbar sympathetic block (LSB) is an established method for the diagnosis and treatment of sympathetically mediated pain of the lower extremities. The local anesthetic block can produce marked pain relief of long duration and is used as part of a comprehensive treatment plan to provide analgesia and facilitate functional restoration in patients with CRPS. Patients with peripheral vascular insufficiency due to small vessel occlusion can also be treated effectively with LSBs.

The American Society of Anesthesiologists (ASA) Task Force on Chronic Pain Management published a 2010 Practice Guideline on recommendations regarding sympathetic blocks: "The use of sympathetic blocks may be considered to support the diagnosis of sympathetically mediated pain. They should not be used to predict the outcome of surgical, chemical, or radiofrequency sympathectomy." It recommended that LSBs be used as components of the multimodal treatment of CRPS.

A. Anatomy

The lumbar sympathetic chain is comprised of two to five paired ganglia containing both pre- and postganglionic fibers which project to the lower limbs and pelvis. The ganglia are frequently located along the anterolateral aspect of the inferior one-third of the L2 vertebrae, L2-L3 disc space, and superior third of the L3 vertebrae (Fig. 16.1). The cell bodies of the neurons that travel to the lumbar sympathetic ganglia lie in the anterolateral region of the spinal cord from T11 to L2, with variable contributions from T10 to L3.

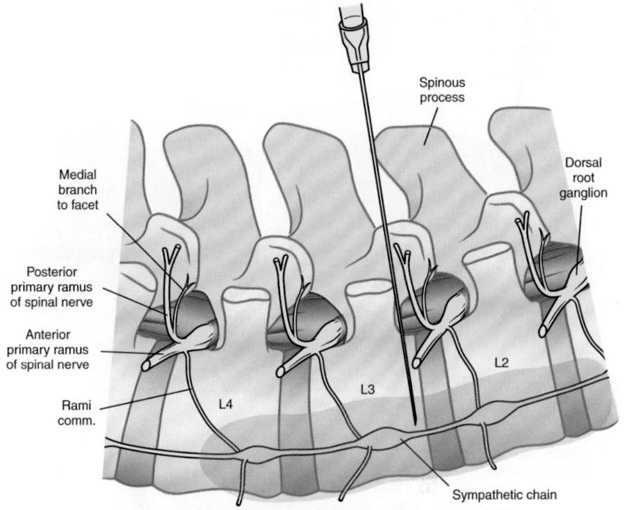

FIGURE 16.1 Lumbar sympathetic block. (From Lumbar sympathetic block and neurolysis. In: Rathmell JP. *Atlas of Image-Guided Intervention in Regional Anesthesia and Pain Medicine.* Philadelphia, PA: Wolters Kluwer 2012:176-186.)

The preganglionic fibers leave the spinal canal with the corresponding spinal nerve, join the sympathetic chain as white rami communicantes, and then synapse with the appropriate ganglion. The postganglionic fibers exit the chain to join the diffuse perivascular plexus around the iliac and femoral arteries or via the gray rami communicantes to join the spinal nerves that form the lumbar and lumbosacral plexus. The sympathetic and somatic nerves are separated by the psoas muscle and fascia.

B. Indications

The indications for lumbar sympathetic nerve blocks (LSB) include the sympathetically mediated pain syndromes CRPS type 1 and 2, neuropathic lower limb pain, acute herpes zoster infection, Raynaud phenomenon, hyperhidrosis, frostbite, vascular insufficiency, and rectal tenesmus secondary to cancer.

C. Technique

The most commonly used technique is a fluoroscopically guided paradiscal approach that requires the patient be placed in a prone position with a pillow under the lower abdomen and iliac crest to reduce lumbar lordosis. The fluoroscope is then used to identify the L2, L3, and L4 levels. Subsequently the L2-L3 disc space is squared, thereby avoiding the segmental artery and vein which tend to lie anterior to the middle third of the vertebral body. The fluoroscope is then rotated ipsilateral oblique, such that the L3 transverse process overlies the L3 vertebral body (typically 20-30 degrees). The skin and subcutaneous tissues are anesthetized with 1-2 mL of 1% lidocaine. A 22-gauge 5- to 7-in spinal needle (7-8 in for obese patients) is advanced coaxially toward the anterolateral aspect of the L3 body. The needle should be kept over the lateral margin of the vertebral body until bone is gently contacted. An anterior-posterior (AP) view is used to confirm contact

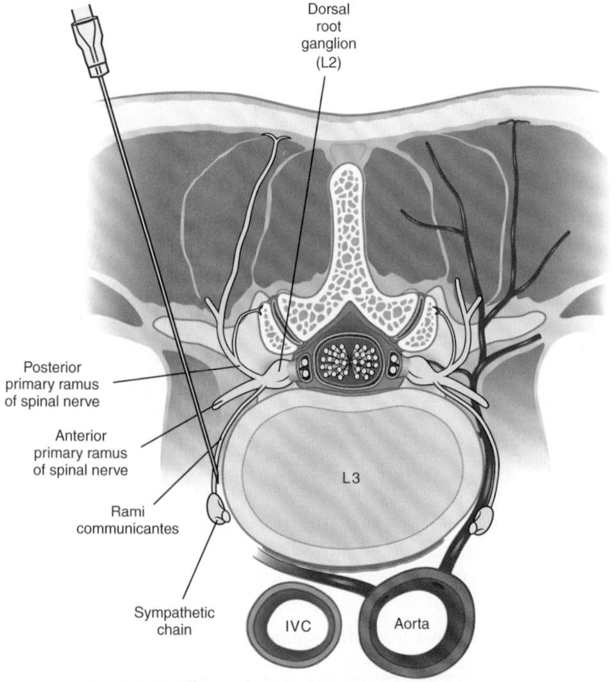

FIGURE 16.2 Axial diagram of lumbar sympathetic block. A single needle passes over the transverse process, and the tip is in position adjacent to the lumbar sympathetic ganglia over the anteromedial surface of the L3 vertebral body. (From Lumbar sympathetic block and neurolysis. In: Rathmell JP. *Atlas of Image-Guided Intervention in Regional Anesthesia and Pain Medicine*. Philadelphia, PA: Wolters Kluwer 2012:176-186.)

with the vertebral body rather than the transverse process. In the lateral view the spinal needle is advanced to the anterior one-third of the vertebral body. Proper needle position is verified in the AP projection, where the needle tip should lie medial to the lateral margin of the vertebral body (Figs. 16.2-16.4). Once the needle is in position, aspiration to detect intravascular needle placement is carried out followed by confirmation with contrast injection (iohexol 180 mg/mL or its equivalent). Then incremental injection of local anesthetic (15-20 mL of 0.25% bupivacaine) or 10% phenol or 50%-100% ethyl alcohol in the case of a neurolytic block is administered.

Signs of successful sympathetic blockade in the lower extremities include venodilation and skin temperature rise (monitored in both lower extremities). A rise of temperature of 1°C without rise in the temperature in the contralateral limb should be considered as a successful sympathetic block.

D. Complications

Significant and potentially toxic levels of local anesthetic can result from placement of the needle into a blood vessel and intravascular injection during a LSB.

Genitofemoral nerve injury or so-called L1 neuralgia can result from LSB neurolysis. There is sparse evidence in the literature regarding

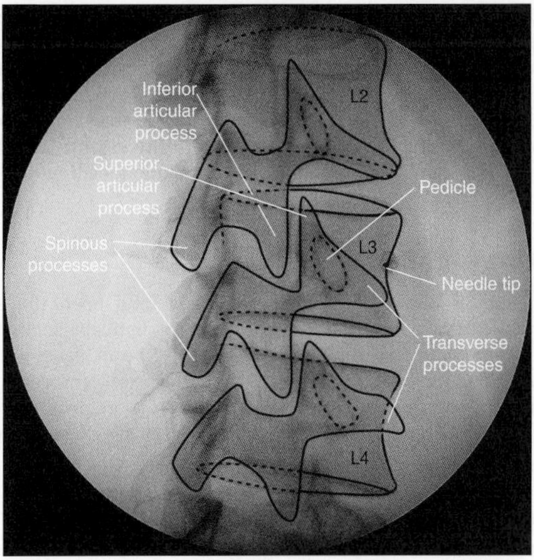

FIGURE 16.3 Oblique radiograph of the lumbar spine during lumbar sympathetic block. A needle passes cephalad to the transverse process of L3 to lie anterolateral to the L3 vertebral body. (From Lumbar sympathetic block and neurolysis. In: Rathmell JP. *Atlas of Image-Guided Intervention in Regional Anesthesia and Pain Medicine.* Philadelphia, PA: Wolters Kluwer 2012:176-186.)

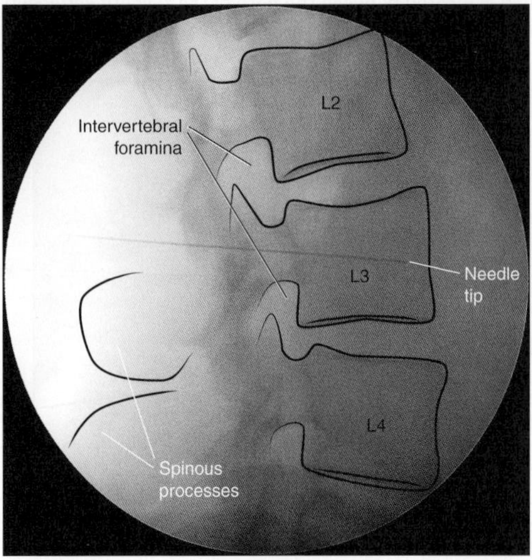

FIGURE 16.4 Lateral radiograph of the lumbar spine during lumbar sympathetic block. A needle is in position over the anterolateral surface of L3. The tip should be positioned over the anterior one-third of the vertebral body in the lateral projection. Note that the foramen and thus the spinal nerve are distant from the path of the needle. (From Lumbar sympathetic block and neurolysis. In: Rathmell JP. *Atlas of Image-Guided Intervention in Regional Anesthesia and Pain Medicine.* Philadelphia, PA: Wolters Kluwer 2012:176-186.)

the incidence of genitofemoral neuralgia postneurolytic LSB, but rates are typically quoted between 5% and 7%. There is evidence to support decreased incidence when targeted LSB at L2 is performed. Intrathecal or epidural injection is also possible particularly when needle placement is at the midvertebral level; local anesthetic solution may travel posteriorly into a tunnel beneath the dense fascia where the segmental artery and vein are located. Additional complications include bleeding and perforation of viscera.

II. STELLATE GANGLION BLOCK

Stellate ganglion block (SGB) (Fig. 16.5) has long been the standard approach to diagnosis and treatment of sympathetically mediated pain syndromes involving the upper extremity (CRPS) and neuropathic pain syndromes including ischemic neuropathies, herpes zoster, early postherpetic neuralgia, and postradiation neuritis. SGB is therefore an established method for diagnosis and treatment of sympathetically maintained pain of the head, neck, and upper extremity.

A. Anatomy

Four bilateral cervical sympathetic ganglia are anatomically identifiable; blockade of the superior, middle, and intermediate cervical ganglia typically produces inconsistent and incomplete blockade to the head and neck secondary to variable course of sympathetic fibers, as well as inconsistent anatomical position; this makes them of little value in the management of sympathetically mediated pain. In 70%-80% of the population, the inferior cervical ganglia and first thoracic ganglia are fused to form the stellate ganglion, which is located between the base of the seventh cervical transverse process and first rib, lateral to the longus colli muscle, and posterior to

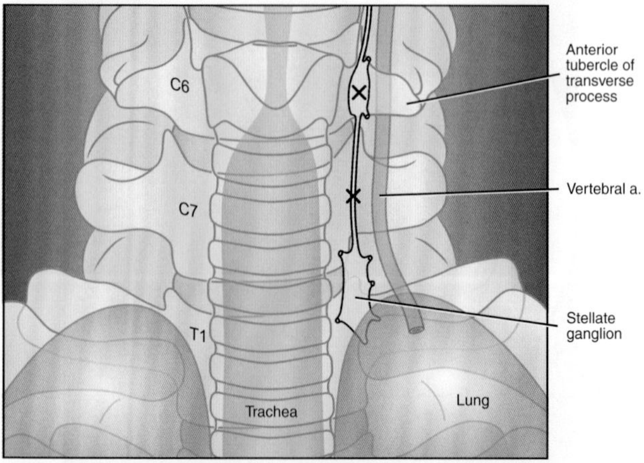

FIGURE 16.5 Anatomy of the stellate ganglion. The stellate ganglion lies over the head of the first rib at the junction of the transverse process and the uncinate process of the T1. It is posteromedial to the cupola of the lung and media to the vertebral artery. The stellate ganglion block is typically carried out at the C6 or C7 levels to avoid a pneumothorax. The *X*s mark the target for needle placement when performing a stellate ganglion block either at C6 or C7. (From Stellate ganglion block. In: Rathmell JP, ed. *Atlas of Image-Guided Intervention in Regional Anesthesia and Pain Medicine*. Philadelphia, PA: Wolters Kluwer 2012:152–161.)

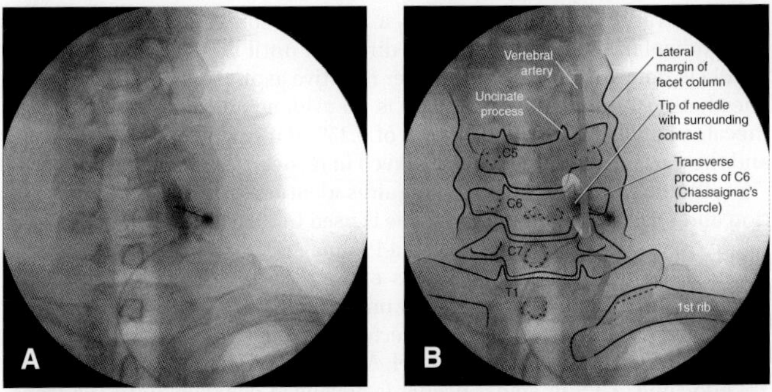

FIGURE 16.6 A. PA radiograph of the cervical spine during stellate ganglion block at C6. The needle is in position at the junction of the C6 transverse process and the vertebral body, just inferior to the uncinate process of C6. Radiographic contrast has been injected and spreads along the anterolateral surface of C6 to reach the adjacent vertebra. **B.** The approximate position of the vertebral artery. (From Stellate ganglion block. In: Rathmell JP, ed. *Atlas of Image-Guided Intervention in Regional Anesthesia and Pain Medicine*. Philadelphia, PA: Wolters Kluwer 2012:152–161.)

the vertebral artery. The preganglionic sympathetic fibers for the head and neck arise from the upper five thoracic spinal nerves while the upper limb from T2 to T6 (Fig. 16.6).

B. Indications

The indications for SGB are similar to those of lumbar sympathetic nerve block which include CRPS types I and II, vascular insufficiency, hyperhidrosis, acute herpes zoster, and frostbite. Additional indications include accidental intra-arterial injection of a drug, cardiac arrhythmia, angina, vascular headache, and facial pain.

C. Technique

Several approaches to SGB are well described in the literature with success rates ranging from 15% to 100%. Success is defined as achieving a chosen temperature threshold typically a temperature increase in the ipsilateral hand of between 1°C and 3°C. It should be noted that development of a Horner syndrome while indicative of cephalic sympathetic block does not signify sympathetic interruption of the arm at the C6 level. Generally the C7 level is considered to be the preferred level for SGB due to its closer proximity to the ganglion; however, at this level, the vertebral artery is uncovered in contrast to C6 where the artery travels posterior to Chassaignac tubercle. If this level is chosen, care must be taken to maintain a more medial needle position on the transverse process.

The non–image-guided technique requires a comprehensive understanding of neck anatomy. After application of standard monitors, the patient is placed in a supine position facing directly forward with a pillow under the upper back and lower neck to hold the neck in slight extension. The cricoid cartilage is palpated to identify the C6 level. The skin crease caudal to the thyroid corresponds to the C6 transverse process in 71% of cases and can be used as an additional landmark. Subsequently Chassaignac tubercle at C6 is identified by palpation. The trachea and carotid artery are palpated by placing the index and middle finger between the sternocleidomastoid muscle and trachea. The carotid is gently retracted, and after infiltration of local anesthetic, a 22-gauge spinal needle is advanced perpendicular to the skin in an AP direction until bone is contacted. The needle is then withdrawn 2 mm; after negative aspiration, 0.5-1 mL of local anesthetic is administered. If there is no evidence of intravascular, intrathecal, or epidural spread, 5-10 mL of 0.25% bupivacaine is administered, and the patient should then be observed in recovery for at least 30 minutes.

The fluoroscopic approach requires identical preprocedural preparation and positioning. The fluoroscope is used to identify the C6 and C7 vertebrae, as well as the trachea using a PA image. The C6 or C7 levels maybe selected; however, if the C7 level is chosen, the final position of needle should be maintained more medial on the transverse process in order to avoid inadvertent puncture of the vertebral artery which overlies the base of the transverse process at this level. After local infiltration with 1-2 mL of 1% lidocaine, a 1.5-in spinal needle is advanced coaxially until the transverse process is contacted using repeated PA imaging; the needle is then withdrawn 2 mm. After negative aspiration contrast (iohexol 180 mg/mL or its equivalent) is injected, ideally contrast spread should cover the C6-T2 levels (Fig. 16.6).

Ultrasound guidance initially described by Kapral et al. (1995) allows for direct visualization of anatomical structures including the esophagus, thyroid gland, vertebral artery, pleura, nerve roots, longus colli muscle, and fascial planes (Fig. 16.7). Real-time spread of local anesthetic can also be observed. Optimal positioning can vary according to provider preference and includes supine, so-called sloppy or modified lateral decubitus, and lateral decubitus. A linear probe 3-12 MHz is placed lateral to trachea at the C6 level; the carotid sheath, the longus colli muscle, and the anterior tubercle (Chassaignac tubercle) are identified. The target is the fascial plane between the lateral aspect of the longus colli muscle posteriorly and the carotid sheath anteriorly.

D. Complications

Inadvertent puncture of the vertebrae at low doses may result in dizziness, light-headedness, and hypotension; higher doses can result in coma, seizures,

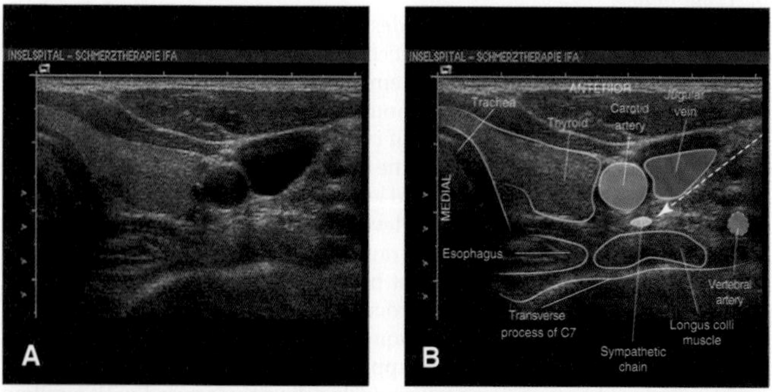

FIGURE 16.7 Anatomy relevant to the stellate ganglion as seen on ultrasound. **A.** Transverse (short-axis) ultrasound view at the level of the transverse process of C7. **B.** Labeled image showing the vertebral artery seen anterior to the echogenic transverse process at the level of C7. The vertebral artery cannot be seen clearly at C6 on ultrasound as it lies posterior to the echogenic transverse process within the foramen transversarium. The *dotted line* shows the optimal trajectory of the needle using an in plane approach. (From Stellate ganglion block. In: Rathmell JP, ed. *Atlas of Image-Guided Intervention in Regional Anesthesia and Pain Medicine*. Philadelphia, PA: Wolters Kluwer 2012:152–161.)

and respiratory depression related to direct effects of local anesthetic on the medullary and pontine centers. Trauma to the inferior thyroid artery can contribute to retropharyngeal hematoma after SGB. The incidence of spread of local anesthetic to adjacent structures including the recurrent laryngeal nerve, phrenic nerve, and brachial plexus increased with increasing volume of injectate. Consequences can include hoarseness (10% with 10 mL volume, 80% with 20 mL volume), shortness of breath, and upper extremity weakness, respectively. Bilateral SGB should not be performed as it could cause bilateral recurrent laryngeal nerve blocks and lead to loss of laryngeal reflexes and respiratory compromise. Puncture of the pharynx, trachea, or esophagus is possible. Puncture of the dome of the lung or thoracic duct can result in pneumo- or chylothorax.

III. CELIAC PLEXUS BLOCK

Neurolytic celiac plexus block (NCPB) is among the most widely applicable of all neurolytic blocks. NCPB has a long-lasting benefit of 70%-90% in patients with pancreatic and other intra-abdominal malignancies by denervation of the abdominal viscera except for the left colon and pelvic viscera. Neurolysis of the celiac plexus or splanchnic nerves can produce dramatic pain relief, reduce or eliminate the need for supplemental analgesics, and improve quality of life in patient with pancreatic cancer and other intra-abdominal malignancies. The long-term benefit of NCPB particularly those with chronic pancreatitis is debatable.

A. Anatomy

The celiac plexus contains both sympathetic fibers arising from T5 to T12 and parasympathetic fibers from the vagus nerve. The plexus, comprised between one and five ganglia, is located retroperitoneally at approximately T12-L1; it is separated from the vertebral column by the crux of the diaphragm and overlies the aorta at L1.

Sympathetic innervations to the abdominal viscera arise from the anterolateral horn of the spinal cord between T5 and T12 levels. Nociceptive information from the abdominal viscera is carried by afferents that accompany the sympathetic nerves. Presynaptic sympathetic fibers travel from the thoracic sympathetic chain toward the ganglion, traversing over the anterolateral aspect of the inferior thoracic vertebrae as the greater (T5-T9), lesser (T10-T11), and least (T12) splanchnic nerves. These presynaptic fibers travelling via the splanchnic nerves synapse with the sympathetic ganglia over the anterolateral surface of the aorta surrounding the origin of the celiac and mesenteric arteries (Fig. 16.8). Postsynaptic fibers from the celiac ganglia innervate all the abdominal viscera, with the exception of the descending colon, sigmoid colon, rectum, and pelvic viscera.

B. Indications

Pain originating from the structures in the upper abdomen including the pancreas, diaphragm, liver, spleen, gall bladder, stomach, ascending and proximal transverse colon, adrenal glands, kidney, abdominal aorta, and mesentery are relayed through the celiac plexus. Neurolytic block of the celiac plexus is indicated in the management of malignant, metastatic, and chronic nonmalignant visceral pain secondary to the abovementioned structures. The most common application is to treat pain associated particularly with pancreatic cancer.

C. Technique

There are three primary approaches described in the literature to execute a celiac plexus block, the classic retrocrural approach, antecrural

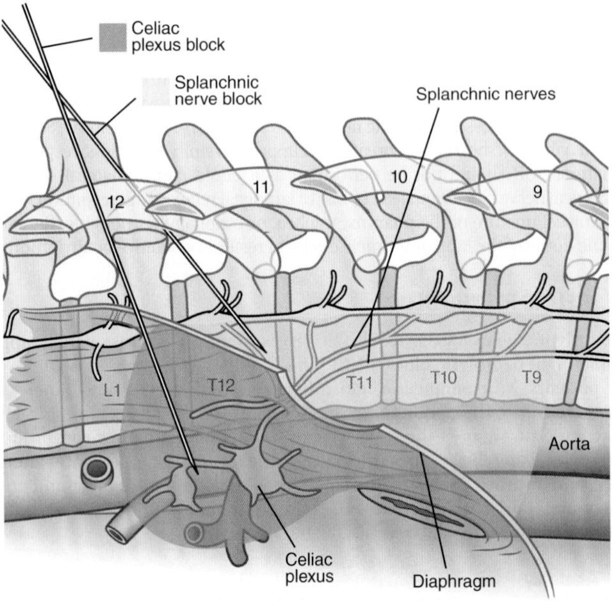

FIGURE 16.8 Anatomy of the celiac plexus and splanchnic nerves. Celiac plexus block using the transcrural approach places the local anesthetic or neurolytic solution directly on the celiac ganglion anterolateral to the aorta. The needles pass directly through the cura of the diaphragm en route to the celiac plexus. In contrast, for splanchnic nerve blocks, the needles remain posterior to the diaphragmatic cura in close apposition to the T12 vertebral body. *Shading* indicates the pattern of solution spread for each technique. (From Celiac plexus block and neurolysis. In: Rathmell JP, ed. *Atlas of Image-Guided Intervention in Regional Anesthesia and Pain Medicine*. Philadelphia, PA: Wolters Kluwer 2012:162–175.)

or transcrural approach, and transaortic technique. All three techniques require prone positioning.

For both the retrocrural and transcrural approaches, the L1 vertebral body is identified using imaging, most commonly fluoroscopy or computed tomography (CT); needle insertion is at the lower border of the 12th rib, 7 cm lateral to the midline and cephalad to the transverse process of the L1 vertebral body. In the transcrural approach, the tip of the needle is then advanced toward the anterolateral border L1 vertebral body. The C-arm is then rotated to the lateral projection, and the needle is advanced to lie 2-3 cm anterior to the anterior margin of L1. A fluid-filled syringe is then attached, and the apparatus is advanced until loss of resistance is felt indicating passage through the anterior wall of the aorta into retroperitoneal fat. The needle tip should be medial to the lateral border of the L1 vertebral body in the AP view. Final needle position is confirmed by injecting 1-2 mL of radiographic contrast (iohexol 180 mg/mL) under live fluoroscopy. The contrast should layer over the anterior surface of the aorta and appear pulsatile. If the contrast spreads to both sides of midline over the anterior surface of the aorta, then only a single needle is necessary; otherwise the same technique is performed on the contralateral side (Figs. 16.9-16.11).

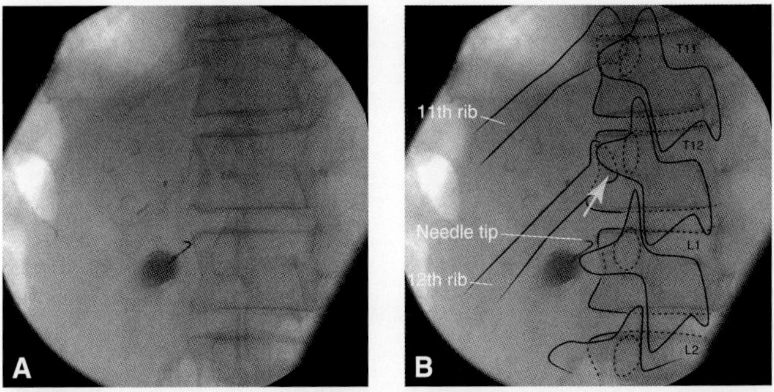

FIGURE 16.9 A. Oblique radiograph of the spine during a celiac plexus block. A needle passes from left oblique angle to lie over the anterolateral surface of the superior aspect of the L1 vertebral body. It passes superior to the transverse process of the L1 and inferomedial to the 12th rib. **B.** The *white arrow* indicates the final needle position for splanchnic nerve block. (From Celiac plexus block and neurolysis. In: Rathmell JP, ed. *Atlas of Image-Guided Intervention in Regional Anesthesia and Pain Medicine.* Philadelphia, PA: Wolters Kluwer 2012:162–175.)

In the retrocrural technique or splanchnic nerve block, the spinal needle is advanced caudal to the 12th rib and cephalad to the transverse process of L1 toward the anterolateral surface of the T12 vertebral body. In this technique, needles must be placed on both sides. After bone is contacted, in the retrocrural approach, the C-arm is rotated to a lateral projection, and the needle is advanced to lie in the anterior one-third of the T12 vertebral body on lateral view. In AP view, the needle tip should be just medial to the lateral border of the T12 vertebral body.

In all three approaches, appropriate caudal spread of contrast should be verified. 50%-100% alcohol or 10% phenol can be utilized to perform a neurolytic block. If alcohol is chosen, 5-10 mL of 0.25% bupivacaine should be administered 5 minutes before introduction of alcohol as it can produce

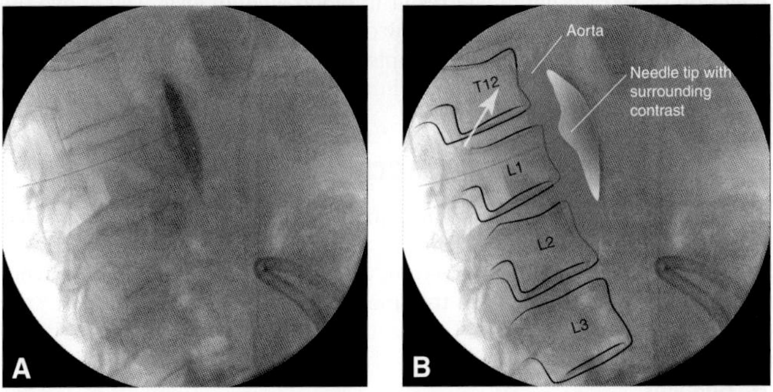

FIGURE 16.10 A. Lateral radiograph of the spine during celiac plexus block. A single needle is in final position over the anterolateral surface of the aorta, ~2 cm anterior to the vertebral body of L1. Radiographic contrast has been injected. **B.** The *white arrow* indicates the final needle position for splanchnic nerve block. (From Celiac plexus block and neurolysis. In: Rathmell JP, ed. *Atlas of Image-Guided Intervention in Regional Anesthesia and Pain Medicine.* Philadelphia, PA: Wolters Kluwer 2012:162–175.)

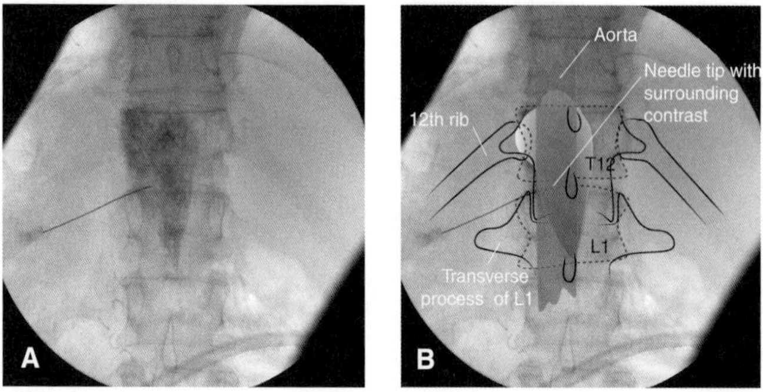

FIGURE 16.11 A. AP radiograph of the spine during celiac plexus block. A single needle has been inserted from a left oblique approach and is in final position over the anterolateral surface of the aorta. Radiographic contrast has been injected followed by 20 mL of 0.25% bupivacaine. **B.** The approximate position of the aorta is shown. (From Celiac plexus block and neurolysis. In: Rathmell JP, ed. *Atlas of Image-Guided Intervention in Regional Anesthesia and Pain Medicine.* Philadelphia, PA: Wolters Kluwer 2012:162–175.)

severe pain. Total volume injected is often cited at 20, 10 mL per side though smaller volumes maybe used in the retrocrural approach.

D. Complications

Complication rates associated with NCPB vary according to the technique utilized. Orthostatic hypotension may occur in 1%-5% of patients and can last up to 5 days postprocedures; incidence is more frequent with retroperitoneal techniques. Sympathetic blockade of the bowel can result in diarrhea; treatments include oral hydration and antidiarrheal medications. Retroperitoneal hemorrhage is a rare but described complication of celiac plexus block; patients with both back pain and orthostatic hypotension should be admitted for serial hematocrit measurements. Backache can result from local trauma, injury to the lumbar plexus, or irritation of the retroperitoneal structures from administration of alcohol. Intravascular injection of 100% ethanol will result in blood alcohol level well above the legal limit for intoxication but below the danger of severe alcohol toxicity. Transient motor paralysis and paraplegia have also been reported. This is thought to result from spasm of the lumbar segmental arteries that perfuse the spinal cord.

IV. SUPERIOR HYPOGASTRIC BLOCK

The sympathetic nervous system is involved in the pathophysiology that leads to a number of different chronic pain conditions, including pain arising from the bladder, uterus, rectum, vagina, and prostate. Superior hypogastric block is useful for the treatment of chronic pain arising from the pelvic viscera.

A. Anatomy

The superior hypogastric plexus is located in the subserous fascia between the bifurcations of the common iliac arteries; it is a continuation of the celiac and inferior mesenteric plexuses (L4-S1). The plexus extends from the lower one-third of the fifth lumbar vertebral body to the upper third of the first sacral vertebral body. The plexus carries sympathetic afferents and postganglionic efferent fibers from the lumbar sympathetic chain, as well as parasympathetic fibers that arise from S2 to S4. Sympathetic nerves passing through the plexus innervate the pelvic viscera, including the bladder, uterus, rectum, vagina, and prostate.

B. Indications

The superior hypogastric plexus supplies visceral innervations to the majority of pelvic structures including the descending colon, rectum, and internal genitalia with the exception of the ovaries and fallopian tubes. Blockade of this plexus first described by Plancarte (1990) can provide pain relief for both malignant and nonmalignant pelvic pain. Temporary block may be useful in better defining the source of pain. More often, superior hypogastric neurolysis is used to treat intractable pelvic visceral pain associated with malignancy. Patients with locally invasive cancer involving the proximal vagina, uterus, ovaries, prostate, and rectum that are associated with pelvic pain may gain significant pain relief from this approach.

C. Techniques

In the prone position, the fluoroscope is positioned 25-35 degrees ipsilateral oblique and 25-35 degrees cephalad to identify the L5-S1 disc space; the needle target is the anterolateral margin of the lumbosacral junction. Once the C-arm is aligned, there is a small triangular window through which the needle must pass to reach the anterolateral margin of the lumbosacral junction. The triangle is bounded superiorly by the transverse process of L5, laterally by the iliac crest and medially by the L5-S1 facet joint. The needle entry site is typically located at 5-7 cm lateral to midline at the level of the L4-L5 disc space. The needle is advanced under fluoroscopic guidance to lie anterolateral to the L5-S1 intervertebral disc or the inferior margin of the L5 vertebral body. A transdiscal approach has also been described in the literature in which the needle transects the anterolateral portion of the L5-S1 disc to achieve needle placement at the anterolateral margin of the lumbosacral junction (Figs. 16.12-16.14).

After negative aspiration, to avoid injection into iliac arteries, 2-3 mL of contrast is administered to verify appropriate needle position. In the AP view, contrast spread is limited to the midline; in lateral imaging, a smooth posterior contour indicates contrast deposition anterior to the psoas fascial plane. Similar to NCPB, neurolysis of the superior hypogastric plexus can be carried out with 10% phenol or 100% alcohol; total volume, however, is smaller, 6-8 mL.

D. Complications

There has been no reported evidence of neurologic complications associated with this block; however, acute ischemia of foot has been described, thought to be related to possible dislodgement of an atherosclerotic plaque from the iliac artery. Additionally, needle trauma can result in retroperitoneal hemorrhage.

V. GANGLION IMPAR BLOCK

Visceral pain in the perineal area associated with or without malignancies may be effectively treated with a block or neurolysis of the ganglion impar.

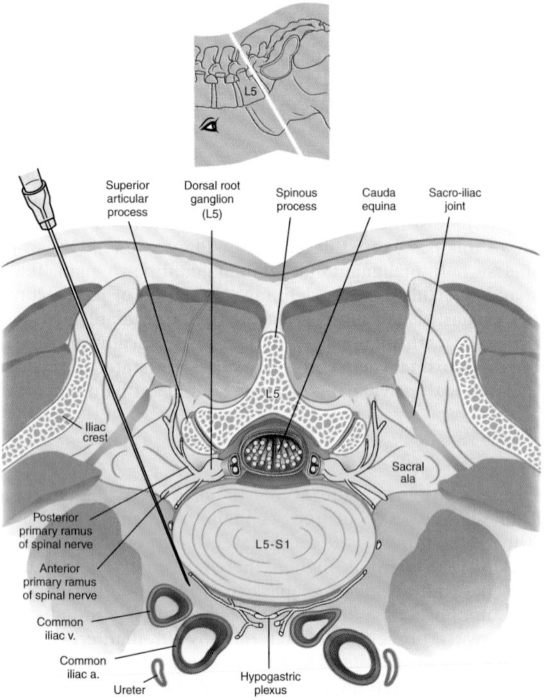

FIGURE 16.12 Axial diagram of the superior hypogastric plexus block. Needles are advanced from either side over the junction between the sacral ala and the superior articular process of S1 to position the needle tips over the anterolateral surface of the L5-S1 disc space. The *inset* shows the plane and orientation of the axial diagram. (From Superior hypogastric block and neurolysis. In: Rathmell JP, ed. *Atlas of Image-Guided Intervention in Regional Anesthesia and Pain Medicine*. Philadelphia, PA: Wolters Kluwer 2012:187-195.)

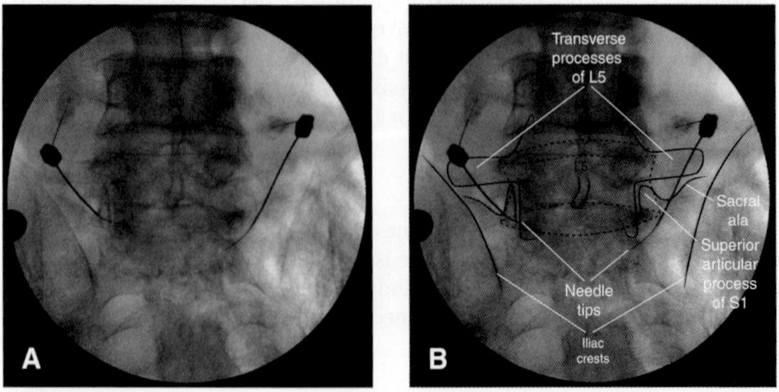

FIGURE 16.13 A. Anteroposterior radiograph of the lumbosacral spine during the superior hypogastric plexus block. Two needles pass obliquely over the sacral ala, where they join with the superior articular processes of S1. **B.** The needle tips are in position over the anterolateral surface of the L5-S1 intervertebral disc. (From Superior hypogastric block and neurolysis. In: Rathmell JP, ed. *Atlas of Image-Guided Intervention in Regional Anesthesia and Pain Medicine*. Philadelphia, PA: Wolters Kluwer 2012:187-195.)

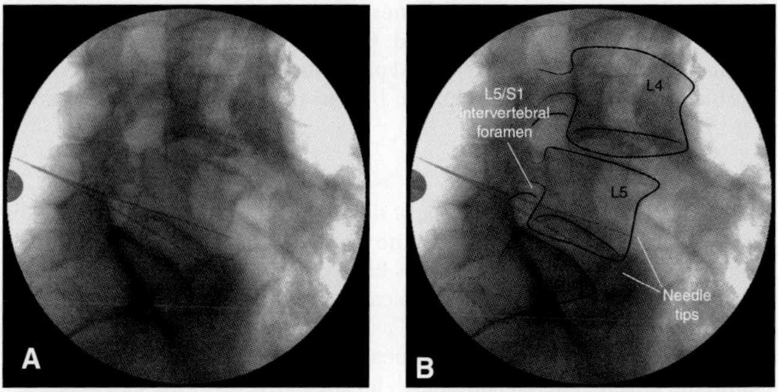

FIGURE 16.14 A. Lateral radiograph of the lumbosacral spine during superior hypogastric plexus block. Two needles are in position over the anterolateral surface of the lumbosacral junction. **B.** The needle tips are aligned with the anterior vertebral margin in lateral projection. (From Superior hypogastric block and neurolysis. In: Rathmell JP, ed. *Atlas of Image-Guided Intervention in Regional Anesthesia and Pain Medicine.* Philadelphia, PA: Wolters Kluwer 2012:187-195.)

Patients who benefit from the block frequently present with a vague, poorly localized pain that is frequently accompanied by a sensation of burning and urgency. However, the clinical value of the block is unclear, because the published experience is limited.

A. Anatomy

The ganglion impar or Walther ganglion is a single retroperitoneal structure which marks the end of the paired sympathetic chains. The location of the ganglion impar is at the level of the sacrococcygeal joint in approximately 18% of patients and can be as far caudally as the coccyx. The ganglion impar block has been used to treat persistent perineal pain as a result of malignancy and treatment-resistant coccydynia.

B. Indications

Ganglion impar blockade is indicated in the management of sympathetically mediated perineal pain often characterized by a burning sensation and sense of urgency in the perineal region. Etiologies are varied and may be related to benign causes such as chronic prostatitis or chronic proctitis, malignancies, or idiopathic. Ganglion impar is also used treat persistent coccydynia; however, its efficacy is debatable.

C. Technique

In the transcoccygeal approach, after the patient is placed in a prone position, fluoroscopy is used to identify the sacrococcygeal junction. A 20-gauge 1.5-in spinal needle is inserted through the sacrococcygeal ligament in the midline and advanced until the needle tip is just posterior to the rectum and anterior to the anterior portion of the sacrum. After negative aspiration, contrast medium is injected; a comma pattern indicates appropriate retroperitoneal spread.

A second approach involves inserting a 22-gauge 3.5-in bent spinal needle through the anococcygeal ligament. It is directed under fluoroscopic guidance to contact bone midline at or near the sacrococcygeal junction.

For diagnostic blocks, local anesthetic alone is used. For neurolytic blocks, phenol 6% is recommended. Cryoablation of the ganglion impar has also been described for repeated procedures via a transsacrococcygeal approach in a patient with chronic benign pain after abdominoperineal resection.

D. Complications

Although there is always the risk of damaging adjacent structures to the ganglion impar, there have been no complications reported from this technique. Plancarte and associates have reported one case in which epidural spread of contrast within the caudal canal was observed. Although published experience is limited and criteria to predict success or failure is unavailable, patients with poorly localized perineal pain, with a burning character, are considered candidates for the block.

Selected Readings

Agarwal-Kozlowski K, Lorke D, Habermann CR, et al. CT-guided blocks and neuroablation of the ganglion impar (Walther) in perineal pain. *Clin J Pain.* 2009;27(7):570-576.

Benzon H, Raja SN, Liu S, Fishman S, Cohen SP. *Essentials of Pain Medicine.* 3rd ed. Philadelphia, PA: Elsevier Saunders; 2011.

Boas RA. Sympathetic nerve blocks: in search of a role. *Reg Anesth Pain Med.* 1998;32(3):292-305.

Brown DL, Bulley CK, Quiel E. Neurolytic celiac plexus block for pancreatic cancer pain. *Anesth Analg.* 1987;66:869-873.

Carron H, Litwiller R. Stellate ganglion block. *Anesth Analg.* 1975;54(5):567-570.

Cha YD, Lee SK, Kim TJ, et al. The neck crease as a landmark of Chassaignac's tubercle in the stellate ganglion block: anatomical and radiological evaluation. *Acta Anaesthesiol Scand.* 2002;46:100-102.

Eisenberg E, Carr DB, Chalmers TC. Neurolytic celiac plexus block for treatment of cancer pain: a meta-analysis. *Anesth Analg.* 1995;80:290-297.

Elias M. Cervical sympathetic and stellate ganglion blocks. *Pain Physician.* 2000;3(3):294-304.

Erdine S, Ucel A, Celik M, Talu GK. Transdiscal approach for hypogastric plexus block. *Reg Anesth Pain Med.* 2003;28(4):304-308.

Hardy PAJ, Wells JCD. Extent of sympathetic blockade after stellate ganglion block with bupivacaine. *Pain.* 1989;36:193-196.

Hayakawa J, Kobayashi O, Murayama H. Paraplegia after intraoperative celiac plexus block. *Anesth Analg.* 1997;84(2):447-448.

Ischia S, Luzzani A, Ischia A, Faggion S. A new approach to the neurolytic block of the celiac plexus: the transhepatic technique. *Pain.* 1983;16:333-341.

Kanazi GE, Perkins FM, Thakur R, Dotson E. New techniques for superior hypogastric plexus block. *Reg Anesth Pain Med.* 1999;24(5):473-476.

Kapral S, Krafft P, Gosch M, et al. Ultrasound imaging for stellate ganglion block: direct visualization of puncture site and local anesthetic spread: a pilot study. *Reg Anesth.* 1995;20(4):323-328.

Kroll CE, Schartz B, Gonzalez-Fernandez M, et al. Factors associated with outcome after superior hypogastric plexus neurolysis in cancer patients. *Clin J Pain.* 2013;30(1):55-62.

Love MA, Varklet VL, Wisley BL. Cryoablation: a novel approach to neurolysis of the ganglion impar. *Anesthesiology.* 1998;88:1391-1393.

Mercadante S, Nicosia F. Celiac plexus block: a reappraisal. *Reg Anesth Pain Med.* 1998;23(1):37-48.

Narouze S. Ultrasound guided stellate ganglion block: safety and efficacy. *Curr Pain Headache Rep.* 2014;18:424.

Plancarte R, Amescua C, Patt RB, Aldrete JA. Superior hypogastric plexus block for pelvic cancer pain. *Anesthesiology.* 1990;73(2):236-239. doi:10.1097/00000542-199008000-00008.

Raj's Practical Management of Pain: Neurolysis of Sympathetic Axis for Cancer Pain Management. 4th ed. Philadelphia, PA: Mosby Elsevier 2008:923-925.

Rocco AG, Palombi D, Raeke D. Anatomy of the lumbar sympathetic chain. *Reg Anesth.* 1995;201(1):13-19.

Sayson SC, Ramamurthy S, Hoffman J. Incidence of genitofemoral nerve block during lumbar sympathetic block: comparison of two lumbar injection sites. *Reg Anesth.* 1997;22(6):569-574.

Schurmann M, Gradl G, Wizgal I, et al. Clinical and physiologic evaluation of stellate ganglion blockade for complex regional pain syndrome type 1. *Clin J Pain.* 2001;17:94-100.

Toshniwal G, Dureja GP, Prashanth SM. Transsacrococcygeal approach to Ganglion impar block for management of chronic perineal pain: a prospective observational study. *Pain Physician.* 2007;10:661-666.

17

Lumbar Diskography and Intradiscal Treatments

Ping Jin, Susie S. Jang,
and Christopher Gilligan

The intervertebral disk is composed of the nucleus pulposus (NP), the annulus fibrosus (AF), and the vertebral endplates (VE). The vertebral body lies above and below the disk. On the posterior side, the disk is supported by two zygapophysial (also called facet) joints. The healthy disk is avascular, and its nutrition depends on diffusion via the AF and the VE. The NP itself has no blood supply.

In the normal intervertebral disk, sensory nerves innervate the outermost third of the annulus. In the degenerated disk, this innervation is deeper, and can extend into the NP. Histological studies have shown disk immunoreactivity to inflammatory mediators in the degenerated disk, such as substance P, prostaglandin E2, interleukins, and tumor necrosis factor. Inflammatory mediators and immune cells may provoke disk degeneration in addition to being present in the setting of established disk degeneration. Pain may be triggered by chemical and mechanical sensitization of these dorsal annular nociceptors. Other studies have shown that the end-plates are also innervated and are capable of generating pain if injured.

Based on CT-diskography studies, the annular tear is frequently implicated as the basis for discogenic pain. The emphasis lies more on the extent of the annular tear than on disk degeneration. Sachs developed the "Dallas Diskogram Scale," a four-point scale that specifies the degree of disk degeneration. Grade 0 indicates a disk in which the contrast agent remains entirely in the NP. Grades 1 through 3 indicate tears in which the contrast agent extends to the inner, outer, and beyond outer sections, respectively, of the AF. Later, the scoring system was modified and grades 4 and 5 were added. A Grade 4 tear reveals contrast that spreads >30 degrees around the circumference of the disk. Grade 5 tears include a grade 3 or 4 tear that has completely ruptured through the outer layers, with contrast seen in the epidural space.

Diskography was used in studies to determine the prevalence of "discogenic pain" in patients experiencing low back pain. The results of these studies vary widely. In one of the most cited studies, Schwarzer et al. found the incidence of internal disk disruption (defined in his study by positive diskography) to be 39% in 92 patients with chronic low back pain.

Holt was the first to question the validity of diskography in a study published in 1968. He found false-positive results in 37% of 30 asymptomatic subjects. One confounding factor in his study was that all participants were volunteer prisoners. Many other authors have raised concerns about the validity of diskography, especially because of the high rate of false-positive results in both healthy and diseased disks. Nevertheless, a meta-analysis of those false-positive studies using the Spine Intervention Society Standard suggests that diskography has a specificity of 0.94 when precise patient selection criteria are applied.

The clinical utility of diskography remains controversial. While some still use provocation diskography to identify symptomatic disk for surgical fusion, others have questioned the usefulness of this test in predicting surgical outcome. In addition, a recent retrospective case-control study suggested that patients undergoing diagnostic diskography have accelerated disk degeneration.

Intradiscal electrothermal therapy (IDET) is a minimally invasive procedure that offers a treatment option to a small subset of patients with discogenic low back pain. Provocation diskography is used to identify symptomatic disks prior to IDET. Because of conflicting evidence about its efficacy, the use of IDET has dramatically declined in the past decade. Several other intradiscal intervention techniques have emerged, including percutaneous disk decompression (PDD) procedures. Among these, the percutaneous plasma disk decompression (nucleoplasty), which uses radiofrequency energy to reduce NP volume and thereby intradiscal pressure, has been shown to be effective for treating patients with contained disk protrusion and associated radicular pain (Fig. 17.1).

I. PROVOCATION DISKOGRAPHY/DISK STIMULATION

A. Definitions

The singular purpose of disk stimulation is to test the hypothesis that an intervertebral disk is causing a patient's back pain. The procedure is performed by inserting a needle into the NP of the target disk and injecting contrast agent, gradually increasing pressure within the disk to provoke pain.

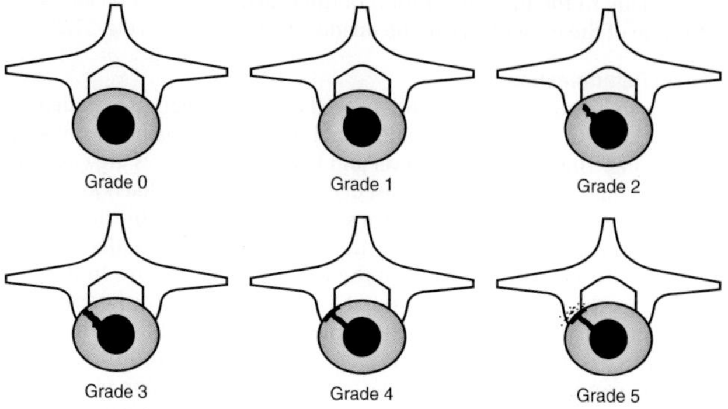

FIGURE 17.1 Modified Dallas discography criteria. (From nonimplantable interventions in chronic pain management: Part II. In: Urman RD, Vadielvu N, eds. *Pocket Pain Medicine*. Philadelphia, PA: Wolters Kluwer; 2011.)

B. Patient Selection

Suitable patients for this procedure are those with chronic low back pain, with or without pseudoradicular referral pain, which has not responded to conservative measures, and for which minimally invasive treatments of the facet joints and the sacroiliac joints are not effective. Imaging studies with computed tomography/magnetic resonance imaging (CT/MRI) shows only nonspecific findings of disk degeneration, such as reduced height and loss of hydration. High-intensity zones, seen on T2-weighted MRI images, in the posterior annulus indicating annular tear and/or granulation tissue is often found in nonsymptomatic patients as well. The implementation of provocative diskography is only advisable as preparation for a possible interventional treatment.

C. Contraindications

1. Pregnancy
2. Local infection at injection site
3. Systemic infection
4. Use of anticoagulants

D. Procedure

1. Provocation diskography is performed in an appropriate procedure suite under strict sterile conditions. Intravenous (IV) antibiotics are administered 30 minutes before the intervention. Antibiotics are also added to the contrast used for intradiscal injection; the concentration is typically between 1 and 3 mg/mL (eg, 1 mg/mL cefazolin).
2. IV sedation with midazolam and fentanyl is appropriate, but caution must be used to avoid over-sedation. The patient must be alert enough to communicate unusual pain/neurological symptoms, such as nerve root irritation and caudal equina injury, to avoid complications. Because diskography relies on patient's feedback during the procedure, excessive sedation makes the interpretation difficult and unreliable.
3. The patient is positioned prone on an x-ray permeable table. The skin of the low back and the gluteal region is prepped, preferably with a solution containing both chlorhexidine and alcohol. Full surgical gowning is required for the interventionalist(s), including surgical caps and gowns, masks, and sterile gloves. After the injection point has been identified, the patient and C-arm are covered with a sterile drape and cover respectively. Due to the limited rotation of the C-arm, it should be located on the side of the patient where the needle will be inserted (Fig. 17.2).

E. Level Determination

The levels to be examined are chosen based on a combination of patient history, physical examination, and additional information gained from CT or MRI imaging. The symptomatic level and two adjacent levels are examined, serving as controls. Typically, the least degenerated or more likely asymptomatic levels are studied first. The patient should be blinded to the disk level.

The C-arm is first positioned with the direction of the radiation beam parallel to the superior endplate of the lower vertebral body. In the disks above L5-S1, the C-arm is then rotated ipsilaterally until the lateral aspect of superior articular process (SAP) overlies the axial middle of the disk to be punctured, and the disk height is at its maximum. In this projection, the needle can be inserted coaxially, parallel to the direction of the radiation beam and brought into position. The target for entering the AF is the lateral-middle side of the disk, just lateral to the lateral edge of the SAP. At the L5-S1 level, the iliac crest often does not allow access to the disk using the coaxial approach. The fluoroscopy tube is rotated until the lateral edge of the SAP of S1 is positioned approximately 25% over the posterior to anterior distance of the vertebral body.

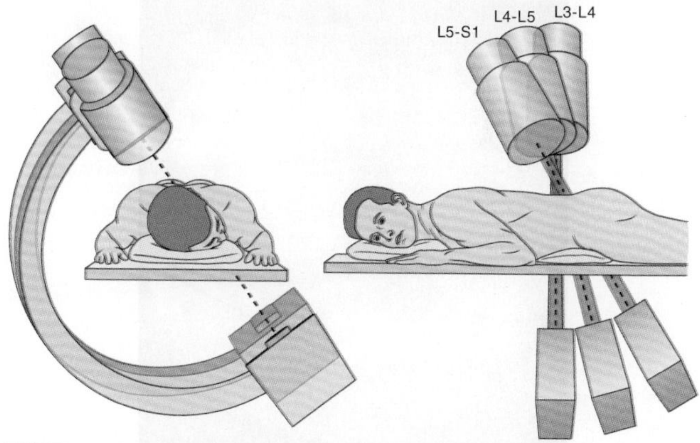

FIGURE 17.2 Position for lumbar diskography. The patient is placed prone with the head turned to one side. The C-arm is rotated 25-35 degrees obliquely and centered on the disk space to be studied. The C-arm is then angled in a cephalad direction that will vary from patient to patient, depending on the disk to be studied and each patient's degree of lumbar lordosis. In general, the L3/L4 disk lies close to the axial plane and requires no angulation to align the VE, the L4/L5 disk requires 0-15 degrees of cephalad angulation, and the L5/S1 disk requires 25-35 degrees of cephalad angulation. (Reprinted with permission from Rathmell J. *Atlas of Image-Guided Intervention in Regional Anesthesia and Pain Medicine.* 2nd ed. Philadelphia, PA: Wolters Kluwer; 2011:135.)

F. Needle Positioning

A new needle is used for each disk to be examined. After anesthetizing the skin and the subcutaneous tissue liberally, a one-needle or a two-needle technique can be used to approach the disk. In a two-needle technique, a 20-G needle is advanced over the lateral edge of the SAP. A 25-G hollow needle is then inserted through this needle and into the AF until it reaches the middle of the nucleus. The two-needle technique may help reduce the incidence of diskitis, and allows entering the disk with a small-diameter needle, which may help prevent the incidence of iatrogenic disk degeneration.

The needle is carefully advanced to optimal positioning, which is the middle of the disk's nucleus. To reach this point, when positioned beyond the SAP, the needle passes through the intervertebral foramen in the vicinity of the ventral ramus. In case of paresthesia, the needle must be repositioned. A strong resistance is felt as the needle passes through the annulus. The needle is pushed through the annulus to the center of the disk. The needle's progress is followed in various projections, first in AP and then in lateral projection. Ideally, after placement, the needle is situated in the middle of the disk's nucleus, as seen in the AP as well as in the lateral projection (Fig. 17.3).

G. Disk Stimulation

After verification of the correct needle position, the stylet is removed and the needle is connected to a contrast agent delivery system that can measure the intradiscal pressure (manometry). The rate of infusion of the contrast agent should not exceed 0.05 mL/s. This rate ensures a static flow and avoids higher dynamic peak pressure. A false-positive response can be triggered by high peak pressures. It is important that the disk expected to be most painful is stimulated last. The patient remains blinded to which disk is being stimulated (Fig. 17.4).

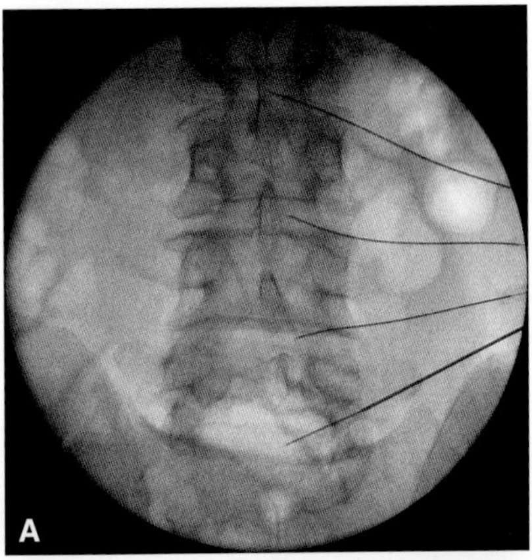

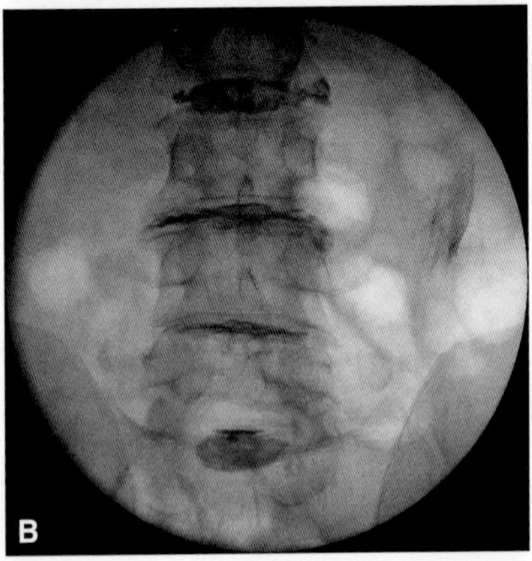

FIGURE 17.3 A. AP radiograph of the lumbar spine with needles in final position for lumbar diskography at the L2/L3, L3/L4, L4/L5, and L5/S1 levels. All needles are positioned within the central one-third of the intervertebral disk. **B.** AP radiograph of the lumbar spine following lumbar diskography at the L2/L3, L3/L4, L4/L5, and L5/S1 levels. Disk height is normal at the L2/L3 level and minimally reduced at the L3/L4, L4/L5, and L5/S1 levels. Discogenic pain was suspected based on persistence of low back pain and loss of T2-weighted signal on MRI within the central disk at the L3/L4 and L4/L5 levels (not shown). The L2/L3 diskogram has the characteristic bilobed appearance of normal contrast spread within the NP, with a small volume of contrast extending into the AF on the right. The L3/L4 and L4/L5 diskograms have diffuse linear spread of the dye to the limits of the AF on both left and right sides. The L5/S1 diskogram also appears normal. The circular appearance of the contrast is caused by the normal lumbar lordosis. The axis of the L5/S1 disk is tilted in a cephalad-to-caudad direction relative to the x-ray path. Note that the call for diskography at four adjacent levels is extremely uncommon. In this case, provocation produced symptoms at the L3/L4 and L4/L5 levels and the L5/S1 level was asymptomatic. The L2/L3 disk was then tested as an adjacent control above the symptomatic levels and produced no pain on provocation. Thus the symptomatic levels based on provocative diskography were L3/L4 and L4/L5 alone. (Reprinted with permission from Lumbar discography and indiscal treatment techniques. In: Rathmell J, ed. *Atlas of Image-Guided Intervention in Regional Anesthesia and Pain Medicine*. 2nd ed. Philadelphia, PA: Wolters Kluwer; 2011:142.)

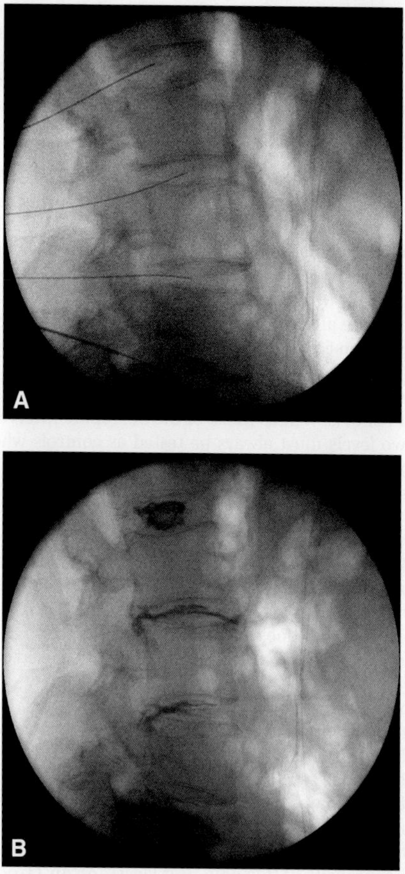

FIGURE 17.4 A. Lateral radiograph of the lumbar spine with needles in final position for lumbar diskography at the L2/L3, L3/L4, L4/L5, and L5/S1 levels. All needles are positioned within the central one-third of the intervertebral disk. **B.** Lateral radiograph of the lumbar spine following lumbar diskography at the L2/L3, L3/L4, L4/L5, and L5/S1 levels. Disk height is normal at the L2/L3 level and minimally reduced at the L3/L4, L4/L5, and L5/S1 levels. Discogenic pain was suspected based on persistence of low back pain and loss of T2-weighted signal on MRI within the central disk at the L3/L4 and L4/L5 levels (not shown). The L2/L3 diskogram has the characteristic bilobed appearance of normal contrast spread within the NP, without any contrast extension into the AF. The L3/L4 and L4/L5 diskograms have diffuse linear spread of the dye to the limits of the AF. There is greater anterior extension of the contrast at the L3/L4 level and the L4/L5 level with contrast extending all the way to the limits of the annulus posteriorly at both levels. The L5/S1 diskogram also appears normal. The axis of the L5/S1 disk is tilted in a cephalad-to-caudad direction relative to the x-ray path. Note that the call for diskography at four adjacent levels is extremely uncommon. In this case, provocation produced symptoms at the L3/L4 and L4/L5 levels, and the L5/S1 level was asymptomatic. The L2/L3 disk was then tested as an adjacent control above the symptomatic levels and produced no pain on provocation. Thus the symptomatic levels based on provocative diskography were L3/L4 and L4/L5 alone. (Reprinted with permission from Lumbar discography and indiscal treatment techniques. In: Rathmell J, ed. *Atlas of Image-Guided Intervention in Regional Anesthesia and Pain Medicine.* 2nd ed. Philadelphia, PA: Wolters Kluwer; 2011:141.)

1. **The following parameters are carefully monitored during the injection of the contrast solution:** the opening pressure (OP), that is, the pressure at which contrast is first visible in the disk; the provocation pressure, that is, the pressure at which complaints of pain arise; and the peak pressure or the final pressure at the end of the procedure. Ideally, pressure, volume, and provocation details are recorded at 0.5-mL increments, with additional notation made for the aforementioned events.
2. The procedure, at each level, is continued until one of the following events:
   a. Concordant pain, 6 or greater on the NRS, is reproduced.
   b. The volume infused reaches 3.0 mL. (Up to 4 mL may be injected into a very degenerated discus when pressures remain <15 psi.)
   c. The pressure rises to 50 psi above OP in disks with a Grade 3 annular tear.
   d. If contrast leaks through the outer annulus or through the endplates, one may not be able to pressurize the disk to a pressure sufficient to test the disk sensitivity. In these cases, rapid manual injection may be acceptable, but must be noted as such.
3. **Assessment criteria:** The guidelines of the IASP (International Association for the Study of Pain), as well as those of the SIS (Spine Intervention Society), state that two levels must always be tested as controls when performing provocation diskography (except if the target disk is that of L5-S1). A disk is only considered to be positive if concordant pain can be induced at the target level, and if the control levels were negative for provocation of pain.
   a. Overestimation of discogenic pain due to a false-positive response to provocative diskography is possible. Asymptomatic disks, with over-pressurization, may become painful. The diagnosis of discogenic pain can only be made if there is reproduction of concordant pain resulting from a pressure that does not produce pain in a normal disk.
   b. The international (IASP and SIS) guidelines are based on these operational criteria:
      1. Absolute discogenic pain:
         a. Stimulation of target discus reproduces concordant pain.
         b. The intensity of this pain is at least 7 on an 11-point NRS scale.
         c. The pain is reproduced by a pressure of <15 psi above the OP.
         d. Stimulation of the two adjacent disks is not painful.
      2. Highly probable discogenic pain:
         a. Stimulation of target discus reproduces concordant pain.
         b. The intensity of this pain is at least 7 on an 11-point NRS scale.
         c. The pain is reproduced by a pressure of <15 psi above the OP.
         d. Stimulation of one of the adjacent disks is not painful.
      3. Discogenic pain:
         a. Stimulation of target discus reproduces concordant pain.
         b. The intensity of this pain is at least 7 on an 11-point NRS scale.
         c. The pain is reproduced by a pressure of <50 psi above the OP.
         d. Stimulation of the two adjacent disks is not painful.
      4. Possible discogenic pain:
         a. Stimulation of target discus reproduces concordant pain.
         b. The intensity of this pain is at least 7 on an 11-point NRS scale.
         c. The pain is reproduced by a pressure of <50 psi above the OP.
         d. Stimulation of one of the adjacent disks is not painful, and stimulation of another discus is painful at a pressure >50 psi above the OP, and the pain is discordant.

II. INTRADISCAL INTERVENTION PROCEDURES

Several minimally invasive intradiscal procedures have been developed to treat discogenic pain, with or without radicular pain. Broadly, these procedures can be categorized as decompression (Dekompressor, nucleoplasty), annuloplasty (IDET, biacuplasty), or a combination of both.

III. PERCUTANEOUS DISK DECOMPRESSION

There is a clear overlap of the clinical signs of discogenic axial low back pain and the symptoms of nerve root compression due to disk herniation. Inflammatory responses and mechanical factors (nerve root compression) act together to cause pain.

The differences between conservative treatment and operative discectomy are not demonstrated in the long term. Operative discectomy is nonetheless utilized on a large scale, which is due to a more rapid reduction in symptom complaints when compared with conservative treatments. The disadvantages are the operative and anesthesia risks, along with the risk of epidural adhesions, which are associated with the so-called postlaminectomy syndrome, or the failed back surgery syndrome.

Otherwise, the indications for operative discectomy include larger disk protrusions and extrusions that show signs of nerve root compression on MRI. Smaller, focal protrusions without nerve root compression appear to be less apt to resorb spontaneously and have a less favorable natural course; in other words, these small hernias often produce long-term pain symptoms with a slow spontaneous recovery.

Over the years, the aforementioned considerations have led to various percutaneous, minimally invasive intradiscal techniques directed at the mechanical factor of disk herniation. Most of these techniques, in contrast to the surgical discectomy, have the common goal of decompressing the nucleus so that there is a change in volume and an accompanying reduction in the pressure on the nerve roots. These techniques are applicable to the "contained" hernia.

A. Intradiscal Electrothermal Therapy

IDET was first introduced by Saal et al. in 1999 as a treatment for discogenic back pain. The procedure consists of percutaneous insertion of a thermocoil into the discus, along the internal aspect of the posterior annulus, under fluoroscopic guidance. The distal portion of the catheter is heated at 80°C-90°C. Early observational studies showed efficacy, but later controlled studies demonstrated only modest efficacy. It fails to benefit 50% of the patients treated but can provide clinically meaningful pain relief for the remainder. As noted previously, use of IDET has declined precipitously in recent years.

1. **Indications**
   a. Low back pain, not responsive to other more conservative treatment.
   b. Discogenic pain as determined by provocation diskography.
   c. Severely degenerated disk (>50% height loss) may not respond well.
2. **Complications:** IDET is a safe procedure if performed correctly. Case reports of cauda equina injury appear to be due to technical error and not recognizing nerve injury symptoms during the procedure. Catheter tip shearing is possible with forceful manipulation.
3. **Techniques:**
   a. IV sedation titrated to maintain patient feedback.
   b. Technique to access the disk is the same as for diskography.
   c. After the skin is infiltrated with local anesthetics, a 17-gauge introducer is inserted into the disk under fluoroscopic guidance. Once in the nucleus, the tip of the introducer should be slightly medial to the pedicle in the AP view, and in the center of the nucleus in the lateral view.

d. Next, the electrode is inserted. The final position of the electrode should be at the interface between the outer nucleus and inner annulus (or more peripherally within the annulus). Final electrode position must be checked in both AP and lateral views to ensure it remains inside the disk. The proximal mark of the electrode should have exited the introducer (to prevent heating of the introducer).

Once the electrode is at a satisfactory position, heating the distal part of it is achieved using an ElectroThermal Spine System generator. The temperature is incrementally increased automatically to achieve a target temperature of 80°C-90°C for 6-8 minutes.

It is important to maintain the maximum temperature of at least 80°C for optimal results.

A slight increase in baseline pain is normal. But any unusual pain, such as radicular pain, should be addressed by adjusting electrode position or temperature.

After heating, the electrode is removed. Antibiotic mixed in contrast medium is injected through the introducer.

Patient can be discharged home after meeting the appropriate discharge criterion.

B. Nucleoplasty

This decompression method utilizes "coblation," in which a high-energy plasma field is generated with a bipolar radiofrequency probe. This plasma field breaks molecular bonds. For this reason, the technique is also called plasma disk decompression (PDD). Tissue can be evaporated in this way at relatively low temperatures (40°C-70°C). However, the plasma field can only arise in conductive medium. In practice, this means that the treatment is not effective in a dehydrated disk.

1. Techniques:
- **a.** IV sedation titrated to maintain patient feedback.
- **b.** Technique to access the disk is the same as for diskography.
- **c.** After a 16-gauge needle has been positioned in the nucleus, the probe is inserted into the nucleus. The probe is then moved back and forth and rotated intradiscally. In this way, six or more tunnels are made in the nucleus, and the intradiscal pressure drops.
- **d.** After the probe is removed, antibiotic mixed in contrast medium is injected through the introducer.
- **e.** The patient can be discharged home after meeting the appropriate discharge criterion.

C. Biacuplasty

Intradiscal biacuplasty is a technology that involves heating the posterior annulus. This is achieved by concentrating radiofrequency between the ends of two straight probes, which allows for relatively even heating. A larger area can be treated by internally cooling the electrodes.

Positioning and setup is consistent with prior procedures. Two 18-gauge electrodes are inserted via introducers and placed bilaterally in the posterior annulus. Radiofrequency energy and its resultant temperature are monitored, and gradually increased to 50°C over 7-8 minutes, and a final heating at 50°C for additional 7 minutes. It is important that the patient is not too sedated during this portion of the procedure, so that he or she may communicate with the physician.

Selected Readings

Aprill C, Bogduk N. High-intensity zone: a diagnostic sign of painful lumbar disc on magnetic resonance imaging. *Br J Radiol.* 1992;65(773):361-369.

Carragee EJ, Don AS, Hurwitz EL, Cuellar JM, Carrino JA, Herzog R. 2009 ISSLS Prize Winner: does discography cause accelerated progression of degeneration changes in the lumbar disc: a ten-year matched cohort study. *Spine (Phila Pa 1976).* 2009;34(21):2338-1345.

Derby R, Howard MW, Grant JM, Lettice JJ, Van Peteghem PK, Ryan DP. The ability of pressure-controlled discography to predict surgical and nonsurgical outcomes. *Spine (Phila Pa 1976).* 1999;24(4):364-371.

Holt EP Jr. The question of lumbar discography. *J Bone Joint Surg Am.* 1968;50(4): 720-726.

Pauza KJ, Howell S, Dreyfuss P, Peloza JH, Dawson K, Bogduk N. A randomized, placebo-controlled trial of intradiscal electrothermal therapy for the treatment of discogenic low back pain. *Spine J.* 2004;4(1):27-35.

Saal JA, Saal JS. Intradiscal electrothermal therapy for the treatment of chronic discogenic low back pain. *Clin Sports Med.* 2002;21(1):167-187.

Saal JA, Saal JS. Intradiscal electrothermal treatment for chronic discogenic low back pain: prospective outcome study with a minimum 2-year follow-up. *Spine (Phila Pa 1976).* 2002;27(9):966-973.

Sachs BL, Vanharanta H, Spivey MA, et al. Dallas discogram description. A new classification of CT/discography in low-back disorders. *Spine (Phila Pa 1976).* 1987;12(3):287-294.

Schwarzer AC, Aprill CN, Derby R, Fortin J, Bogduk N. The relative contributions of the disc and zygapophyseal joint in chronic low back pain. *Spine (Phila Pa 1976).* 1994;19(7):801-806.

18 Spinal Cord Stimulation

Dermot P. Maher and George Hanna

Despite introduction of novel therapies and refinement of existing treatments for painful conditions, a significant population of patients remains refractory to pharmacological, surgical, and more conventional pain management strategies. In such cases, pain physicians may offer patients more advanced treatment alternatives. Neuromodulation is a term that is now widely used to refer to treatment modalities that lead to the alteration of nerve activity through targeted delivery of a stimulus, such as electrical stimulation or chemical agents. Electrical stimulation of the dorsal columns of the spinal cord is one form of neuromodulation, more commonly called spinal cord stimulation (SCS). SCS is well studied and has become a widely utilized therapy for the treatment of conditions including complex regional pain syndrome (CRPS), failed back surgery syndrome (FBSS) with neuropathic features, radiculopathy, HIV-associated neuropathy, painful diabetic peripheral neuropathy, vascular claudication, angina refractory to medical treatment, Raynaud phenomenon-associated pain, and for selected patients with axial spinal pain. Evidence for the effectiveness of SCS for the treatment of these painful conditions is derived from a series of high-quality clinical trials and systematic reviews. There is ongoing debate about the role of SCS for the treatment of cancer-associated pain, abdominal/visceral pain, pain derived from brachial plexus avulsion, pain associated with spasticity, postherpetic neuralgia, and phantom limb/postamputation pain. Currently, SCS is not recommended for nonspecific low back pain or back pain with radiculitis in the setting of a prolapsed intervertebral disc.

I. MECHANISM OF ACTION

Several mechanisms have been postulated to explain the observed reduction in pain in patients treated with dorsal column electrical stimulation via electrodes placed in the posterior epidural space. Prior to the first reported successful treatment of intractable pain with an intrathecal electrode in 1967, the "gate control theory" was put forward by Wall and Melzack in 1965. This theory holds that application of nonpainful, electrical stimulation of the large myelinated Aβ fibers, which rapidly conduct efferent and afferent signals involved in cutaneous mechanoreception, will inhibit conduction of nociceptive signals in lightly myelinated Aδ and nonmyelinated C fibers. The gate control theory has often been invoked to explain how SCS produces analgesia, by substituting a nonnoxious electrical sensation that "closes the gate" preventing noxious stimuli from being transmitted to the brain. However, the gate control theory has fallen out of favor as our understanding of the neurobiology of nociception has grown.

Several alternative theories for the underlying mechanism of action of SCS have also been advanced based on clinical observations and basic science research. There is evidence that SCS therapy modulates both ascending and descending pathways by altering the concentration of certain neurotransmitters in the dorsal horn, including norepinephrine, serotonin, acetylcholine, and γ-amino-butyric acid (GABA). The phenotypic expression of receptors on neurons in the dorsal columns may also be altered by tonic electrical stimulation. Electrical stimulation can also produce analgesia through direct suppression of the hyperexcitable state of the wide-dynamic range (WDR) neurons. The observed decrease in peripheral vascular pain and refractory angina observed with SCS therapy has been postulated to arise from stimulation of release of vasodilating substances such as calcitonin gene–related peptide and nitric oxide.

The analgesic mechanism of action of specific dorsal root ganglion (DRG) stimulation appears to be direct action on abnormally functioning DRG cell bodies. Newer stimulation modalities, such as burst waveform and high-frequency SCS (10 kHz), may provide analgesia by similar mechanisms as conventional stimulation or may have unique mechanisms. Most of these observed effects of electrical stimulation are derived from animal models, and the role that each mechanism plays in producing analgesia in humans receiving SCS therapy remains unclear.

II. INDICATIONS AND EVIDENCE

The optimal candidates for SCS are those with persistent and disabling pain in one or more extremity that has failed to respond to more conservative treatment, including patients with pain due to peripheral nerve injury, chronic radiculopathy, or ischemia associated with small vessel peripheral vascular disease (PVD). Patients with axial lumbosacral pain have also been treated successfully with SCS. Those with abdominal or pelvic pain, thoracic pain, or pain in the head and neck from any cause are less likely to respond to traditional SCS. With placement of epidural electrodes and use of conventional stimulation parameters, producing stimulation in these areas can be difficult or impossible. The rapid evolution of new techniques like peripheral nerve stimulation, high-frequency stimulation, and DRG stimulation holds promise for treatment of a wider array of painful conditions. DRG appears especially promising for patients with focal neuropathic pain.

Generally, patients should have well-managed comorbidities and a psychological profile that does not preclude surgical intervention or the long-term management of an active implanted medical device. Patients with untreated anxiety or depression and those with major psychiatric comorbidities have poor outcomes: less likelihood of gaining satisfactory pain reduction and greater likelihood of device removal early after placement. It is important to keep in mind that studies of higher quality, for example, prospective studies, those with longer follow-up, and those with multicenter enrollment, tend to report lower analgesic benefit once adjusted for other factors. As with many treatments for chronic pain, there remains a select population that is refractory to SCS therapy. Patient responses to neuropathic pain medications or sympathetic nerve blocks do not reliably predict SCS outcomes.

FBSS/postlaminectomy pain syndrome is persistent low back pain and/or extremity pain following spine surgery. One prospective trial randomized 50 subjects with FBSS to either SCS or reoperation. The authors reported a higher percentage of subjects having a decrease in pain of at least 50% and increased satisfaction with therapy in the SCS group compared to those randomized to reoperation (47% vs 12%). In the same study, which permitted group crossover, 54% of subjects initially randomized to receive reoperation crossed over to SCS compared to 21% of subjects initially randomized to SCS who crossed over to reoperation. Forty-three percent of those who crossed over to SCS achieved successful pain relief, whereas 0% of those who crossed over to reoperation achieved successful pain relief. Subjects randomized to reoperation were also utilizing significantly greater amounts of opioids compared to the SCS group. Reanalysis of the same data demonstrated that the use of SCS was more cost-effective than reoperation (US $48 357 for SCS vs US $105 928 for reoperation in a treatment as intended analysis). A second prospective trial randomized 100 subjects with FBSS with neuropathic radicular leg pain to either SCS or conventional medical management (CMM). At 6 months, 48% of SCS subjects and 9% of CMM subjects had achieved a reduction of leg pain of at least 50%. Between 6 and 12 months, 10% of SCS subjects crossed over to CMM and 73% of CMM subjects crossed over to SCS. At 12 months after post-hoc adjustment for crossover, 34% of SCS subjects and 7% of CMM achieved the same degree of pain relief. Secondary outcomes such as improved leg and back pain relief, quality of life, and functional capacity, as well as treatment satisfaction were also higher in the SCS group. This study also noted that 32% of subjects experienced some sort of SCS complication during the 12-month study period. The use of high-frequency SCS (10 000 Hz) has been compared to conventional SCS (50-100 Hz) for the treatment of both "back pain." Unfortunately, this study failed to distinguish the responses of the enrolled subjects with FBSS vs other causes of back pain. This leaves meaningful comparison to prior data challenging. However, the cohort of subjects with "back pain" from a heterogeneous group of diagnoses did achieve a pain reduction of 67% for high-frequency SCS vs 44% for conventional SCS. Minor improvements in Oswestry Disability Index (ODI) and a significant decrease in average daily opioid consumption were also noted in the high-frequency SCS group compared to the conventional SCS group. Weaknesses of that trial included the fact that patients could easily identify which therapy they were receiving.

CRPS is a neuropathic pain syndrome defined by the Budapest Criteria. In a prospective study, 36 subjects with CRPS were randomized in a 2:1 ratio to either physiotherapy in addition to SCS or to physiotherapy alone. At 6 months, there were no observed differences between the groups. However, at 2-year follow-up, there was a decrease in observed visual analog scale (VAS) pain intensity (–3.0 vs 0.0 cm), global perceived effect (43% vs 6% reporting "much improved"), improved pain rating on the McGill Pain Questionnaire, and quality-of-life dimension of the Nottingham Health Profile. However, there was no observed improvement in functional status. At a 5-year follow-up of the same cohort, there was a nonsignificant trend toward a reduced pain intensity in the SCS group (–2.5 vs –1.0 cm). Ninety-five percent of the SCS subjects indicated that they would undergo the treatment again for the same result. There were no differences in quality of life or other indices at 5 years. At the 5-year follow-up, 42% of subjects had undergone reoperation for an SCS complication. This series of publications raises the concerning issue that SCS therapy may lose effectiveness over time. The use of high-frequency SCS has been reported to be effective for "extremity pain," but, as noted, the existing literature fails to identify the individual pain etiologies, such as CRPS.

Painful diabetic peripheral neuropathy occurs at a rate of 15%-50% among diabetics with a higher reported incidence in patients with non–insulin-dependent diabetes. A prospective trial randomized 60 subjects in a 2:1 ratio to receive either CMM or CMM in addition to SCS. At 6 months, 60% of subjects in the SCS group and 5% in the CMM group reported at least a 50% reduction in pain. Forty percent of subjects in the SCS group reported increased sleep at 6 months, compared to 5% in the CMM group. The quality-of-life indices increased significantly in the SCS group and actually decreased in the CMM group. The SCS group was noted to have three device-related complications requiring minor revisions. Neither group experienced an increase in diabetic management complications. In a second prospective trial, 36 subjects were randomized in a 2:1 ratio to receive either CMM or CMM in addition to SCS. At 6 months, 59% of subjects had at least a 50% reduction in pain compared to 7% in CMM. The average decrease in VAS pain score was 3.1 in the SCS group compared to 0 in the CMM group. In the SCS group, 22% of subjects completely eliminated analgesic medications, 32% were able to decrease their analgesic medications, and 55% reported no change. In the CMM group, 64% remained on the same analgesic regimen, while the remainder increased their utilization. The efficacy of the SCS decreased during a 24-month follow-up.

The treatment of vascular claudication and cardiogenic/ischemic visceral pain with SCS therapy has been evaluated in randomized controlled trials and is the subject of several literature reviews. Three prospective studies followed 239 subjects; 128 of whom were treated with SCS therapy. One hundred and nine subjects treated with SCS had PVD and 19 subjects had refractory angina pectoris (rAP). The mean reduction in VAS pain was observed to be 3.4 for rAP subjects and 3.3 for PVD subjects. The use of SCS for rAP and cardiogenic visceral pain is safe in the setting of an implanted pacemaker with or without a cardiac defibrillator if both devices are programmed in bipolar mode, the SCS frequency is 20 Hz, and EKG monitoring is used during reprogramming of either device. In such cases, close communication and coordination with a cardiac electrophysiologist is essential.

III. TECHNICAL CONSIDERATIONS

At present, there are several choices of available devices that are made by several different manufacturers including Boston Scientific, Medtronic, Abbott, and Nevro. Each system varies by the types of lead, implanted pulse generators (IPGs), programming characteristics, and stimulator functionality (conventional frequency vs high frequency vs various pulse waveforms vs various pulse densities).

Two types of epidural leads are available; paddle leads and cylindrical leads. Paddle leads are flat and wide with insulation on one side and electrical contacts on the opposite side. Paddle leads must be placed by laminectomy or laminotomy except in the case of one manufacturers percutaneously placed paddle lead, and they have the advantage of producing an efficient unidirectional electrical field. Cylindrical leads may be inserted percutaneously through an epidural needle. They generate a less efficient electrical field circumferentially around the lead. The use of multiple percutaneous leads is frequently used to direct current to attain optimal coverage. The ability of percutaneous leads to be removed without spine surgical intervention makes them the most reasonable option for use in SCS trials.

There are three primary types of power supplies that are available to which the leads may be connected. Primary cells are the largest of the IPG types and have an average life span of ~4-5 years, although the life span may be shorter depending on device programming and utilization. Rechargeable IPGs have lithium-ion batteries and have a life span of ~8-10 years. Radiofrequency IPGs are not limited by battery life span but require an external power supply, which may present a patient inconvenience and cause skin irritation. IPGs utilized in high-frequency stimulation consume power at a much higher rate and require more frequent charging (typically daily). Conversely, DRG stimulation uses ~5% of the power of conventional SCS. Power consumption is a major consideration in choosing appropriate hardware for the purposes of patient comfort/satisfaction and the cost of IPG revisions. The IPG is generally implanted in the lower abdominal area, the lumbar area, or the posterior superior gluteal area. The patient should be able to access the area easily with his or her hand to make any necessary adjustments or to charge the device.

The use of an SCS trial period decreases, but does not prevent, therapeutic failures after permanent implantation. During the trial, stimulator leads are percutaneously placed in the dorsal epidural space using sterile technique and fluoroscopic guidance. The leads are passed through an epidural needle that is typically inserted at a relatively shallow angle to skin to allow for optimal lead navigation. For conventional SCS trials, the patient remains responsive to assess the area of paresthesia mapping achieved by the trial lead placement and to monitor for adverse events during epidural access and lead positioning.

For conventional SCS, final location of the leads is dependent on the site of the pain and the delivered paresthesia coverage. The following landmarks are only for orientation as interindividual variance can be considerable. Careful intraoperative mapping is needed for optimal coverage. In general, for upper extremity pain, the SCS lead tip should be between C2 and C5. The shoulder area is notoriously difficult to achieve adequate paresthesia mapping. Occipital neuralgia may require placement around C1-C2 subcutaneously. Chest pain requires lead tip placement at T1-T2. Low back pain requires lead tip placement at T8-T10, and lower extremity pain requires the lead tips to be around T9-T10. Pelvic pain may be addressed with multiple leads placed in a retrograde position within the sacrum or through the S2-S4 foramina. The entry point is generally at least two spinal levels below the intended final lower lead position. Although these are commonly reported positions, the exact final position of an SCS lead for conventional SCS depends on the individual patient's intraoperative paresthesia mapping. A trial of high-frequency SCS, in which patients will typically not feel paresthesias, utilizes a consistent radiographically determined location for two-lead placement, and patient interaction is not used for the purposes of analgesic coverage. It is advisable to have the patient remain interactive in order to report any adverse events during epidural access and lead placement.

Once the trial lead(s) are in place and secured to the skin with adhesives or skin sutures, the patient is instructed to be as active as possible in their usual environment except for bending and twisting movements that may cause trial lead migration. We find a catheter fixation device such as a StayFIX to be the most reliable dressing for fixation of a trial lead to the patient's skin. The length of the trial is variable by physician and by country. Too short of a trial increases the risks of a false-negative trial, and too long a trial may increase the risk of infection. The average reported trial length in the literature is 3-7 days for conventional SCS and 7 days for high-frequency SCS. A trial is generally considered positive if the patient experiences a decrease in pain of at least 50%. Additional benefit may be observed with increased functionality or decreased analgesic consumption. Following a successful trial with no other contraindications, a patient may be offered to proceed with a permanent implant of an SCS device.

There are several methods described for conversion of a trial lead to an implanted system. The most common practice is to undergo a "percutaneous lead" trial. During the trial, the leads are only anchored to the skin with either adhesive or, in some cases, small skin sutures. Following the trial, the lead position is documented and the lead is removed and discarded regardless of trial outcome. On a separate occasion, the patient is taken to the operating room for a permanent implant in the same location. Alternatively, the patient may undergo an "implanted lead" trial in the operating room, in which the lead is placed and then anchored to the supraspinous fascia via a small incision using nonabsorbable suture. An extension cable is then connected to the lead and tunneled away from the back incision. Following a successful trial, the patient returns to the operating room and the extension cable is disconnected and discarded. The lead is connected to a subcutaneously implanted IPG. The "percutaneous lead" trial method has the advantage of not requiring a surgical incision, which could complicate trial interpretation, avoiding two operations, and decreasing the risk of infection. It has the disadvantage of requiring purchase and placement of two sets of leads and introduces the potential for lead placement in a nonidentical position. The "implanted lead" trial method has the advantage of decreased cost from not requiring two sets of leads and ensuring identical lead placement for both the trial and permanent phase. It has the theoretical disadvantage of increasing the risk of infection and requiring two operations. A final type of conversion from trial to permanent implant requires the use of percutaneously inserted leads followed by surgical insertion of a paddle lead via a laminectomy or laminotomy. The addition of a laminectomy or laminotomy to a trial adds a significant degree of pain and can confuse the trial outcome making this method infrequently utilized.

IV. COMPLICATIONS

Many technical problems can arise with placement and long-term management of a permanent SCS. Consensus guidelines regarding best practices to reduce the rate and severity of SCS complications have been published. The incidence of severe neurologic injury, including spinal cord and nerve root injury, following SCS placement is reported to be very low.

The incidence of superficial infections has been reported to be between 2.5% and 12%. The risk of progression of a superficial infection to meningitis or an epidural abscess is believed to be extremely rare (<0.1%). Some physicians have reported effective management of superficial infections with antibiotics and incision and drainage of the infected tissue. However, complete resolution of infections, in most circumstances, requires complete removal of hardware and antibiotic therapy. Any change in neurological exam warrants immediate removal of the hardware, infectious disease consultation, and possible neurosurgical consultation. The routine use of antibiotics prior to trial lead placement and prior to skin is incision for permanent implant surgery is well accepted. Ongoing antibiotics during the trial or for several days following permanent implantation is practiced by some providers but widely debated.

No reports of epidural hematomas were reported in large case series of percutaneous leads. The incidence of epidural hematomas following paddle placements in a case series of over 44 000 was noted to be 0.19% with over half the reported cases exhibiting persistent neurologic deficits.

The incidence of cerebrospinal fluid leak has been reported to be 0.3%-0.5%. Dural puncture with a large Tuohy needle will almost certainly cause a postdural puncture headache. Many physicians will abandon the procedure and ask the patient to return in 2 weeks for a repeat procedure in order to allow adequate time to recover from any headache symptoms.

The most frequently reported adverse events are equipment related and are generally related to discomfort near the hardware. The incidence of non–life-threatening events has been reported in the literature including lead migration (7%-21%), lead damage (6%-9%), and malfunction or failure of equipment (4.5%-10%). Lead dysfunction may occur months and even years after device placement. The incidence of lead migration may be mitigated by placing the needle for epidural access at a relatively low angle, careful technique for lead anchoring including placing the tip of the anchor through the fascia, use of a tension relief loop, and instructing the patient to avoid excessive twisting or flexion of the low back following permanent placement. The use of a soft cervical collar is advocated by some physicians for use in patients with cervical stimulators for at least the first 4 weeks following implant. Lead damage may result in an electric shock-like sensation. The patient may also experience failure of analgesia if a lead is not functioning properly due to migration or a fracture. The IPG is a rare source of hardware failure.

V. FUTURE DIRECTIONS

Neuromodulation for the treatment of chronic pain is a rapidly evolving aspect of pain medicine. Development of new technologies such as high-frequency stimulation, burst stimulation, and DRG stimulation have reported efficacy superior to that of conventional neurostimulation. It is encouraging that newly developed therapies are being rigorously tested for efficacy and safety. Increased use of rigorous trial designs including effective blinding and the use of sham controls will improve our knowledge of which therapies are effective for which groups of patients. Further, comparison of different modalities in comparative effectiveness trials will offer better guidance for both physicians and patients about which technology will provide the most benefit for a given patient.

Selected Readings

Cameron T. Safety and efficacy of spinal cord stimulation for the treatment of chronic pain: a 20-year literature review. *J Neurosurg.* 2004;100:254-267.

de Vos CC, Meier K, Zaalberg PB, et al. Spinal cord stimulation in patients with painful diabetic neuropathy: a multicentre randomized clinical trial. *Pain.* 2014;155:2426-2431.

Deer TR, Mekhail N, Provenzano D, et al. The appropriate use of neurostimulation of the spinal cord and peripheral nervous system for the treatment of chronic pain and ischemic diseases: the Neuromodulation Appropriateness Consensus Committee. *Neuromodulation.* 2014;17:515-550, discussion 550.

Deer TR, Mekhail N, Provenzano D, et al. The appropriate use of neurostimulation: avoidance and treatment of complications of neurostimulation therapies for the treatment of chronic pain. Neuromodulation Appropriateness Consensus Committee. *Neuromodulation.* 2014;17:571-597, discussion 597-598.

Deer TR, Thomson S, Pope JE, Russo M, Luscombe F, Levy R. International neuromodulation society critical assessment: guideline review of implantable neurostimulation devices. *Neuromodulation.* 2014;17:678-685, discussion 685.

Foreman RD, Linderoth B. Neural mechanisms of spinal cord stimulation. *Int Rev Neurobiol.* 2012;107:87-119.

Kapural L, Yu C, Doust MW, et al. Novel 10-kHz high-frequency therapy (HF10 therapy) is superior to traditional low-frequency spinal cord stimulation for the treatment of chronic back and leg pain: the SENZA-RCT randomized controlled trial. *Anesthesiology*. 2015;123:851-860.

Kemler MA, De Vet HC, Barendse GA, Van Den Wildenberg FA, Van Kleef M. The effect of spinal cord stimulation in patients with chronic reflex sympathetic dystrophy: two years' follow-up of the randomized controlled trial. *Ann Neurol*. 2004;55:13-18.

Kemler MA, de Vet HC, Barendse GA, van den Wildenberg FA, van Kleef M. Effect of spinal cord stimulation for chronic complex regional pain syndrome Type I: five-year final follow-up of patients in a randomized controlled trial. *J Neurosurg*. 2008;108:292-298.

Kemler MA, Reulen JP, Barendse GA, van Kleef M, de Vet HC, van den Wildenberg FA. Impact of spinal cord stimulation on sensory characteristics in complex regional pain syndrome type I: a randomized trial. *Anesthesiology*. 2001;95:72-80.

Kinfe TM, Pintea B, Link C, et al. High frequency (10 kHz) or burst spinal cord stimulation in failed back surgery syndrome patients with predominant back pain: preliminary data from a prospective observational study. *Neuromodulation*. 2016;19:268-275.

Kinfe TM, Pintea B, Vatter H. Is spinal cord stimulation useful and safe for the treatment of chronic pain of ischemic origin? A review. *Clin J Pain*. 2016;32:7-13.

Kriek N, Groeneweg JG, Stronks DL, Huygen FJ. Comparison of tonic spinal cord stimulation, high-frequency and burst stimulation in patients with complex regional pain syndrome: a double-blind, randomised placebo controlled trial. *BMC Musculoskelet Disord*. 2015;16:222.

Kumar K, Hunter G, Demeria D. Spinal cord stimulation in treatment of chronic benign pain: challenges in treatment planning and present status, a 22-year experience. *Neurosurgery*. 2006;58:481-496, discussion 481-496.

Kumar K, Taylor RS, Jacques L, et al. Spinal cord stimulation versus conventional medical management for neuropathic pain: a multicentre randomised controlled trial in patients with failed back surgery syndrome. *Pain*. 2007;132:179-188.

Lamer TJ, Deer TR, Hayek SM. Advanced innovations for pain. *Mayo Clin Proc*. 2016;91:246-258.

Liem L. Stimulation of the dorsal root ganglion. *Prog Neurol Surg*. 2015;29:213-224.

Linderoth B, Foreman RD. Physiology of spinal cord stimulation: review and update. *Neuromodulation*. 1999;2:150-164.

Mekhail NA, Mathews M, Nageeb F, Guirguis M, Mekhail MN, Cheng J. Retrospective review of 707 cases of spinal cord stimulation: indications and complications. *Pain Pract*. 2011;11:148-153.

Melzack R, Wall PD. Pain mechanisms: a new theory. *Science*. 1965;150:971-979.

Meyerson BA, Cui JG, Yakhnitsa V, et al. Modulation of spinal pain mechanisms by spinal cord stimulation and the potential role of adjuvant pharmacotherapy. *Stereotact Funct Neurosurg*. 1997;68:129-140.

North RB, Kidd DH, Farrokhi F, Piantadosi SA. Spinal cord stimulation versus repeated lumbosacral spine surgery for chronic pain: a randomized, controlled trial. *Neurosurgery*. 2005;56:98-106, discussion 106-107.

North RB, Kidd D, Shipley J, Taylor RS. Spinal cord stimulation versus reoperation for failed back surgery syndrome: a cost effectiveness and cost utility analysis based on a randomized, controlled trial. *Neurosurgery*. 2007;61:361-368, discussion 368-369.

Rudiger J, Thomson S. Infection rate of spinal cord stimulators after a screening trial period. A 53-month third party follow-up. *Neuromodulation*. 2011;14:136-141, discussion 141.

Slangen R, Schaper NC, Faber CG, et al. Spinal cord stimulation and pain relief in painful diabetic peripheral neuropathy: a prospective two-center randomized controlled trial. *Diabetes Care*. 2014;37:3016-3024.

Smits H, van Kleef M, Joosten EA. Spinal cord stimulation of dorsal columns in a rat model of neuropathic pain: evidence for a segmental spinal mechanism of pain relief. *Pain*. 2012;153:177-183.

Taylor RS, Van Buyten JP, Buchser E. Spinal cord stimulation for chronic back and leg pain and failed back surgery syndrome: a systematic review and analysis of prognostic factors. *Spine (Phila Pa 1976)*. 2005;30:152-160.

Truin M, van Kleef M, Verboeket Y, Deumens R, Honig W, Joosten EA. The effect of Spinal Cord Stimulation in mice with chronic neuropathic pain after partial ligation of the sciatic nerve. *Pain*. 2009;145:312-318.

van Beek M, Slangen R, Schaper NC, et al. Sustained treatment effect of spinal cord stimulation in painful diabetic peripheral neuropathy: 24-month follow-up of a prospective two-center randomized controlled trial. *Diabetes Care.* 2015;38(9): e132-e134.

Zhang TC, Janik JJ, Grill WM. Mechanisms and models of spinal cord stimulation for the treatment of neuropathic pain. *Brain Res.* 2014;1569:19-31.

19 Peripheral Nerve Blocks

Mark J. Young

I. OCCIPITAL NERVE BLOCK

A. Indications

Diagnosis and treatment of occipital neuralgia; treatment of cluster headache, chronic daily headache, and cervicogenic headache.

B. Equipment and Position

Alcohol prep, 27- or 30-gauge needle, and local anesthetic with or without steroid. The patient sits with head flexed forward to expose the occiput.

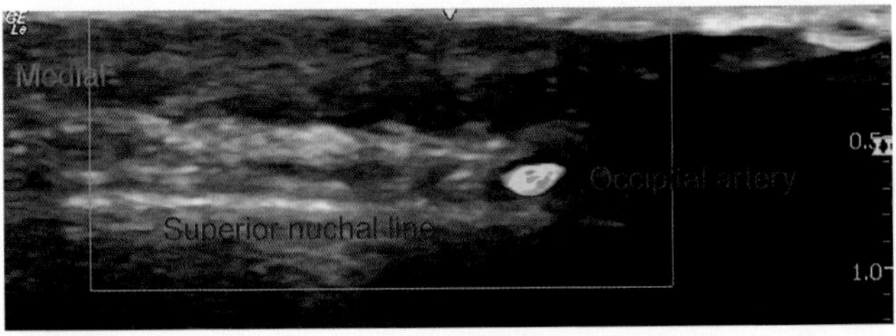

FIGURE 19.1 Occipital nerve block. Probe oriented transversely along the superior nuchal line. Occipital artery is seen with pulsation on Doppler.

C. Technique

The injection is performed along the superior nuchal line, one-third the distance from occipital protuberance to the mastoid process and medial to the palpated occipital artery. Other localization techniques include ultrasonography (Fig. 19.1) and nerve stimulation. The nerve can also be targeted more proximally between the obliquus capitis inferior muscle and the semispinalis capitis muscles.

D. Complications

Temporary numbness is common. Nerve damage, bruising, and hematoma are possible. Ensure the needle does not traverse the foramen magnum or a bone defect, which may be present after neurosurgery.

E. Considerations

Therapies for refractory occipital neuralgia include peripheral nerve stimulation, pulsed radiofrequency, and botulinum toxin injection. The lesser occipital nerve, which lies inferolateral along the nuchal line closer to the mastoid process, may be blocked simultaneously.

II. TRIGEMINAL NERVE BRANCH BLOCKS

A. Indications

Suspected trigeminal neuralgia; atypical facial pain; herpes zoster in the V1, V2, or V3 distribution.

B. Equipment and Position

For V1 peripheral nerve branches: alcohol prep and a 27- or 30-gauge needle. For V2/V3 nerve blocks: fluoroscope, chlorhexidine prep, sterile drape, and a 22-gauge spinal needle. The patient is positioned supine.

C. Technique

1. Pain in Ophthalmic (V1) Division

Rather than targeting the entire V1 division, we block peripheral nerve braches. For pain in the forehead, we generally block the supraorbital and supratrochlear nerves together. The brow is prepared with alcohol swabs. The supraorbital foramen is palpated at the 12 o'clock position of the supraorbital rim. A block needle is then inserted superior to the foramen, and local anesthetic with or without steroid is deposited after negative aspiration. The supratrochlear nerve is blocked superior to the supratrochlear notch, which can be palpated along the supraorbital rim about 1 cm medial to the supraorbital notch. Usually a single needle entry site can be used for both blocks.

2. Pain in Maxillary (V2) and Mandibular (V3) Divisions

The patient is positioned with mouth slightly open. Using fluoroscopic guidance, a spinal needle is inserted below the zygomatic arch and through the coronoid notch of the mandible. After contacting the lateral pterygoid plate, the needle is withdrawn slightly. Injecting at this location can block both V2 and V3 branches together. Walking the needle anteriorly and superiorly until falling off of the plate and into the pterygopalatine fossa can isolate the maxillary (V2) branch, though the sphenopalatine ganglion is often blocked simultaneously with this approach. Redirecting posteriorly and inferiorly may isolate the mandibular (V3) branch.

D. Complications

Complications include facial numbness, weakness in chewing, facial droop (from V3 motor branch blockade), local anesthetic toxicity, hemorrhage, and anesthesia dolorosa after neuroablative procedures. With coronoid approaches, injury to the eustachian tube has been reported.

E. Considerations

The entire trigeminal nerve (including V1, V2, and V3) can be blocked at the gasserian (trigeminal) ganglion. In the classic approach to this block, a needle is advanced just lateral to the corner of the mouth and directed to the foramen ovale.

III. SPHENOPALATINE GANGLION BLOCK

A. Indications

Atypical facial pain, migraine headache, cluster headache, and posttraumatic headaches.

B. Equipment

Cotton-tipped applicators that feature a plastic, hollow shaft and lidocaine.

C. Technique

In the transnasal approach, local anesthetic is applied to cotton-tipped applicators that have a plastic hollow shaft. The applicators are advanced along the lateral border of the middle turbinate until resistance is met at the back wall of the sinus. Additional anesthetic is dripped over the applicator and through the shaft to keep the tip moistened with local anesthetic. Applicators are then left in place for 20-30 minutes to increase local anesthetic absorption.

D. Complications

Epistaxis, bitter taste due to local anesthetic, and throat numbness. Patients should avoid eating and drinking until symptoms resolve.

E. Considerations

Intraoral and lateral (coronoid) approaches to this block have also been described.

IV. SUPRASCAPULAR NERVE BLOCK

A. Indications

Chronic shoulder pain; acute pain from arthroscopic shoulder surgery; alternative to interscalene block when contraindicated (eg, severe pulmonary disease, contralateral diaphragmatic compromise).

B. Equipment

Fluoroscope or ultrasound depending on technique, chlorhexidine prep, sterile drape, and a 22-gauge spinal needle.

C. Techniques

1. Landmark Technique

In Meier's technique, the ipsilateral arm is placed on the contralateral shoulder. A line from the medial scapular spine to the lateral acromion is bisected, and the needle entry site is 2 cm superior and 2 cm medial from this point. The needle is inserted in a 45μ latero-caudal direction with 30μ ventral inclination. Bone of the supraspinous fossa is contacted; the needle is slightly withdrawn; and the medication is injected after negative aspiration. In this approach, the needle does not enter the suprascapular notch.

2. Fluoroscopically Guided Technique

The patient is in prone position, and the fluoroscope is angled until the suprascapular notch is visualized. The needle is directed parallel to the beam of the fluoroscope just inferior to the notch until contacting bone and then walked superiorly until just entering the notch, being careful to avoid pneumothorax. Negative aspiration and nonvascular contrast flow help ensure proper position before delivering local anesthetic with or without steroid.

3. Ultrasound Guided Technique

A linear probe is aligned parallel along the superior aspect of the scapular spine. The probe is first directed caudal (toward the floor) and then gradually tilted anteriorly until the suprascapular notch is identified. The nerve is identified within the notch and under the superior transverse scapular ligament (Fig. 19.2). Occasionally, the suprascapular artery can be identified by visual pulsations or by color flow Doppler. Using an in-plane technique, the needle is advanced in close proximity to the nerve without entering the pleura before injecting.

D. Complications

Pneumothorax.

E. Considerations

Additional approaches (eg, stimulation-guided techniques) have been described. Ultrasound guidance enables real-time visualization of the nerve, vascular structures, and pleura.

V. INTERCOSTAL NERVE BLOCK

A. Indications

Chronic chest wall pain (eg, postthoracotomy pain); acute pain management (eg, after chest surgery and in the setting of rib fractures).

B. Equipment and Position

Fluoroscope or ultrasound depending on technique, chlorhexidine prep, sterile drape, and a 22-gauge spinal needle. Patient position varies, though most often patients are prone.

C. Technique

1. Landmark Technique

A common target site for the nerve is the angle of the rib with the patient lying prone. Due to cutaneous overlap, we generally target three or more

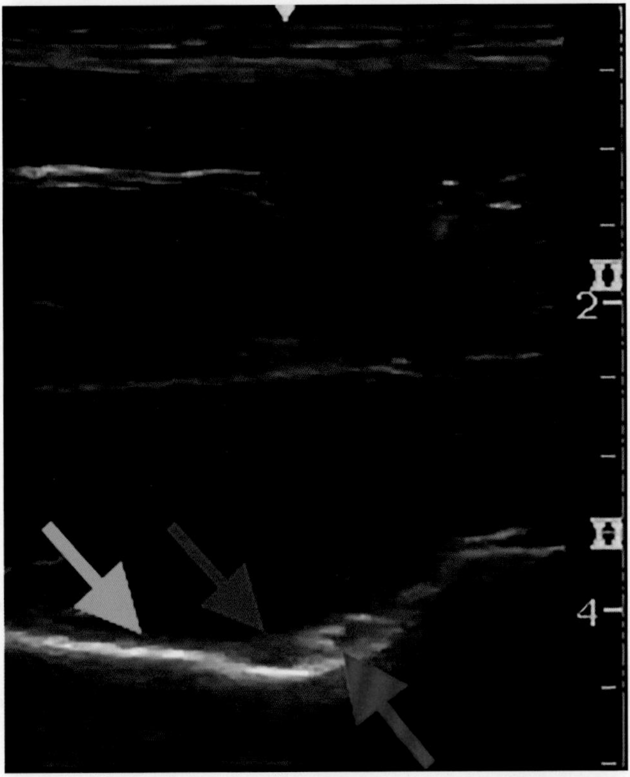

FIGURE 19.2 Suprascapular nerve block. *Green arrow* indicates scapula. *Red arrow* indicates superior transverse scapular ligament. *Blue arrow* indicates suprascapular nerve within the suprascapular notch. Above these structures are supraspinatus and trapezius muscles.

nerves to treat chest wall pain. A spinal needle is advanced toward the rib overlying the nerve that corresponds to the affected area until bone is contacted. The needle is then carefully walked off bone inferiorly until minimally (2 mm) deep to the posteroinferior rib edge. After negative aspiration, local anesthetic with or without steroid is injected.

2. Fluoroscopy Guided Technique

With an anterior-posterior view, the needle is advanced in trajectory view until contacting the angle of the rib. During this portion, the needle always overlies the rib to prevent inadvertent lung puncture. The needle is then repositioned similar to the landmark technique. Contrast injection can demonstrate spread along the subcostal groove and rule out intravascular uptake.

3. Ultrasound Guided Technique

Generally, the target remains inferior to the rib at the angle. The three intercostal muscle layers and the pleura are visualized, and the needle

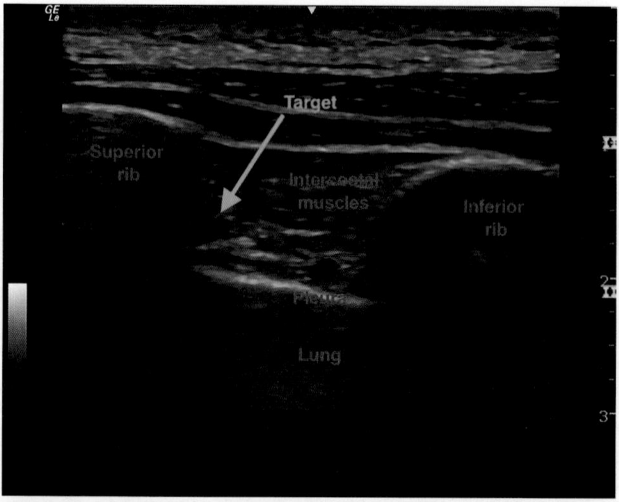

FIGURE 19.3 Intercostal nerve block. The target for this block is inferior to the rib and between the internal and innermost intercostal muscles.

tip is advanced between the internal and innermost intercostal muscles (Fig. 19.3).

D. Specific Complications

Pneumothorax and local anesthetic toxicity. There is significant systemic absorption of local anesthesia from this block, so caution must be used to prevent toxicity.

E. Considerations

Another common site for blockade is at the posterior-axillary line, just proximal to the mid-axillary line where the lateral cutaneous branches divide from the intercostal nerves.

VI. ILIOINGUINAL AND ILIOHYPOGASTRIC NERVE BLOCK

A. Indications

Chronic pain after surgery in the lower abdomen (eg, inguinal herniorrhaphy), nerve entrapment, and acute pain management after some lower abdominal wall and groin surgeries.

B. Equipment

Ultrasound (depending on technique), chlorhexidine prep, sterile drape, and a 25-gauge needle.

C. Technique

1. Landmark Technique

The ilioinguinal (II) and iliohypogastric (IH) nerves are targeted 2 cm cephalad and medial to the anterior superior iliac spine (ASIS). A needle is advanced perpendicular to the skin until two "pops" are appreciated. These "pops" represent penetration through fascia investing the external and internal oblique muscles, respectively. Local anesthetic with or without steroid is injected.

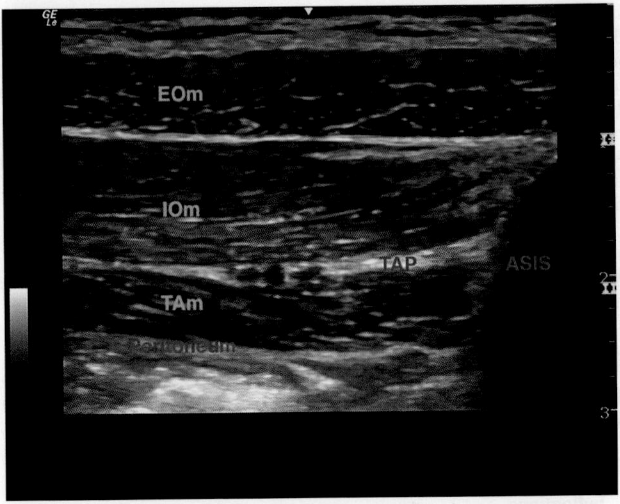

FIGURE 19.4 Ilioinguinal and iliohypogastric nerve block. The target is just deep to the fascial layer between the internal oblique muscle (IOm) and transversus abdominal muscle (TAm). The external oblique muscle (EOm) lies superficial to the internal oblique muscles (IOm), while peritoneum lies deep to the transversus abdominal muscle (TAm).

2. Ultrasound Guided Technique

The probe is placed in a transverse oblique position with the lateral end over the ASIS and the medial end directed toward the umbilicus. In this area, the II nerve is lateral, closer to the ASIS, while the IH nerve is medial (Fig. 19.4). An echogenic block needle is advanced to the transversus abdominis plane (TAP) between the internal oblique and the transversus abdominis muscle.

D. Complications

Peritoneal perforation and intravascular injection. The deep circumflex iliac artery also traverses the TAP in the area of the ASIS.

E. Considerations

There is often overlap in cutaneous coverage between the neighboring ilioinguinal and iliohypogastric nerves, so it is common to block both nerves simultaneously. However, a selective ultrasound-guided technique has been described. Ultrasound guidance may improve efficacy and avoid complications.

VII. PUDENDAL NERVE BLOCK

A. Indications

Diagnose and treat pudendal neuralgia; treat chronic perineal pain involving the genitalia or the anorectal area.

B. Equipment

Fluoroscope, chlorhexidine prep, sterile drape, and a 22- or 25-gauge spinal needle.

C. Technique

This procedure is often performed with fluoroscopic guidance. Patients are positioned prone, and the skin over the ipsilateral buttock is prepared sterilely. The ischial spine is initially visualized in an anteroposterior view, and slight ipsilateral oblique angulation then optimizes the target by separating it from the overlapping pelvic brim. A spinal needle is advanced to the ischial spine in trajectory view until contacting bone and then slightly withdrawn. After a reassuring contrast spread pattern without vascular uptake, local anesthetic with or without steroid is delivered.

D. Specific Complications

Perineal paresthesia, loss of bowel or bladder control, sciatic nerve paresthesia, and neuropathy (eg, foot drop).

E. Considerations

Ultrasound-guided techniques have been described, but the deep position of the nerve makes ultrasound visualization relatively challenging. In a randomized study, ultrasound was not superior to fluoroscopy for this block.

VIII. LATERAL FEMORAL CUTANEOUS NERVE BLOCK

A. Indications

Diagnosis and treatment of meralgia paresthetica; analgesia for anterolateral thigh procedures such as skin graft harvesting.

B. Equipment

Ultrasound (depending on technique), sterile prep, and a 25 or 27-gauge needle.

C. Technique

1. Landmark Technique

A block needle is advanced into the thigh at a position 2 cm medial and 2 cm caudal to the ASIS until a pop sensation is appreciated representing penetration through the fascia lata. Local anesthetic with or without steroid is then injected in a fan pattern.

2. Ultrasound Guided Technique

The nerve is identified inferomedial to the ASIS, often between the fascia lata and fascia iliaca at a depth <1 cm. A block needle is advanced to the nerve using an in-plane technique before aspirating and then injecting.

D. Complications

Perforation of the peritoneum; perforation of the spermatic cord in males.

E. Considerations

The course of this sensory nerve is quite variable, which may confer an advantage of ultrasound guidance over the landmark technique.

IX. GENICULAR NERVE BLOCK

A. Indications

Chronic knee pain from osteoarthritis.

B. Equipment

Fluoroscope, chlorhexidine prep, sterile drape, and a 22 or 25-gauge spinal needle.

C. Technique

There are three target points: the junction of the femur and superior epicondyle laterally (1) and medially (2) and the junction of the tibia and inferior epicondyle medially (3). First, needles are inserted in an antero-posterior view at these locations. Needles are then advanced posteriorly in a lateral view until halfway between the anterior and posterior extent of the femur or tibia shaft cortex, respectively. Initial blocks are diagnostic. If beneficial, radiofrequency ablation, either conventional or cooled, can be utilized for long-term pain relief.

D. Complications

Infection, nerve damage.

E. Considerations

Although there are additional genicular nerves, only the three targeted are felt to have relatively precise and easily accessible locations. The origin and location of all genicular nerves is an area of ongoing investigation, and this work may soon lead to refinements in block technique.

ACKNOWLEDGMENT

The author thanks Dr. Raj Doshi for reviewing this chapter.

Selected Readings

Chan CW, Peng PWH. Suprascapular nerve block. *Reg Anesth Pain Med.* 2011;36(4):358-373.

Choi WJ, Hwang SJ, Leem JG, et al. Radiofrequency treatment relieves chronic knee osteoarthritis pain: a double-blind randomized controlled trial. *Pain.* 2011;152:481-487.

Franco CD, Buvaedran A, Petersohn JD, et al. Innervation of the anterior capsule of the human knee: implications for radiofrequency ablation. *Reg Anesth Pain Med.* 2015;40(4):363-368.

Jankovik D, Peng P, eds. *Regional Nerve Blocks in Anesthesia and Pain Therapy.* 4th ed. Switzerland: Springer; 2015.

Narouze SN, ed. *Atlas of Ultrasound-Guided Procedures in Interventional Pain Management.* New York, NY: Springer; 2011.

Peng PWH, Narouze S. Ultrasound-guided interventional procedures in pain medicine: a review of anatomy, sonoanatomy, and procedures. Part I: nonaxial structures. *Reg Anesth Pain Med.* 2009;34(5):458-474.

Price DJ. The shoulder block: a new alternative to interscalene brachial plexus blockade for the control of postoperative shoulder pain. *Anaesth Intensive Care.* 2007;35:575-581.

Waldman SD, ed. *Atlas of Pain Management Injection Techniques.* 3rd ed. Philadelphia, PA: Saunders; 2012.

20 Implanted Spinal Drug Delivery Systems

Dermot P. Maher and George Hanna

The delivery of pharmacologic agents to the intrathecal (IT) space to treat pain rapidly emerged from the discovery that specific ligand receptors are present in high density on the first-order neurons in the dorsal horn that relay pain signals from the point of injury to the brain. Spinal delivery of opioids is aimed at improving pain relief while minimizing the risk of intolerable systemic side effects. IT opioids, local anesthetics, and other agents are now commonly used in patients for whom adequate analgesia cannot be achieved with systemic medications. Technological advances have led to implanted pump systems that can reliably deliver intrathecal medication, increasing both patient benefit and safety. Battery-powered externally programmable pumps are commonly used, but nonprogrammable gas-driven pumps are also available.

I. MECHANISM OF ACTION

The presence of opioid receptors within the dorsal horn of the spinal cord has proven to be a useful analgesic target. The receptors are anatomically located on the outermost and most accessible aspect of the posterior spinal cord. Agonist binding to opioid receptors at the spinal cord level reduces presynaptic primary afferent excitability, reduces presynaptic release of substance P and calcitonin gene–related peptide (CGRP), and suppresses excitatory amino acid postsynaptic potentials. This reduces the frequency and magnitude of pain signals that reach higher centers producing potent analgesic effects when opioids are administered intrathecally.

Several other medications have been administered through implanted drug delivery systems (IDDS). The presence of axonal sodium channels provides a scientific foundation for the clinical application of continuous IT infusion of local anesthetics, such as bupivacaine, to block the propagation of action potentials. Multiple synaptic receptor classes have been identified on wide dynamic range neurons, which are also located in the pharmacologically accessible posterior spinal columns. IT clonidine has been demonstrated to bind to α-adrenergic receptors on both pre- and postsynaptic afferent fibers in the dorsal column. IT ziconotide binds to presynaptic N-type calcium channels also in the dorsal column.

II. OVERVIEW OF IT PHARMACOLOGY

A. Morphine

At present, preservative-free morphine is currently the only opioid approved by the U.S. Food and Drug Administration (FDA) for IT use for the treatment of chronic pain. The equianalgesic potency of IT morphine is believed to be ~300 times that of oral morphine, although this can vary in opioid-tolerant individuals. The typical starting daily dose is 0.5 mg for opioid-naive patients and 1 mg for opioid-tolerant patients with a maximum daily dose of 15 mg. The evidence for the use of IT morphine for chronic cancer pain is derived from a series of high-quality clinical trials and systematic reviews. A prospective trial randomized 143 subjects with cancer pain to either comprehensive medical management (CMM) or IT morphine via an IDDS. 84.5% of IDDS subjects were able to achieve a clinically relevant reduction in pain compared to 70.8% of CMM subjects. IDDS subjects were able to achieve a >20% reduction in their pain more frequently than CMM (57.7% vs 27%). A second prospective observational study of 119 subjects with cancer pain demonstrated that IDDS with IT morphine had an overall success rate, defined as a 50% reduction in numeric analog scale pain, use of systemic opioids, or opioid complication severity index, in 83%, 90%, 85%, and 91% of subjects at months 1, 2, 3, and 4 following implant, respectively.

The data regarding the use of intrathecal morphine for noncancer pain are not as robust. A prospective observational study performed a trial of IT morphine in 25 subjects and noted a benefit in 16, all of whom underwent surgical placement of an IDDS. The subjects were then followed for an average of 29 months. The average visual analog scale (VAS) pain reduction at 6 months was 67.5%, and the average final VAS pain reduction was 57.5%. Two of the original 16 subjects failed to achieve therapeutic relief from IT morphine alone and required additional IT medications. Two additional subjects had the IDDS explanted due to intolerable side effects. Other studies designed to examine IT morphine for chronic noncancer pain had significant methodologic flaws.

IDDS are capable of delivering any water-soluble opioid, including morphine, hydromorphone, fentanyl, sufentanil, methadone, and meperidine. All IT opioids produce similar side effects that are well described in the medical literature. The most common problems associated with IT opioid therapy include nausea, vomiting, pruritus, urinary retention, and constipation. Less common side effects may include respiratory depression, sedation, opioid-induced hyperalgesia, endocrine abnormalities (in particular, sexual dysfunction), and edema. The loss of libido or amenorrhea may be seen with initiation of therapy but may then resolve. Finally, all opioids demonstrate a loss of analgesic function with time due to the development of tolerance.

B. Hydromorphone

Hydromorphone is not FDA approved for IT use at the time of this publication. Through extensive off-label use and study, it has gained widespread use in clinical practice, and consensus guidelines have elevated it to a first-line IDDS medication for nociceptive pain. Hydromorphone is believed to be approximately five times as potent as an equivalent dose of morphine. The typical starting daily dose is 0.25 mg with a maximum daily dose of 4 mg. There are no high-quality studies describing its independent use in IDDS. The hydrophilic nature of morphine and hydromorphone make them excellent candidates for IDDS as there is a decreased opportunity for extradural side effects and greater intrathecal spread.

C. Fentanyl and Sufentanil

Neither of these synthetic potent opioids is FDA approved for IT use at the time of this publication. Consensus guidelines rate these medications as third-line alternatives. Fentanyl is believed to be ~75-125 times as potent as morphine. The typical starting daily dose of fentanyl is 100 µg with a maximum daily dose of 1500 µg. Sufentanil is believed to be 500-1000 times as potent as morphine. The typical starting daily dose of sufentanil is 1 µg with a maximum daily dose of 15 µg. Doses of 40 µg IT sufentanil have been reported to produce transient diffuse muscle spasm, mimicking seizure activity. There is some suggestion in published studies that these lipophilic opioids may be more useful for segmental, rather than diffuse analgesia, as there spread within the CAF from the point of injection is less than that of the more hydrophilic opioids morphine and hydromorphone. There are no high-quality studies describing their independent use in IDDS.

The use of methadone and meperidine through an IDDS has been described but is not commonly practiced.

D. Bupivacaine

Preservative-free bupivacaine is not FDA approved for IT use currently. However, it has gained widespread clinical use, especially when compounded with IT opioid mixtures. Consensus guidelines characterize bupivacaine as a second-line medication. The typical starting daily dose is around 48 mg with a maximum daily dose of 300 mg. The utility of bupivacaine is as an adjuvant to IT opioid therapy. In a double-blind trial, subjects with nonmalignant pain and IDDS in place were randomized to receive either opioid therapy (hydromorphone or morphine) or opioid therapy in addition to 4-8 mg daily bupivacaine. The combination group reported improvements in quality of life and a nonsignificant improvement in pain. This study was likely hindered by a low bupivacaine dose as other retrospective studies have demonstrated a more encouraging response. Small retrospective studies suggest an analgesic benefit with higher doses of intrathecal bupivacaine with the rare occurrence of bupivacaine-related side effects. Rarely observed side effects attributable to IT bupivacaine include transient paresthesias, motor blockade, and gait impairment.

E. Clonidine

Clonidine is not FDA approved for intrathecal use for the treatment of chronic pain. It has unique properties in the treatment of neuropathic pain and has gained acceptance as a second-line adjuvant medication. The typical starting daily dose of clonidine is 50 µg with a maximum daily dose of 1.5 mg. In a prospective observational study, 31 subjects with cancer pain unresponsive to IT morphine via an IDDS had clonidine added to their infusion solution. Seventy-one percent of subjects were able to achieve at least a 50% decrease in pain. Fifty-nine percent of these subjects were able to achieve a similar level of pain relief for an average of 16 months. Clonidine is highly lipophilic and may produce systemic side effects such as a modest (30%) decrease in both blood pressure and heart rate. Although it does not produce respiratory depression, it can induce transient sedation. Rebound hypertension may also occur with sudden discontinuation.

F. Ziconotide

Ziconotide is FDA approved for intrathecal use for the treatment of chronic pain. Like clonidine, it has demonstrated efficacy in the treatment of neuropathic pain including complex regional pain syndrome, HIV-associated neuropathy, painful diabetic neuropathy, postherpetic neuralgia, and central pain syndromes including poststroke pain, multiple sclerosis, and spinal cord injury. It is currently recommended as a first-line agent for neuropathic pain and a third-line agent for nociceptive pain. The typical starting daily dose is 1.4 μg with a maximum daily dose of 19 μg. A prospective study of 111 subjects with either cancer-related pain or HIV-associated neuropathy randomized subjects in a 2:1 ratio to receive IT ziconotide or placebo. Ziconotide caused a statistically significant decrease in VAS of 53.1% vs only 18.1% in the placebo group. Also noted in this study was that ziconotide produced significantly more vestibular effects including somnolence, confusion, urinary incontinence, and fever compared to placebo. The authors attributed this to blockade of N-channels in the granular cell layer of the cerebellum. They also noted that this could be avoided with a lower starting dose and less frequent dose titration. Another prospective study randomized 220 subjects to receive either IT ziconotide or placebo for the treatment of heterogeneous chronic pain conditions. The ziconotide-treated subjects had a significantly decreased VAS compared to placebo (14.7% vs 7.2%). This study also confirmed that many of the vestibular effects can be mitigated, but not entirely eliminated, with a lower starting dose and slower titration. Abrupt discontinuation of ziconotide therapy appears to be safe. Side effects that were noted in blinded prospective studies include dizziness, nystagmus, nausea, postural hypotension, abnormal gait, and memory impairment. Decreasing the infusion rate was noted to generally assuage these side effects. The dose-limiting and frequent side effects associated with IT ziconotide have limited its clinical use.

The commonly accepted practice for dosing of IT medications is to start with either a pure opioid regimen or a regimen that combines medications. Use of single IT agents is the exception and not the rule. There are multiple well-conducted studies evaluating the safety and efficacy of combination therapy.

III. PATIENT SELECTION

Candidates for IT therapy may be experiencing malignant, neuropathic, nociceptive pain, or a combination of these types of pain. The selection of appropriate candidates for continuous IT medication delivery systems is a major factor in predicting therapeutic outcomes. Patients must have demonstrated that they are experiencing continued pain despite maximal conservative medical therapy or that such therapy caused unacceptable side effects. In general, patients should have relatively well-managed comorbidities and a psychological profile that does not preclude surgical intervention or the long-term management of implanted hardware. The patients should not have any coagulopathies, either from intentional medication use or malignancy-related coagulopathy that would complicate surgical placement or predispose the patient to subcutaneous, epidural, or intradural hematomas. Patients should not have an allergy to any of the planned medications to be utilized. The absence of cerebrospinal fluid (CSF) flow is a relative contraindication as low CSF flow may predispose the patient to catheter tip granuloma formation but not necessarily a poor analgesic result. A life expectancy of <3 months is a relative but not an absolute contraindication to placement; less invasive and more cost-effective measures may offer equivalent analgesic benefit and a shorter recovery.

The final aspect of patient selection is a favorable response to an IT medication trial. Most physicians conduct a trial with percutaneous insertion of an intrathecal catheter and titration of intrathecal medication in a monitored inpatient setting. Other methods of conducting a trial include a single-shot spinal injection with close observation for analgesic benefit or analgesic infusion via an epidural catheter. A positive trial is generally considered a decrease in pain of at least 50%. Additional benefit may be observed with increases in functionality or decreased analgesic medication consumption. An unsuccessful trial is a contraindication to a permanent implantation. Physicians must be mindful of placebo effect and bias by both the physician and the patient to overreport trial success. Longer trials of at least 3-5 days may decrease the chances of a false positive. There is no documented proof of superiority of one trial method over another. Following a successful trial and barring other contraindications, a patient may be offered a permanent implant of an IDDS

IV. NONPHARMACOLOGICAL COMPLICATIONS

Many technical problems may arise with placement and long-term management of a permanent IDDS. Consensus guidelines have been developed to minimize the risk of potential complications. Numerous texts detail the surgical placement of IDDS. As with any surgical procedure, complications such as bleeding and infection are present. Infections at the pump insertion site are relatively common. Some physicians have reported effective management of superficial infections with antibiotics and incision and drainage of the infected tissue. However, complete resolution of infections, in many circumstances, requires complete removal of hardware and antibiotic therapy. Any change in neurological exam warrants immediate removal of the hardware, infectious disease consultation, advanced imaging to delineate the location and extent of infection, and possible neurosurgical consultation. The routine use of antibiotics during the trial, the permanent implant, and for 3-5 days following implantation is routinely practiced but widely debated. Reimplantation following an infection is usually delayed for 3 months after the completion of antibiotic therapy. Bleeding at the pump pocket may create a hematoma that requires surgical drainage. Bleeding at the catheter insertion site may produce devastating epidural or subdural hematomas. Seromas may also form but are generally benign and do not need to be addressed surgically. Necrosis and skin perforations can also occur, especially in cachectic or poorly nourished patients and should be surgically treated.

The device may be placed under general anesthesia, a field block with local anesthesia, or spinal anesthesia. Accessing the intrathecal space under general anesthesia carries the same significant risk of unrecognized neurologic injury as other neuraxial techniques performed under general anesthesia. Spinal cord injury has also been reported during catheter placement under general anesthesia. Determination of the placement of the pump in the lower abdomen must be done prior to patient positioning as attempting an unmarked placement in the lateral position is notoriously difficult and will often result in the pump being placed too far laterally.

A rare but serious complication is the formation of an inflammatory mass such as a granuloma at the catheter tip. Consensus guidelines for the detection and management of catheter tip granulomas are available. The development of granulomas can lead to spinal cord or nerve root compression. Granulomas may manifest as a new neurologic deficit, a new pain presentation, or loss of IDDS effectiveness. MRI of the spinal cord is indicated if neurologic symptoms occur in these patients.

In general, IDDS administer a precise amount of medication to the CSF and then rely on diffusion and CSF movement to further disperse medications. Special situations, such as pain in a specific dermatome or the use of lipophilic opioids or bupivacaine, have led some to thread the catheter tips to spinal levels higher than the lumbar cistern. However, development of catheter tip granulomas causing potential neurologic compromise have led some to recommend against cephalad tip placement, except in very select circumstances.

A CSF leak may occur after violation of the thecal sac, including following intrathecal catheter placement. This may lead to the development of a post-dural puncture headache requiring a fluoroscopically guided blood patch. Fluoroscopic guidance is recommended in order to avoid catheter damage during blood patch.

Catheter-related complications occur in 25% of patients and may include kinking, obstruction, disconnection, dislodgement, breaks, and migration. Several procedural techniques may limit catheter malfunction including confirmation of CSF flow, anchoring to the supraspinous ligament using an anchoring device, inserting the catheter via a shallow paramedian approach, and use of fluoroscopy and contrast to confirm placement. Finally, a strain relief loop distal to the fixation device may limit migration and dislocation.

V. CONCLUSIONS

Implanted spinal drug delivery systems are a useful tool for the delivery of multiple medications, alone or in combination, directly to the central nervous system for the alleviation of pain in those who have failed to improve with less invasive treatments. Successful use of IDDS requires careful selection of each patient and the medication to be used and a high level of vigilance from the time of surgical implantation through the entire course of treatment to minimize complications.

Selected Readings

Deer TR, Levy R, Prager J, et al. Polyanalgesic Consensus Conference—2012: recommendations to reduce morbidity and mortality in intrathecal drug delivery in the treatment of chronic pain. *Neuromodulation.* 2012;15:467-482; discussion 482.

Deer TR, Prager J, Levy R, et al. Polyanalgesic Consensus Conference—2012: consensus on diagnosis, detection, and treatment of catheter-tip granulomas (inflammatory masses). *Neuromodulation.* 2012;15:483-495; discussion 496.

Deer TR, Prager J, Levy R, et al. Polyanalgesic Consensus Conference 2012: recommendations for the management of pain by intrathecal (intraspinal) drug delivery: report of an interdisciplinary expert panel. *Neuromodulation.* 2012;15:436-464; discussion 464-466.

Hassenbusch SJ, Gunes S, Wachsman S, Willis KD. Intrathecal clonidine in the treatment of intractable pain: a phase I/II study. *Pain Med.* 2002;3:85-91.

Kumar K, Bodani V, Bishop S, Tracey S. Use of intrathecal bupivacaine in refractory chronic nonmalignant pain. *Pain Med.* 2009;10:819-828.

Kumar K, Kelly M, Pirlot T. Continuous intrathecal morphine treatment for chronic pain of nonmalignant etiology: long-term benefits and efficacy. *Surg Neurol.* 2001;55:79-86; discussion 86-88.

Mironer YE, Haasis JC, Chapple I, Brown C, Satterthwaite JR. Efficacy and safety of intrathecal opioid/bupivacaine mixture in chronic nonmalignant pain: a double blind, randomized, crossover, multicenter study by the National Forum of Independent Pain Clinicians (NFIPC). *Neuromodulation.* 2002;5:208-213.

Raphael JH, Duarte RV, Southall JL, Nightingale P, Kitas GD. Randomised, double-blind controlled trial by dose reduction of implanted intrathecal morphine delivery in chronic non-cancer pain. *BMJ Open.* 2013;3.

Rauck RL, Cherry D, Boyer MF, Kosek P, Dunn J, Alo K. Long-term intrathecal opioid therapy with a patient-activated, implanted delivery system for the treatment of refractory cancer pain. *J Pain.* 2003;4:441-447.

Rauck RL, Wallace MS, Leong MS, et al. A randomized, double-blind, placebo-controlled study of intrathecal ziconotide in adults with severe chronic pain. *J Pain Symptom Manage.* 2006;31:393-406.

Smith TJ, Staats PS, Deer T, et al. Randomized clinical trial of an implantable drug delivery system compared with comprehensive medical management for refractory cancer pain: impact on pain, drug-related toxicity, and survival. *J Clin Oncol.* 2002;20:4040-4049.

Staats PS, Yearwood T, Charapata SG, et al. Intrathecal ziconotide in the treatment of refractory pain in patients with cancer or AIDS: a randomized controlled trial. *JAMA.* 2004;291:63-70.

21 Infusion Therapies

Michael Hermann, Rebecca L. Wu, and George Hanna

I. LIDOCAINE AND MEXILETINE

A. Mechanism of Action and Pharmacology

The local anesthetic, lidocaine, and mexiletine, a congener of lidocaine, block sodium channels and are also antiarrhythmic drugs. Clinically, their effects result from selective sodium channel blockade with inhibition of action potential propagation along nerves. The use of systemic lidocaine for pain management was first described 1961 by Bartlett and Hutaserani who used intraoperative lidocaine infusions for postoperative pain relief. Subsequent studies have demonstrated that lidocaine may have utility in controlling different types of pain as outlined below. Local anesthetics have been used specifically for neuropathic pain. Animal studies suggested that lidocaine may selectively suppress ectopic discharges, a core feature of neuropathic pain, while maintaining normal nerve function. Mexiletine also has a similar effect.

Further research has demonstrated that the mechanism of lidocaine is complex and the blockade of abnormal ectopic discharges is only one potential mechanism of pain control. In addition, multiple sodium channels have been elucidated, specifically tetrodotoxin-sensitive (TTX-S) and TTX-resistant (TTX-R) sodium channels in the dorsal root ganglion (DRG), with TTX-R having a particular role in pain and pain modulation. The role of lidocaine effects on these channels is still being examined, and studies indicate that IV lidocaine is useful for treatment of neuropathic pain associated with a variety of chronic conditions. Of note, while the half-life of lidocaine is short (2 hours), the beneficial effects can last for weeks. However, other studies show conflicting results, and further research is necessary to better define efficacy.

B. Uses in Specific Populations

1. **Perioperative period:** Lidocaine infusions have been used intraoperatively for a variety of surgeries, most commonly abdominal. Lidocaine has been associated with decreased postoperative pain scores, lower postoperative opioid use, faster return of bowel function, and decreased hospital stay. Other uses include orthopedic, cardiac, urologic, gynecologic, spine, and otolaryngology surgeries.
2. **Outpatient treatment:** Lidocaine infusions have also been routinely used on an outpatient basis to treat a variety of chronic pain conditions.
   a. **Central and peripheral neuropathic pain:** Lidocaine and mexiletine have been extensively used to treat neuropathic pain. Current evidence suggests that lidocaine and mexiletine are superior to placebo in multiple studies.
   b. **Fibromyalgia:** Lidocaine infusions have been used to treat fibromyalgia with effects lasting for weeks.
   c. **Cancer pain:** Infusions of lidocaine may be beneficial in opioid-resistant cancer pain.
   d. **Chronic regional pain syndrome (CRPS) I and II:** The role of lidocaine and mexiletine is evolving. One study demonstrates an improved response to cool stimuli.
   e. **Other uses:** Postherpetic neuralgia (intravenous and topical), residual limb pain, adolescent pain, chronic daily headache, and neuropathic pain from stroke and spinal cord injury pain.

C. Dosing

1. **Lidocaine**
   a. **Intraoperative:** Induction and bolus doses vary; however, multiple studies have demonstrated minimal to no complications with intraoperative use. Dosing length varies between immediate cessation to continuing up to 48 hours after surgery; however, there is likely no outcome difference by continuing the infusion beyond 60 minutes after surgery.
   b. **Outpatient:** Various amounts of lidocaine have been used; however, infusions are usually 5 mg/kg over 30 minutes to 1 hour (Table 21.1).
2. **Mexiletine:** Usually used if the patient has a positive response to lidocaine. Dosing ranges from 400 to 1200 mg/day.

D. Routes of Administration

1. **Systemic:** Lidocaine is most often given as an IV infusion; however, the subcutaneous route (bolus dose or infusion) and topical routes are also

TABLE 21.1 Intravenous Lidocaine Dosing for Pain Management

Type	Bolus Dose	Infusion Dose	Infusion Duration
Intraoperative	1.5-2 mg/kg	1.5-2 mg/kg/h	Beginning of surgery to immediately after closure to 48 h.
Outpatient	Optional, usually not performed	Up to 5 mg/kg	30-60 min

available. The plasma concentration is the determining factor of effectiveness, not route of administration.

2. Mexiletine is given as an oral drug.

E. Adverse Effects

1. Common side effects of lidocaine and mexiletine are similar to those of other local anesthetics and include nausea, vomiting, diarrhea, abdominal pain, dizziness, tingling, numbness, perioral symptoms, metallic taste, and dry mouth (McCarthy et al., 2010; Mooney et al., 2014, Vigneault et al., 2011). Lidocaine infusions typically have an increased incidence of these effects compared to oral mexiletine (McCarthy et al., 2010).
2. Serious side effects of local anesthetic toxicity including cardiac arrhythmias and seizures; however, these have not been reported in large meta-analyses.
3. Allergic reactions are another potential side effect. Lidocaine is an amide local anesthetic, and most local anesthetic allergic reactions are associated with the ester class of local anesthetics.

II. KETAMINE INFUSION

A. Mechanism of Action and Pharmacology

Ketamine is a noncompetitive antagonist of the *N*-methyl-D-aspartic acid (NMDA) receptor. One of the main advantages of ketamine as a hypnotic drug is its dual amnestic and analgesic properties. In addition, ketamine preserves spontaneous ventilation and pharyngeal and laryngeal reflexes. Ketamine also has a favorable hemodynamic profile secondary to central sympathetic stimulation and induced catecholamine release.

B. Uses in Specific Populations

1. **Perioperative period:** Many studies have found ketamine infusions to be an effective analgesic adjunct in the acute perioperative setting. When given with a loading dose, ketamine infusion rates of 1-6 μg/kg/min have been found to have analgesic, opioid-sparing, and antihyperalgesic properties.
2. **Outpatient treatment:**
   a. **Neuropathic pain:** Evidence from multiple studies (all with study-design limitations) suggests that ketamine may be effective in treating central and peripheral neuropathic pain. Two randomized controlled studies with 9 and 10 patients, respectively, found IV ketamine infusions to be effective in central pain after spinal cord injury. The latter study found a 50% reduction in VAS pain scores for spontaneous and ongoing pain during the ketamine infusion. Several other randomized trials have found IV ketamine infusions to be equally effective in treating peripheral neuropathic pain, such as in patients with chronic phantom limb pain.
   b. **Peripheral nerve injury and postherpetic neuralgia (PHN):** Few studies have analyzed ketamine use in peripheral nerve injury and PHN. One randomized controlled trial with eight patients showed ketamine infusions reduced spontaneous pain, pain evoked by nonnoxious stimulation, and wind-up-like pain. Another randomized controlled trial with 20 patients with nerve injury pain showed a reduction in ongoing and evoked pain.
   c. **Fibromyalgia:** Some studies have shown that ketamine infusions reduce muscular pain at rest in fibromyalgia patients. However, one

study found that a short-term ketamine infusion does not provide long-term pain relief for patients with fibromyalgia.

d. **Cancer Pain:** Although few randomized controlled trials have been performed, preliminary studies have shown ketamine infusions to be an effective adjunct to opioid analgesics in treatment of chronic cancer pain. One randomized study of cancer patients with pain unrelieved by morphine found that ketamine infusions reduced pain up to 180 minutes after the infusion ended.

e. **CRPS:** Many studies, both nonrandomized and randomized, have investigated the effect of ketamine infusion in CRPS patients. Overall, ketamine infusions appear to be a promising treatment. Although ketamine has a strong analgesic effect during short-term infusions in CRPS, the prolonged effect of ketamine following infusion therapy is more ambiguous. There is some evidence that long-term infusion therapy (ie, up to 14 days) may be associated with pain relief lasting up to 3-6 months following treatment in a subset of individuals.

C. Dosing

Subanesthetic doses of ketamine are commonly used during infusion therapies. Intraoperative ketamine infusions used as adjuncts for intra- and postoperative pain traditionally range from 5 to 15 μg/kg/min. In outpatient settings for treatment of chronic pain, doses studied have ranged from 0.15 to 0.5 mg/kg for therapies lasting from 10 minutes to a few hours daily over a course of several days.

D. Routes of Administration

Ketamine infusion therapies can be administered intravenously and subcutaneously.

E. Adverse Effects

The most common side effects of ketamine are increased secretions and dissociative symptoms such as hallucinations, anxiety, paranoia, and memory deficits. Hypersalivation can be prevented or treated with an antisialagogues such as atropine or glycopyrrolate, and psychedelic side effects can be minimized with the use of benzodiazepines.

III. DEXMEDETOMIDINE INFUSION

A. Mechanism of Action and Pharmacology

Dexmedetomidine is an α-2 agonist with a high selectivity for α-2 compared to α-1 (α-2: α-1 activity is 1620:1, compared to 220:1 for clonidine). Dexmedetomidine's selectivity for the α-2 receptor may explain its stronger sedative and analgesic effects compared to clonidine. It appears to exert its analgesic effects at supraspinal sites and the spinal cord level.

B. Uses in Specific Populations

1. **Perioperative period:** Several randomized controlled trials have found that α-2 agonists, including dexmedetomidine infusions, reduce postoperative opioid consumption, pain intensity, and nausea.
2. **Outpatient treatment:** The role of dexmedetomidine infusions in the outpatient setting to treat chronic pain has not been studied as extensively. One randomized controlled study in 7 healthy volunteers found that a dexmedetomidine infusion reduced pain measured by a cold pressor test (subjects immersed their hand into ice water for 1 minute and then pain was evaluated).

C. Dosing
There are no standardized doses for dexmedetomidine infusions. In the randomized controlled study analyzing the analgesic effects of dexmedetomidine, an initial 10-minute infusion of 6 μg/kg/h was used followed by a 50-minute infusion rate of 0.2-0.6 μg/kg/h.

D. Routes of Administration
Dexmedetomidine infusions are given intravenously.

E. Adverse Effects
Potential serious adverse effects of dexmedetomidine include hypotension and bradycardia. Although the respiratory effects of dexmedetomidine are controversial, it is generally accepted that it causes minimal respiratory depression.

IV. BISPHOSPHONATE INFUSION

A. Mechanism of Action and Pharmacology
Bisphosphonates are pyrophosphate analogues and are traditionally used to treat bone disorders such as osteoporosis and Paget disease by inhibiting osteoclastic bone resorption. Recent studies have shown that via inhibition of osteoclasts and other cells involved in modulation of bone pain, bisphosphonates may have a role in treatment of chronic bone pain and CRPS.

B. Uses in Specific Populations
1. **CRPS:** Several randomized trials (though all with small sample sizes) have studied the effect of bisphosphonates on CRPS pain. One study with 11 patients found IV infusion of pamidronate to improve CRPS-associated pain (measured with the VAS) hyperhidrosis, vasomotor changes, and joint stiffness. Two other studies, with 23 and 29 patients, respectively, also found IV infusion of pamidronate to significantly reduce pain and improve physical function in patients with CRPS. Not only has pamidronate been found to be effective, but IV ibandronate has also been found to improve the symptoms of CRPS. A recent randomized, controlled study with 82 patients found that IV infusion of another bisphosphonate, neridronate, significantly reduced pain and improved functional status.

C. Dosing
There is no standardized dosing of IV bisphosphonate infusions. Studies analyzing pamidronate have used a wide range of IV infusion rates: ranging from 30 mg over 4 hours daily for 3 days, 1 mg/kg/d over 3 hours for 3 days, and 60 mg/d over 4 hours for 3 days).

D. Routes of Administration
Bisphosphonate infusions are given intravenously.

E. Adverse Effects
Bisphosphonates have few serious adverse effects. Side effects are usually well tolerated and include mild flulike symptoms or a transient acute phase reaction (eg, fever, myalgias, arthralgias) lasting 24-72 hours, which can be treated with NSAIDS. Another potential adverse effect is musculoskeletal pain. Although not noted in CRPS patients receiving bisphosphonate infusion therapy, osteonecrosis of the jaw has been reported as a serious potential adverse effect in patients receiving chronic IV bisphosphonate treatment for bone malignancies.

V. PHENTOLAMINE

A. Mechanism of Action and Pharmacology

Sympathetically mediated pain was originally coined by Roberts in 1986 when describing CRPS. Sympathetically mediated pain occurs through a variety of mechanisms including sprouting within the dorsal root. Other conditions such as invasive cancer, cancer, spinal cord injury, and fibromyalgia have also been suspected to have sympathetically mediated components. Invasive sympathetic blocks are used to treat intractable pain, and it has been surmised that phentolamine acts through a similar mechanism by attenuating sympathetic outflow.

B. Uses in Specific Populations

1. **Chronic neuropathic pain:** Studies evaluating the effectiveness of phentolamine are quite limited; some efficacy has been suggested for control of chronic neuropathic pain. Peak pain relief varies from shortly after completion of the infusion to several days later.

C. Dosing

IV 25-75 mg over 30 minutes. A preinfusion bolus may be administered for hypotension prevention.

D. Routes of Administration

Phentolamine for chronic pain has been evaluated as an intravenous infusion.

E. Adverse Effects

Evidence is sparse; however, side effects can include nasal stuffiness, dizziness, wheezing, hypotension, tachycardia, and/or arrhythmias.

Selected Readings

Akoplan AA, Souslova V, England S, et al. The tetrodotoxin-resistant sodium channel SNS has a specialized function in pain pathways. *Nat Neurosci.* 1999;2:541-548.

Attal N, Gaudé V, Brasseur L, et al. Intravenous lidocaine in central pain: a double-blind placebo-controlled psychophysical study. *Neurology.* 2000;54:564-574.

Baranowski AP, De Courcey J, Bonello E. A trial of intravenous lidocaine on the pain and allodynia of postherpetic neuralgia. *J Pain Symptom Manage.* 1999;17:429-433.

Bartlett EE, Hutaserani O. Xylocaine for the relief of postoperative pain. *Anesth Analg.* 1961;40:288-295.

Bhattacharya A, Gurnani A, Sharma PK, Sethi AK. Subcutaneous infusion of ketamine and morphine for relief of postoperative pain: a doubleblind comparative study. *Ann Acad Med Singapore.* 1994;23:456-459.

Blaudszun G, Lysakowski C, Elia N, Tramer MR. Effect of perioperative systemic α-2 agonists on postoperative morphine consumption and pain intensity: systematic review and meta-analysis of randomized controlled trials. *Anesthesiology.* 2012;116:1312-1322.

Breuer B, Pappagallo M, Ongseng F, Chen CI, Goldfarb R. An open-label pilot trial of ibandronate for complex regional pain syndrome. *Clin J Pain.* 2008;24:685-689.

Chabal C, Russell LC, Burchial KJ. The effect of intravenous lidocaine, tocainide, and mexiletine on spontaneously active fibers originating in rat sciatic neuromas. *Pain.* 1989;38:333-338.

Chan AK, Cheung CW, Chong YK. Alpha-2 agonists in acute pain management. *Expert Opin Pharmacother.* 2010;11:2849-2868.

Correll GE, Maleki J, Gracely EJ, Muir JJ, Harbur RE. Subanesthetic ketamine infusion therapy: a retrospective analysis of a novel therapeutic approach to complex regional pain syndrome. *Pain Med.* 2004;5:263-275.

Cortet B, Flipo RM, Coquerelle P, Duquesnoy B, Delcambre B. Treatment of severe, recalcitrant reflex sympathetic dystrophy: assessment of efficacy and safety of the second generation bisphosphonate pamidronate. *Clin Rheumatol.* 1997;16:51-56.

Devor M, Jänig W, Michaelis M. Modulation of activity in dorsal root ganglion neurons by sympathetic activation in nerve-injured rats. *J Neurophysiol.* 1994;71:38-47.

Devor M, Wall PD, Catalan N. Systemic lidocaine silences ectopic neuroma and DRG discharges without blocking nerve conduction. *Pain.* 1992;48:261-268.

Duvulder JER, Ghys L, Dhondt W, Rolly G. Neuropathic pain in a cancer patient responding to subcutaneously administered lignocaine. *Clin J Pain.* 1993;9: 220-223.

Eichenberger U, Neff F, Sveticic G, et al. Chronic phantom limb pain: the effects of calcitonin, ketamine, and their combination on pain and sensory thresholds. *Anesth Analg.* 2008;106:1265-1273.

Eide PK, Jorum E, Stubhaug A, Bremnes J, Breivik H. Relief of post-herpetic neuralgia with the N-methyl-D-aspartic acid receptor antagonist ketamine: a double-blind, cross-over comparison with morphine and placebo. *Pain.* 2004;58:347-354.

Eide PK, Stubhaug A, Stenehjem AE. Central dysesthesia pain after traumatic spinal cord injury is dependent on N-methyl-D-aspartate receptor activation. *Neurosurgery.* 1995;37:1080-1087.

Finnerup NB, Biering-Sørensen F, Johannesen IL, et al. Intravenous lidocaine relieves spinal cord injury pain: a randomized controlled trial. *Anesthesiology.* 2005;102:1023-1030.

Galer BS. Peak pain relief is delayed and duration of relief is extended following intravenous phentolamine infusion. *Reg Anesth.* 1995;20:444-447.

Galer BS, Harle J, Rowbotham MC. Response to intravenous lidocaine infusion predicts subsequent response to oral mexiletine: a prospective study. *J Pain Symptom Manage.* 1996;12:161-167.

Gamal G, Helaly M, Labib YM. Superior hypogastric block: transdiscal versus classic posterior approach in chronic pelvic pain. *Clin J Pain.* 2006;22:544-547.

Gottrup H, Bach FW, Juhl G, Jensen TS. Differential effect of ketamine and lidocaine on spontaneous and mechanical evoked pain in patients with nerve injury pain. *Anesthesiology.* 2006;104:527-537.

Graven-Nielsen T, Aspegren Kendall S, Henriksson KG, et al. Ketamine reduces muscle pain, temporal summation, and referred pain in fibromyalgia patients. *Pain.* 2000;85:483-491.

Hall JE, Uhrich TD, Barney JA, Arain SR, Ebert TJ. Sedative, amnestic, and analgesic properties of small-dose dexmedetomidine infusions. *Anesth Analg.* 2000;90:699-705.

Jahangir SM, Islam F, Aziz L. Ketamine infusion for postoperative analgesia in asthmatics: a comparison with intermittent meperidine. *Anesth Analg.* 1993;76:45-49.

Jung HS, Joo JD, Jeon YS, et al. Comparison of an intraoperative infusion of dexmedetomidine or remifentanil on perioperative haemodynamics, hypnosis and sedation, and postoperative pain control. *J Int Med Res.* 2011;39:1890-1899.

Kastrup J, Angelo H, Peterson P, Dejgård A, Hilsted J. Treatment of chronic painful diabetic neuropathy with intravenous lidocaine infusion. *Br Med J (Clin Res Ed).* 1986;292:173.

Khan JS, Yousuf M, Victor JC, Sharma A, Siddiqui N. An estimation for an appropriate end time for an intraoperative intravenous lidocaine infusion in bowel surgery: a comparative meta-analysis. *J Clin Anesth.* 2016;28:95-104.

Kosharskyy B, Almonte W, Shaparin N, Pappagallo M, Smith H. Intravenous infusions in chronic pain management. *Pain Physician.* 2013;16:231-249.

Kubalek I, Fain O, Paries J. Kettaneh A, Thomas M. Treatment of reflex sympathetic dystrophy with pamidronate: 29 cases. *Rheumatology.* 2001;40:1394-1397.

Kvarnstrom A, Karlsten R, Quiding H, Gordh T. The analgesic effect of intravenous ketamine and lidocaine on pain after spinal cord injury. *Acta Anaesthesiol Scand.* 2004;48:498-506.

Liu X, Chung K, Chung JM. Ectopic discharges and adrenergic sensitivity of sensory neurons after spinal nerve injury. *Brain Res.* 1999;849:244-247.

Maillefert JF, Chatard C, Owen S, Peere T, Tavernier C, Tebib J. Treatment of refractory reflex sympathetic dystrophy with pamidronate. *Ann Rheum Dis.* 1995;54:687.

Mao J, Chen LL. Systemic lidocaine for neuropathic pain relief. *Pain.* 2000;87:7-17.

Martinez-Lavin M. Fibromyalgia as a sympathetically maintained pain syndrome. *Curr Pain Headache Rep.* 2004;8:385-389.

McCarthy GC, Megalla SA, Habib AS. Impact of intravenous lidocaine infusion on postoperative analgesia and recovery from surgery: a systematic review of randomized controlled trials. *Drugs.* 2010;70:1149-1163.

McLachlan EM, Jänig W, Devor M, Michaelis M. Peripheral nerve injury triggers noradrenergic sprouting within dorsal root ganglia. *Nature.* 1993;363:543-546.

Mercadante S, Arcuri E, Tirelli W, Casuccio A. Analgesic effect of intravenous ketamine in cancer patients on morphine therapy: a randomized, controlled, double-blind, crossover, double-dose study. *J Pain Symptom Manage.* 2000;20:246-252.

Mooney JJ, Pagel PS, Kundu A. Safety, tolerability, and short-term efficacy of intravenous lidocaine infusions for the treatment of chronic pain in adolescents and young adults: a preliminary report. *Pain Med.* 2014;15:820-825.

Nagy I, Woolf CJ. Lignocaine selectively reduces C fibre-evoked neuronal activity in rat spinal cord in vitro by decreasing N-methyl-D-aspartate and neurokinin receptor-mediated post-synaptic depolarizations; implications for the development of novel centrally acting anesthetics. *Pain.* 1994;64:59-70.

Noppers I, Niesters M, Swartjes M, et al. Absence of long-term analgesic effect from a short-term S-ketamine infusion on fibromyalgia pain: a randomized, prospective, double blind, active placebo-controlled trial. *Eur J Pain.* 2011;15:942-949.

Owen H, Reekie RM, Clements JA, Watson R, Nimmo WS. Analgesia from morphine and ketamine. A comparison of infusions of morphine and ketamine for postoperative analgesia. *Anaesthesia.* 1987;42:1051-1056.

Peixoto RD, Hawley P. Intravenous lidocaine for cancer pain without electrocardiographic monitoring: a retrospective review. *J Palliat Med.* 2015;18:373-377.

Raja SN, Rolf-Detlef T, Davis KD, Campbell JN. Systemic alpha-adrenergic blockade with phentolamine: a diagnostic test for sympathetically maintained pain. *Anesthesiology.* 1991;74:691-698.

Raphael JH, Southall J, Treharne GJ, Kitas GD. Efficacy and adverse effects of intravenous lignocaine therapy in fibromyalgia syndrome. *BMC Musculoskelet Disord.* 2002;3:1-8.

Roberts WJ. A hypothesis on the physiological basis for causalgia and related pains. *Pain.* 1986;24:297-311.

Rowbotham MC, Davies PS, Verkempinck C, Galer BS. Lidocaine patch: double-blind controlled study of a new treatment method for post-herpetic neuralgia. *Pain.* 1996;65:39-44.

Schafranski MD, Malucelli T, Machado F, et al. Intravenous lidocaine for fibromyalgia syndrome: an open trial. *Clin Rheumatol.* 2009;28:853-855.

Schwartzman RJ, Alexander GM, Grothusen JR, Paylor T, Reichenberger E, Perreault M. Outpatient intravenous ketamine for the treatment of complex regional pain syndrome: a double-blind placebo controlled study. *Pain.* 2009;147:107-115.

Sharma S Rajagopal MR, Palat G, Singh C, Haji AG, Jain D. A phase II study to evaluate use of intravenous lidocaine for opioid-refractory pain in cancer patients. *J Pain Symptom Manage.* 2009;37:85-93.

Shir Y, Cameron LB, Raja SN, Bourke DL. The safety of intravenous phentolamine administration in patients with neuroleptic pain. *Anesth Analg.* 1993;76:1008-1011.

Sorensen J, Bengtsson A, Backman E, Henriksson KG, Bengtsson M. Pain analysis in patients with fibromyalgia, effects of intravenous morphine, lidocaine and ketamine. *Scand J Rheumatol.* 1995;24:360-365.

Stubhaug A, Breivik H, Eide PK, Kreunen M, Foss A. Mapping of punctuate hyperalgesia around a surgical incision demonstrates that ketamine is a powerful suppressor of central sensitization to pain following surgery. *Acta Anaesthesiol Scand.* 1997;41:1124-1132.

Tremont-Lukats IW, Hutson PR, Backonja MM. A randomized, double-masked, placebo-controlled pilot trial of IV lidocaine infusion for relief of ongoing neuropathic pain. *Clin J Pain.* 2006;22:266-71.

Varenna M, Adami S, Rossini M, et al. Treatment of complex regional pain syndrome type I with neridronate: a randomized, double-blind, placebo-controlled study. *Rheumatology.* 2013;52:534-542.

Vickers ER, Cousins MJ. Neuropathic orofacial pain. Part 2. Diagnostic procedures, treatment guidelines, and case reports. *Aust Endod J.* 2000;26:53-63.

Vigneault L, Turgeon AF, Côté D, et al. Perioperative intravenous lidocaine infusion for postoperative pain control: a meta-analysis of randomized controlled trials. *Can J Anaesth.* 2011;58:22-37.

Virtanen R, Savola JM, Saano V, Nyman L. Characterization of selectivity, specificity, and potency of medetomidine as alpha 2-adrenoreceptor agonist. *Eur J Pharmacol.* 1988;150:9-14.

Wallace MS, Ridgeway BM, Leung AY, Gerayli A, Yaksh TL. Concentration-effect relationship of intravenous lidocaine on allodynia of complex regional pain syndrome types I and II. *Anesthesiology.* 2000;92:75-83.

Wu H, Sultana R, Taylor KB, Szabo A. A prospective randomized double-blinded pilot study to examine the effect of botulinum toxin type A injection versus Lidocaine/Depomedrol injection on residual and phantom limb pain: initial report. *Clin J Pain.* 2012;28:108-112.

Yan BM, Myers RP. Neurolytic celiac plexus block for pain control in unresectable pancreatic cancer. *Am J Gastroenterol.* 2007;102:430-438.

Yasukawa M, Yasukawa K, Kamiizumi Y, Yokoyama R. Intravenous phentolamine infusion alleviates the pain of abdominal visceral cancer, including pancreatic carcinoma. *J Anesth.* 2007;21:420-423.

22 Neurosurgical Interventions for Pain

Benjamin L. Grannan

I. GENERAL CONSIDERATIONS

A. Timing and Patient Selection

Although neurosurgical advances have led to less invasive and even reversible interventions for the treatment of pain, neurosurgery should only be considered after medical therapies and temporary anesthetic interventions (eg, injections, nerve blocks) have been considered and exhausted. The appropriate timing of referral for neurosurgical evaluation depends upon the etiology and severity of the pain, the patient's personal disposition toward surgical intervention, and the patient's comorbidities and life expectancy. When performed under the correct clinical circumstances and with appropriate expectations about the probable outcome, neurosurgical procedures for pain can be highly successful and can often lead to drastic improvements in quality of life. Neurosurgical interventions carry significant risk, and some of these interventions may cause new neurologic deficits in order to gain pain relief. Patient selection for a given intervention, however, is not trivial and the likelihood of benefit can be uncertain. It is critical that the neurosurgeon shares expectations about the most probable outcomes with the patient and other clinicians involved in care of the patient in order to achieve optimal patient satisfaction.

B. Treatment Modalities

Historically, most neurosurgical procedures for pain have consisted of tissue resection or ablation, permanently removing or destroying a neurological structure involved in the underlying aberrant pain signaling. Examples of such procedures include trigeminal ganglion resection or ablation for trigeminal neuralgia or spinothalamic tract ablation for unilateral pain associated with invasive cancer. Microvascular decompression, the microsurgical technique used to eliminate vascular compression of the trigeminal nerve, remains a highly utilized and effective option for treatment of trigeminal neuralgia. A similar technique (albeit much less commonly) is used to treat glossopharyngeal neuralgia. More recently, neurosurgical options have expanded to include neuromodulatory approaches which leverage the use electrical stimulation through implanted electrodes connected to indwelling pulse generators. Neuromodulatory interventions decrease pain transmission and/or perception by delivering stimulation to either narrow targets (eg, dorsal root ganglion stimulation, dorsal anterior cingulate gyrus) or to broader anatomic areas (eg, multilevel epidural spinal cord stimulation [SCS]). In this chapter, the major pain pathologies amenable to at least one of these treatment modalities are discussed.

II. TRIGEMINAL NEURALGIA

A. Diagnostic Considerations

Trigeminal neuralgia is characterized by episodes of lancinating pain in one or multiple sensory distributions of the trigeminal nerve. Pain episodes can occur spontaneously but can also be triggered by movements of face musculature or minor tactile stimulation. Trigeminal neuralgia has a median age of onset in the late 50s and tends to have a female predominance (5.9 female compared to 3.4 male annual age-adjusted incidence).[1,2] Trigeminal neuralgia is often divided into two subtypes: type 1 is described as the classic lancinating electric pain that tends to be episodic, whereas type 2 has a more constant and often burning component, although episodic pain is still often present. Determining the appropriate surgical intervention, if any, requires identifying trigeminal neuralgia and its subtype correctly and excluding other facial pain diagnoses (eg, atypical facial pain, postherpetic neuralgia, nervus intermedius neuralgia, glossopharyngeal neuralgia, trigeminal neuropathic pain, or temporomandibular joint syndrome) through careful history taking. Since the diagnosis is largely made based upon the patient history, helpful questionnaires have been developed to aid in clinical diagnosis (see Oregon Health & Science University Public Diagnostic Platform: https://neurosurgery.ohsu.edu/tgn.php).[3] Although the exact pathophysiology of trigeminal neuralgia remains uncertain, it has been frequently proposed in the literature that vascular compression of the root entry zone of the trigeminal complex is the underlying causal process. Studies linking preoperative imaging and intraoperative evidence of neurovascular compression contain equivocal support for this theory.[4,5]

B. Microvascular Decompression

Microvascular decompression remains the preferred treatment for trigeminal neuralgia when medication is either not effective or not tolerated. Other options should be considered, however, in patients with significant medical comorbidities or in patients who are particularly averse to surgical intervention.[6] The procedure is performed under general anesthesia and consists of a suboccipital craniotomy to surgically access the cerebellopontine angle for decompression of the trigeminal nerve at its root entry zone. While the surgical technique varies, a common approach is to implant multiple synthetic pledgets between the nerve and any abutting arterial (typically the superior cerebellar artery) or venous structures. Hospital stay is typically 2-3 days in duration. Patients often experience immediate facial pain relief following surgery and long-term pain relief without the assistance of medications is cited at ~70%.[1,7] The procedure can be performed safely but does carry some risks such as cerebrospinal fluid leak (2.5%), severe facial sensory loss (1.6%), severe hearing loss (1.1%), and mortality (0.2%).[1,8]

C. Percutaneous Treatments

Radiofrequency and balloon compression rhizotomy are two percutaneous approaches for the treatment of trigeminal neuralgia that can be considered in patients who are averse to surgical intervention, not good surgical candidates from a medical perspective, or who have recurrent trigeminal neuralgia despite prior microvascular decompression. Both procedures are minimally invasive, provide immediate relief, and can be performed in under 1 hour. They are often safely done as ambulatory surgery, without the need for inpatient hospitalization.

Radiofrequency rhizotomy is performed by percutaneously introducing a radiofrequency probe through the foramen ovale under fluoroscopic guidance such that retro-gasserian trigeminal fibers can be reached and ablated by the probe. With the patient under sedation, the electrode is introduced into the initial position and low-level electrical stimulation is administered. During this testing, the patient is asked to confirm that the induced sensory disturbances match the distribution of his or her trigeminal neuralgia pain. This provides verification of the appropriate positioning of the electrode. Ablation of ophthalmic segment trigeminal fibers via this technique is generally avoided due to the risk of corneal hypoesthesia and subsequent corneal abrasion. Radiofrequency rhizotomy results in immediate pain relief in over 90% of patients and durable pain relief has been reported at nearly 60% of patients at 5-year follow-up.[9] A rare but notable side effect of this procedure is anesthesia dolorosa which is estimated to occur in 0.8% of cases.[9]

Balloon compression rhizotomy similarly involves percutaneous access of the gasserian ganglion and retrogasserian nerve fibers via the foramen ovale. A Fogarty balloon catheter containing x-ray contrast is introduced into this space under fluoroscopic guidance and then expanded to compress the trigeminal complex for several minutes. Balloon compression rhizotomy also has high rates of immediate and long-term success. In one large series, pain recurrence was found to be 19.2% and 31.9% at 5 and 10.7 years, respectively. In this same cohort, there were no instances of anesthesia dolorosa or corneal anesthesia.[10] Rates of immediate sensation disturbances are high in this procedure and can be long standing in 5%-40% of cases.[11] Also, this procedure can be performed for ophthalmic division trigeminal neuralgia since it has a low rate of corneal desensitization.

D. Radiosurgery

Several options are available for delivery of radiation therapy to the trigeminal ganglion and/or nerve for treatment of trigeminal neuralgia. These include Gamma Knife, CyberKnife, and linear accelerator therapies. While radiosurgery does not provide immediate pain relief, initial pain improvement (at 1-2 months) occurs in 70%-90% of cases.[11] The procedure is typically well tolerated but is associated with facial sensory disturbances.[12] Radiosurgery provides a good treatment option for surgically averse patients, patients who are poor medical surgical candidates, and patients with recurrent trigeminal neuralgia despite prior interventions.

There are no meaningful comparative studies to help understand which among the numerous available ablative techniques available to treat trigeminal neuralgia is superior. Because of the high, durable success of microvascular decompression, this approach is most often used for patients who have failed medical treatment and whose comorbid medical conditions do not prevent safely proceeding with open neurosurgical intervention.

III. SPINAL INTERVENTIONS FOR NEUROPATHIC PAIN

A. Dorsal Root Entry Zone Lesioning

Patients suffering from neuropathic pain due to a peripheral nerve injury with deafferentation pain (eg, nerve root avulsion or brachial plexus injury) may benefit from dorsal root entry zone (DREZ) lesioning. It is theorized that that loss of peripheral afferent pain signaling in the setting of peripheral nerve injury leads to dysregulation of second order afferent neurons within the substantia gelatinosa of the dorsal horn. These neurons reside just deep to the entry zone of the dorsal nerve rootlets as they enter the spinal cord; lesioning them eliminates their aberrant painful signaling to cortical sensory domains.[13] Given the nature of the procedure, patients with pain restricted to one or two dermatomes tend to respond better to the procedure than patients with more widespread pain syndromes.[14]

The procedure is performed with the patient under general anesthesia in the prone position. Laminectomies are performed at and surrounding the level of injury and a durotomy is made to visualize the spinal cord and the DREZ. An area of avulsion can often be directly visualized. Atrophic nerve rootlets are also suggestive of the injured level. Radiofrequency ablation with a Nashold electrode is the typical technique used for lesioning. The electrode is placed orthogonally into the DREZ to a depth of 1-3 mm and is powered to a temperature of 75°C for 15-20 seconds.[15] Depending on the targeted area, which includes flanking levels to compensate for the 1-2 spinal cord level span of Lissauer tract, several tens of ablations can be performed sequentially.[16]

In patients with brachial plexus injury or nerve root avulsion pain, DREZ lesioning has been shown to significantly improve pain symptoms in 60%-90% of patients.[17-19] The procedure has shown only occasional efficacy in patients suffering chronic pain in the setting of spinal cord injury, spasticity, postherpetic neuralgia, and destructive malignancies. The major adverse outcome from DREZ lesioning is paresthesia which is most often a temporary phenomenon.[14]

B. Spinal Cord Stimulation

SCS is a neuromodulatory technique that provides epidural stimulation to dorsal columns, typically at the mid to low thoracic levels, through an implanted stimulating electrode array connected to an indwelling pulse generator. This has become a common intervention for chronic neuropathic pain, especially in the setting of failed back surgery syndrome and complex regional pain syndrome. Efficacy of SCS has been rigorously studied in multiple randomized control studies which have demonstrated improved short- and long-term pain control compared to medical management.[20] More recently, the use of high-frequency stimulation (10 kHz) has demonstrated superior pain control to conventional SCS.[21,22] Future efforts dedicated to optimizing stimulation paradigms, including closed-loop technologies, hold promise for additional improvement in pain control outcomes from SCS. For more in-depth discussion of spinal cord stimulation, see Chapter 18.

IV. CANCER PAIN

A. Cordotomy

Spiller and Martin first introduced the concept of cordotomy, or the destruction of the spinothalamic tract, for chronic pain in 1912.[23] The procedure is most appropriate for patients with localized, unilateral nociceptive pain and is most commonly performed in cancer patients with intractable unilateral pain (eg, hemipelvic pain from pelvic metastases). The surgery can either be performed through a percutaneous approach at the C1-C2 spinal level or through an open surgical approach at the upper thoracic spinal cord. Pain-mediating afferent fibers enter the spinal cord and synapse in the substantia gelatinosa ipsilateral to the side of the painful stimulus. Postsynaptic afferent fibers then decussate and join the contralateral ascending spinothalamic tract. The decussation can occur over 2-5 spinal levels.[24] Because of this, the level of ablation must be sufficiently rostral to the level of the painful stimulus in order to ensure adequate ablation. Cervical cordotomy at C1-C2 can achieve reliable control of pain below the C5 level, and a thoracic cordotomy at T4 can achieve reliable pain control below the T10 level.[25] Anterior horn cells controlling level-specific motor control are located deep and medial to the spinothalamic tract and are at risk of injury during ablation. Anterior horn cells at high cervical and thoracic levels do not control critical motor function which is another reason these are areas targeted by this approach. However, interneurons controlling respiratory drive within the high cervical spinal cord are at risk. For this reason, bilateral cervical cordotomies are rarely performed since bilateral injury to these interneurons can result in Ondine's curse, a life-threatening sleep-related apnea phenomenon.

Following cordotomy, ~90% of patients experience immediate pain relief, and 50%-60% continue to experience pain after 1 year follow-up.[26] Open cordotomy achieves comparable rates of pain relief (93% immediate and 54%-64% at 1 year).[27-29] Cordotomy is not as effective when used to treat nonmalignant sources of pain (~20% pain relief). Adverse outcomes of the procedure include mirror pain (temporary pain on contralateral side of body that is similar in nature to the initial pain syndrome), temporary bowel and bladder dysfunction, ataxia, and temporary weakness.

B. Implantable Drug Delivery Pumps

Pumps can be surgically implanted for the purpose of continuous, programmable intrathecal drug delivery. The pump is implanted in the soft tissue of the abdominal wall and is connected to a catheter which is tunneled subcutaneously and through the interspinous lumbar space and into the thecal sac. Compared to surgical procedures such as cordotomy, implantable systems may not be appropriate in patients with short life expectancies or barriers to receiving follow-up care which is necessary for pump refill and battery change. When compared to intensive standard medical management of pain, intrathecal drug delivery achieve higher rates of reported pain improvement (84.5% vs 70.8%) and has also been associated with survival benefit and decreased rates of suppressed mental status and fatigue, which often result from oral opioid therapy.[30] For more in-depth discussion of intrathecal drug delivery, see Chapter 20.

V. AFFECTIVE PAIN

A. Cingulotomy

Ablation of the cingulate gyrus for treatment of refractory pain syndrome was first developed by Foltz and White at the University of Washington. Building upon observations made in patients who had undergone prefrontal lobotomies, they utilized the anterior cingulotomy for patients whose pain was largely affective with "prominent emotional factors".[31] Technically, the procedure consists of making a series of radiofrequency thermocoagulation lesions within the dorsal anterior cingulate gyrus.[32]

Cingulotomy initially was offered only for cancer-related nociceptive pain but additional studies have showed comparable rates of pain relief in both cancer and noncancer pain syndromes (65.3% and 68%, respectively).[33] Adverse side effects of the procedure include confusion, disorientation, decrements in executive function, seizure, and personality changes, which are infrequent and often are transient.[33,34]

VI. NEUROMODULATION FOR PAIN

A. Deep Brain Stimulation

Deep brain stimulation (DBS) to the stereotactic implantation of a multicontact stimulation macroelectrode to a subcortical brain target. It is commonly used for the treatment of movement disorders but DBS has also been used in off-label fashion for chronic pain. Many brain areas have been targeted for refractory brain syndromes including thalamic nuclei (most commonly the ventroposterior lateral nucleus), anterior cingulate cortex, and the periaqueductal and periventricular gray (PAG/PVG).[35,36] Levy et al. reviewed all outcome reports for DBS for pain and found that 50% of patients, across all indications, experienced long-term pain relief.[37] Of note, ventroposterior lateral stimulation was associated with 56% long-term success when used for neuropathic pain but achieved 0% efficacy when used for nociceptive pain. Conversely, PAG/PVG stimulation achieved better outcomes when applied for nociceptive pain (59%) compared to neuropathic indications (23%).[37] The dorsal anterior cingulate gyrus has also been a target for neuropathic pain and preliminary analysis of a heterogeneous treatment population (failed back surgery syndrome, post-stroke, spinal cord injury, brachial plexus injury) showed statistically significant improvement in functional status and pain scale assessments at ~1-year follow-up.[38]

B. Motor Cortex Stimulation

Continuous stimulation of the primary motor cortex through epidural stimulation of the brain has been reported for treatment of intractable pain syndromes in which other treatment options remain limited, such as thalamic postinfarct pain syndromes, neuropathic facial pain, and other chronic, neuropathic pain syndromes.[37,39] It is thought that motor cortical stimulation inhibits thalamic hyperactivity, which can be present in neuropathic pain syndromes.[40] The procedure consists of preoperative fMRI to identify motor cortex representation of anatomic area affected by the pain. In the operating room, standard neuronavigation is used to place a stimulating electrode over the targeted area of the motor cortex in the epidural space. This is followed by a trial stimulation period in which the stimulating parameter space is explored and confirmed to be effective before the indwelling pulse generator is implanted. Pain relief rates are ~60%-70% in both facial pain and post-stroke pain syndromes. Adverse outcomes associated with motor cortex stimulation are rare but include intracranial hemorrhage and seizure.[37]

VII. CONCLUSIONS

There are a wide range of neurosurgical procedures that can be used to treat refractory pain. These procedures range from microsurgical neurovascular decompression in the setting of trigeminal neuralgia to neuromodulatory techniques such as DBS and spinal cord stimulation. Ablative procedures such as DREZ lesioning for neuropathic pain in the setting of brachial plexus avulsion or cordotomy for intractable cancer pain offer relief of symptoms in patients who may not have other reasonable options. Effective use of neurosurgery for pain management requires careful patient selection tailored to specific pain pathophysiology and overall prognosis.

References

1. Barker FG, Jannetta PJ, Bissonette DJ, Larkins MV, Jho HD. The long-term outcome of microvascular decompression for trigeminal neuralgia. *N Engl J Med.* 1996;334(17):1077-1083. doi: 10.1056/NEJM199604253341701.
2. Katusic S, Williams DB, Beard M, Bergstralh EJ, Kurland LT. Epidemiology and clinical features of idiopathic trigeminal neuralgia and glossopharyngeal neuralgia: similarities and differences, Rochester, Minnesota, 1945-1984. *Neuroepidemiology.* 1991;10(5-6):276-281. doi: 10.1159/000110284.
3. OHSU. TGN—Public Diagnostic Platform. https://neurosurgery.ohsu.edu/tgn.php
4. Baldwin NG, Sahni KS, Jensen ME, Pieper DR, Anderson RL, Young HF. Association of vascular compression in trigeminal neuralgia versus other "facial pain syndromes" by magnetic resonance imaging. *Surg Neurol.* 1991;36(6):447-452. doi: 10.1016/0090-3019(91)90158-6.
5. Revuelta-Gutierrez R, Martinez-Anda JJ, Coll JB, Campos-Romo A, Perez-Peña N. Efficacy and safety of root compression of trigeminal nerve for trigeminal neuralgia without evidence of vascular compression. *World Neurosurg.* 2013;80(3-4):385-389. doi: 10.1016/j.wneu.2012.07.030.
6. Slavin KV, Nersesyan H, Colpan ME, Munawar N. Current algorithm for the surgical treatment of facial pain. *Head Face Med.* 2007;3(1):30. doi: 10.1186/1746-160X-3-30.
7. Sindou M, Leston J, Decullier E, Chapuis F. Microvascular decompression for primary trigeminal neuralgia: long-term effectiveness and prognostic factors in a series of 362 consecutive patients with clear-cut neurovascular conflicts who underwent pure decompression. *J Neurosurg.* 2007;107(6):1144-1153. doi: 10.3171/JNS-07/12/1144.
8. McLaughlin MR, Jannetta PJ, Clyde BL, Subach BR, Comey CH, Resnick DK. Microvascular decompression of cranial nerves: lessons learned after 4400 operations. *J Neurosurg.* 1999;90(1):1-8. doi: 10.3171/jns.1999.90.1.0001.
9. Kanpolat Y, Savas A, Bekar A, Berk C. Percutaneous controlled radiofrequency trigeminal rhizotomy for the treatment of idiopathic trigeminal neuralgia: 25-year experience with 1600 patients. *Neurosurgery.* 2001;48(3):524-534. doi: 10.1097/00006123-200103000-00013.
10. Skirving DJ, Dan NG. A 20-year review of percutaneous balloon compression of the trigeminal ganglion. *J Neurosurg.* 2001;94(6):913-917. doi: 10.3171/jns.2001.94.6.0913.
11. Bick SKB, Eskandar EN. Surgical treatment of trigeminal neuralgia. *Neurosurg Clin N Am.* 2017;28(3):429-438. doi: 10.1016/j.nec.2017.02.009.
12. Wolf A, Kondziolka D. Gamma knife surgery in trigeminal neuralgia. *Neurosurg Clin N Am.* 2016;27(3):297-304. doi: 10.1016/j.nec.2016.02.006.
13. Nashold BS, Ostdahl RH. Dorsal root entry zone lesions for pain relief. *J Neurosurg.* 1979;51(1):59-69. doi: 10.3171/jns.1979.51.1.0059.
14. Piyawattanametha N, Sitthinamsuwan B, Euasobhon P, Zinboonyahgoon N, Rushatamukayanunt P, Nunta-Aree S. Efficacy and factors determining the outcome of dorsal root entry zone lesioning procedure (DREZotomy) in the treatment of intractable pain syndrome. *Acta Neurochir (Wien).* 2017;159(12):2431-2442. doi: 10.1007/s00701-017-3345-3.
15. Schulder M. *Handbook of Stereotactic and Functional Neurosurgery.* S.l.: CRC Press; 2019.
16. Eli I, Konrad P, Niemat J. Ablative procedures for neuropathic pain. In: Shaffrey CI, Couldwell WT, Berger MS, Harbaugh R, eds. *Neurosurgery Knowledge Update: A Comprehensive Review.* New York: Thieme; 2015:300-307. https://www.thieme-connect.de/products/ebooks/book/10.1055/b-003-122078. Accessed January 17, 2020.
17. Thomas DG, Jones SJ. Dorsal root entry zone lesions (Nashold's procedure) in brachial plexus avulsion. *Neurosurgery.* 1984;15(6):966-968. doi: 10.1227/00006123-198412000-00040.
18. Tomás R, Haninec P. Dorsal root entry zone (DREZ) localization using direct spinal cord stimulation can improve results of the DREZ thermocoagulation

procedure for intractable pain relief. *Pain.* 2005;116(1-2):159-163. doi: 10.1016/j.pain.2005.03.015.
19. Samii M, Moringlane JR. Thermocoagulation of the dorsal root entry zone for the treatment of intractable pain. *Neurosurgery.* 1984;15(6):953-955.
20. Grider J, Manchikanti L, Carayannopoulos A, et al. Effectiveness of spinal cord stimulation in chronic spinal pain: a systematic review. *Pain Physician.* 2016;19(1):E33-E54.
21. Al-Kaisy A, Van Buyten J-P, Smet I, Palmisani S, Pang D, Smith T. Sustained effectiveness of 10 kHz high-frequency spinal cord stimulation for patients with chronic, low back pain: 24-month results of a prospective multicenter study. *Pain Med.* 2014;15(3):347-354. doi: 10.1111/pme.12294.
22. Kapural L, Yu C, Doust MW, et al. Comparison of 10-kHz high-frequency and traditional low-frequency spinal cord stimulation for the treatment of chronic back and leg pain. *Neurosurgery.* 2016;79(5):667-677. doi: 10.1227/NEU.0000000000001418.
23. Spiller WG. The treatment of persistent pain of organic origin in the lower part of the body by division of the anterolateral column of the spinal cord. *JAMA.* 1912;LVIII(20):1489. doi: 10.1001/jama.1912.04260050165001.
24. Kanpolat Y, Ugur HC, Ayten M, Elhan AH. Computed tomography-guided percutaneous cordotomy for intractable pain in malignancy. *Neurosurgery.* 2009;64(3 Suppl):187-193; discussion ons193-194. doi: 10.1227/01.NEU.0000335645.67282.03.
25. Jones B, Finlay I, Ray A, Simpson B. Is there still a role for open cordotomy in cancer pain management? *J Pain Symptom Manage.* 2003;25(2):179-184. doi: 10.1016/s0885-3924(02)00689-9.
26. Konrad P. Dorsal root entry zone lesion, midline myelotomy and anterolateral cordotomy. *Neurosurg Clin N Am.* 2014;25(4):699-722. doi: 10.1016/j.nec.2014.07.010.
27. Cowie RA, Hitchcock ER. The late results of antero-lateral cordotomy for pain relief. *Acta Neurochir (Wien).* 1982;64(1-2):39-50. doi: 10.1007/bf01405617.
28. Piscol K. [Open spinal operations (anterolateral cordotomy and commissural myelotomy) in modern treatment of pain (author's transl)]. *Langenbecks Arch Chir.* 1976;342:91-99. doi: 10.1007/bf01267353.
29. White JC, Sweet WH, Hawkins R, Nilges RG. Anterolateral cordotomy: results, complications and causes of failure. *Brain.* 1950;73(3):346-367. doi: 10.1093/brain/73.3.346.
30. Smith TJ, Staats PS, Deer T, et al. Randomized clinical trial of an implantable drug delivery system compared with comprehensive medical management for refractory cancer pain: impact on pain, drug-related toxicity, and survival. *J Clin Oncol.* 2002;20(19):4040-4049. doi: 10.1200/JCO.2002.02.118.
31. Foltz EL, White LE. Pain "relief" by frontal cingulumotomy. *J Neurosurg.* 1962;19:89-100. doi: 10.3171/jns.1962.19.2.0089.
32. Agarwal N, Choi PA, Shin SS, Hansberry DR, Mammis A. Anterior cingulotomy for intractable pain. *Interdiscip Neurosurg.* 2016;6:80-83. doi: 10.1016/j.inat.2016.10.005.
33. Sharim J, Pouratian N. Anterior cingulotomy for the treatment of chronic intractable pain: a systematic review. *Pain Physician.* 2016;19(8):537-550.
34. Cohen RA, Kaplan RF, Moser DJ, Jenkins MA, Wilkinson H. Impairments of attention after cingulotomy. *Neurology.* 1999;53(4):819-824. doi: 10.1212/wnl.53.4.819.
35. Hosobuchi Y, Adams JE, Linchitz R. Pain relief by electrical stimulation of the central gray matter in humans and its reversal by naloxone. *Science.* 1977;197(4299):183-186. doi: 10.1126/science.301658.
36. Russo JF, Sheth SA. Deep brain stimulation of the dorsal anterior cingulate cortex for the treatment of chronic neuropathic pain. *Neurosurg Focus.* 2015;38(6):E11. doi: 10.3171/2015.3.FOCUS1543.
37. Levy R, Deer TR, Henderson J. Intracranial neurostimulation for pain control: a review. *Pain Physician.* 2010;13(2):157-165.
38. Boccard SGJ, Fitzgerald JJ, Pereira EAC, et al. Targeting the affective component of chronic pain. *Neurosurgery.* 2014;74(6):628-637. doi: 10.1227/NEU.0000000000000321.
39. Tsubokawa T, Katayama Y, Yamamoto T, Hirayama T, Koyama S. Chronic motor cortex stimulation for the treatment of central pain. *Acta Neurochir Suppl (Wien).* 1991;52:137-139. doi: 10.1007/978-3-7091-9160-6_37.
40. Tsubokawa T, Katayama Y, Yamamoto T, Hirayama T, Koyama S. Treatment of thalamic pain by chronic motor cortex stimulation. *Pacing Clin Electrophysiol.* 1991;14(1):131-134. doi: 10.1111/j.1540-8159.1991.tb04058.x.

23 Complications Associated With Interventional Pain Treatment

James P. Rathmell

I. OVERVIEW

Complications can arise in the course of any type of medical treatment, and the common interventions used to treat acute and chronic pain are no exception. The best approach to preventing adverse outcomes during the majority of interventional treatments is to have detailed knowledge of the anatomy of the adjacent structures that lie near the target site for each intended treatment and a clear understanding of how the technique has been devised to minimize the risk of harm to those structures. Needle placement for many pain procedures is now best carried out with the use of image guidance, and the widespread availability of fluoroscopy and ultrasonography has increased both the precision and the safety of many techniques. When complications do arise, prompt recognition and treatment can often prevent serious sequelae.

II. COMPLICATIONS ASSOCIATED WITH EPIDURAL, FACET JOINT, AND SACROILIAC INJECTION

Serious complications associated with epidural, facet joint, and sacroiliac joint injections are rare. Nerve injury, infection, death/brain damage, headache, and increased pain/no relief have all been reported. In the past decade, there has been an alarming increase in the number of claims associated with pain interventions carried out at the level of the cervical spine. Injuries in those cases were often severe and related to direct needle trauma to the spinal cord, most often resulting in permanent disabling spinal cord injuries. Traumatic spinal cord injury was more common in patients who received sedation or general anesthesia and in those who were unresponsive during the procedure. Pain medicine claims have increased in number and severity over time. In addition, there are significant concerns about the neurotoxic potential of the corticosteroid preparations. Neurotoxicity, neurologic injury, and the pharmacological effects of corticosteroids have all been reported as complications following epidural, facet joint, and sacroiliac corticosteroid injections.

A. Neurotoxicity

The intrathecal injection of neurotoxic substances can result in inflammation of the meninges with or without direct neural injury in the form of arachnoiditis or cauda equina syndrome. Arachnoiditis is an inflammatory condition of the meninges that can extend to the underlying neural structures. Cauda equina syndrome is a descriptive term that refers to neurologic signs and symptoms that arise from dysfunction of the cauda equina. This is characterized by bilateral leg pain, saddle hypoesthesia, lower extremity weakness, and bowel, bladder, and sexual dysfunction. While cauda equina syndrome is most often seen in association with compressive lesions (eg, a tumor or large central disc herniation), similar symptoms can occur with severe arachnoiditis.

Concern regarding the potential for neurotoxicity associated with epidural steroid injections stems from reports of arachnoiditis that arose during the course of repeated intrathecal injections administered for the treatment of multiple sclerosis. Only one case of documented arachnoiditis has been reported following epidural steroid injection for sciatica complicated by a traumatic tap; the symptoms resolved following subsequent discectomy. There is limited evidence that any of the components of the available corticosteroid preparations are neurotoxic. There was much controversy around the risk of arachnoiditis following epidural methylprednisolone acetate in Australia during the 1990s. This led some practitioners to use Celestone Chronodose (betamethasone 5.7 mg, as betamethasone sodium phosphate 3.9 mg [in solution] and betamethasone acetate 3 mg [in suspension] per mL in an aqueous vehicle; Schering-Plough, Kenilworth, NJ, USA) for epidural injection. This product contains sodium phosphate monobasic, disodium edetate, benzalkonium chloride, and water. However, a study in sheep demonstrated arachnoiditis in animals receiving 2 mL or more of this preparation intrathecally. More recently, practitioners have moved to the use of the potent, soluble steroid dexamethasone for epidural use; a recent study in rodents found no evidence of arachnoiditis or neural injury following intrathecal administration of this agent.

It is not clear that intrathecal injection of any of the available corticosteroid preparations will cause harm. However, it is important to realize that, despite their widespread use for epidural injection, neither the United States Food and Drug Administration nor any other regulatory agency labels these steroid preparations for epidural use. Prompted by increasing reports of harm, in 2014, the FDA issued a Drug Safety Communication describing a label change to warn of rare but serious neurologic problems after epidural corticosteroid injections for pain. The most prudent approach is to use all means available to avoid intrathecal injection. A local anesthetic test dose prior to steroid injection can rule out intrathecal placement. Use of radiographic guidance and injection of radiographic contrast can also be used to confirm epidural localization of the injectate. In those patients where a dural puncture occurs during needle placement, it is prudent to consider abandoning the procedure.

B. Neurologic Injury

Direct injury to the spinal nerves or the spinal cord can occur during epidural injection. The most common form of nerve injury is persistent paresthesia. Injury to the spinal cord can occur when the needle enters the substance of the spinal cord (Fig. 23.1). Surprisingly, needle penetration into the cord is not always catastrophic and may even occur without the patient reporting symptoms. More significant injury occurs if there is bleeding in the spinal cord or if injectate is placed into the parenchyma of

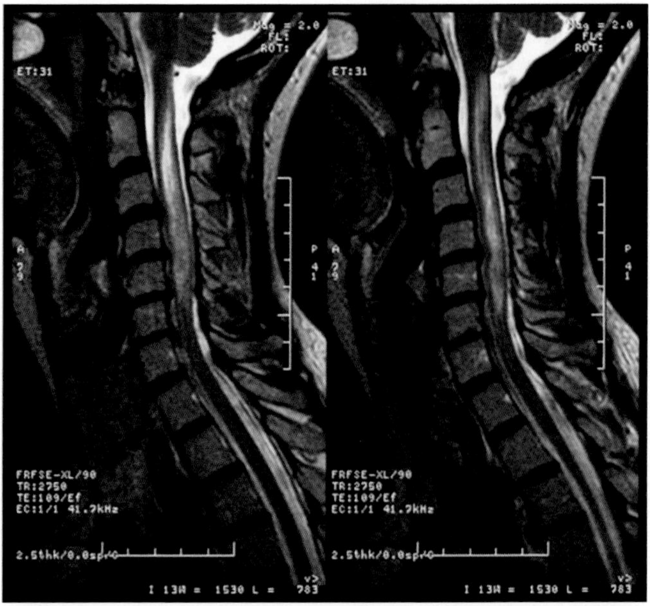

FIGURE 23.1 T2-weighted magnetic resonance image of the cervical spine immediately following cervical interlaminar epidural steroid injection. Increased signal within the substance of the cord and new onset of bilateral upper and lower extremity neurologic deficits suggests direct injection within the parenchyma of the spinal cord.

the spinal cord. Neural injury during epidural steroid injection, particularly at the level of the cervical spine, can result in permanent, disabling spinal cord injuries, with direct needle trauma as the predominant cause.

The risk of direct injury to the spinal cord is greatest when epidural injection is carried out at the high lumbar, thoracic, or cervical levels, where the spinal cord lies directly anterior to the path of the advancing needle. Cases of spinal cord injury following cervical epidural steroid injections conducted with fluoroscopic guidance have also been reported. The details of use of fluoroscopy were not given in these cases. In both cases, the patients received sedation. The authors postulate that these patients failed to report any symptoms due to the level of sedation. Neurologic injury has also been reported with cervical epidural steroid injections in unsedated patients, particularly those with marked stenosis of the central spinal canal. Direct injury to the spinal cord could occur even without dural puncture when narrowing or obliteration of the epidural space is present.

Fluoroscopy offers some protection against neural injury. The position of the needle in the AP view can be kept midline as it is advanced, eliminating the risk of lateral deviation and injury to the nerve roots or the spinal nerve. The primary means of detecting penetration of the epidural space remains the loss-of-resistance to injection as the needle is advanced, but a lateral view on fluoroscopy can be used to assure that the needle tip is at the level of the posterior border of the bony spinal canal. Once the tip of the needle appears to be in good position in both AP and lateral views, injection of a small volume of radiographic contrast can be used to assure that the injectate is within the epidural space. Most reports describe the immediate onset of severe pain in one or both lower extremities reported by awake patients receiving epidural injections who went on to develop spinal cord injuries. Thus, minimizing sedation is an important measure—the patient should be alert enough to respond to paresthesias induced by needle contact with neural structures and the practitioner should be alert to indications that these are occurring. In the majority of cases, there is probably little more than supportive care that can be offered to those patients who do suffer neural injury in the course of epidural injection.

III. PHARMACOLOGIC EFFECTS OF CORTICOSTEROIDS

The administration of exogenous corticosteroids can lead to hypercortisolism and suppression of the adrenal cortex's normal production of endogenous glucocorticoids. Cushing syndrome occurs as the result of excessive endogenous cortisol production by the adrenal cortex and results in a characteristic pattern of obesity associated with hypertension. Prolonged administration of exogenous glucocorticoids can result in similar manifestations and is termed cushingoid syndrome. The long-acting corticosteroid preparations used for epidural steroid injection slowly release the active steroid over 1-3 weeks. Fluid retention and weight gain, increased blood pressure, and congestive heart failure have been reported after epidural steroid injections and may be more likely in those with a history of previous congestive heart failure or chronic diuretic use. Cushingoid side effects have been reported even after a single epidural administration of corticosteroid.

Epidural administration of long-acting corticosteroid preparations leads to prompt, marked, and prolonged suppression of serum cortisol levels. After 80 mg of epidural methylprednisolone acetate, ACTH and plasma cortisol levels are depressed from 1 to 21 days after treatment, and the ability of exogenous ACTH to raise plasma cortisol levels is reduced over the same interval. Three epidural injections of 80 mg of triamcinolone acetate given at weekly intervals reduce ACTH and serum cortisol levels starting within 45 minutes of the first injection; levels are nearly normal 30 days following the last injection. There is no specific treatment for the adrenal suppression that follows epidural injection of corticosteroid; however, it seems prudent to consider coverage with an additional dose of exogenous steroid in those undergoing major surgery in the weeks following epidural steroid injection.

Glucocorticoid administration reduces the effect of insulin and results in increased blood glucose levels and insulin requirements in diabetics for 48-72 hours. A single caudal epidural injection of triamcinolone acetonide results in an increase in serum insulin levels and a suppression of serum glucose response to insulin within 24 hours, returning to normal after 1 week. Glucose levels in diabetic patients should be monitored closely during the week following any type of long-acting steroid. Patients need to be informed that adjustment of insulin dose may be required, particularly if they have any history of brittle diabetes.

IV. BLEEDING COMPLICATIONS

Similar to single-shot epidural placement for surgical anesthesia, epidural injection for pain treatment carries the risk of intraspinal bleeding. Significant bleeding within the epidural space can cause compression of neural elements potentially resulting in paraplegia or quadriplegia. Both epidural and subdural hematomas have been reported following epidural steroid injections in patients without any apparent coagulopathy, but most reports stem from patients who had been taking anticoagulants. The risks and considerations regarding neuraxial blockade in patients receiving anticoagulation are similar in those receiving the injections for treatment of pain to those who are receiving epidural anesthesia or perioperative epidural analgesia. Relevant guidelines have been published by the American Society of Regional Anesthesia and Pain Medicine. Epidural injection of steroids should be avoided in patients who are anticoagulated with systemic anticoagulants (eg, Coumadin or heparin) or potent antiplatelet agents (eg, clopidogrel or ticlopidine). However, nonsteroidal anti-inflammatory drugs (NSAIDs), including aspirin, do not appear to increase the risk of epidural hematoma formation associated with epidural injection.

V. INFECTIOUS COMPLICATIONS

Injection therapy for pain treatment carries a small risk of both superficial and deep infection, including neuraxial infection such as epidural abscess. Both superficial and deep infections have been reported after injection therapies for pain including epidural steroid injections, facet injections, and trigger point injections. The most worrisome and potentially devastating infectious complication is epidural abscess. Abscess formation within the epidural space can occur without injection or instrumentation of the spinal canal. Spontaneous epidural abscess occurs more commonly in diabetic patients. Common presenting symptoms include paralysis (80%), localized spinal pain (89%), radicular pain (57%), and chills and fever (67%). The erythrocyte sedimentation rate (ESR) is always elevated. *Staphylococcus aureus* is the most common organism isolated. Meningitis and osteomyelitis have also been reported. Epidural abscess often requires surgical decompression and may result in permanent motor and sensory deficits.

Similar to epidural infections, the majority of cases of septic arthritis of the facet and sacroiliac joints occur in the absence of injection or instrumentation. Following intra-articular facet injection, septic arthritis in the facet joints can extend to involve the paraspinous muscles and the epidural space.

Considerations regarding sterile technique and use of disinfectant solutions are similar to those recommended for single-shot regional anesthetic techniques performed in the perioperative period. Most experts recommend the use of an iodine-based skin preparation solution, routine use of sterile drapes and gloves, and strong consideration of routine use of face masks and hats. Routine use of preprocedure antibiotics does not appear to be warranted in the majority of single-shot spinal and perispinal injections. Pain practitioners should establish written postprocedural guidelines for their patients that include a clear description of the signs and symptoms of evolving infection and a clear process for contacting pain clinic personnel.

VI. COMPLICATIONS ASSOCIATED WITH TRANSFORAMINAL INJECTIONS

There have now been numerous reports of complications associated with both cervical and lumbar transforaminal injection of steroids. The most concerning risk of transforaminal injection involves unintentional intravascular injection of the steroid solution, with a reported incidence of 19% during cervical transforaminal injections. The observed vascular injections seem to have been intravenous and no adverse outcomes occurred. Intravenous injection is an innocuous event during transforaminal injection; particulate steroid injected intravenously will be carried away from the site of inflammation, thus reducing any local anti-inflammatory effect. In contrast, intra-arterial injection is far less common, but the effects may lead to catastrophic neurologic injury.

In the cervical spine, the vertebral artery, the ascending cervical artery, and the deep cervical artery each furnish spinal branches that enter the intervertebral foramina. These spinal branches supply the vertebral column but also give rise to radicular arteries that accompany the dorsal and ventral roots of the spinal nerves. Not infrequently, anterior radicular arteries are of significant caliber and reinforce the anterior spinal artery. Such reinforcing arteries can occur at any cervical level but appear to be more common at lower cervical levels. If particulate steroid is injected within a reinforcing radicular artery during transforaminal injection, infarction of the cervical spinal cord could ensue. The vertebral artery lies anterior to the cervical intervertebral foramina and should not be encountered in a carefully executed transforaminal injection. However, radicular arterial branches arising from the vertebral artery can also join the arterial supply that reaches the anterior spinal artery; it is possible that injectate placed within a radicular artery during a transforaminal injection could reach the vertebral artery via retrograde flow through an arterial anastomosis. If particulate steroid reaches the vertebral artery during transforaminal injection, infarction of the regions of the brain supplied by the posterior circulation including the cerebellum could ensue.

Minor complications occur in about 9% of lumbar transforaminal injections. Transient headaches (3%), increased back pain (2%), facial flushing (1%), increased leg pain (0.6%), and vasovagal reaction (0.3%) were the most frequently reported. These complications are similar to those associated with lumbar interlaminar and caudal injections. The major complications associated with lumbar transforaminal injections involve the reinforcing radicular artery, known as the artery of Adamkiewicz. Although this artery typically arises at thoracic levels, in 1% of individuals, this artery arises as low as L2, and more rarely as low as the sacral levels. In those with a low-lying radicular artery, the artery can be entered during lumbar transforaminal injections. There have been two reports of complications that likely resulted from direct injection into this vessel.

Published guidelines for the conduct of transforaminal injections are designed to guard against these complications. The needle must be accurately and correctly placed using radiographic guidance. Once the needle has been placed, a test dose of contrast medium should be injected and its flow carefully monitored *during* injection, using "live" or "real-time" fluoroscopy with or without digital subtraction. Under normal circumstances, the injectate should flow around the target nerve and into the lateral epidural space. Simultaneously, but more critically, this test dose of contrast shows if intravascular injection occurs. Close attention is required to notice if the injection is intra-arterial. The rapid flow through arteries means that intra-arterial contrast medium will appear only fleetingly. This event is unlikely to be captured by postinjection spot films. The flow of contrast medium must be monitored using continuous fluoroscopy throughout the injection.

Neurologic complications of transforaminal injections are often catastrophic. They are immediately obvious with the onset of spinal weakness and numbness. Their recognition requires no special investigations. Magnetic resonance imaging (MRI) of the spinal cord and hindbrain serves only to identify the location and extent of the neurologic damage (Fig. 23.2). Immediate treatment is with ventilatory and cardiovascular support as

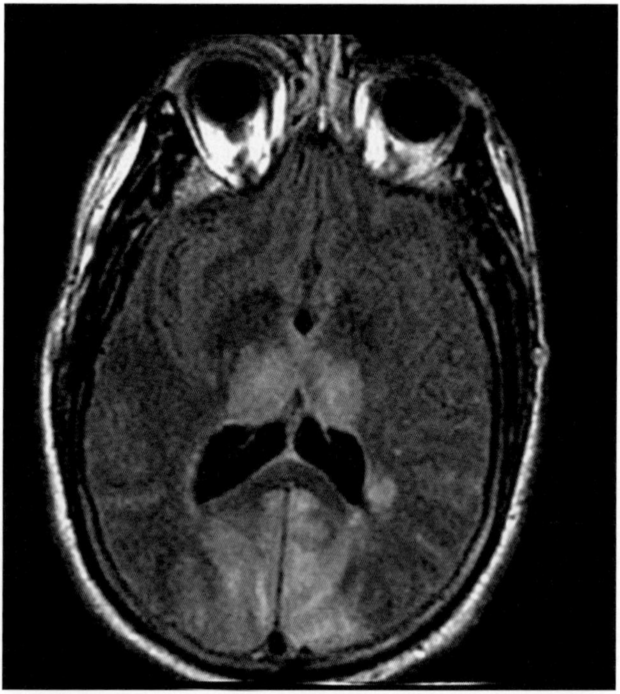

FIGURE 23.2 Cerebrovascular accident following intra-arterial injection of particulate steroid within the vertebral artery. Axial MRI (T1 FLAIR sequence) of the brain demonstrating massive bilateral stroke in the distribution of the posterior cerebral circulation.

needed, and subsequent management and rehabilitation follow standard protocols for spinal cord injury or stroke.

VII. COMPLICATIONS ASSOCIATED WITH IMPLANTABLE DEVICES

Spinal cord and peripheral nerve stimulation (SCS) and intrathecal drug delivery systems (IDDS) using implantable devices are now commonly used in the treatment of chronic pain, with the pain physician typically assuming the role of the surgeon. A range of complications can occur with these implantable devices, some related to the technical aspects of surgical placement and others related to the management of the patient after implantation. Device-related care consisted of surgical device procedures and IDDS maintenance. Severity of injury was greater in IDDS maintenance claims (56% death or severe permanent injury) than in surgical device procedures (26%). Death and brain damage in IDDS maintenance claims resulted from medication administration errors; spinal cord injury resulted from delayed recognition of granuloma formation. The most common damaging events for surgical device procedures were infections, inadequate pain relief, cord trauma, retained catheter fragments, and subcutaneous hygroma. In an independent analysis, damaging events included IDDS refill errors (eg, subcutaneous administration of medication, reprogramming errors), intraoperative nerve damage, and postoperative infection (eg, epidural abscess, meningitis). High-severity outcomes included nerve damage (eg, paraplegia) and death. Medium-severity outcomes included drug reactions (eg, respiratory arrest from opioid overdose) and the need for reoperation. For both IDDS and SCS, deficits in technical skill were the most common contributing factor to injury, followed by deficits in clinical judgment, communication, and documentation. Implanted devices used for pain management involve a significant risk of morbidity and mortality. Proper education of providers and patients is essential. Providers must acquire the technical skills required for implantation and refilling of these devices and the clinical skills required for the identification and management of complications, such as intrathecal granuloma. Proper patient selection and clear communication between the provider and the patient about these possible complications are of paramount importance.

Selected Readings

Abrecht CR, Greenberg P, Song E, et al. A contemporary medicolegal analysis of implanted devices for chronic pain management. *Anesth Analg.* 2017;125:1761-1768.

FDA Drug Safety Communication: FDA requires label changes to warn of rare but serious neurologic problems after epidural corticosteroid injections for pain. Issued April 23, 2014. http://www.fda.gov/downloads/Drugs/DrugSafety/UCM394286.pdf. Last accessed June 14, 2016.

Field J, Rathmell JP, Stephenson JH, et al. Neuropathic pain following cervical epidural steroid injection. *Anesthesiology.* 2000;93:885-888.

Fitzgibbon DR, Posner KL, Caplan RA, et al. Chronic pain management: American Society of Anesthesiologists Closed Claims Project. *Anesthesiology.* 2004;100:98-105.

Fitzgibbon DR, Stephens LS, Posner KL, et al. Injury and liability associated with implantable devices for chronic pain. *Anesthesiology.* 2016;124:1384-1393.

Horlocker TT, Wedel DJ, Benzon H, et al. Regional anesthesia in the anticoagulated patient: defining the risks (the second ASRA Consensus Conference on Neuraxial Anesthesia and Anticoagulation). *Reg Anesth Pain Med.* 2003;28:172-197.

Huntoon MA. Anatomy of the cervical intervertebral foramina: vulnerable arteries and ischemic neurologic injuries after transforaminal epidural injections. *Pain.* 2005;117(1–2):104-111.

Kay J, Findling JW, Raff H. Epidural triamcinolone suppresses the pituitary-adrenal axis in human subjects. *Anesth Analg.* 1994;79:501-505.

Knight CL, Burnell JC. Systemic side effects of extradural steroids. *Anaesthesia.* 1980;35:593-594.

Narouze S, Benzon HT, Provenzano DA, et al. Interventional spine and pain procedures in patients on antiplatelet and anticoagulant medications: guidelines from the American Society of Regional Anesthesia and Pain Medicine, the European Society of Regional Anaesthesia and Pain Therapy, the American Academy of Pain Medicine, the International Neuromodulation Society, the North American Neuromodulation Society, and the World Institute of Pain. *Reg Anesth Pain Med.* 2015;40:182-212.

Nelson DA. Dangers from methylprednisolone acetate therapy by intraspinal injection. *Arch Neurol.* 1988;45:804-806.

Pollak KA, Stephens LS, Posner KL, et al. Trends in pain medicine liability. *Anesthesiology.* 2015;123:1133-1134.

Rathmell JP, Aprill C, Bogduk N. Cervical transforaminal injection of steroids. *Anesthesiology.* 2004;100(6):1595-1600.

Rathmell JP, Benzon HT, Dreyfuss P, et al. Safeguards to prevent neurologic complications after epidural steroid injections: consensus opinions from a multidisciplinary working group and national organizations. *Anesthesiology.* 2015;122:974-984.

Rathmell JP, Lake T, Ramundo MB. Infectious risks of chronic pain treatments: injection therapy, surgical implants, and intradiscal techniques. *Reg Anesth Pain Med.* 2006;31:346-352.
Rathmell JP, Michna E, Fitzgibbon DR, et al. Injury and liability associated with cervical procedures for chronic pain. *Anesthesiology.* 2011;114:918-926.
Tang HJ, Lin HJ, Liu YC, et al. Spinal epidural abscess—experience with 46 patients and evaluation of prognostic factors. *J Infect.* 2002;45:76-78.
Ward A, Watson J, Wood P, et al. Glucocorticoid epidural for sciatica: metabolic and endocrine sequelae. *Rheumatology.* 2002;41:68-71.

24 Fluoroscopy and Radiation Safety

M. Alice Vijjeswarapu and
James P. Rathmell

I. OVERVIEW

Pain practitioners have come to rely on fluoroscopy and, to a lesser but growing extent on computed tomography (CT), to facilitate image-guided pain treatment techniques. Fluoroscopy and CT employ ionizing radiation to produce x-rays needed for imaging. Understanding the physics and biology of ionizing radiation will help pain practitioners minimize radiation exposure to their patients, other practitioners, and themselves during image-guided injections. The basic elements of the fluoroscopy unit are illustrated in Figure 24.1. X-rays emanate from an x-ray tube, which is typically positioned beneath the table and the patient to minimize radiation exposure. X-rays pass through the table and patient to strike the input phosphor of the image intensifier. X-rays are then converted to visible light and are detected by an output phosphor that transfers the signal to a digital camera for visual monitor display. The size and shape of the x-ray beam as well as C-arm variation relative to the patient can be adjusted to maximize image quality and minimize radiation dose.

The advent of fluoroscopy units that can rotate around the patient and reconstruct the images in multiple planes has blurred the distinction between CT-fluoroscopy and traditional CT. These CT-fluoroscopy units yield data that can rival the quality of conventional CT, at a cost of increased radiation dose. In most instances, the superior anatomic information provided does not warrant the routine use of these advanced imaging modalities (see below for discussion of radiation doses). Patients undergoing high-risk procedures, in which small variations in anatomy can alter the risk/benefit ratio of a given technique, may benefit from CT-fluoroscopy or conventional CT guidance.

II. BASIC RADIATION PHYSICS

X-rays with high frequency have enough energy to remove electrons from an atom and are termed ionizing radiation. This process yields free radicals that can lead to harmful biological effects. In radiography, x-rays that penetrate the body without effect emerge to strike an image intensifier, where they are converted to visible light and displayed on a monitor or transferred to film.

Several factors and definitions are central to the basic understanding of radiation safety. Biological effects of ionizing radiation are proportional to

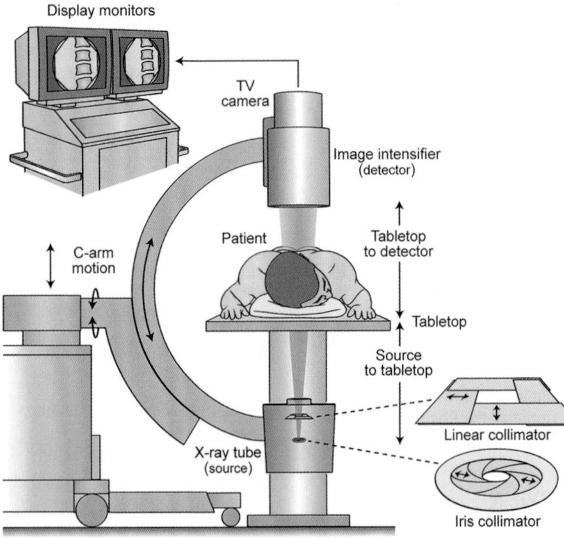

FIGURE 24.1 Diagram of the components of a typical fluoroscopy unit. (Reprinted with permission from Rathmell JP. *Atlas of Image-guided Intervention in Regional Anesthesia and Pain Medicine.* 2nd ed. Philadelphia, PA: Lippincott Williams & Wilkins; 2012.)

the time of radiation exposure. Radiation exposure is inversely proportional to the square of the distance from the radiation source. Radiation exposure is the ability of x-rays to ionize air and is measured in Roentgens (R). The amount of energy absorbed per unit mass at a specific point is called absorbed radiation dose, measured in Gray or Rads. The absorbed dose of different types of radiation creates different levels of biologic damage and is thus measured in Sieverts (Sv). The units used to express radiation exposure are listed in Table 24.1. For x-rays, 1 Roentgen (R) ~ 1 Rad ~ 1 Rem.

Electrical input to the x-ray tube generates x-rays that are varied in number and energies. Increased current applied to the x-ray tube (expressed as milliamps or mA) results in more x-rays that strike the image intensifier and a darker image. Lengthening the exposure time will also increase the number of x-rays reaching the image intensifier, thus variations in current and exposure time are expressed as mAs (mA × seconds). Increased voltage (expressed as kilovoltage peak or kVp) applied to the x-ray tube results in x-ray emission at higher energy levels (ie, with greater ability to penetrate). In general, high kVp (75-125 kVp) and low mA (50-1200 mA) are employed for fluoroscopy with short exposure times. This

TABLE 24.1 Units Used to Express Radiation Exposure and Dose

Term	Traditional Units	SI Units	Conversion
Exposure	Roentgen (R)	Coulomb/kg (C/kg)	1 R = 2.5 × 10^{-4} C/kg
Radiation absorbed dose	rad	Gray (Gy)	100 rad = 1 Gy
Radiation equivalent in man	rem	Sievert (Sv)	100 rem = 1 Sv

TABLE 24.2 Annual Maximum Permissible Radiation Doses

Area/Organ	Annual Maximum Permissible Dose
Thyroid	0.5 mSv (50 rem)
Extremities	0.5 mSv (50 rem)
Lens of the eye	0.15 mSv (15 rem)
Gonads	0.5 mSv (50 rem)
Whole body	0.05 mSv (5 rem)
Pregnant women	0.005 mSv to fetus (0.5 rem)

Data from the National Council on Radiation Protection and Measurements (NCRP). *Report No. 116. Limitation of Exposure to Ionizing Radiation.* Bethesda, MD: NCRP Publications; 1993.

optimizes image quality while minimizing radiation exposure. High kVp/low mA combinations expose the patient to significantly less radiation than low kVp/high mA combinations. Modern fluoroscopy units typically employ automatic brightness control (ABC), which adjusts kVp and mA to yield optimal brightness and contrast.

X-rays generated during fluoroscopy produce ionizing radiation that have potentially significant biological effects. Small doses of ionizing radiation produce molecular changes that can manifest as cancerous transformation over time. Exposure to low doses of ionizing radiation is likely inconsequential because normal cellular mechanisms repair the damage. The International Committee on Radiation Safety Protection (ICRP) has produced estimates of maximum permissible dose (MPD) of annual radiation to various organs (Table 24.2). Exposure below these levels is unlikely to lead to any significant effects, but the ICRP recommends that workers should not receive more than 10% of the MPD.

Use of fluoroscopy for interventional procedures grew rapidly during the late 1980s, leading to increased concerns about radiation exposure. In 1994, the U.S. Food and Drug Administration (FDA) issued a public health advisory about serious radiation-related skin injuries resulting from some fluoroscopic procedures. Today's equipment and techniques have reduced the risks of radiation exposure dramatically. Radiation exposure during a typical epidural steroid injection with fluoroscopy, assuming the practitioner is at least 1 m from the x-ray tube, has been reported to be as low as 0.03 mR. In contrast, the entrance skin exposure during fluoroscopy ranges from 1 to 10 R per minute. A typical chest radiograph leads to a skin entrance exposure of 15 mR. Thus, 1 minute of continuous fluoroscopy at 2 R per minute is equivalent to the exposure of 130 chest radiographs. Minimum target organ radiation doses that lead to pathologic effects are shown in Table 24.3. Radiation dermatitis still occurs in fluoroscopists with

TABLE 24.3 Minimum Target Organ Radiation Doses to Produce Organ Pathologic Effects

Organ	Dose (rad)	Dose (Gy)	Results
Eye lens	200	2	Cataract formation
Skin	500	5	Erythema
	700	7	Permanent alopecia
Whole body	200-700	2-7	Hematopoietic failure (4-6 weeks)
	700-5000	7-50	Gastrointestinal failure (3-4 days)
	5000-10 000	50-100	Cerebral edema (1-2 days)

TABLE 24.4 Comparative Radiation Doses for Common Diagnostic X-ray and Fluoroscopic Procedures

X-Ray—Chest	0.1 mSv (10 mrem)
X-Ray—Mammography	0.42 mSv (42 mrem)
X-Ray—Skull	0.1 mSv (10 mrem)
X-Ray—Cervical Spine	0.2 mSv (20 mrem)
X-Ray—Lumbar Spine	6 mSv (600 mrem)
X-Ray—Upper GI	6 mSv (600 mrem)
X-Ray—Abdomen (kidney/bladder)	7 mSv (700 mrem)
X-Ray—Barium Enema	8 mSv (800 mrem)
X-Ray—Pelvis	0.6 mSv (60 mrem)
X-Ray—Hip	0.7 mSv (70 mrem)
X-Ray—Dental Bitewing/Image	0.005 mSv (0.5 mrem)
X-Ray—Extremity (hand/foot)	0.005 mSv (0.5 mrem)
Fluoroscopy[a], intermittent, for example for lumbar transforaminal or facet injection	0.007-0.03 mSv (0.7-3 mrem)
Fluoroscopy[a], high dose	(3-6 fold the radiation exposure of standard dose)
Fluoroscopy[a], continuous, pulsed mode	0.2-1 mSv/minute of exposure (20-100 mrem/minute of exposure)
Fluoroscopy[a], continuous	2-10 mSv/minute of exposure (200-1000 mrem/minute of exposure)
Fluoroscopy[a], continuous, high dose	10-20 mSv/minute of exposure (1000-2000 mrem/minute of exposure)
Fluoroscopy[a], continuous, digital subtraction	20-40 mSv/minute of exposure (2000-4000 mrem/minute of exposure)
Computed Tomography—Head	2 mSv (200 mrem)
Computed Tomography—Chest	7 mSv (700 mrem)
Computed Tomography—Abdomen/Pelvis	10 mSv (1000 mrem)
Computed Tomography—Extremity	0.1 mSv (10 mrem)
Computed Tomography—Angiography (heart)	20 mSv (2000 mrem)
Computed Tomography—Angiography (head)	5 mSv (500 mrem)
Computed Tomography—Spine	10 mSv (1000 mrem)
Computed Tomography—Whole Body	10 mSv (1000 mrem)
Computed Tomography—Cardiac	20 mSv (2000 mrem)

[a]Fluoroscopy exposure values are approximate and vary widely based on the region of the body examined and the body habitus of each patient. The values presented are extrapolated from data provided by Philips Medical Systems for the Pulsera 9-in. mobile C-arm and the following references: Wagner AL. Selective lumbar nerve root blocks with CT fluoroscopic guidance: technique, results, procedure time, and radiation dose. *AJNR Am J Neuroradiol.* 2004;25:1592-1594; Mahesh M. The AAPM/RSNA physics tutorial for residents. Fluoroscopy: patient radiation exposure issues. *RadioGraphics.* 2001;21:1033-1045.

Data adapted from American Nuclear Society. Radiation dose chart. http://www.new.ans.org/pi/resources/dosechart/. Accessed January 9, 2011.

unknown long-term consequences. Estimates of the relative radiation dose to the patient during use of fluoroscopy in comparison to other common diagnostic radiologic procedures are shown in Table 24.4.

III. MINIMIZING PATIENT RADIATION EXPOSURE

A. Minimize Dose and Time

Practitioners using ionizing radiation should adhere to the ALARA principle ("As Low As Reasonably Achievable"), combining optimal technique and shielding to minimize patient and personnel exposure. All ionizing radiation has some biological effect and cannot be considered absolutely safe. Thus, radiographs should be used only when necessary, and the dose and exposure time should be limited. Dose is a factor of both the number of x-rays (proportional to mA × seconds of exposure) and the energy of the x-rays (proportional to kVp). As mentioned above, modern fluoroscopy units employ ABC, which automatically controls mA and kVp settings to optimize brightness and contrast while minimizing dose. However, when using fluoroscopy in manual mode (eg, to increase penetration in an obese patient), the kVp should be increased while minimizing mA. For an equivalent increase in exposure, the mA must be doubled, whereas the kVp must be raised only 15%. When using ABC mode, the only element under practitioner control is the exposure time, which should be minimized. Short pulses of exposure rather than continuous exposure should be employed whenever feasible. Continuous fluoroscopy in the form of movies (cineradiography) and digital subtraction exposes patients to markedly higher doses than brief spot images or pulse mode (Table 24.4). Pulse mode produces brief, periodic spot images separated by an interval without exposure (eg, a new image is displayed one to two times per second). Pulse mode can reduce overall exposure dramatically and is suitable for procedures in the pain clinic where continuous fluoroscopy is needed (eg, while threading an epidural catheter or spinal cord stimulation lead; see Fig. 24.2).

B. Optimize the Position of the X-ray Tube

Radiation exposure to the patient is best minimized by ensuring optimal distance between patient and the x-ray tube (Fig. 24.3). When the x-ray tube is positioned close to the patient, a small area of skin will be exposed to radiation. However, the dose that this smaller area will be exposed to is much higher. When the tube is positioned further from the patient, a larger

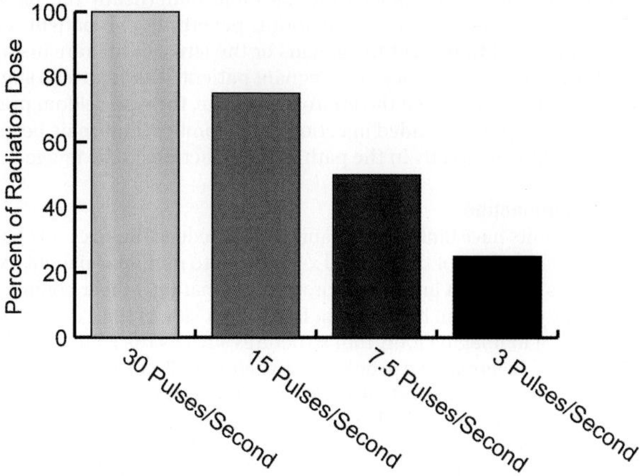

FIGURE 24.2 Effect of pulsed fluoroscopy on radiation dose (patient entrance skin dose). For example, by switching from continuous fluoroscopy (typically 30 pulses/second) to 15 pulses per second, dose savings of nearly 22% are achieved. (Adapted from Mahesh M. The AAPM/RSNA physics tutorial for residents. Fluoroscopy: patient radiation exposure issues. *RadioGraphics*. 2001;21:1033-1045. Copyright © 2001 Radiological Society of North America.)

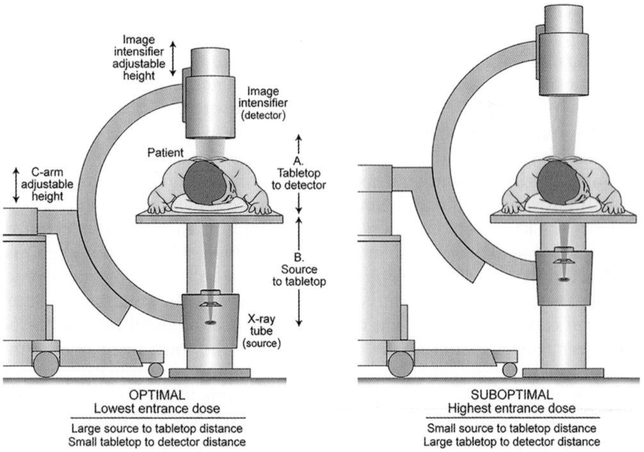

FIGURE 24.3 Optimal spacing between the x-ray source and the patient to minimize radiation exposure. (Reprinted with permission from Rathmell JP. *Atlas of Image-guided Intervention in Regional Anesthesia and Pain Medicine.* 2nd ed. Philadelphia, PA: Lippincott Williams & Wilkins; 2012.)

area is exposed to a smaller dose of radiation. The x-ray tube should be positioned as far from the patient as possible, without including unnecessary structures in the field of view.

C. Employ Shielding Whenever Possible

The use of lead shielding can prevent exposure of regions adjacent to the area that is to be imaged from being exposed to any ionizing radiation. Small lead shields can be placed on the table underneath the patient, directly in front of the x-ray beam before it penetrates the patient. Lead shields can be used to protect the gonads or the fetus, in the rare instance where fluoroscopy is necessary in a pregnant patient. Although lead shields should be readily available in the fluoroscopy suite, they are seldom practical for use during image-guided injection of the lumbosacral spine because the shield would lie directly in the path of the structures to be imaged.

D. Employ Collimation

Fluoroscopy units have built-in mechanisms that reduce the size and change the shape (collimation) of the emitted x-ray beam to minimize patient exposure. All units have both linear and circular collimation. Linear collimation employs shutters that can be moved in from either side of the exposure field and are helpful in imaging long, thin structures such as the spine (Fig. 24.4). Circular or "iris" collimation can be helpful when a small, circular area is being imaged (Fig. 24.5). Collimation can exclude areas of greatly varying radiodensity by reducing the range of densities included in the field. For instance, imaging the thoracic spine can be difficult due to large density differences between the spine and the adjacent air-filled lungs. Linear collimation to limit the field to the spine itself will dramatically improve the image quality. Likewise, imaging in the cervical spine presents the same difficulties when the air on either side of the neck is included in the x-ray field (see Fig. 24.4). Linear or circular collimation (see Fig. 24.5) can be used to limit the field and

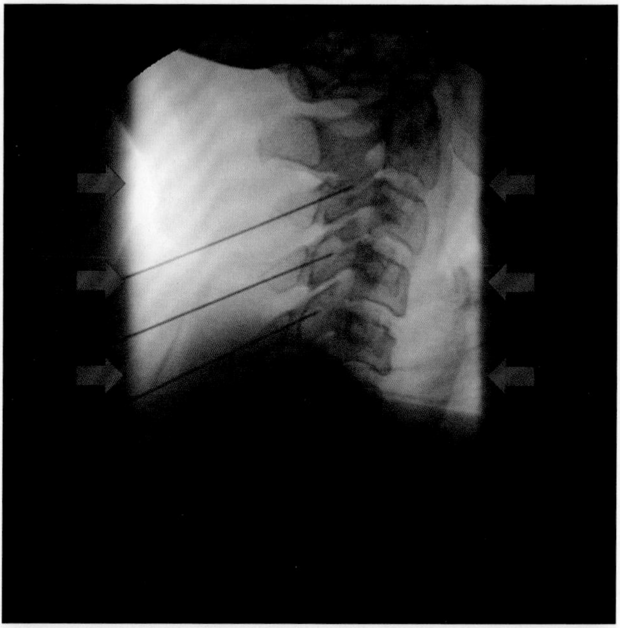

FIGURE 24.4 Use of adjustable (linear) collimator to decrease radiation exposure to the patient, while improving image resolution by decreasing the range of tissue density included in the image field. (Reprinted with permission from Rathmell JP. *Atlas of Image-guided Intervention in Regional Anesthesia and Pain Medicine*. 2nd ed. Philadelphia, PA: Lippincott Williams & Wilkins; 2012.)

improve image quality while reducing radiation exposure. Modern fluoro units may also allow for electronic magnification of the area of interest. Magnification allows better visualization of a smaller area, but leads to increased radiation exposure as the system increases output to compensate for losses in gain. To minimize the dose to the patient, the largest field of view in conjunction with the tightest collimation, should be employed.

IV. MINIMIZING PRACTITIONER EXPOSURE

A. Employ Proper Shielding

Only the personnel needed to conduct the procedure should be in the fluoroscopy suite, and all personnel should be shielded with lead aprons before use of fluoroscopy begins. The practitioner using the fluoroscopy unit should alert everyone in the room that he or she is about to begin and ensure that personnel are shielded. Routine use of thyroid shields can minimize the long-term risk of thyroid cancer. Although protective lead gloves can reduce the exposure of the hands to radiation, they can produce a false sense of security. When leaded gloves are employed and the practitioner's hands are in the field of exposure, units with ABC will increase output to compensate for the radiodense leaded gloves and negate their protective effects by increasing scatter radiation. The practitioner's hands should be kept out of the x-ray field should at all times. Protective eyeglasses are available that dramatically reduce eye exposure during fluoroscopy. Leaded eyewear is recommended for practitioners who

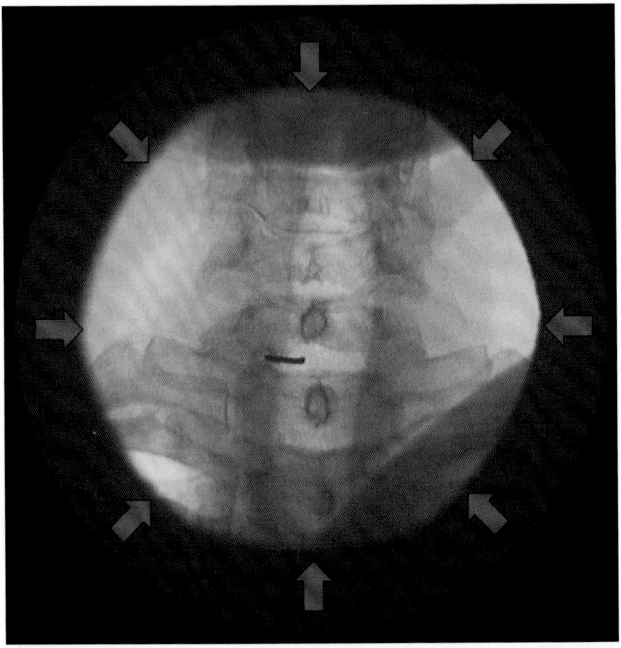

FIGURE 24.5 Use of adjustable (iris) collimator to limit the field to the area of interest reduces radiation exposure to the patient and improves image resolution by decreasing the range of tissue density included in the image field. (Reprinted with permission from Rathmell JP. *Atlas of Image-guided Intervention in Regional Anesthesia and Pain Medicine.* 2nd ed. Philadelphia, PA: Lippincott Williams & Wilkins; 2012.)

accumulate monthly readings on collar badges above 400 mrem (4 Sv), more commonly seen in settings such as the interventional cardiology suite.

B. Practitioner Position

Practitioners must understand the geometry of the radiation path as it passes from the x-ray tube to the image intensifier and adopt positions that minimize exposure during fluoroscopy (Fig. 24.6). The dose drops proportionally to the square of the distance from the x-ray source. Thus, increasing distance from the x-ray tube is the first means to minimize exposure. When injecting contrast under continuous or live fluoroscopy, using an intravenous extension tube and taking a step back from the table also reduces exposure. When the x-ray tube is rotated to obtain a lateral image, the practitioner should step completely away from the table or move to the same side of the image intensifier. Inverting the C-arm so the x-ray tube is above the table and the image intensifier is below the table is a means used by some practitioners to increase the C-arm's range of lateral movement beyond the typical 45-55 degrees allowed by the unit. This practice dramatically increases exposure to both patient and practitioner by bringing them in close proximity to the x-ray source and increasing scatter radiation.

C. Optimizing Image Quality

As mentioned above, modern fluoroscopy units use ABC, which adjusts mA and kVp to optimize image brightness and contrast while minimizing

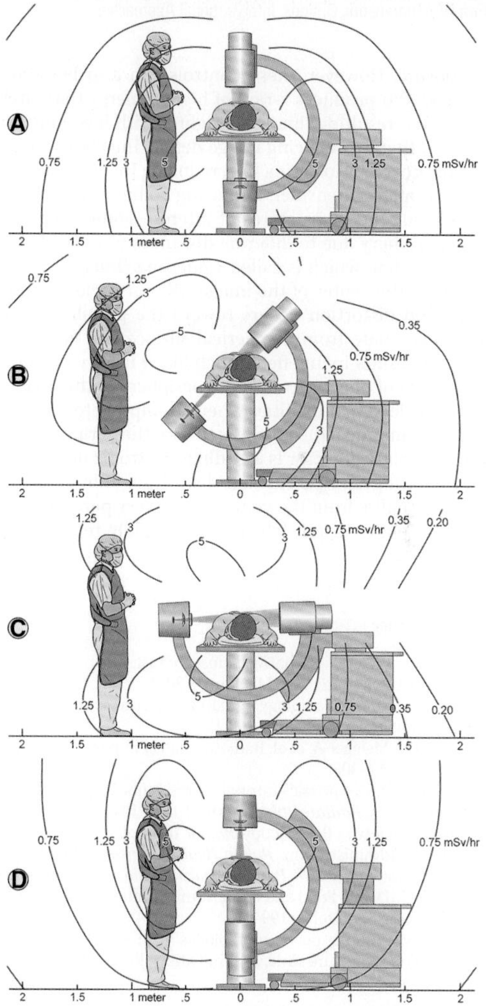

FIGURE 24.6 Radiation exposure dosage during fluoroscopy. **A.** During routine use in the anterior-posterior plane, the x-ray tube (source) should be positioned below the patient and the detector above the patient to minimize radiation exposure to both the patient and the practitioner. **B.** The oblique projection results in markedly increased exposure to the practitioner. **C.** During use in the lateral projection, the practitioner should step completely behind the x-ray tube (source) to minimize radiation exposure. When it is necessary to work close to the patient during lateral fluoroscopy, the practitioner should step away from the x-ray tube and move to the side of the table opposite the x-ray tube to minimize exposure. **D.** Radiation exposure to both patient and practitioner is dramatically increased when the x-ray tube (source) is inverted above the patient. Some practitioners invert the C-arm to allow for more extreme lateral angle (eg, rotation beyond 35-45 degrees oblique to the side opposite the C-arm is not possible without inverting the C-arm on some units). Radiation exposure can be reduced by rotating the patient on the table and keeping the x-ray source below the table. (Illustration by courtesy of Koninklijke Philips N.V. based on radiation exposure data for the Pulsera 9-inch mobile C-arm, from Rathmell JP, ed. *Atlas of Image-Guided Intervention in Regional Anesthesia and Pain Medicine*. 2nd ed. Philadelphia, PA: Lippincott Williams & Wilkins; 2012.)

radiation exposure. However, these controls can also be adjusted separately. Increased kVp produces x-rays of higher energy that attenuate less within tissues. The resulting image is brighter with less contrast between different tissues, thereby reducing image detail. The clarity of small structures can be improved by lowering kVP, reducing the distance between the patient and the image intensifier, and using collimation to limit the field of exposure to only those structures of interest. Fluoroscopic images are darker at the periphery due to differing distances from the focusing point to the outer phosphor, which is called vignetting. Thus, placing the structure of interest in the center of the image will also yield maximum image detail. Pincushion distortion occurs toward the periphery of the image because x-rays emanate from a spherical surface and are detected on a flat surface. This results in an effect much like a fisheye camera lens with a splaying outward of objects toward the periphery of the image. Pincushion distortion can lead to difficulties when attempting to advance a needle using a coaxial technique if the needle is toward the periphery of the image. An electronic flat plate detector is a gridlike electronic detector that eliminates both vignetting and pincushion distortion. This detector provides optimum image quality from the center to the very peripheral portions of each image. Flat plate digital detectors are rapidly replacing traditional image intensifiers.

Suggested Readings

American Nuclear Society. Radiation dose chart. http://www.new.ans.org/pi/resources/dosechart/. Accessed January 9, 2011.

Berlin L. Malpractice issues in radiology: radiation-induced skin injuries and fluoroscopy. *AJR Am J Roentgenol.* 2001;178:153-157.

Fishman SM, Smith H, Meleger A, et al. Radiation safety in pain medicine. *Reg Anesth Pain Med.* 2002;27:296-305.

Mahesh M. The AAPM/RSNA physics tutorial for residents. Fluoroscopy: patient radiation exposure issues. *RadioGraphics.* 2001;21:1033-1045.

Norris TG. Radiation safety in fluoroscopy. *Radiol Technol.* 2002;73:511-533.

U.S. Food and Drug Administration. *Public Health Advisory: Avoidance of Serious X-ray Induced Skin Injuries to Patients During Fluoroscopically-guided Procedures.* Rockville, MD: U.S. Food and Drug Administration, Center for Devices and Radiological Health; September 1994.

Wagner AL. Selective lumbar nerve root blocks with CT fluoroscopic guidance: technique, results, procedure time, and radiation dose. *AJNR Am J Neuroradiol.* 2004;25:1592-1594.

25 Outcome Data and Interventional Pain Medicine

Mark C. Bicket

I. INTRODUCTION

Outcome data for interventional pain medicine is essential to the interpretation of clinical research studies, the delivery of evidenced-based medicine, and understanding the latest advances in big data. Yet many questions exist regarding the manner in which outcome data are obtained, which, depending on the answer, change the interpretation of results. Fundamental topics such as the categories, characteristics, and bias relevant to outcome data set the stage for topics specific to the field of pain medicine. These include nuances that distinguish outcome data relevant to pain, measurement of pain in special populations, and outcome data in clinical trials.

II. TYPES OF OUTCOME DATA

Outcomes for pain medicine, as well as all other areas of research, exist as one of the following types:

A. **Dichotomous** data are defined by an outcome with only one of two possible responses. Examples include Yes/No. Other types of outcome data can be recoded to dichotomous outcomes by establishing a cut point for ordinal (ie, "moderate" or worse vs less than "moderate") or continuous data (ie, ≥50% vs <50%).

B. **Categorical** data are defined by groupings with more than two possible responses, but without an order or rank. Examples include a pain quality response of "sharp," "stabbing," or "burning"; or race response of "African American," "Hispanic," or "Other."

C. **Ordinal** data are defined by groupings with more than two possible responses, with a defined order or rank. Most nonnumeric pain measurement scales measure outcomes as ordinal data. For example, an ordinal pain rating may use the responses of "none," "mild," "moderate," "intense," or "extreme."

D. **Continuous** data are defined by an outcome measured by a number or numeric quantity. For example, the 100-mm Visual Analog Scale (VAS) provides a continuous measurement of pain intensity.

E. **Time-to-event** data are defined by a measurement of time within a defined period until an event occurs. For example, measuring the time from analgesic initiation until a patient reports meaningful reduction in pain provides time-to-event data. In other fields, these data are commonly known as **survival data**.

III. CHARACTERISTICS OF OUTCOME DATA

Five characteristics are needed to define outcome data completely and should be enumerated in research protocols, clinical studies, and other investigations.

A. **Domain** to be measured. For example, pain intensity, pain quality, pain behaviors, or pain interference represent different domains relevant to pain.
B. **Specific measurement** such as the tool, instrument, scale, or technique is used to define the measurement. For example, NRS, VAS, Patient-Reported Outcome Measurement Information System (PROMIS) pain interference 6b form, or use of rescue medication.
C. **Specific metric** used to characterize results. Examples include:
   1. Absolute or final value
   2. Change over time (final value minus baseline)
   3. Percentage (change or change over time)
   4. Probability (P) or odds (O). $P = O/(1 + O)$ while $O = P/(1 - P)$.
D. **Method of aggregation** used to summarize the data. For example, mean, median, proportion with decrease in VAS by ≥50%, odds ratio, or relative risk.
E. **Time point** at which measurement takes place. For example, 6 hours after injection, 1 week after intervention, or 3 months from baseline.

IV. BIAS IN OUTCOME DATA

The quality of measurement in pain, as in other areas of medicine, is a critical issue dependent on error, validity, and reliability.

A. **Error**
   1. A measured value for pain represents the true value of pain plus measurement error (ie, measured value for pain = true value for pain + measurement error). The goal of measurement is to minimize error as much as possible.
   2. Error represents bias, defined as the systematic component of error, plus random error (ie, measurement error = systematic bias + random error).
B. **Validity** describes the degree to which an instrument measures what it is supposed to measure. When measurement error is low, validity is high and the measure values more closely approximately true values.
C. **Reliability** describes the degree to which a measurement demonstrates consistent results when repeated measurements are taken. When random error is low, reliability is high.
   1. **Test-retest** reliability compares measurements made by the same person at two different, but closely related, points in time. Metrics include percentage of overall agreement and kappa coefficient.

V. SPECIAL FEATURES OF OUTCOME DATA IN PAIN MEDICINE

Pain medicine presents a number of special features that must be taken into consideration when measuring outcome data whether in clinical practice, research studies, or quality improvement projects.

A. As a **subjective** experience, pain resists conventional attempts for accurate quantification into an objective measure.
   1. Despite imperfectly measuring pain, numeric values such as the Numeric Rating Scale (NRS) or Verbal Rating Scale (VRS) attempt to simplify measurement and demonstrate widespread use in clinical practice.
   2. Advances in functional magnetic resonance imaging (fMRI) may lead to the adoption of neurologic signatures to improve detection and reduce measurement error of physical pain in the near future.

B. The **multidimensional** nature of the pain experience fails to be captured when measurement is limited to pain intensity. The sensory, emotional, and cognitive dimensions of the pain experience make a single, unifying summary measure difficult to obtain.
   1. Instruments such as the McGill Pain Questionnaire and the Brief Pain Inventory assess multiple dimensions of a person's pain experience.

C. As a **dynamic** and **complex** process, pain presents challenges to some patients when they attempt to assign numbers to describe pain.

D. **Overlap** of pain with other sensations (paresthesias) and emotions (anxiety, depression) may make separation of these entities difficulty for patients reporting pain.

E. **Variation** in pain reports by level of activity requires clinicians to assess pain at rest, with activity, or during other meaningful events.

F. **Memory** of past events is needed to permit measurement and assessment of pain in most patients.

G. **Mismatch** may occur between reports of pain intensity, behavior, and interference for patients, and all domains are related, relevant, but distinct outcomes.

VI. OUTCOME MEASUREMENT IN SPECIAL POPULATIONS

Pain measurement in special populations requires different tools, instruments, and techniques that takes into account the specific characteristics of these groups.

A. **Children, neonates, and infants** all experience pain that merits assessment and measurement, with multiple instruments available depending on developmental stage.
   1. The **Neonatal Infant Pain Scale (NIPS)** scores six observed behaviors in preterm and full-term neonates. NIPS indicators include facial expression, cry, breathing patterns, arms, legs, and arousal state, with score range of 0-7 (crying scores 0, 1, or 2 points).
   2. The **Wong-Baker FACES Pain Rating Scale**, in which a person self-selects one of six faces best corresponding to the level of pain, is appropriate to use for children ages 3 and older.

B. Cognitively compromised patients may have pain despite inability to alter facial expressions due to stroke, dementia, or mental illness.
   1. The **Iowa Pain Thermometer Scale** consists of a shaded thermometer with six words and response options permitting scores from 0 to 12, which measures pain in cognitively impaired as well as normal adults.
   2. Instruments measuring pain in advanced dementia generate a pain score based on behaviors such as facial expressions, verbalizations, body movements, changes in activity patterns, and mental status.

VII. OUTCOME DATA FOR PAIN

The subjective and multidimensional nature of pain, as well as clinical overlap of associated conditions, results in a number of different outcomes with potential relevance to pain clinical trials. As a result, significant heterogeneity in the outcomes measured in clinical trials for pain exists, which hinders efforts to compare outcomes among treatments and populations.

A. **IMMPACT guidelines**, sponsored by the Initiative on Methods, Measurement, and Pain Assessment in Clinical Trials (IMMPACT), address the lack of standardization regarding outcomes in pain trials. The group provides consensus reviews and recommendations regarding the conduct of clinical research. Core outcome domains for chronic pain trials include:
   1. **Pain** domains such as pain intensity, rescue analgesic use, concomitant pain treatments, pain quality, and temporal aspects of pain
   2. **Physical functioning** domains such as activities of daily living, ability to work, and disease-specific measures of physical functioning (ie, Oswestry Disability Index for chronic low back pain).
   3. **Emotional functioning** domains such as anxiety, depression, sleep disturbance, and fatigue.
   4. **Participant ratings of improvement and satisfaction with treatment** such as the Patient Global Impression of Change (PGIC).
   5. **Symptoms and adverse events** specific to the intervention under study should include open-ended questions and active capture of safety outcomes.
   6. **Participant disposition** should detail the flow of patients per Consolidated Standards of Reporting Trials (CONSORT) guidelines.

B. **Primary vs secondary outcomes** in clinical trials should be clearly enumerated *a priori* at time of trial registration on a public site such as ClinicalTrials.gov. A single primary outcome defined by five characteristics (see III. Characteristics of outcome data) should be expected for high-quality clinical trials.

C. **Minimal important difference (MID)** represents the smallest difference in an outcome score that patients perceive to be beneficial. Determination of a change in value that is clinically meaningful to patients is not always straightforward. Different values may be obtained when comparing MID between two different individuals or between two different populations. Additionally, MID for an individual may differ from the MID for a population.

D. **Patient-reported outcomes (PROs)** measure the effect of pain on outcomes that are reported by and most relevant to patients. Besides clinical trials, PROs are relevant to health care organizations, patients, and routine clinical practice. The National Institutes of Health funded PROMIS provides reliable, precise measures of PROs at no cost for physical, mental, and social well-being.
   1. PROMIS Physical health domains relevant to pain include pain intensity, pain interference, pain behavior, pain quality, physical function, and sleep disturbance.
   2. PROMIS Mental health domains relevant to pain include depression, anxiety, and substance abuse.
   3. PROMIS Social health domains relevant to pain include ability to participate in social roles and activities.

VIII. CONCLUSIONS

The potential for significant and sustained improvement in measuring and treating pain has never been greater. Tracking relevant domains related to pain using validated and reliable instruments moves beyond the limitations of single numeric value measures of pain intensity. Incorporation of outcome data, including PROs, into both clinical trials as well as the routine clinical practice of pain medicine serves as a more inclusive approach to addressing the various facets of life impacted by a person's pain.

Selected Readings

Dansie EJ, Turk DC. Assessment of patients with chronic pain. *Br J Anaesth.* 2013;111(1):19-25.

Dworkin RH, Turk DC, Farrar JT, et al. Core outcome measures for chronic pain clinical trials: IMMPACT recommendations. *Pain.* 2005;113:9-19.

Gordis L. *Epidemiology*, 5th ed. Philadelphia, PA: Saunders; 2014.

Landis JR, Koch GG. The measurement of observer agreement for categorical data. *Biometrics.* 1977;33:159.

Turk DC, Dworkin RH, Burke LB, et al. Developing outcome measures for pain clinical trials: IMMPACT recommendations. *Pain.* 2006;125:208-215.

Witkin LR, Farrar JT, Ashburn MA. Can assessing chronic pain outcomes data improve outcomes? *Pain Med.* 2013;14(6):779-791.

SECTION V

Therapeutic Options: Nonpharmacologic/ Noninterventional Approaches

26

Behavioral Treatments for Chronic Pain*

Matthew A. Roselli, Michael E. Schatman, and Ronald J. Kulich

I. INTRODUCTION

Chronic pain affects ~100 million Americans[1] and is often associated with disability, comorbid mental health conditions, and substance use disorders. Chronic pain treatments informed only by the biomedical model unfortunately yield only modest and temporary benefits for some patients or, at worst, cause harm both to the patient and society. Due to the complexity of chronic pain, treatment is arguably best grounded in the biopsychosocial model and delivered by an interdisciplinary team of providers in collaboration with the patient.

This chapter presents an overview of behavioral interventions for chronic pain that can be particularly effective when psychological and behavioral obstacles to functional improvement are present (eg, pain catastrophizing, pain-related anxiety and fear, and learned helplessness). These interventions, including operant behavioral therapy, cognitive-behavioral therapy (CBT), acceptance and commitment Therapy, and mindfulness meditation, now constitute a group of evidence-based nonpharmacologic therapies that are considered first-line treatments for people suffering from chronic pain prior to prescribing opioid analgesics.[2]

II. HISTORY

In order to provide a historical perspective, and for the sake of organization, the three main behavioral models of pain treatment will be presented in chronological order of their development and application to chronic pain.

*Excerpts of this chapter adapted from Roselli M. Psychosocial interventions for chronic pain. Social Work CE Institute: FOCUS Continuing Education Courses. National Association of Social Workers–MA Chapter, May 2018.

A. Operant Behavioral

Operant behavioral is the application of the principles of operant conditioning to pain treatment, first introduced by Wilbert Fordyce and colleagues in the late 1960s.[3]

B. Cognitive-Behavioral Therapy

CBT is a combination of behavioral interventions, cognitive restructuring of maladaptive thoughts, pain psychoeducation, and coping strategies.[4]

C. Mindfulness- and Acceptance-Based Treatments

1. Mindfulness-based stress reduction (MBSR): an 8-week training in mindfulness meditation, combining education and multiple forms of meditative practice[5]
2. Acceptance and Commitment Therapy (ACT): a form of CBT that combines acceptance and mindfulness interventions with values-based behavioral change[6]

Additionally, the application of motivational interviewing (MI) to chronic pain patients will be presented, as it is not uncommon for patients in pain (who may view their pain as a strictly physical problem) to be ambivalent or resistant to engaging in behavioral therapy or active forms of treatment, such as exercise. MI skills can help guide clinicians in difficult interactions with patients, offering the insight that an empathic, accepting clinician who is willing to explore and resolve this ambivalence with the patient is more likely to facilitate change than is a confrontational, directive approach.

III. DSM-5 CHANGES: SOMATIC SYMPTOM DISORDER

It may be worth noting the significant changes that the 5th edition of the Diagnostic and Statistical Manual of Mental Disorders[7] introduced to the category of somatic symptom and related disorders. Multiple previous diagnoses applicable to patients with somatic symptoms as a main focus of clinical attention were combined into one diagnosis. Conditions that were previously referred to as somatization disorder, pain disorder, and undifferentiated somatoform disorder are now all labeled as a somatic symptom disorder. These changes were intended to address the confusion that medical providers with limited mental health training encountered in their efforts to diagnose patients. Additionally, the change shifts the focus away from the concept of unexplained medical symptoms and toward an assessment of the degree to which a patient's thoughts, feelings, and behaviors regarding his or her somatic symptoms are disproportionate or excessive. Key diagnostic criteria include having one or more somatic symptom (that may or may not be associated with a medical condition) and persistence of more than 6 months, along with at least one of the following: disproportionate and persistent thoughts about the seriousness of symptoms, significant anxiety regarding health or pain symptoms, and/or excessive time and energy devoted to these symptoms or health concerns (can be mild, moderate, or severe, depending on the number of these symptoms).

IV. PSYCHOLOGICAL FACTORS THAT IMPACT PAIN AND FUNCTION

Researchers have identified many psychological factors that influence the course of chronic pain and therefore help guide both assessment and treatment. Keefe and colleagues identified seven key psychological factors that most affect individuals with chronic pain.[8] Three factors contribute to increased pain, distress, and disability and are thus targets for intervention: (1) pain catastrophizing, involving excessive focus on pain and negative thoughts about current or future pain symptoms or health status, (2) pain-related anxiety and fear, which are often associated with excessive avoidance behaviors,[9] and (3) learned helplessness, manifested as patients ceasing efforts to improve their pain and function following repeated exposure to pain from which escape is deemed impossible. Another four factors contribute to improvements in pain, distress, and disability and are often goals for treatment: (1) self-efficacy—a person's belief in his or her ability to take action and accomplish a given goal, (2) readiness to change—drawn from the stages of change model,[10] whereby a patient becomes willing to actively engage in new, more adaptive responses to his or her pain, (3) pain coping strategies—active, intentional, and problem-focused activities that help patients live with pain and other challenges, and (4) acceptance—an attitude of openness and receptivity toward pain, described in behavioral terms as consisting of two parts: *activity engagement* (taking part in meaningful activities even in the presence of pain) and *pain willingness* (suspending efforts to escape or avoid pain if they are not helpful or are interfering with life activities).

Additionally, there are several behavioral health issues that significantly impact pain and disability and accordingly should also be assessed and treated, most notably insomnia, obesity, and tobacco use. Up to 88% of chronic pain patients present with complaints of impaired sleep.[11] This can be due to unmanaged pain, an underlying sleep disorder (such as sleep apnea or restless legs syndrome), or psychophysiologic insomnia. Some of these issues may have predated the pain condition and contributed to the development of chronic pain. Treating the underlying sleep disorders, through either behavioral interventions or treatment by a sleep physician (or both), will improve pain treatment outcomes.[11] CBT and ACT have both been applied to insomnia and can be incorporated into the chronic pain treatments covered later in this chapter.[12,13] Excess weight also has a negative impact on musculoskeletal pain.[14] Behavioral interventions for weight loss combined with nutrition counseling and exercise programs should be considered as part of the treatment plan in these cases. Lastly, tobacco use has been shown to increase the risk of developing chronic pain and is associated with increased pain, disturbance of mood, and increased disability.[15–17] Smoking cessation should therefore be recommended for all patients with chronic pain. Behavioral interventions, with or without medication assistance, should be included in a comprehensive treatment plan. Again, CBT and ACT have both been applied to smoking cessation and can be incorporated into treatment.

V. BEHAVIORAL HEALTH INTERVENTION FOR PATIENTS UTILIZING OPIOID MEDICATIONS

Behavioral health professionals often play an important role in the assessment and monitoring of a patient's risk for opioid misuse or diversion as well as providing interventions to improve medication adherence. An opioid risk assessment includes a thorough psychosocial pain assessment, including substance use history and any previous aberrant medication behavior, as well as standardized measures of risk of opioid misuse (such as the Screener and Opioid Assessment for Patients with Pain-Revised [SOAPP-R],[18] the Current Opioid Misuse Measure [COMM],[19] and the Opioid Risk Tool [ORT]).[20] The reasons for a patient's utilization of medications in a manner other than that prescribed vary widely and warrant careful consideration, ranging from "misuse" (eg, taking an extra dose when in exacerbated pain) to "self-medication" (eg, unconsciously attempting to treat a mood disorder with pain medication) to an opioid use disorder, all of which require different interventions from the treating clinicians. MI, presented later in this chapter, has been demonstrated to be effective for reducing the risk of prescription opioid misuse and improving self-efficacy, motivation to change, and depression.[21]

VI. OPERANT BEHAVIORAL THERAPY

Behavioral interventions for chronic pain date back ~50 years, and the interventions from these early approaches are still applicable to treatment today. Wilbert Fordyce presented the application of operant conditioning to chronic pain in his book *Behavioral Methods for Chronic Pain and Illness*.[22] Fordyce proposed a radically different view of pain treatment, opting to analyze and treat pain as a set of *behaviors* rather than symptoms, which allows for an analysis of the environmental reinforcers of both *pain behavior* (eg, grimacing or lying down) and *well behavior*. For example, if a patient's spouse offers additional affection (positive reinforcement) or relief from undesirable household chores (negative reinforcement) in response to his or her pain behaviors, these behaviors will continue, leading to increased pain and disability. On the other hand, if a spouse reinforces continued activity irrespective of pain, the patient is more likely to remain functional and better adjusted to his or her pain condition. Treatment aims to change these environmental contingencies so that all well behaviors are reinforced (eg, by medical providers, fellow patients, and family) and pain behaviors are no longer reinforced, thereby leading to their extinction.

Goal setting is an important first step in an operant approach, and the goals are ideally functional in nature ("walking for one hour without stopping") rather than symptom focused ("reducing my pain from a 6 to a 2"). Goals should be linked in some way to the patient's values and motivation in order to assure that they are intrinsically reinforcing. To maximize treatment outcome, goals should also be specific ("going out to dinner once per week") rather than general ("seeing my friends more often"), realistic rather than excessive, and time-limited rather than open-ended.

After goals are set, patients are guided to gradually increase their physical function over the course of treatment through the creation of quota-based activity schedules, in which they commit to increasing amounts of activities based on numerical goals (eg, number of steps per day or number of minutes on an exercise bike). They are instructed to meet, and not exceed, the quota regardless of the status of their pain symptoms. Patients are thereby learning to base their activity on numerical goals rather than on pain symptoms and accordingly pace themselves more adaptively. Quota-based exercise has been shown to improve pain, disability, and fear of movement in chronic pain patients.[23]

In an operant approach, family and friends of the patient are educated on the program and underlying principles and instructed to reinforce any of the patient's functional gains and to discontinue both offering reprieve from the patient's daily tasks and paying excessive attention to his or her pain complaints. Patients are also instructed to take their pain medications on a time-contingent schedule rather than on an as-needed basis in response to pain, reducing the likelihood of medications becoming negative reinforcers of pain complaints or behaviors. Throughout treatment, education is provided on the difference between "hurt" and "harm," with "hurt" referring to any pain sensation that can be experienced and worked through and "harm" representing a pain sensation indicative of damage being done to the body. Through this process, patients learn to stop fearing "hurt" and to persist in tasks even in its presence. The operant behavioral approach can be successful in group settings in which a team of clinicians is offering reinforcement along with other patients who are making similar progress, although the principles and interventions apply to individual treatment as well.

VII. COGNITIVE-BEHAVIORAL THERAPY

Shortly following the initial application of the operant model to chronic pain, developments in the mental health field, most notably cognitive therapy, and advances in the understanding of pain perception led to the development of CBT for chronic pain. CBT is based on the conceptualization that pain and the associated functional impairment are influenced not only by patients' physical pathology but also by their emotional state, thoughts regarding their pain, and their behavioral responses to pain. CBT provides education and adaptive coping strategies aimed at improving function, reducing pain, and improving mood and distress. CBT protocols for pain vary on the specific combination of interventions included, but they share the same cognitive-behavioral conceptualization of the patient. A course of CBT may include some or all of the following: goal setting; psychoeducation regarding pain, relaxation, and stress-management strategies; activity pacing (and/or quota-based activity); and cognitive interventions to address maladaptive thoughts, beliefs, and attitudes and improve emotional distress.

CBT offers patients pain psychoeducation on the range of factors that influence pain perception, which can serve as an introduction and rationale for treatment and as a way to begin to shift the patients' perspectives on their pain symptoms. The gate control theory of pain[24] (and subsequent principles of neuroplasticity) offers patients the insight that their perception of pain is not solely determined by the signals being sent from the pain site up the spinal cord to the brain but also by information coming from the brain down the spinal cord. The theory states there are "gates" along the spinal cord that amplify the pain signal when open or attenuate the pain signal when closed. Examples of this theory can be offered to the patient for discussion, such as soldiers who are injured in battle and barely notice any pain due to their intense focus on the task at hand but once returned to safety become suddenly aware of significant pain. The clinician can emphasize that gate control theory does not assert that all pain is psychogenic but rather that pain is a complex phenomenon that takes place in *the nervous system* and is under the influence of a range of factors, including physical, cognitive, emotional, behavioral, and social.[25] The clinician invites the patient to take inventory of what factors are contributing to his or her pain in order to identify targets for treatment.

Patients are taught that specific thoughts regarding pain, such as catastrophizing or excessive attention to pain, contribute to its intensity, as can emotional states such as sadness, anxiety, fear, stress, and anger. On the other hand, when attention is focused outside the body on an engaging activity, pain perception can decrease significantly or stop altogether without any change in pathophysiology. Thoughts reflective of self-efficacy, such as pain being manageable or knowing there is a way to cope with it, can decrease pain perception as well; the same is true for positive emotional states and relaxation. Behavioral factors, such as level of activity and health habits (diet, weight, sleep, tobacco, or other drug use), also influence pain levels. Finally, patients are taught that social factors play a role in pain perception as well. Having minimal support or friends and family who are overprotective and pain focused make matters worse, whereas positive social support, including people who encourage reasonable activity, are helpful in reducing pain and its impact.[26] This discussion leads to insight into the complex nature of their pain and results in enhanced motivation to engage in CBT.

Most patients recognize that any life stress, including that associated with having chronic pain, increases their perceptions of pain. The mechanism may be any combination of muscle tension, increased inflammation in the body, excessive attention to pain, or tendency toward negative cognitions, all of which result from too much time spent in the "fight or flight" mode. Education on the sympathetic and parasympathetic nervous systems is helpful to explain the connection between stress and pain. Physiological explanations of the pain-stress connection can destigmatize and normalize the process of emotions increasing or causing pain, making patients more willing to learn to address the stress in their lives.

Relaxation training can help patients cope more effectively with pain and the associated anxiety and stress. These techniques were developed to reduce muscle tension, increase feelings of self-efficacy, and reduce the intensity of pain. Examples of formal relaxation techniques include diaphragmatic breathing, progressive muscle relaxation, guided imagery, and meditation. Additional stress reduction strategies may include healthy sleep habits, proper nutrition, regular exercise, development and maintenance of positive social connections, and enjoyable or meaningful activities.

It is common for patients with chronic pain to become fixated in maladaptive activity patterns, which can take two forms: (1) persistent activity avoidance, leading to deconditioning, stiffness, boredom, and depression, or (2) behavioral overpacing followed by pain and extended sedentary periods. Both of these patterns will lead to increased pain and a decline in physical functioning over time. Quota-based activity scheduling, covered in the operant behavioral section, can help patients in the first category slowly regain function in small, defined increments. Patients in the second category can often benefit from work on time-based activity pacing, which helps them maintain relatively consistent levels of activity and resist the urge to push through any one task to the point of excessive pain. Patients learn to engage in an activity for a predetermined period of time that may involve pain at a manageable level, followed by a brief period of rest, and then a return to the activity. As with quota-based activity, patients learn to associate their activity with time instead of pain. Through this new pattern, pain and overall function are likely to improve.

Cognitive distortions are consistent errors in patterns of thinking that lead to negative emotions and maladaptive behavior.[27] With an understanding of pain perception, clinicians are additionally aware of which distortions lead to increase pain and disability. Common cognitive distortions seen in chronic pain treatment include but are not limited to catastrophizing (previously discussed), black-and-white thinking (eg, "Either I have this dose of medication or I'll be in bed"), and overgeneralization (eg, "I tried physical therapy a few times 10 years ago and it was too painful; I don't want to do that again"). Cognitive restructuring involves patients first becoming aware of their automatic negative thoughts, beliefs, and attitudes and their impact on their emotional state and behavior. They are then asked to challenge and reality-test these thoughts, weighing the evidence supporting and contradicting their validities. Finally, patients are guided to develop more adaptive thoughts, such as those expressing a sense of control over pain or beliefs about pain being manageable, and then encouraged to notice the new thoughts' effects. Through a course of CBT, patients become progressively more skilled at identifying cognitive distortions, challenging them, and developing more adaptive alternatives, leading to improved mood, function, and pain.

There is evidence that CBT for chronic pain is effective for a range of pain conditions, including back pain, headaches, and orofacial pain. CBT has statistically significant effects on pain and disability and moderate effects on mood and catastrophizing when compared to treatment as usual. When compared to active control conditions, there are significant effects on catastrophizing and disability.[28] Given CBT's additional evidence base for a range of mental health conditions and substance use disorders, patients presenting with such comorbidities may benefit the most from a course of CBT that addresses both conditions concomitantly by the same clinician rather than treating one condition first or having two separate providers. For example, a protocol for an integrated CBT intervention for comorbid post-traumatic stress disorder (PTSD) and chronic pain demonstrated promise in a pilot study and is under further investigation.[29]

One challenge for research on CBT for chronic pain is the variation in interventions delivered across different studies. As shown in this section, CBT for pain is a collection of interventions that in practice can be effectively tailored to the individual patient, but in research, the varied protocols can make it unclear which interventions are active, which may be inert, and by what mechanisms change occurs. Ehde and colleagues accordingly summarize future directions for CBT for pain: "More research is needed to advance the field from the question 'Does it work?' to the question 'Why, for whom, and under what circumstances does it work?'".[30]

VIII. MINDFULNESS MEDITATION

Before presenting ACT, a form of CBT that includes mindfulness practices, mindfulness meditation as a standalone treatment for chronic pain will be presented. Mindfulness can be defined as "the awareness that emerges through paying attention on purpose, in the present moment, and nonjudgmentally"[31] (p. 145). This quality of attention can be cultivated through formal meditation practice (sitting, lying down, or walking) or through informal practices such as being mindful during daily activities (eg, washing dishes). Mindfulness originated in Buddhist meditation practice thousands of years ago. Its application in Western medicine to a range of conditions, including chronic pain, depression, and anxiety, began in the late 1970s with the 8-week MBSR program.[32]

There are several attitudinal foundations of mindfulness that are cultivated through practice.[32] An attitude of nonjudgment involves stepping out of one's habitual tendency to judge internal and external experiences quickly (as pleasant, unpleasant, or neutral) and then react accordingly (approach, avoid, or ignore) and alternatively taking the stance of an impartial witness. "Beginner's mind" refers to the capacity to approach every moment as if it were completely new, with openness and curiosity, as a beginner would with any new activity, as opposed to using ideas and concepts to quickly filter and process experience. While patients with chronic pain understandably engage in many efforts to reduce their pain, mindfulness poses the challenge of doing the exact opposite. Acceptance is an active willingness to be with experiences as they are and, as mentioned, both refrain from unsuccessful avoidance behaviors and engage in life activities even in the presence of pain. Mindfulness meditation is an opportunity to repeatedly practice acceptance every time a challenge (such as pain or related emotions) arises during the meditation. The more this attitude is practiced in formal meditation, the more readily it can be applied to experiences of pain in daily life.

Mindfulness training can include instructions for focusing attention on the five senses, the sensation of breath in the nostrils or abdomen, the sensations experienced in the body as a whole, as well as mindful walking and yoga practice. The patient is encouraged to practice acknowledging and accepting any other objects that enter awareness and then returning his or her focus to breathing or a body part. The technique of counting breaths can be useful as a means of maintaining focus during breathing meditation. Mindfulness meditation practiced by patients with chronic pain has been demonstrated to lead to pain reduction, improvements in mood and anxiety, and increased acceptance of pain.[33] Mindfulness training is an effective, standalone intervention for chronic pain and can also be incorporated into ACT interventions.

IX. ACCEPTANCE AND COMMITMENT THERAPY

ACT is a form of CBT that combines acceptance and mindfulness processes with commitment to behavioral change processes to increase psychological flexibility.[34] Psychological flexibility can be defined as "the ability to be in the present moment with full awareness and openness to our experience, and to take action guided by our values".[35] It is composed of six key processes: acceptance, cognitive defusion, contact with the present moment, self as context, values, and committed action.[35] This section will present these processes and the associated interventions.

ACT often begins with helping a patient discover the costs of excessive avoidance of his or her pain in order to lay the foundation for the process of acceptance. The therapist explores with the patient the results of the strategies they have used to attempt to control and avoid pain, most often leading to the realization that although they may be effective in the short term (eg, "I stay in bed and the pain settles down"), they are often ineffective or harmful in the long term ("My pain is feeling worse now and I have lost connection with important people in my life"). Following this realization, acceptance interventions can be introduced, which may include increasing values-based activities even in the presence of pain, mindfulness meditations, or introducing metaphors that can shift one's perspective to an accepting stance. One example is the "tug of war with a monster" metaphor, in which the therapist invites the patient to consider that his or her struggle with their pain is tantamount to playing tug-of-war with a monster. The patient is pulling the rope harder and harder to defeat his or her pain without success, while the most helpful approach is often to drop the rope and let go of this struggle, freeing up one's energy for other activities.

ACT includes strategies to create cognitive defusion, or psychological distance, from maladaptive thoughts. "Cognitive fusion" refers to excessive use of language that leads to inflexible, avoidant behavioral patterns,[35] such as pain catastrophizing, leading to excessive rest. Rather than directly challenging these thoughts and creating alternative thoughts, as discussed in the CBT approach, cognitive defusion techniques allow patients to gain distance from them and view them as simply words, sounds, or images that may or may not warrant a behavioral response. Examples include repeating a thought over and over again until it loses its meaning and impact, adding the phrase "I notice I am having the thought that" before an unhelpful thought, or saying a playful "thank you, mind" after an unhelpful thought.

Two other mindfulness processes in ACT are maintaining contact with the present moment and cultivating a sense of self-as-context. In contrast to being fused with thoughts about the past ("I used to be able to run 5 miles") or future ("I'll never work again"), patients are taught strategies such as focusing on their five senses at various points throughout the day or engaging in routine daily activities (eg, washing dishes) with full awareness of their senses. When a patient is fused with a rigid sense of personal identity, referred to as "self as content" (ie, "I am a construction worker; I don't want to do anything else"), interventions that create a sense of self-as-context lead to more flexible behaviors, such as the pursuit of alternative forms of employment or training. Examples include mindfulness exercises that emphasize a sense of a continuous observer of one's experience as well as metaphors such as the mind being like the sky and clouds, with the sky representing the observing self that is always there in the background and the clouds representing the thoughts, emotions, and physical sensations that constantly come and go.[36]

Patients who have struggled with chronic pain for many years have often spent inordinate amounts of their time and energy on pain reduction to the point that they have lost sight of other factors that might be determinants of quality of life. ACT includes a strong focus on the values clarification process. Values and desired qualities of action and life directions are chosen, such as being a loving parent or a supportive friend. Patients are often guided through an exercise that asks them to identify values in key life domains (eg, work and social), rank the relative importance of each domain to them, and rate the consistency which with they have been living that value in the past month.[36] This process creates a discrepancy between what is valued to the patient and how he or she is currently living, which can increase motivation to work toward one's goals.

Committed action is the final process of ACT, whereby patients are willing to move in the direction of their values on a consistent basis while utilizing acceptance and mindfulness skills to navigate any potential obstacles to action. It involves a similar goal setting process as that mentioned in the operant behavioral section but with an ongoing connection with the other five ACT processes. A classic ACT metaphor, "Passengers on the Bus,"[35] can be introduced to patients to target committed action as well as values, acceptance, and defusion. Patients are asked to imagine themselves driving their bus toward their values and goals even when there are difficult "passengers" such as pain and anxiety present rather than pulling the bus over to the side of the road or engaging in a fight whenever the passengers show up. The goal of ACT is to help patients accept and stop fighting with their passengers, thereby allowing them to maintain their focus on their values and goals along the road ahead.

ACT for chronic pain has shown similar effectiveness to CBT. A systematic review of 10 ACT for pain RCTs concluded that ACT led to improvements in pain intensity, sick leave usage, pain disability, physical function, depression, anxiety, and life satisfaction.[37] There has been only one published study that has compared CBT to ACT for chronic pain patients, and both groups showed similar improvements in function, mood, and anxiety, with ACT participants expressing greater satisfaction with care.[38] One strength of ACT is that it clearly defines the processes that moderate treatment outcomes, which offers a path forward for refining and improving treatments.[39]

X. MOTIVATIONAL INTERVIEWING

Patients with chronic pain may present to treatment as more motivated to engage in *passive* treatments aimed at reducing their symptoms than in *active* forms of treatment, such as learning new coping strategies or exercise. If patients view their pain as strictly medical issues without any associated psychosocial or behavioral factors, they will be understandably ambivalent about or resistant to engaging in behavioral therapy and learning different ways to cope with their pain. Mental health and medical professionals should be prepared to meet patients in their current stage of change and work patiently toward developing shared goals of treatment.

MI offers a framework for helping resistant or ambivalent patients progress toward healthy behavioral change and better self-management of symptoms. MI is a directive, patient-centered style of counseling that supports behavioral change by helping patients explore and resolve their ambivalence.[40] It was originally developed as an intervention for substance use disorders but has been applied to other mental health and medical issues that often co-occur with chronic pain, including anxiety, depression, PTSD, and obesity. In studies of MI for chronic pain patients, MI combined with exercise was shown to improve pain, self-efficacy, anxiety, happiness, and mobility[41] and help patients adhere to exercise programs[42] and was effective for reducing the risk of prescription opioid misuse and improving self-efficacy, motivation to change, and depression.[21]

MI operates on several key assumptions regarding how people progress toward making behavioral changes. Motivation is a state of readiness to change that fluctuates from one time and situation to another and is *not* a fixed, innate character trait. Motivation is due at least in part to interpersonal interactions and accordingly can be influenced through effective counseling. A confrontational style in the clinician will produce resistance, while an empathic stance is more likely to bring out self-motivational responses and create conditions for change. MI assumes that ambivalence to change is normal and expected and that it is the clinician's role to explore and help resolve these competing feelings.[31] A therapist using MI matches his or her intervention to the current motivation level of the patient. For example, relaxation skills training can be an effective intervention for a patient who is prepared to learn new coping skills but is ineffective for a patient who is actively resistant to behavioral interventions.

MI has four guiding principles that the therapist brings to patient interactions: empathy, developing discrepancy, rolling with resistance, and supporting self-efficacy. Taking an empathic stance toward patients means actively expressing an understanding and acceptance of their perspectives. This is necessary to create a relationship in which patients may begin to consider change. Clinicians seek to raise awareness of the discrepancy between the patient's current behavior (which may include avoiding work out of fear of increased pain) and the way the patient would like his or her life to be (a satisfying, productive career). In MI, the clinician should strive to refrain from directly arguing for change, as such an approach prompts the patient to argue against change, thereby reducing its likelihood. Instead, clinicians attempt to roll with any resistance that develops in the session and shift their approaches as needed to avoid unproductive arguments and maintain alliances with their patients. Lastly, the clinician aims to create and support self-efficacy, which, as previously discussed, is a key factor in creating positive outcomes.

In MI, therapists attempt to elicit and reinforce "change talk" from the patient, which refers simply to any statement that is reflective of the possibility of change. Examples from chronic pain patients may include desire to change ("I would like to learn better strategies to manage my pain"), ability to enact change ("I could get a gym membership and figure out a time to exercise"), reasons for change ("I should reduce my medications because they are really making me foggy"), or their commitment to change ("I will practice my meditation three times this week"). Any form of change talk increases the likelihood that change will occur.[43]

Strategies to elicit change talk may include engaging the patient in a discussion of their values and motivations, as well as identification of short-term, achievable goals. Another technique is having patients rate the importance of change, their confidence in their ability to change, and their readiness to change on a scale of 1-10, with follow-up questions such as "Why did you choose that number and not lower?" and "What would it take to move one number higher?" The responses to these questions represent forms of change talk to highlight and explore. Exploring a decisional balance is another strategy, in which the patient is asked to list pros and cons of making a change or staying in the same place. With patients considering reducing their dosages of opioid medications, they might be able to identify the improved energy, cognitive function, and mood that will potentially result from an opioid reduction and become more willing to attempt such change. The identified cons of reducing their medications, such as lack of confidence in ability to cope with pain and anxiety, can also be targets for skills training, pain coping strategies, and anxiety management.

XI. CONCLUSIONS AND FUTURE DIRECTIONS

Chronic pain is a complex, biopsychosocial condition with a significant public health and economic impact. Approaching this condition strictly from a biomedical perspective has had adverse effects for patients and for society, with the prescription opioid epidemic of the previous decade and the early years of this one perhaps being the most visible example. Patients with chronic pain should be consistently offered nonopioid and nonmedication treatments that can help them maintain their qualities of life and function. While the behavioral interventions outlined in this chapter have been demonstrated to be beneficial, many patients are unable to access them due to multiple factors, including limits on insurance coverage, lack of patient knowledge, limited availability of mental health professionals trained in chronic pain treatment, and lack of physician knowledge. In addition to further dissemination of knowledge to mental health professionals, the use of telemedicine for pain services, including behavioral health, has demonstrated promise in improving access to care and outcomes.[44] Hopefully with improved insurance coverage of these services, behavioral treatments may become more widely accessible. Broader application of the techniques that have been discussed may indeed represent a glimmer of hope for American pain medicine.

References

1. Institute of Medicine. *Relieving Pain in America: A Blueprint for Transforming Prevention, Care, Education and Research.* Washington, DC: The National Academies Press; 2011.
2. Dowell D, Haegerich TM, Chou R. CDC guideline for prescribing opioids for chronic pain—United States, 2016. *MMWR Recomm Rep.* 2016;65(1):1-49.
3. Fordyce WE, Fowler RS Jr, Lehmann JF, DeLateur BJ. Some implications of learning in problems of chronic pain. *J Chronic Dis.* 1968;21(3):179-190.

4. Bobey MJ, Davidson PO. Psychological factors affecting pain tolerance. *J Psychosom Res.* 1970;14(4):371-376.
5. Kabat-Zinn J. An outpatient program in behavioral medicine for chronic pain patients based on the practice of mindfulness meditation: theoretical considerations and preliminary results. *Gen Hosp Psychiatry.* 1982;4(1):33-47.
6. McCracken LM. Learning to live with the pain: acceptance of pain predicts adjustment in persons with chronic pain. *Pain.* 1998;74(1):21-27.
7. American Psychiatric Association. *Diagnostic and Statistical Manual of Mental Disorders.* 5th ed. Washington, DC: American Psychiatric Association; 2013.
8. Keefe FJ, Rumble ME, Scipio CD, Giordano LA, Perri LM. Psychological aspects of persistent pain: current state of the science. *J Pain.* 2004;5(4):195-211.
9. Vlaeyen JS, Linton SJ. Fear-avoidance and its consequences in chronic musculoskeletal pain: a state of the art. *Pain.* 2000;85(3):317-332.
10. Prochaska JO, DiClemente CC, Norcross JC. In search of how people change: applications to addictive behaviors. *Am Psychol.* 1992;47:1102-1114.
11. Finan PH, Goodin BR, Smith MT. The association of sleep and pain: an update and a path forward. *J Pain.* 2013;14(12):1539-1552.
12. Trauer JM, Qian MY, Doyle JS, Rajaratnam SMW, Cunningham D. Cognitive therapy for chronic insomnia: a systematic review and meta-analysis. *Ann Intern Med.* 2015;163:191-204.
13. Hertenstein E, Thiel N, Külz AK, et al. Quality of life improvements after acceptance and commitment therapy in nonresponders to cognitive behavioral therapy for primary insomnia. *Psychother Psychosom.* 2014;83(6):371-373.
14. Walsh TP, Arnold JB, Evans AM, Yaxley A, Damarell RA, Shanahan EM. The association between body fat and musculoskeletal pain: a systematic review and meta-analysis. *BMC Musculoskelet Disord.* 2018;19(1):233.
15. Ditre JW. *Tobacco Smoking and Chronic Pain: Complex Interactions and Novel Treatment Considerations.* 2014. https://www.gmuace.org/documents/events/ditre.pdf. Accessed September 20, 2018.
16. Shi Y, Weingarten TN, Mantilla CB, Hooten WM, Warner DO. Smoking and pain: pathophysiology and clinical implications. *Anesthesiology.* 2010;113(4):977-992.
17. Mikkonen P, Leino-Arjas P, Remes J, Zitting P, Taimela S, Karppinen J. Is smoking a risk factor for low back pain in adolescents? *Spine.* 2008;33(5):527-532.
18. Butler SF, Fernandez K, Benoit C, Budman SH, Jamison RN. Validation of the revised screener and opioid assessment for patients with pain (SOAPP-R). *J Pain.* 2008;9(4):360-372.
19. Butler SF, Budman SH, Fernandez KC, et al. Development and validation of the current opioid misuse measure. *Pain.* 2007;130(1-2):144-156.
20. Webster LR, Webster RM. Predicting aberrant behaviors in opioid-treated patients: preliminary validation of the opioid risk tool. *Pain Med.* 2005;6(6):432-442.
21. Chang Y, Compton P, Almeter P, Fox CH. The effect of motivational interviewing on prescription opioid adherence among older adults with chronic pain. *Perspect Psychiatr Care.* 2015;51(3):211-219.
22. Fordyce WE. *Behavioral Methods for Chronic Pain and Illness.* Saint Louis, MO: Mosby; 1976.
23. Kernan T, Rainville, J. Observed outcomes associated with a quota-based exercise program on measures of kinesiophobia in patients with chronic low back pain. *J Orthop Sports Phys Ther.* 2007;37(11):679-687.
24. Melzack R, Wall PD. Pain mechanisms: a new theory. *Science.* 1965;150:971-979.
25. Otis JD. *Managing Chronic Pain: A Cognitive-Behavioral Therapy Approach Therapist Guide.* Oxford, UK: Oxford University Press; 2007.
26. Che X, Cash R, Chung S, Fitzgerald PB, Fitzgibbon BM. Investigating the influence of social support on experimental pain and related physiological arousal: a systematic review and meta-analysis. *Neurosci Biobehav Rev.* 2018;92:437-452.
27. Beck JS. *Cognitive Behavior Therapy: Basics and Beyond.* New York, NY: The Guilford Press; 2011.
28. Williams AC, Eccleston C, Morley S. Psychological therapies for the management of chronic pain (excluding headache) in adults. *Cochrane Database Syst Rev.* 2012;(11):CD007407.
29. Otis JD, Keane TM, Kerns RD, Monson C, Scioli E. The development of an integrated treatment for veterans with comorbid chronic pain and posttraumatic stress disorder. *Pain Med.* 2009;10(7):1300-1311.

30. Ehde DM, Dillworth TM, Turner JA. Cognitive-behavioral therapy for individuals with chronic pain: efficacy, innovations, and directions for research. *Am Psychol.* 2014;69(2):153-166.
31. Kabat-Zinn J. Mindfulness-based interventions in context: past, present, and future. *Clin Psychol Sci Pract.* 2003;10(2):144-156.
32. Kabat-Zinn J. *Full Catastrophe Living: Using the Wisdom of Your Body and Mind to Face Stress, Pain and Illness.* New York, NY: Bantam Books; 2013.
33. Chiesa A, Serretti A. Mindfulness-based interventions for chronic pain: a systematic review of the evidence. *J Altern Complement Med.* 2011;17(1):83-93.
34. Hayes SC, Strosahl KD, Wilson KG. *Acceptance and Commitment Therapy: The Process and Practice of Mindful Change.* New York, NY: The Guildford Press; 2012.
35. Harris R. *ACT Made Simple: An Easy-To-Read Primer on Acceptance and Commitment Therapy.* Oakland, CA: New Harbinger; 2009.
36. Dahl JC, Wilson KG, Luciano C, Hayes SC. *Acceptance and Commitment Therapy for Chronic Pain.* Oakland, CA: Context Press; 2005.
37. Hann KEJ, McCracken LM. A systematic review of randomized controlled trials of acceptance and commitment therapy for adults with chronic pain: outcome domains, design quality, and efficacy. *J Contextual Behav Sci.* 2014;(3):217-227.
38. Wetherell JL, Afari N, Rutledge T, et al. A randomized, controlled trial of acceptance and commitment therapy and cognitive-behavioral therapy for chronic pain. *Pain.* 2011;152(9):2098-2107.
39. McCracken LM, Vowles KE. Acceptance and commitment therapy and mindfulness for chronic pain: model, process, and progress. *Am Psychol.* 2014;69(2): 178-187.
40. Rollnick S, Miller WR. *Motivational Interviewing in Health Care: Helping Patients Change Behavior.* New York, NY: The Guildford Press; 2008.
41. Tse MM, Vong SK, Tang SK. Motivational interviewing and exercise programme for community-dwelling older persons with chronic pain: a randomised controlled study. *J Clin Nurs.* 2013;(22):1843-1856.
42. Jones KD, Burckhardt CS, Bennett JA. Motivational interviewing may encourage exercise in persons with fibromyalgia by enhancing self-efficacy. *Arthritis Care Res.* 2004;(51):864-867.
43. Strang J, McCambridge J. Can the practitioner correctly predict outcome in motivational interviewing? *J Subst Abuse Treat.* 2004;27(1):83-88.
44. Vorenkamp KE. Improving pain care through telemedicine: future or folly? *Pain Med.* 2016;17(6):997-998.

27 Physical Therapy

Danielle L. Sarno

Rehabilitation programs for patients with pain aim to restore function, prevent pain recurrence, and assist patients in returning to activity participation. Functional restoration involves improving performance of physical skills as well as maximizing integration of skills into the patient's social and physical environments. When pain impairs a patient's optimal functional ability, including work participation, or inhibits a patient's independence in activities of daily living, a referral to physical therapy (PT) is appropriate. Treatment with PT aims to reduce disability and suffering by reducing pain and increasing tolerance to movement.

I. PHYSICAL THERAPY EVALUATION

The PT program is individualized to fit the needs and abilities of the patient. Rehabilitation prescriptions are based upon medical and functional evaluations, noting the patient's diagnoses, relevant medical comorbidities, functional impairments, functional goals, frequency of treatment, and risk factors. The physical therapist uses this information as well as information from a comprehensive musculoskeletal examination to design an appropriate treatment program.

A thorough PT evaluation involves identifying impairments contributing to pain, learning about the patient's goals and preferences, recording baseline measurements of impairments and activity restriction, establishing baseline exercise tolerance, and identifying barriers to activity and participation. The musculoskeletal evaluation includes test of active and passive movement, tissue palpation, end range testing, repeated movements, and sustained postures. The physical therapist evaluates the patient's postural alignment, body mechanics, willingness to move, and movement patterns to gain an understanding about the patient's general mobility. Information regarding the ability to perform activities required for return to activity, including work participation, is provided by functional performance tests and task analysis. A functional capacity evaluation (FCE) may be performed to evaluate an individual's capacity to perform work activities related to his or her participation in employment. Aerobic fitness may be determined from a bicycle or treadmill test. Based upon the PT evaluation, an individualized rehabilitation program can be developed, including exercise, coping, and education.

II. PHYSICAL THERAPY INTERVENTION/PAIN MANAGEMENT

A. PT Treatment should have an observable endpoint associated with:

1. Restoration of optimal physical functioning
2. Reduction of the impact of pain on the patient's life, or reduced disability
3. Resolution of treatable impairments that interfere with normal function and work participation
4. Prevention of future occurrences
5. Improvement of the patients' knowledge of independent pain management

B. Components of PT intervention for pain include:

1. Education/self-management techniques
2. Active modalities (eg, therapeutic exercise)
3. Passive modalities (eg, thermotherapy, cryotherapy, electrical stimulation, therapeutic ultrasound, and joint and soft tissue mobilization)

C. Education and Self-management

Educating patients and teaching self-management techniques lead to increased self-reliance. Self-reliance increases patients' participation in the therapy process and contributes to improved outcomes. Educating patients about their diagnoses helps to clarify misconceptions and reduce fear they may have of worsening their condition with movement. For example, for mechanical low back pain, it has been shown that bed rest/inactivity longer than 48 hours can worsen the initial injury. Inactivity leads to weakening of the core muscles, which contributes to poor posture and compensated movements, which can further exacerbate pain. Therefore, education about this concept and learning exercises with the guidance of a physical therapist can help ease patients back into their usual daily activities or exercise routine. When patients understand their diagnoses and agree with the goals of intervention, they are more likely to be compliant with the intervention offered.

D. Therapeutic Exercise

Exercise for therapeutic purposes is defined as the systematic, planned performance of bodily movements, postures, or physical activities. Regular exercise improves general fitness and the perception of well-being and is associated with lower incidence of depression, fatigue, and insomnia in patients with chronic pain. The exercise program is individualized by mutual goal setting, which helps to maximize patient satisfaction and exercise compliance. For patients with chronic pain, individually designed exercise programs with regular practitioner follow-up are associated with improvement in pain and function. Randomized controlled trials have demonstrated that supervision and adequate compliance are associated with positive outcomes for exercise interventions for patients with chronic low back pain. The 2018 Lancet Low Back Pain Series Working Group provides strong support for exercise in the treatment of chronic low back pain.

Exercise therapy may improve range of motion and muscle conditioning to increase the degree of stability and function as well as improve pain control. A recent meta-analysis of core stability exercise vs general exercise for chronic low back pain revealed that core stability exercise was more effective than general exercise in the short term for decreasing pain and increasing back-specific functional status in patients with low back pain.

1. Elements of exercise programs include:
   a. *Specific exercises* related to movement control, spinal stabilization, direction of movement, submaximal strengthening, specific mobility/flexibility, and symptom reduction
   b. *Global exercises* including aerobic conditioning, general strength training, endurance training, general stretching, and exercises related to coordination, agility, and balance
   c. *Coping* including cognitive restructuring, reduction of fear of moving, clarification of misconceptions, self-management, and self-efficacy
   d. *Education* regarding anatomy, pathomechanics, body mechanics, postural alignment, exercise technique, kinesthetic awareness, exercise progression, activity modification, and pacing

An exercise program may include specific exercises alone, specific and global exercises, or mostly global exercises. This depends upon the purpose of the therapy (the patient's and clinician's goals for the exercise intervention) and the stage of management (acute, subacute, or chronic pain, or the physiologic status of the tissue, such as inflammation and tissue irritability associated with acute pain or reduced tissue irritability and increased exercise tolerance associated with subacute pain). To facilitate program compliance, the physical therapist develops a program that matches the patient's baseline exercise and pain tolerance.

A main goal of therapeutic exercise is to regain physical function, so the exercises often imitate functional movements. For example, functional progress can be made through gait training using a mirror to promote symmetrical motion or through correcting improperly used muscles, restoring normal muscle length and postural alignment, and working on strength and endurance to balance muscle groups around major joints.

For patients with chronic musculoskeletal conditions, such as chronic low back pain, fibromyalgia, and myofascial pain syndrome, exercise is an essential part of the rehabilitation program. The effectiveness of regular physical activity has been demonstrated in clinical trials for people with chronic pain. Basic science studies testing different exercise protocols reveal that exercise-induced analgesia involves activation of central inhibitory pathways. Analgesia associated with exercise is found to be promoted by opioid, serotonin, and NMDA mechanisms acting in the rostral ventromedial medulla.

It is essential for patients to continue performing the exercises they learned during the formal course of PT. Physical therapists provide patients with a home exercise program, and it is important for members of the pain management team to encourage compliance with this program. As many patients with back pain have issues related to body mechanics and deconditioning, it has been found that high adherence rates to active PT-based exercise programs are associated with significant reduction in disability and pain. Furthermore, getting into the routine of exercise during PT may encourage patients to pursue a more active lifestyle, which improves general health and contributes to pain reduction.

E. Passive Modalities

Passive modalities include physical agents as well as hands-on techniques, such as joint and soft tissue mobilization. There is a wide variety of therapeutic physical agents available for pain management. Physical agents use physical energy for their therapeutic effects. The selection of the appropriate agent is made with consideration of the pain etiology as well as known contraindications to the various modalities. The use of physical agents for pain management should be adjunctive to active therapeutic exercise. Of note, there is insufficient evidence to support the use of passive modalities, and some guidelines advise against the use of certain physical agents due to ineffectiveness. Reliance on passive modalities may lead to increased disability and interference with return to work.

1. Physical agents
   a. Thermotherapy including hot packs, paraffin wax, fluidotherapy, electric heating pads, air-activated wraps, and rice-filled cloth bags
   b. Cryotherapy including ice bags, ice massage, cold compression units, and vapocoolant sprays
   c. Light therapy including laser and monochromatic infrared
   d. Therapeutic ultrasound including continuous (thermal), pulsed (nonthermal), and phonophoresis
   e. Diathermy including shortwave diathermy, continuous shortwave diathermy, and pulsed shortwave diathermy
   f. Electrical current including transcutaneous electrical nerve stimulation (TENS), interferential current, and iontophoresis
   g. Somatosensory desensitization

Some of the more commonly used passive modalities are described in the section that follows.

Thermotherapy is the application of superficial heat, which may be used to increase circulation, enhance healing, increase soft tissue extensibility, decrease stiffness, and control pain.

Cryotherapy is the therapeutic use of cold, which may be used to minimize inflammation, reduce edema, enhance movement, reduce spasticity, and control pain.

Electrical current/stimulation may be used for pain reduction, edema, muscle spasm, and stimulation of muscle contraction. TENS was developed based upon the 1965 gate control theory of pain by Melzack and Wall. High-frequency stimulation is thought to stimulate A-β fibers, "closing the gate," whereas low-frequency stimulation is thought to activate the pain-inhibiting descending pathways. High- and low-frequency TENS may reduce pain and improve range of motion in patients with chronic back pain. TENS also may be effective in the treatment of migraine and tension-type headache. Iontophoresis involves the transmission of medication through the skin by means of electrical stimulation.

Therapeutic ultrasound has both thermal and nonthermal effects. The thermal effects include increased blood flow and increased extensibility of collagenous tissues via alterations in tertiary molecular bonding. Nonthermal (pulsed) ultrasound is used to stimulate cellular activity during acute inflammation and repair. Therefore, therapeutic ultrasound can be used as a thermal agent to increase pain threshold or as a nonthermal agent to facilitate tissue repair. Studies have shown that therapeutic ultrasound may be helpful in managing pain originating from myofascial trigger points (TrPs), muscle spasms, epicondylitis, carpal tunnel syndrome, tendonitis, adhesive capsulitis, prolapsed intervertebral discs, and soft tissue lesions. Phonophoresis involves the transmission of topically applied medications through the skin by means of ultrasound.

Joint mobilization is a technique used to improve joint mobility when the ligamentous and capsular structures limit passive range of motion. Pathologic mechanisms involved in joint contracture development include immobilization, joint trauma, sepsis, degenerative processes, and a variety of disturbances that result in mechanical incongruity of the joint surfaces.

A lesion of the capsule will give rise to limitation of capsular mobility. This decreased mobility will limit the patient's active and passive range of motion and cause pain with movement. Treatment aims to restore normal capsular mobility and, therefore, normal range of motion. Joint mobilization can restore normal capsular extensibility by applying carefully directed forces across the articular surfaces. Collagenous tissues rely heavily on movement to ensure adequate nutrition, as does bone. Joint mobilization can be used to decrease pain by stimulating the type I and II mechanoreceptors. To increase effectiveness, joint mobilization may be combined with ultrasound or heat to make the tissue more extensible.

Soft tissue mobilization includes massage, passive stretching, and manipulation/myofascial techniques, such as myofascial release. Therapeutic massage may reduce pain by increasing local circulation and by stimulating A-β fibers. Studies have shown that massage may be beneficial for patients with subacute and chronic nonspecific low back pain, especially when combined with exercises and education. Myofascial TrP manipulation in combination with passive stretching is thought to inhibit TrPs in muscle, thereby reducing myofascial pain. Desensitization techniques such as tapping, stroking, and massaging the skin are used in the treatment of patients with complex regional pain syndrome (CRPS) to increase their tolerance of touch to the allodynic area. Furthermore, manipulation has been shown to provide long-term benefit for neck pain, headaches, and chronic mechanical spine pain.

F. Coordination With Care Team

Traditionally, the musculoskeletal examination and treatment of tissue structures and biomechanics have been the focus for physical therapists. However, over the last few decades, research has demonstrated the importance of central nervous system processing and psychosocial contributors to pain perception. New concepts for improved multidisciplinary treatment approaches are being developed, emphasizing the biopsychosocial model of chronic pain. An important aspect of a rehabilitation program is collaboration between the physician and the physical therapist. PT goals for patients with chronic pain are to increase function, decrease disability, establish effective pain coping and management skills, and decrease health care utilization in the long term. To achieve these goals, it is recommended that the physical therapist work within a team including behavioral therapists, occupational therapists, psychologists, social workers, and physicians.

III. CONCLUSION

PT is an essential component of multimodal pain management, and physical therapists are important members of the multidisciplinary pain team. An effective PT program reduces pain perception and restores impaired function. Evidence suggests that exercise therapy is an intervention with few adverse events that may improve pain severity and physical function and, therefore, improve quality of life. Therapeutic exercise to address the mechanisms of pain generation and utilizing the biopsychosocial approach to chronic pain in a multidisciplinary pain management setting can help facilitate functional restoration.

ACKNOWLEDGMENTS

The authors gratefully acknowledge the contributions of Theresa H. Michel and Harriët Wittink to previous editions of this chapter.

Selected Readings

Cameron MH. *Physical Agents in Rehabilitation: From Research to Practice.* Philadelphia, PA: WB Saunders; 2003.

Coulombe BJ, Games KE, Neil ER, Eberman LE. Core stability exercise versus general exercise for chronic low back pain. *J Athl Train.* 2017;52(1):71-72.

Fishman SM, Ballantyne JC, Rathmell JP, eds. *Bonica's Management of Pain.* 4th ed. Philadelphia, PA: Lippincott Williams & Wilkins; 2010.

Foster NE, Anema JR, Cherkin D, et al.; Lancet Low Back Pain Series Working Group. Prevention and treatment of low back pain: evidence, challenges, and promising directions. *Lancet.* 2018;391(10137):2368-2383. doi: 10.1016/S0140-6736(18)30489-6.

Geneen LJ, Moore RA, Clarke C, Martin D, Colvin LA, Smith BH. Physical activity and exercise for chronic pain in adults: an overview of Cochrane Reviews. *Cochrane Database Syst Rev.* 2017;1(1):CD011279.

Lima LV, Abner TS, Sluka KA. Does exercise increase or decrease pain? Central mechanisms underlying these two phenomena. *J Physiol.* 2017;595(13):4141-4150.

Physical Therapy Treatments for Chronic Non-Cancer Pain: A Review of Guidelines [Internet]. Ottawa, ON: Canadian Agency for Drugs and Technologies in Health; 2016.

Soer R, van der Schans CP, Groothoff JW, Geertzen JH, Reneman MF. Towards consensus in operational definitions in functional capacity evaluation: a Delphi Survey. *J Occup Rehabil.* 2008;18(4):389-400.

Swinkels A, Cochrane K, Burt A. Exercise interventions for non-specific low back pain: an overview of systematic reviews. *Phys Ther Rev.* 2009;14:247-259.

Wittink H, Michel T, eds. *Chronic Pain Management for Physical Therapists.* 2nd ed. Boston, MA: Butterworth-Heineman; 2002.

28 Myofascial Pain Syndrome and Fibromyalgia: Evaluation and Treatment

Danielle L. Sarno and Gary I. Polykoff

I. OVERVIEW

Myofascial pain syndrome (MPS) and fibromyalgia are common causes of chronic widespread pain. These conditions may be distinguished from each other on the basis of the medical history and physical examination. However, patients may have both conditions at the same time. This chapter reviews the clinical features and management options for MPS and fibromyalgia.

A. Myofascial Pain Syndrome

MPS is a musculoskeletal disorder characterized by the presence of myofascial trigger points (TrPs). A TrP is a localized, sensitive, nodular area in a palpable taut band of skeletal muscle fibers that produces local and referred pain to a zone of reference. TrPs are typically painful with compression and may produce referred pain, motor dysfunction, and autonomic phenomena. MPS may be associated with anxiety and depression as well. MPS often is grouped with other pain syndromes; however, it is distinct from fibromyalgia in that MPS may be focal and is characterized by an active TrP in a skeletal muscle.

MPS may be more common in women, but the evidence is unclear. The etiology of TrPs may include acute focal injury, excessive repetitive motions or muscle overload, psychological stress or tension, or a preexisting tender point. The pathophysiology of MPS is not well understood, but proposed theories include increased acetylcholine release from muscle cell end plates associated with injury or repetitive use causing excessive release of calcium from the sarcoplasmic reticulum, producing contraction of focal sarcomeric units. This idea has led to research involving botulinum toxin injections into TrPs in an attempt to reduce excessive release of acetylcholine. Studies have yielded inconsistent findings.

Local tissue injury, with concomitant elevation of various inflammatory mediators, catecholamines, neurogenic peptides, and cytokines, may lead to sensitization of the nociceptor terminal (ie, peripheral sensitization). In addition, small-fiber, unmyelinated afferents have been found to exhibit retrograde, neurosecretory properties similar to sympathetic fibers, involving a process referred to as neurogenic inflammation. The continual bombardment of primary afferent activity over time can lead to abnormal function and structural changes in the dorsal root ganglia and dorsal horn neurons, known as central sensitization. Clinical manifestations include allodynia, hyperalgesia, temporal summation of pain, and expansion of the receptive field of pain. The pain associated with active TrPs may depend on segmental central sensitization at the level of the spinal cord leading to abnormal muscle irritability, a local twitch response, and pain at rest.

Central neurologic processes are increasingly viewed as an essential factor in chronic pain syndromes. The medial thalamus is the principal relay of nociceptive input to the anterior cingulate cortex, and persistent stimulation of this pathway by pain in peripheral tissues has been demonstrated to change neurons in the cingulate cortex. Persistent pain is associated with long-term changes in the morphology, neurochemistry, and gene expression of the anterior cingulate cortex, which is connected with autonomic arousal, contributing to the maintenance and exacerbation of pain.

A combination of factors, such as poor posture, body asymmetry, lack of exercise, mechanical stressors, radiculopathy, nutritional deficiencies, endocrine dysfunction, sleep disturbances, and psychological factors, may contribute to the development of microtrauma and the symptoms of MPS. Occupational or recreational activities that produce repetitive stress on a specific muscle or muscle group or contribute to "muscle overload" commonly cause chronic stress in muscle fibers, leading to TrPs. Examples of predisposing activities include holding a telephone receiver between the ear and shoulder, prolonged bending over a table, sitting in chairs with poor back support, improper height of arm rests or no arm rests, and moving boxes using improper body mechanics. Acute sports injuries, surgical scars, and tissues under tension frequently found after spinal surgery and hip replacement are additional predisposing factors to the development of TrPs. MPS may be considered either a primary disorder causing local or regional pain syndromes or a secondary disorder that occurs as a consequence of another condition, such as radiculopathy or zygapophyseal joint disorders. Often, there is significant overlap in the clinical presentation of muscle pain disorders. Table 28.1 highlights the broad differential diagnosis of muscle pain.

B. Fibromyalgia

Fibromyalgia or fibromyalgia syndrome (FMS) is a chronic functional illness characterized by chronic widespread musculoskeletal pain of at least 3 months' duration. It is a multisystem disorder associated with fatigue, stiffness, sleep difficulties, cognitive dysfunction, anxiety, and depressed mood or depressive episodes.

Fibromyalgia is six times more common in women than men. Although the exact etiology of fibromyalgia has not been determined, studies have shown that sensitization of the central and peripheral nervous systems play a role in maintaining pain and the other main fibromyalgia symptoms. The pathogenesis of fibromyalgia may be related to abnormal pain processing in peripheral, central, and sympathetic nervous systems and abnormal processing in the hypothalamic-pituitary-adrenal stress response axis. Functional magnetic resonance imaging (MRI) studies have shown that fibromyalgia patients display increased neuronal activation in the insula in comparison to controls when the same low-intensity stimulus is applied to both groups. Patients with fibromyalgia demonstrate augmented sensory processing to the sensation of pain as well as other sensory stimuli. Patients with fibromyalgia also have altered levels of biomarkers associated with pain, particularly glutamate and substance P. Endogenous opioid levels have been shown to be elevated relative to controls, demonstrated through positron emission tomography (PET)–derived μ-receptor

TABLE 28.1 Differential Diagnosis of Muscle Pain

Joint disorders	Zygapophyseal joint disorders Osteoarthritis Loss of normal joint motion
Inflammatory disorders	Polymyositis Polymyalgia rheumatic Rheumatoid arthritis
Neurologic disorders	Radiculopathy Entrapment neuropathy Metabolic myopathy
Regional soft tissue disorders	Bursitis Epicondylitis Tendonitis Cumulative trauma
Discogenic disorders	Degenerative disc disease Annular tears Disc protrusion or herniation
Visceral referred pain	Gastrointestinal Cardiac Pulmonary Renal
Mechanical stress	Postural dysfunction Scoliosis Leg length discrepancy
Nutritional, metabolic, and endocrine disorders	Vitamin deficiency (B_1, B_{12}, D, calcium, folic acid, iron, magnesium) Alcoholic and toxic myopathy Hypothyroidism
Psychological disorders	Depression Anxiety Disordered sleep
Infectious disease	Viral illness Chronic hepatitis Bacterial or viral myositis
Widespread chronic pain	Fibromyalgia

Reprinted from Borg-Stein J. Treatment of fibromyalgia, myofascial pain, and related disorders. *Phys Med Rehabil Clin N Am*. 2006;17(2):491-510, viii.

occupancy. Another theory suggests that activated glial cells (microglia and astrocytes) may underlie the behavioral symptoms of fibromyalgia, known as sickness behaviors. Other researchers propose that patients with fibromyalgia may have extra sensory nerve fibers in tiny muscular valves or "shunts," which form a direct connection between arterioles and venules in the skin. This excess sensory innervation may be related to certain symptoms reported by patients with fibromyalgia, such as hand tenderness and pain.

Genetic factors may contribute to the development of fibromyalgia as certain genotypes have been found to be more likely to develop chronic pain and overall increased sensitivity to pain. Environmental factors/physical or emotional trauma, stress, infections, such as Epstein-Barr virus, Lyme disease, hepatitis C, and parvovirus, may interact with genetic factors to facilitate the development of fibromyalgia. Of note, there is no evidence that fibromyalgia is either autoimmune or infectious in nature. Sleep problems are associated with an increased incidence of fibromyalgia in women. Approximately 25% of patients with fibromyalgia report themselves disabled and are collecting some form of disability payment.

II. EVALUATING THE PATIENT WITH CHRONIC WIDESPREAD PAIN

A. Myofascial Pain Syndrome

1. Clinical Presentation

Patients with MPS often have regional muscle pain, which may be described as dull or aching. Associated symptoms may include limited mobility, weakness of the involved muscle, referred pain, and paresthesias. Pain usually occurs during repetitive activities or during activities requiring sustained postures. Symptoms are exacerbated with digital pressure over tender areas of muscle with reproduction of the patient's usual pain. Symptoms may be relieved with rest or cessation of repetitive activities. Pain may be acute or chronic and pain may persist for weeks or months.

A patient's past medical history may provide helpful clues leading to the diagnosis of MPS. Myofascial pain may be the primary pain generator, or there may be coexisting or underlying structural diagnoses that contribute to muscles having TrPs. Table 28.2 highlights the muscles with TrPs associated with various clinical conditions. It is important to inquire about headaches, migraines, temporomandibular joint (TMJ) dysfunction, and pelvic floor pain, as these may be associated issues. It is recommended to ask about past injury or trauma to the affected area, muscle overuse activities, and history of diagnoses associated with repetitive activities, such as lateral epicondylosis, shoulder impingement, or rotator cuff tendinopathy. Clinicians should inquire about history of herpes zoster infection, surgery, whiplash injury, as well as congenital or acquired skeletal abnormalities, such as scoliosis and leg-length discrepancies.

TABLE 28.2 Clinical Conditions and Muscles Associated with Myofascial Pain

Clinical Condition	Muscles Involved With TrPs
Tension headaches	Upper trapezius, splenius capitis, semispinalis, scalenes, SCM
TMJ	Masseter, temporalis, SCM
Cervical radiculopathy	Upper trapezius, scalenes, levator scapula, teres minor
Thoracic back pain	Lower trapezius, rhomboids, serratus anterior and posterior
Lumbar back pain	Quadratus lumborum, gluteus medius, iliopsoas
Lumbar radiculopathy	Gluteus medius and piriformis
Greater trochanter bursitis	Gluteus medius and piriformis without sciatic entrapment
Coccygodynia	Piriformis and gemelli without sciatic entrapment
Biceps tendinitis	Pectoralis minor, biceps, subscapularis
Rotator cuff tendinitis	Supra- and infraspinatus, teres minor, latissimus dorsi

MTrPs, myofascial trigger points; SCM, sternocleidomastoid; TMJ, temporomandibular joint.

As previously noted, MPS is associated with TrPs. The two types of TrPs are known as active and latent TrPs.

1. An **active TrP** is clinically associated with spontaneous pain in the immediate surrounding tissue and/or to distant sites in specific referred pain patterns. Strong digital pressure on the active TrP exacerbates the patient's spontaneous pain complaint and mimics the patient's familiar pain experience.
2. A **latent TrP** is physically present but is not associated with a spontaneous pain complaint. However, pressure on the latent TrP elicits local pain at the site of the nodule.

Both latent and active MTrPs can be associated with muscle dysfunction, muscle weakness, and a limited range of motion.

Physical examination includes evaluating for asymmetry of muscle groups, skeletal deformities, such as scoliosis, or leg length discrepancies. Identify TrPs by any of the following features: palpable taut band of contracted muscle fibers, spot tenderness of the nodule in the taut band, manual pressure on the tender nodule that reproduces referred pain in a distant area ("target area") that coincides with the patient's pain, and observation of a "local twitch response" (rapid contraction of muscle fibers of the ropy taut band) by visual or tactile methods or induced by needle penetration in the nodule. Manipulation of the TrP/mechanical stimulation is achieved by digital pressure/"snapping" palpation, a flick across the muscle, or needle insertion. When a TrP is palpated, the patient may involuntarily withdraw from contact or vocalize discomfort, which is called a jump sign. Evaluate for limited range of motion due to pain and associated muscle weakness.

2. Diagnostic Criteria

There are no standardized criteria for diagnosis, and diagnostic descriptions vary among experts. The TrP is generally considered the hallmark of MPS. The examiner should find spot tenderness with deep palpation over the TrP and stimulation of the TrP should result in concordant pain with referral of pain to a zone of reference within the affected muscle.

Validating diagnostic criteria for MPS has been challenging for investigators. In a study where experienced clinicians standardized their examination techniques and their approach to interpretation of the findings before participating in a blinded examination, the most reproducible clinical features from among Simons and Travell criteria included finding a tender spot in the proximal or distal third of an affected skeletal muscle, referral of pain to a zone of reference, and reproduction of the patient's usual pain. Poorer reliability was associated with eliciting local tenderness, palpating a taut band, and documenting the local twitch response. In a study designed to validate diagnostic criteria of MPS involving muscles of the upper part of the torso, the most specific discriminators of patients with MPS from healthy controls were painfully restricted range of motion, muscle strength limited by pain, and the pressure pain threshold according to algometry. The neurological examination typically is normal.

Laboratory testing is not required to confirm the clinical diagnosis of MPS. Routine laboratory testing often is obtained to evaluate other possible causes of signs or symptoms, such as complete blood count (CBC), thyroid function testing, and vitamin levels. Whereas no specific lab tests confirm (or refute) a diagnosis of MPS, some tests may be helpful in looking for predisposing conditions, such as hypothyroidism, hypoglycemia, and vitamin deficiencies. Specific tests that may be helpful included CBC, chemistry profile, erythrocyte sedimentation rate (ESR), and levels of vitamins C, B_1, B_6, B_{12}, and folic acid. If clinical features of thyroid disease are present, an assay for thyrotropin may be indicated.

Other testing is performed mostly in research settings, such as electromyography which may show low amplitude (10-50 μV) discharges in the taut band and intermittent high amplitude (up to 500 μV) discharges in painful TrPs. End-plate noise is more prevalent in TrPs than in sites that lie outside of the TrP, but still within the end-plate zone. This observation has been attributed to a spinal reflex as the response is abolished by motor nerve ablation or infusion of local anesthetic. Ultrasound may reveal a local twitch response to palpation, thermography may find a hot spot over the TrP, and microdialysis has shown increased pronociceptive substances, such as bradykinin, substance P, protons, calcitonin gene-related peptide (CGRP), tumor necrosis factor-alpha, interleukin-1 beta, serotonin, and norepinephrine in active TrPs.

B. Fibromyalgia

1. Clinical Presentation

A patient with fibromyalgia typically presents with sleep disturbances, depressed mood, fatigue, stiffness, anxiety, and cognitive disturbances, such as decreased comprehension, memory problems, and difficulty in concentration, organization, and motivation (termed "fibro fog"). Patients also may have headache, TMJ syndrome, irritable bowel syndrome, chronic fatigue syndrome, paresthesias, or genitourinary manifestations, such as pelvic or bladder pain. Patients may be limited in their daily activities and exercise tolerance by both pain and fatigue.

Blood pressure recording for orthostatic hypotension is performed. A thorough joint inspection should be normal. The neurologic examination findings also should be largely normal but may demonstrate slight sensory or motor abnormalities. Mood and affect are noted. By conducting a comprehensive neurologic and musculoskeletal examination, one may rule out superimposed pain generators, such as bursitis, tendinitis, radiculopathy, and TrPs.

2. Diagnostic Criteria

Fibromyalgia is characterized by widespread and long-lasting pain (>3 months) located above and below the waist, bilaterally. The 2010 American College of Rheumatology (ACR) diagnostic criteria include the widespread pain index and symptom severity scale (Tables 28.3 and 28.4). The widespread pain index incorporates symptoms considered to be key features of fibromyalgia, such as fatigue, cognitive symptoms, and somatic symptoms.

- **a.** According to the 2010 ACR diagnostic criteria for fibromyalgia, the patient must have:
  - **i.** a widespread pain index score ≥7 and a symptom severity scale score ≥5
  - **ii.** OR
  - **iii.** a widespread pain index score 3-6 and a symptom severity score ≥9
- **b.** The scoring is based on number and severity of somatic symptoms. In addition,
  - **i.** Symptoms must be present at a similar level for at least 3 months, and
  - **ii.** The patient must not have another disorder that would otherwise explain the pain.

TABLE 28.3 Widespread Pain Index (WPI)

Give 1 point for each of the following areas in which patient had pain in previous week (score range 0-19)

- Shoulder girdle, left
- Shoulder girdle, right
- Upper arm, left
- Upper arm, right
- Lower arm, left
- Lower arm, right
- Hip (buttock, trochanter), left
- Hip (buttock, trochanter), right
- Upper leg, left
- Upper leg, right
- Lower leg, left
- Lower leg, right
- Jaw, left
- Jaw, right
- Chest
- Abdomen
- Upper back
- Lower back
- Neck

c. For reference, the 1990 American College of Rheumatology criteria for classification of fibromyalgia can be seen in Table 28.5.

d. Presence of a second clinical disorder does not exclude the diagnosis of fibromyalgia. Widespread pain and tenderness in ≥11 of 18 tender points had 88.4% sensitivity and 81.1% specificity for classification of fibromyalgia.

TABLE 28.4 Symptom Severity (SS) Scale[a]

	Score
Determine level of severity for fatigue, waking unrefreshed, and cognitive symptoms over the previous week; for each symptom, score as	• 0—no problem • 1—slight or mild problems (generally mild or intermittent) • 2—moderate, considerable problems (often present) • 3—severe, pervasive, life-disturbing problems (continuous)
For somatic symptoms in general, score as	• 0—no symptoms • 1—few symptoms • 2—moderate number of symptoms • 3—great deal of symptoms

[a]SS scale score is the sum of the severity of the three symptoms (fatigue, waking unrefreshed, cognitive symptoms) plus the extent (severity) of somatic symptoms in general; the final score is between 0 and 12.

TABLE 28.5 1990 American College of Rheumatology Criteria for Classification of Fibromyalgia

- **History of widespread pain meeting all of the following criteria:**
  - Pain in left side of body
  - Pain in right side of body
  - Pain above waist
  - Pain below waist (may be low-back pain)
  - Axial skeletal pain (cervical spine, anterior chest, thoracic spine, or low back)
  - Widespread pain present at least 3 months
- **Pain in at least 11 of 18 tender points on digital palpation** (performed with an approximate force of 4 kg [10 lb per square inch])

e. Laboratory testing is not required to confirm the clinical diagnosis of fibromyalgia. However, routine laboratory testing often is obtained to evaluate other possible causes of signs or symptoms, such as CBC, erythrocyte sedimentation rate (ESR), C-reactive protein (CRP), creatine kinase, metabolic panel, and thyroid function testing. Routine testing for antinuclear antibodies (ANA) or rheumatoid factor is not recommended unless history and physical examination are suggestive of an autoimmune disorder or initial inflammatory indices (ESR and/or CRP) are abnormal. Additional laboratory testing or radiographic testing may be indicated based on the clinical evaluation, such as ferritin, iron-binding capacity and percentage of saturation, and vitamin D levels.

f. Neuropsychological testing is reserved for patients with severe cognitive impairment and patients who need reassurance that they are not developing dementia. Furthermore, as patients often report feeling unrefreshed by their sleep, it may be useful to screen for sleep apnea. If positive, may refer for overnight polysomnogram.

III. TREATMENT PRINCIPLES

A. Myofascial Pain Syndrome

A comprehensive, systematic, multidisciplinary approach to treatment is recommended, including follow-up with an experienced provider who makes strategic use of physical modalities and medications. Although there is limited evidence of efficacy of most treatments, commonly advised initial interventions include muscle strengthening and stretching exercises, and application of cold spray over the TrP, followed by gentle massage of the TrP and stretching of the affected muscle (the "spray and stretch" technique). A complication of untreated and progressive MPS is long-standing physical inactivity that may lead to cardiovascular disease.

1. Pharmacologic Management

Nonsteroidal anti-inflammatory drugs (NSAIDs) may be a useful adjunct to an active exercise-based treatment of MPS. However, no randomized placebo-controlled clinical trials exist to support the efficacy of NSAIDs in this condition. Muscle relaxants may provide benefit to patients with MPS. For example, cyclobenzaprine, tizanidine, methocarbamol, baclofen, metaxalone, or orphenadrine may be indicated as an adjunct to physical therapy (PT) for the relief of muscle spasm associated with acute, painful musculoskeletal conditions. Potential side effects must be taken into account. In contrast to low-dose cyclobenzaprine (5 mg three times daily), a higher dose (10 mg three times daily) is associated with more somnolence, dizziness, and dry mouth. Anticonvulsants, serotonin-norepinephrine reuptake inhibitors, tricyclic antidepressants, and topical diclofenac, or lidocaine (patch or gel) also may provide adjunctive pain relief. Goals of pharmacologic management are to reduce pain and address comorbidities, such as sleep disorders and depression, in order to facilitate participation in an active exercise program. Opioid analgesics are not recommended for treatment of this condition.

2. Interventional Treatments/Trigger Point Injections

In combination with other therapies, interventional techniques can be an effective adjunct in the multidisciplinary management of patients with MPS. In the treatment of MPS, other than TrP injections, interventional procedures (eg, epidural steroid injections, sacroiliac joint injections, and medial branch blocks) usually are not employed. However, at times, myofascial pain is associated with or caused by other underlying conditions. For example, lumbar myofascial pain also may have some component of lumbar facet arthropathy. Lumbar medial branch blocks and radiofrequency denervation, alone or in combination with the other therapies (eg, muscle relaxants), may work together to relieve myofascial pain.

TrP injections should be individualized for both the patient and the clinician. The diagnostic skill required to find active TrPs depends on palpation ability, training, and clinical experience. Typically, a 5/8-in 25 gauge needle is adequate for superficial muscles. For small muscles, such as facial muscles, a 1-in 30-gauge needle is sufficient. For larger muscles, a 1-in or 1.5-in 25-gauge needle is appropriate.

After the patient is relaxed, the TrP is located. The TrP is ascertained by gentle pressure from the end of a fingertip applied at regular 1 cm intervals. The patient is observed closely during the palpation. For active TrPs, each muscle has a characteristic elicited referred pain pattern that often is familiar to the patient. When questioned, the patient will respond that this pressure reproduces the usual pain and may describe painful sensations at a site slightly distant to the point under the examiner's finger.

Once the TrP has been located, the skin is marked and cleaned. When the needle is advanced to the TrP, a local twitch response may be elicited. Of note, a local twitch response is not always observed despite significant improvement of myofascial pain with TrP injections. Other findings that may help determine the needle entrance to the TrP are the patient's confirmation of reproduction of the usual pain pattern and the clinician's sensation of increased resistance as the needle is advanced from normal muscle tissue to the taut band. Various techniques are used for TrP injections. One common technique is performed in the following manner: after negative aspiration for blood, 1 mL of injectate (eg, lidocaine 1%) is administered and then, needling is performed in a fanlike manner/to the 4 quadrants surrounding the TrP for ~5 seconds. Although local anesthetic offers no long-term benefit, it may make the procedure less uncomfortable. Needling without the use of anesthetic or saline solution is known as dry needling. Clinicians may use acupuncture needles to minimize pain and tissue injury. The needle is inserted in the TrP using a swift tap, the muscle and surrounding fascia are probed with an up and down motion of the needle in a clockwise direction, and the needle may be left in place for 1-2 minutes for full therapeutic benefit.

The greatest risk of treatment of the patient with MPS is related to TrP injections in the thoracic area. Due to the proximity of the lung to the upper trapezius, scalene, and rhomboid muscles, the clinician must be aware of the potential for pneumothorax as a result of TrP injection in these areas. The use of long (>1 in), small-gauge needles should be avoided in these areas as long, thin needles can easily bend once they are inserted into the muscle, and the tip can puncture the pleura. Short (<1 in) needles should be used for TrP injections anywhere near the apex of the lung. In addition, the needle should be directed away from structures at risk for inadvertent puncture. To provide additional proprioceptive feedback during the injection, grasping the muscle between the thumb and forefinger will allow the clinician to palpate the thickness of the tissue to be injected. Thin patients or those with reduced lung capacity from underlying diseases are particularly at risk, so the clinician should use extra precautions when performing TrP injections in these patients, such as ultrasound guidance.

Dry needling should not be performed in the following scenarios: a patient who has a needle phobia, a patient who is unable or unwilling to give consent, a patient with a history of an abnormal reaction to needling or injection, a patient on anticoagulant therapy, or a patient with thrombocytopenia. Dry needling should not be performed in an area with lymphedema, recent surgery, or any sign of infection.

The effectiveness of the needling procedure may be explained by local structural damage to the TrP as a result of repeated passes of the needle. There may be disruption of abnormal muscle fibers or nerve endings that make up the sensory and motor aspects of the feedback loop, which may be responsible for TrP activity. Needling may cause a local release of intracellular potassium, which may disrupt nerve conduction. Typically, several local needling applications over a period of weeks or months are needed to obtain significant benefit. Some clinicians have found usefulness in the injection of botulinum toxin A, but there is conflicting evidence to support use of botulinum toxin A for myofascial pain. Acupuncture may improve quality of life in patients with MPS as well.

3. Rehabilitation Approaches

PT is an important part of the comprehensive management plan. A physical therapist may improve the patient's posture and body mechanics, provide education about proper ergonomics, relaxation techniques, and may utilize TrP massage, massage with ice ("ice stroking"), postisometric relaxation, reciprocal inhibition, and other therapeutic modalities, such as heat/ultrasound, and various forms of muscle and nerve stimulation. As noted above, the "spray and stretch" technique may provide at least temporary relief. A coolant, such as fluoromethane vapocoolant spray, is applied over the TrP in line with the involved muscle fibers, from the TrP to a reference point at a 45-degree angle at 4 in per second 3-4 times, while the area is gently stretched.

PT techniques that focus on correction of muscle shortening by targeted stretching, strengthening of affected muscles, and correction of aggravating postural and biomechanical factors are considered to be the most effective treatment of MPS. The goal for the treatment of MPS is to engage patients in active therapy to prevent the development of a debilitating chronic pain syndrome and to improve functioning.

Manual therapy, such as Osteopathic Manipulative Treatment (OMT), also may be beneficial for patients with MPS. Therefore, a referral to a Doctor of Osteopathy (D.O.) who specializes in OMT is recommended, if the patient is interested in manual therapy. Other forms of manual therapy are performed by chiropractors and physical therapists.

4. Psychological Therapies

Cognitive behavioral therapy (CBT) is the psychological approach that focuses on changing dysfunctional beliefs or "schemas" by which individuals process, store, and act on information. For individuals with chronic pain to successfully participate in a functionally oriented rehabilitation approach, they need to understand and believe the following:

- **a.** The nature of the pain has been thoroughly evaluated, and there is no cure for the pain (ie, surgery or another procedure).
- **b.** The rehab approach involving physical activity and conditioning will increase functional capabilities and eventually reduce suffering.
- **c.** The hurt engendered through physical conditioning will not cause harm.
- **d.** Reinjury or worsening of the painful condition is unlikely, and it is the individual's best interest to become more functional.

In a function restoration program, the physical therapist educates and guides the patient through a progressive physical reconditioning regimen. The physician periodically reevaluates the patient, provides reassurance, and adjusts medications to facilitate involvement in the program. Concurrently, the psychologist provides training in stress management, pacing, and pain coping strategies. A group setting helps to normalize the reactions and experience of the patient and provides social support and encouragement by peers. A cognitive-behavioral, functional restoration approach is particularly effective for chronic MPS as it is clear that increased activity in patients with MPS will not cause harm and will lead to long-term benefit. Hypnosis or mindfulness meditation guided by a psychologist specializing in chronic pain may be beneficial as well.

B. Fibromyalgia

Treatment of MPS and fibromyalgia is similar as evidence supports the role of exercise, CBT, education, and social support in the management of both MPS and fibromyalgia, although the evidence is limited. The objectives of treatment are to reduce pain, improve sleep, restore physical function, maintain social interaction, reestablish emotional balance, as well as reduce the need for expensive health care resources. It is important to note that inconsistencies between treatment guidelines have been reported and a guideline consensus meeting has been recommended to reduce the inconsistencies and synthesize recommendations. As fibromyalgia is a heterogeneous disorder with varying symptoms, symptom intensity, stress responses, and coping patterns, there is a need for future research and guidelines to consider matching treatments with subgroup characteristics.

1. General management principles
- **a.** Treatment strategy should incorporate principles of self-management using a multimodal approach, including nonpharmacologic strategies with active patient participation.
- **b.** Encourage patients to identify specific goals regarding health status and quality of life and to pursue as normal a life pattern as possible.

2. *Tailor approach based on individual symptoms, with close monitoring and regular follow-up, especially in early stages of management.*

3. Of note, injections or surgical interventions for pain specifically related to fibromyalgia are not indicated. Noninvasive procedures have been examined for patients with chronic widespread pain. For example, transcranial magnetic stimulation (TMS) of the prefrontal cortex can cause changes in acute pain perception and alleviation of depression. However, TMS often is not covered by insurance.

1. Pharmacologic Management

Pharmacologic management should be guided by symptoms and may require a combination of medications. Of note, authors of a Cochrane review (2018) conclude that there is limited evidence to support or refute the use of combination pharmacotherapy due to few, large, high-quality trials comparing combination pharmacotherapy with monotherapy for fibromyalgia. Pharmacologic treatment guidelines include the following:

a. Start at a low dose and titrate upward as needed.

b. Evaluate regularly to assess efficacy and side effects.

Three medications are currently approved by the FDA for the treatment of pain related to fibromyalgia—the amine reuptake inhibitors duloxetine and milnacipran and the membrane stabilizer pregabalin. However, many medications are used off-label. One approach to pharmacologic management in fibromyalgia includes targeting three main symptoms, such as pain, insomnia, and depression.

All categories of antidepressant medications are used to treat pain and other symptoms in patients with fibromyalgia. Antidepressants may improve pain, fatigue, and depressed mood in patients with fibromyalgia. Amitriptyline, a tricyclic antidepressant, has the most supporting evidence for fibromyalgia. Low-dose amitriptyline (10-25 mg nightly) is widely used in patients with fibromyalgia and is thought to help improve the patient's sleep cycle. Nortriptyline, another TCA, is an option as well. As with all TCAs, there is a need to monitor for suicidality since overdose with this class of drugs is lethal. Duloxetine (60 mg/d), a selective serotonin-norepinephrine reuptake inhibitor (SNRI), may reduce pain in patients with fibromyalgia.

Antiepileptic medications may be effective for their pain-modulating properties. Pregabalin and gabapentin are ligands for the $\alpha 2\delta$ subunit of voltage-gated calcium channels. These medications have been shown to have antihyperalgesic/anti-allodynic, anxiolytic, and anticonvulsant activity in animal models. They reduce the release of neurochemicals, including glutamate, norepinephrine, and substance P. Pregabalin 150 to 600 mg/d in divided doses has been shown to improve symptoms of fibromyalgia, particularly in reducing the severity of body pain, improving quality of sleep, and reducing fatigue. Gabapentin may reduce pain in fibromyalgia.

In a patient with fibromyalgia with three prominent symptoms, such as pain, insomnia, and depression, the use of either pregabalin in combination with duloxetine may be appropriate. However, as there is limited research published regarding this regimen, this is considered clinically experimental, should be tailored to the individual patient, and the patient must be monitored for safety.

Cyclobenzaprine (5-20 mg nightly), a muscle relaxant structurally related to tricyclic antidepressants, may improve symptoms of fibromyalgia, while very low doses may improve restorative sleep. Other muscles relaxants may be tried, as previously mentioned in the MPS management section of this chapter. NSAIDs have not been shown to be effective as monotherapy for fibromyalgia. Opioids do not seem to be effective in ameliorating the symptoms of fibromyalgia and are not recommended for treatment of this condition. For patients with severe pain that is unresponsive to other treatments, a therapeutic trial with a weak opioid such as tramadol may be considered. Prior to starting opioid-based therapy, it is important to have a discussion with the patient regarding a defined end point and a defined target dose, and a clear opioid contract should be signed.

As the pain amplification of central sensitization can be inhibited or attenuated by *N*-methyl-D-aspartate (NMDA) receptor antagonists, two NMDA receptor antagonists, ketamine and dextromethorphan, have been studied in patients with fibromyalgia. Both were found to improve spontaneous pain and allodynia, although risk of adverse effects need to be considered and more studies are needed to examine the long-term benefit.

Recent studies are examining the potential role of low-dose naltrexone (4.5 mg oral daily) as a management option related to the central nervous system gliopathy hypothesis.

2. Interventional Treatments

Although there are no injections or surgical procedures specifically indicated to manage the chronic widespread pain associated with fibromyalgia, there may be coexisting issues, such as arthritis or bursitis which may respond to injection therapy. When MPS and fibromyalgia coexist, TrP injections may be beneficial. TMS of the prefrontal cortex has been studied in patients with fibromyalgia as TMS can cause changes in acute pain perception and may alleviate depression.

3. Rehabilitation Approaches

Aerobic exercise has been shown to be more effective than various other interventions for patients with fibromyalgia. A supervised aerobic exercise training program may improve global well-being and physical function in patients with fibromyalgia. Exercise with self-management education seems to be more effective than education alone for improvement of quality of life. Patients with fibromyalgia should participate in a graded exercise program of their choice. Moderate to high-intensity resistance training may improve physical function, pain, tenderness, and fatigue in women with fibromyalgia. Aquatic exercise may increase muscle strength and reduce stiffness in adults with fibromyalgia but may not have clinically important benefit in improving pain or function.

As noted for the treatment of MPS, manual therapy, such as OMT, may be beneficial for patients with fibromyalgia as well.

4. Psychological Therapies

As discussed previously for patients with MPS, CBT may help reduce fear of pain and activity, as well as reduce disability and fatigue in patients with fibromyalgia. Psychological evaluation and/or counseling may be helpful for patients with fibromyalgia, which is often associated with psychological distress. Psychological treatment and participation in a functional restoration program may improve pain, sleep issues, function, and depression in patients with fibromyalgia.

Additional options to consider for a comprehensive management plan include mind-body therapies such as biofeedback, relaxation training, yoga, Tai chi, meditation, hypnosis, instruction in self-control strategies, group discussion, behavioral treatment, autogenic training, stress management, and electroacupuncture.

IV. CONCLUSION

In conclusion, although our understanding of the disease process is evolving and there are increased therapeutic options, diagnosing and treating patients with chronic widespread pain continue to be challenging. For the management of MPS and fibromyalgia, a multimodal approach, including pharmacologic and nonpharmacologic therapies, such as PT, psychosocial support, and education, is employed to achieve the best results.

Selected Readings

Arnold LM, Clauw DJ, McCarberg BH; FibroCollaborative. Improving the recognition and diagnosis of fibromyalgia. *Mayo Clinic Proc.* 2011;86(5):457-464.

Benzon HT, Rathmell JP, Wu CL, et al. *Practical Management of Pain.* 5th ed. Philadelphia, PA: Elsevier Mosby; 2014.

Borg-Stein J. Treatment of fibromyalgia, myofascial pain, and related disorders. *Phys Med Rehab Clin North Am.* 2006;17(2):491-510.

Borg-Stein J, Iaccarino MA. Myofascial pain syndrome treatments. *Phys Med Rehab Clin North Am.* 2014;25(2):357-374.

Clauw DJ. Fibromyalgia: an overview. *Am J Med.* 2009;122(12):3.

Frontera WR, Silver JK, Rizzo TD. *Essentials of Physical Medicine and Rehabilitation.* Philadelphia, PA: Hanley & Belfus; 2008.

Goldenberg DL. Diagnosis and differential diagnosis of fibromyalgia. *Am J Med.* 2009;122(12):14-21.

Macfarlane GJ, Kronisch C, Dean LE, et al. EULAR revised recommendations for the management of fibromyalgia. *Ann Rheum Dis.* 2017;76(2):318-328.

Mense S, Simons DG, Russell IJ. *Muscle Pain: Understanding Its Nature, Diagnosis, and Treatment.* Philadelphia, PA: Lippincott Williams & Wilkins; 2001.

Shah JP. Integrating dry needling with new concepts of myofascial pain, muscle physiology, and sensitization. In: Audette JF, Bailey A, eds. *Integrative Pain Medicine. Contemporary Pain Medicine (Integrative Pain Medicine: The Science and Practice of Complementary and Alternative Medicine in Pain Management).* New Jersey, NJ: Humana Press, 2008.

Shah JP, Gilliams EA. Uncovering the biochemical milieu of myofascial trigger points using in vivo microdialysis: an application of muscle pain concepts to myofascial pain syndrome. *J Bodyw Mov Ther.* 2008;12(4):371-384.

Shah JP, Thaker N, Heimur J, Aredo JV, Sikdar S, Gerber L. Myofascial trigger points then and now: a historical and scientific perspective. *PM R.* 2015;7(7):746-761.

Simons DG, Travell JG, Simons LS, Travell JG. *Myofascial Pain and Dysfunction: The Trigger Point Manual.* Baltimore, MD: Williams & Wilkins; 1999.

Thieme K, Mathys M, Turk DC. Evidenced-based guidelines on the treatment of fibromyalgia patients: are they consistent and if not, why not? Have effective psychological treatments been overlooked?. *J Pain.* 2017;18(7):747-756. doi:10.1016/j.jpain.2016.12.006.

Thorpe J, Shum B, Moore RA, Wiffen PJ, Gilron I. Combination pharmacotherapy for the treatment of fibromyalgia in adults. *Cochrane Database Syst Rev.* 2018;2(2):CD010585.

Woolf CJ. Central sensitization: uncovering the relation between pain and plasticity. *Anesthesiology.* 2007;106(4):864-867.

29 Acupuncture

Lucy Chen

I. INTRODUCTION

Acupuncture is one of the most significant components of the health care system in China for more than 3000 years. It has been practiced all over the world. Over the last few decades, acupuncture has gained increasing popularity and has come under increasing scrutiny in Europe and America, beginning in the 1970s in the United States.

Several events contributed to the interest and the integration of acupuncture into current medical practice. In 1995, the U.S. Food and Drug Administration (FDA) classified acupuncture needles as medical equipment, subject to the same strict quality control standards applied to medical needles, syringes, and surgical scalpels.[1] In 1997, the National Institutes of Health (NIH) organized a Consensus Development Conference on Acupuncture, acknowledging that acupuncture was widely practiced by physicians, dentists, acupuncturists, and other practitioners for relief from or prevention of pain and for various other health conditions. One of the reasons for patients seeking acupuncture treatment is the incidence of adverse effects is substantially lower than that of many drugs and commonly accepted medical procedures.[2] The NIH Office of Alternative Medicine (OAM) later expanded and was renamed the National Center for Complementary and Alternative Medicine (NCCAM), most recently changed to National Center for Complementary and Integrative Health (NCCIH). Many research funds gave to the projects relating to acupuncture treatment for multiple medical and pain conditions. Because of increasing demand from patients for acupuncture and complementary therapies, a substantial amount of data from clinical/laboratory research, and a gradual increase in coverage by insurance, there has been vast progress in health care practitioners' understanding and practicing of acupuncture. In a national survey, Eisenberg et al. found that the number of visits to alternative therapy centers was twice that of visits to primary care physicians and that the money spent on complementary and alternative medicine (CAM) was nearly equal to out-of-pocket expenditures for conventional care.[3] The total out-of-pocket expenditures relating to alternative therapies increased to $33.9 billion in 2009.[4] Third-party reimbursements for alternative therapies also have increased with patient demand. With ever-growing health care costs in the United States, health insurance providers have begun to emphasize preventative measures, particularly in the face of a rapidly aging population. Most medical schools in the United States have included subjects on integrated medicine. Integrative medicine will promote a more holistic, purposeful effort toward maintaining health, contrasting with conventional medicine's interventional approach toward management of disease, and therefore will likely play a vital role in minimizing costs and in improving patient health and satisfaction.

II. THE THEORY OF ACUPUNCTURE TREATMENT

Acupuncture involves the insertion of fine sterilized needles through the skin at specific points, so-called acupoints. According to traditional Chinese medicine, qi (pronounced "chee") is the life force or energy that flows through all living things and influences health on physical, mental, emotional, and spiritual levels. The human health is maintained through a delicate balance of two opposing but inseparable elements: Yin and Yang. Yin represents "cold, slow, and passive elements," whereas Yang represents "hot, exciting, and active elements." Any imbalance of the Yin and Yang system would cause the disruption or blockage the flow of qi and lead to a state of disease or pain. Acupuncture treats disease and disorders by influencing the flow of qi, thereby restoring the normal balance of organ systems. Because qi is thought to flow through specific pathways in a human body, so-called meridians, acupuncture treatment involves placing fine acupuncture needles into the acupoints located along the meridians to treat the disease by strengthening the weak qi and releasing the excessive qi or removing the blockage from the flow of qi, to restore the normal balance of the Yin and Yang system. The human body consists of 12 main meridians and 8 secondary meridians, which run vertically along each side of the body. There are also acupoints located beyond the meridians. There are about 2000 acupuncture points on the human body (including auricular, hand, foot, scalp, etc.).

Before starting the acupuncture treatment, the practitioner will first have to make the diagnosis through evaluation of patients. Diagnostic techniques for traditional Chinese medicine include the following methods: (1) observation of patient's mental status, facial expression, mobility, skin, tongue and coating, urine and stool, etc; (2) auscultation and olfaction of patient voice, breathing, coughing, moaning, smelling odor of the secretion and excretion, etc; (3) inquiring of patient's symptoms; and (4) palpation of radial and ulnar pulses and various part of body related to disease. Acupuncture points are usually chosen based on the practitioner's assessment of the particular imbalance that needs to be restored.

Several sizes of needles are available. Needles can be manipulated in many ways—often by rotating the needle in specific directions or by applying electricity. The sensation of *deqi*—an aching, warm or tingling sensation at the insertion site noted by the patient, is thought to be necessary for the therapeutic effect.

Electroacupuncture (EA) is commonly practiced currently and uses electrical impulses conducted through needles for enhanced stimulation of acupuncture points. Different frequencies of electricity have been shown to have distinct effects and mechanisms of action. Related techniques include moxibustion (burning of herbs to apply heat near acupuncture points), acupressure (stimulation of points without penetration of the skin with needles), and cupping (heat creates a partial vacuum in small jars, which are used to stimulate points with suction). Other variations employ stimulation of acupuncture points using laser and ultrasound.

III. COMPLICATIONS AND SIDE EFFECTS

The 1997 NIH consensus panel on acupuncture stated that the documented occurrence of adverse events in practice of acupuncture has been extremely low. The most commonly reported complication is bruising or bleeding at the needle insertion site (note that there are no specific guidelines on anticoagulation therapy and acupuncture), followed by the incidence of a transient vasovagal response, which resolves quickly and completely with repositioning of the patient. Other rare complications include infection, dermatitis, and broken needle fragments. Minor but significant adverse events were reported (0.13%), including severe nausea and actual fainting; unexpected, severe, and prolonged aggravation of symptoms; prolonged and unacceptable pain and bruising; and psychological and emotional reactions in a large-scale study (34 407 acupuncture treatments).[5] However, since acupuncture is still considered an invasive medical intervention, serious complications such as pneumothorax, hemothorax, internal organ puncture, and pericardial effusion could happen if the treatment is not properly administered.[6] Factors that may contribute to serious complications from acupuncture are similar to other medical treatment: (1) elderly and more fragile patients, (2) debilitated patients with complex comorbidities, and (3) less skilled practitioners. Thus, it is important that the acupuncture licensing and regulation mandate the use of standards of acupuncture training through adopting strict requirement for the knowledge of anatomy and sterile techniques

IV. SCIENTIFIC BASIS

Since the acupuncture has been used to treat many medical conditions, a great deal of research work has been done on the "scientific" basis of acupuncture's effects. Convincing evidence has supported that central nervous system, peripheral nerves, endorphins, neurotransmitters, neurohumoral factors, and other chemical mediators are involved. Different means of acupuncture stimulation elicit different mechanisms of pain inhibition.

A. Central Nervous System

In the most widely accepted acupuncture model, needling of nerve fibers in the muscle sends impulses that activate the spinal cord, midbrain, and hypothalamus-pituitary system. EA at different frequencies could have different effects on the synthesis and release of neuropeptides in the central nervous system. Moreover, a mu-opioid receptor antagonist or antiserum against endorphin blocked acupuncture analgesia induced by EA at 2 Hz but not at 100 Hz.

1. The spinal cord site uses enkephalin and dynorphin to block incoming messages during EA at a low frequency (2-4 Hz). Other neurotransmitters (eg, GABA) are stimulated with high-frequency (50-500 Hz) acupuncture.

2. The midbrain uses enkephalin to activate the raphe descending system, which inhibits the transmission of spinal cord pain through the synergistic effects of serotonin and norepinephrine. Another midbrain circuit bypasses the endorphin-mediated steps during high-frequency EA.
3. At the hypothalamus-pituitary level, the pituitary releases β-endorphin into the blood and cerebrospinal fluid (CFS) to produce distant analgesia. The hypothalamus sends long axons to the midbrain and activates descending analgesia via β-endorphin. This center is activated only with low-frequency not high-frequency EA. Other neurotransmitters in the central nervous system also can be modulated by EA. For example, cholecystokinin-like immune reactivity was increased within the medial thalamic area, and the activity of natural killer cells suppressed by the hypothalamic lesion was enhanced or restored after EA.

B. Peripheral Nerve System

An intact peripheral nervous system appears to be necessary for the analgesic effects of acupuncture as supported by the finding that the analgesic effects can be abolished if the acupuncture site is affected by postherpetic neuralgia or intervened with local anesthetics.

C. Endogenous Opioid Peptides

The following findings from several laboratories support the role of endorphins and a humorally mediated mechanism of EA:

1. The effects of acupuncture are not immediate; analgesia occurs after a 20- to 30-minute induction period, as might be expected in a humorally mediated mechanism. Analgesia persists for 1-2 hours after cessation of acupuncture.
2. Acupuncture led to a significant increase in the endogenous endorphin production, and the effect of acupuncture can be blocked by the opioid receptor antagonist naloxone.
3. Animals genetically deficient in opioid receptors or endorphins show poor acupuncture analgesia. Substances that inhibit endorphin enzymatic degradation enhance acupuncture effects.
4. Acupuncture analgesia can be passed from one animal to a second animal via CSF transfer or via cross-circulation of blood between the two animals. This effect is blocked by naloxone given to **either** animal.

D. Neurotransmitters

The observation that different neurotransmitters (serotonin and norepinephrine, etc.) act as mediators is supported by the following findings:

1. EA at different frequencies (2, 10, or 100 Hz) elicited the analgesic effects and such effects could be at least partially blocked by a serotonin receptor antagonist.
2. When lesions are made in areas of the brain rich in serotonin-releasing cells (eg, the raphe magnus of the brainstem and medial medulla oblongata), acupuncture-induced analgesia is abolished.
3. Agents that block biosynthesis of serotonin (eg, *p*-chlorophenylalanine) block acupuncture analgesia. Agents that block serotonin receptors block acupuncture. Analgesia is enhanced when serotonin levels are increased.
4. EA increases the anandamide (an endogenous cannabinoid) level in inflammatory skin tissues, and local pretreatment with a specific cannabinoid (CB2) receptor antagonist, AM630, significantly attenuated

the antinociceptive effect of EA, suggesting that activation of the CB2 receptor contributes to the analgesic effect of EA on inflammatory pain.

5. The NMDA receptor subunit NR2B was involved in the analgesic effects of EA in pain in the thyroid region by down-regulating the NR2B phosphorylation level.
6. Norepinephrine is implicated as a mediator in studies demonstrating suppression of EA effects via inhibition of the descending adrenergic system with yohimbine and phentolamine.

E. Nitric Oxide

New research suggests that EA induces up-regulation of neuronal nitric oxide/NADPH diaphorase expression in the gracile nucleus in rats. L-Arginine-derived nitric oxide then mediates acupuncture signals through dorsal medulla-thalamic pathways. This may play a major role in central autonomic regulation of somatosympathetic reflex activities, which contribute to acupuncture effects in somatic and visceral pain processing, and cardiovascular regulation. In a clinical study, a total of 40 healthy subjects were equally randomized into acupuncture group and nonacupuncture group. The local nitric oxide (another proposed neurotransmitter) content in those subjects in the acupuncture group was significantly higher than those in the nonacupuncture group, indicating that acupuncture stimulation can up-regulate dermal nitric oxide content.

F. Functional Magnetic Resonance Imaging

The neuroimaging techniques such as functional magnetic resonance imaging (fMRI) and positron emission topographic (PET) scan have made it possible to further understand the acupuncture effects on human brain neuronal activity. Acupuncture treatment with de-qi sensation have showed the attenuation of neuronal activity in periaqueductal gray (PAG), thalamus, hypothalamus, somatosensory cortex, and prefrontal cortex regions in the human brain, which is activated by pain. Compared with manual acupuncture, EA, particularly at a low frequency, produced more widespread fMRI signal changes in the anterior insula area (signal increases) as well as in the limbic and paralimbic structures (signal increases). More interesting findings are that different acupuncture points evoked a signal increase or decrease in specific areas within the central nerve system, suggesting that there might be a correlation between the effects of acupuncture and neuronal changes in the brain. Other studies have also showed that neuronal responses to EA stimulation can be visualized in the rat primary somatosensory cortex using an optical imaging system and each meridian is connected to a representative area in the cerebral cortex suggesting that the meridian system defined in the theories of Chinese medicine might overlap with distinct supraspinal regions. This process may help in understanding the neural mechanisms of acupuncture treatment and meridian phenomena.

V. CLINICAL EVIDENCE

A. Treatment Effect Categories From WHO

In 2003, the World Health Organization (WHO) published a review of all clinical trials up to the year 1999 and determined four categories of disorders treated by acupuncture.[7] Table 29.1 represents the four categories: **(1) the first category:** diseases, symptoms, or conditions for which acupuncture has been proved—through controlled trials—to be an effective treatment; **(2) the second category:** diseases, symptoms, or conditions for which the

TABLE 29.1 WHO Disorders Treated by Acupuncture

Category	Diseases, Symptoms, or Conditions
Category 1[a]	Adverse reactions to radiotherapy and/or chemotherapy
	Allergic rhinitis (including hay fever)
	Biliary colic
	Depression (including depressive neurosis and depression following stroke)
	Dysentery, acute bacillary
	Dysmenorrhea, primary
	Epigastralgia, acute (in peptic ulcer, acute and chronic gastritis, and gastrospasm)
	Facial pain (including cranio-mandibular disorders)
	Headache
	Hypertension, essential
	Hypotension, primary
	Induction of labor
	Knee pain
	Leukopenia
	Low back pain
	Malposition of fetus, correction of
	Morning sickness
	Nausea and vomiting
	Neck pain
	Pain in dentistry (including dental pain and temporomandibular dysfunction)
	Periarthritis of shoulder
	Postoperative pain
	Renal colic
	Rheumatoid arthritis
	Sciatica
	Sprain
	Stroke
	Tennis elbow
Category 2[b]	Abdominal pain (in acute gastroenteritis or due to gastrointestinal spasm)
	Acne vulgaris
	Alcohol dependence and detoxification
	Bell palsy
	Bronchial asthma
	Cancer pain
	Cardiac neurosis
	Cholecystitis, chronic, with acute exacerbation
	Cholelithiasis
	Competition stress syndrome
	Craniocerebral injury, closed
	Diabetes mellitus, non–insulin dependent
	Earache
	Epidemic hemorrhagic fever
	Epistaxis, simple (without generalized or local disease)
	Eye pain due to subconjunctival injection

(*Continued*)

TABLE 29.1 WHO Disorders Treated by Acupuncture (*Continued*)

Category	Diseases, Symptoms, or Conditions
	Female infertility
	Facial spasm
	Female urethral syndrome
	Fibromyalgia and fasciitis
	Gastrokinetic disturbance
	Gouty arthritis
	Hepatitis B virus carrier status
	Herpes zoster, human (alpha) herpesvirus
	Hyperlipemia
	Hypo-ovarianism
	Insomnia
	Labur pain
	Lactation, deficiency
	Male sexual dysfunction, nonorganic
	Ménière disease
	Neuralgia, postherpetic
	Neurodermatitis
	Obesity
	Opium, cocaine, and heroin dependence
	Osteoarthritis
	Pain due to endoscopic examination
	Pain in thromboangiitis obliterans
	Polycystic ovary syndrome (Stein-Leventhal syndrome)
	Postextubation in children
	Postoperative convalescence
	Premenstrual syndrome
	Prostatitis, chronic
	Pruritus
	Radicular and pseudoradicular pain syndrome
	Raynaud syndrome, primary
	Recurrent lower urinary tract infection
	Reflex sympathetic dystrophy
	Retention of urine, traumatic
	Schizophrenia
	Sialism, drug-induced
	Sjögren syndrome
	Sore throat (including tonsillitis)
	Spine pain, acute
	Stiff neck
	Temporomandibular joint dysfunction
	Tietz syndrome
	Tobacco dependence
	Tourette syndrome
	Ulcerative colitis, chronic
	Urolithiasis
	Vascular dementia
	Whooping cough (pertussis)

TABLE 29.1 WHO Disorders Treated by Acupuncture (*Continued*)

Category	Diseases, Symptoms, or Conditions
Category 3[c]	Chloasma
	Choroidopathy, central serous
	Color blindness
	Deafness
	Hypophrenia
	Irritable colon syndrome
	Neuropathic bladder in spinal cord injury
	Pulmonary heart disease, chronic
	Small airway obstruction
Category 4[d]	Breathlessness in chronic obstructive pulmonary disease
	Coma
	Convulsions in infants
	Coronary heart disease (angina pectoris)
	Diarrhea in infants and young children
	Encephalitis, viral, in children, late stage
	Paralysis, progressive bulbar and pseudobulbar

[a]**The first category:** diseases, symptoms, or conditions for which acupuncture has been proved—through controlled trials—to be an effective treatment.
[b]**The second category:** diseases, symptoms, or conditions for which the therapeutic effect of acupuncture has been shown but for which further proof is needed,
[c]**The third category:** diseases, symptoms, or conditions for which there are only individual controlled trials reporting some therapeutic effects, but for which acupuncture is worth trying because treatment by conventional and other therapies is difficult.
[d]**The fourth category:** Diseases, symptoms, or conditions for which acupuncture may be tried provided the practitioner has special modern medical knowledge and adequate monitoring equipment.
Derived from World Health Organization. Acupuncture: review and analysis of reports on controlled clinical trials, 2002. http://apps.who.int/medicinedocs/pdf/s4926e/s4926e.pdf

therapeutic effect of acupuncture has been shown but for which further proof is needed; **(3) the third category:** diseases, symptoms, or conditions for which there are only individual controlled trials reporting some therapeutic effects, but for which acupuncture is worth trying because treatment by conventional and other therapies is difficult; **(4) the fourth category:** diseases, symptoms, or conditions for which acupuncture may be tried provided the practitioner has special modern medical knowledge and adequate monitoring equipment.

Although there is still controversy about the strength of scientific evidence for acupuncture, there have been many recent advances, particularly in relation to acupuncture in the treatment of pain. It is encouraging to see that more controlled, randomized clinical studies of acupuncture have replaced the bulk of anecdotal case reports. The following is a brief discussion of some of these trials on several common clinical pain conditions.

B. Back Pain

Although many medical and interventional treatment options have been developed for *chronic* low back pain, low back pain is associated with high medical expenses and disability and is one of the most common health problems that patients seeking treatment for. Every year, there are about $90 billion in health care expenses spending on patients with back pain problems.[8] Although many medical and interventional treatment options have developed for low back pain treatment, long-term effects remain unsatisfied due to many reasons. Recently, acupuncture has become one of the most frequently used alternative therapies in treating low back pain.

In several randomized placebo-controlled clinical trials, the results indicate that acupuncture was superior to physical therapy regarding pain intensity, pain-related disability, and psychological distress. When compared with sham acupuncture, true acupuncture was also superior in the reduction of psychological stress, improved return to work, quality of sleep, and reduced use of analgesics.[9,10] Such treatment results may be attributed to the factors that acupuncture not only can reduce the pain, but also treat anxiety and depression symptoms through the modulation of multiple neurotransmitters. In a large study involving 1162 patients with chronic low back pain, acupuncture therapy improved low back pain for at least 6 months. The effectiveness of acupuncture was almost twice that of conventional therapy. The cost-effectiveness analysis showed that acupuncture plus routine care was associated with a marked clinical improvement and was relatively cost-effective.[11] Therefore, the clinical practice guideline from American College of Physicians and the American Pain Society for chronic low back pain patients recommend physicians to consider acupuncture as an addition of nonpharmacologic therapy with proven benefits for low back pain.[12,13]

C. Neck and Shoulder Pain

Chronic neck and shoulder pain can be caused by cervical degenerated disc disease, cervical facet joint disease, myofascial pain, and shoulder joint disease. Medications and interventional procedures including surgery as treatments for chronic neck and shoulder pain are not always satisfied by patients. Therefore, acupuncture treatment has commonly been used through an integrative approach to reduce pain symptoms. In one study, the acupuncture treatment reduced chronic pain in neck and shoulders for at least three years with a concomitant improvement in depression, anxiety, sleep quality, pain-related activity impairment, and quality of life.[14,15] Another study compared the treatment effect of acupuncture combining with physical therapy to that of acupuncture or physical therapy alone for patients with neck pain due to neck tension syndrome. All groups showed significant improvement after 10 weeks of treatment, but the group receiving a combination of acupuncture and physical therapy was superior in pain reduction and function disability improvement than other groups with acupuncture or physical therapy alone. The improvements of all groups were maintained ($P < .05$) at the 6 months of follow-up. The data suggest that acupuncture treatment may assist and/or enhance the physiotherapy effect on musculoskeletal rehabilitation for tension neck syndrome.[16] For neck pain induced by cervical spondylosis, one study enrolled 106 subjects and randomly divided these subjects into real acupuncture group and control sham acupuncture group. The effective rate was 75.5% in the acupuncture group and 52.8% in the control group ($P < .05$).[17]

One large-scale clinical trial with a total of 14 161 patients also demonstrates that integrating acupuncture with routine medical care in patients with chronic neck pain may result in both pain improvement and a reduction of disability.[18] In two meta-analysis studies with 10-14 clinical trials included, there was moderate evidence that acupuncture was more effective for pain relief than some types of sham controls or inactive, sham treatments, when measured immediately after the treatment and at short-term follow-up.[19,20]

D. Headache

Treatment for headache disorders has advanced with the developments of many new pharmacological agents, such as selective serotonin receptor agonists like sumatriptan, for migraine headache. There are still some migraine patients who may not achieve adequate therapeutic effect through such treatment. Alternatively, acupuncture has become a new modality of treatment for those patients suffering from tension headache, migraine, and other types of headaches. In a multicenter randomized study with 302 migraine headache patients divided into three groups, acupuncture, minimal acupuncture and waiting list, there is significant effect in those treated with acupuncture and minimal acupuncture as compared to those on the waiting list for treatment.[21] Many other headache studies with either tension headache or migraine headache, with a sample size from 50 to 2022 patients, also showed similar results.[22–31]

For many patients, acupuncture not only has a similar, if not better, efficacy as compared with sumatriptan in preventing full migraine attack but also has unique benefits over sumatriptan-related medications because of its negligible side effects.[28] In a systematic review of 22 trials of 4419 participants, there is consistent evidence that acupuncture provides additional benefit in treatment of acute migraine attacks as compared to routine care only.[32] For chronic tension headache, a study found that acupuncture treatment has statistically significant and clinically relevant short-term (up to 3 months) benefits over control in terms of the number of headache days and pain intensity in 2317 participants. Acupuncture could be a valuable nonpharmacological tool in patients with frequent episodic or chronic tension-type headaches.[33] In a recent review with 27 clinical trials to evaluate the efficacy of acupuncture in the treatment of primary headaches (migraine headache, tension headache, and mixed forms), majority of trials (23 out of 27 trials) showed favorable outcomes in the treatment of headaches using acupuncture.[34] Moreover, the pediatric patient population also benefits from this alternative therapy for headache treatment.[35] Per international cost-effectiveness threshold values, acupuncture is a cost-effective treatment in patients with primary headache.[36]

E. Acupuncture for Other Pain

In many other pain conditions, acupuncture has showed benefit in reducing pain, for example, acupuncture treatment for labor pain. In one study, significantly reduced need of epidural analgesia and a better degree of relaxation have been shown in parturients who received acupuncture during labor. No negative effect on delivery is noted as compared with a control group.[37,38] For acute postoperative pain, several studies have shown that patients who received acupuncture prior to operation had a lower pain level, reduced opioid requirement, a lower incidence of postoperative nausea and vomiting, and lower sympathoadrenal responses.[39–42] On the other hand, acupuncture has been shown to provide some improvement in function and pain relief in the treatment of osteoarthritis of the knee when compared with sham acupuncture or control groups using education.[43] In addition, the benefit of acupuncture treatment in fibromyalgia, rheumatoid arthritis, and chronic lateral epicondylitis (tennis elbow) is supported by several clinical trials.[44–46] Large-scale clinical trials on these pain conditions may be warranted.

F. Acupuncture for Other Medical Conditions

Not only can acupuncture been used for the treatment of pain, but also it can be used to treat many other conditions. Several clinical trials strongly support the therapeutic effect of acupuncture in postoperative nausea and vomiting, either needle acupuncture or applying acupressure to the relevant acupoints, as compared with antiemetics such as droperidol and Zofran (ondansetron).[47–53] There is an increasing number of patients seeking acupuncture treatment for many medical conditions including allergy, asthma, depression, anxiety, obesity, insomnia, cancer-related fatigue, premenstrual syndrome, menopause symptoms, assisted conception and infertility, spinal cord injury, quitting smoking, and detoxification from opioids or other drug addiction.[54–76] Acupuncture can be either a supplement therapy or replacement of their conventional treatments. Medical conditions for which acupuncture can be useful are listed in the WHO for clinical pain conditions recommended for acupuncture above published in 2002.

VI. CHALLENGES OF ACUPUNCTURE TREATMENT

Although many convincing studies on acupuncture have been published in the latest meta-analyses, reviews, and government health agency statements, clinical trials on the efficacy of acupuncture have their unique issues such as individualization, placebo controls, and the crossover design. True blinding of the patient is difficult, and that of the treating acupuncturist is impossible. Nonspecific needling (ie, not at recognized acupuncture sites or at non–site-specific points for the disease in question) can elicit responses that may be similar to responses to active treatment, thereby skewing results and making interpretation difficult.

Several developments in acupuncture study techniques and equipment have occurred over the last several years. A placebo or "sham needle," designed to make the patient feel that the skin is being punctured, was developed in 1998. The needle shaft disappears inside itself and adheres to the skin via a small plastic ring. The plastic ring is then also added to real acupuncture needles for study groups for blinding effect.

However, generalized conclusions are still challenging. This is possible due to (1) the variation in acupuncture points selected, (2) variation in the mode of needle stimulation, (3) treatment duration and intervals between treatments, and (4) diagnosis different in Eastern medicine given the same clinical conditions in Western medicine. In clinical setting, acupuncture treatment is often highly individualized for a given clinical condition, which varies from one practitioner to another.

VII. CONCLUSION

Acupuncture has become increasingly popular in Europe and America as people have become more familiar with this treatment modality. With increasing number of clinical trials on acupuncture treatments providing more information, particularly on the role of acupuncture in clinical pain management, it can be anticipated that acupuncture is likely to play a growing and positive role in pain management.

References

1. Turner JS. The regulation of acupuncture needles by the United States Food and Drug Administration. *J Altern Complement Med.* 1995;1(1):15-16.
2. NIH consensus conference. Acupuncture. *JAMA.* 1998;280(17):1518-1524.
3. Eisenberg DM, Davis RB, Ettner SL, et al. Trends in alternative medicine use in the United States, 1990–1997, results of a follow-up national survey. *JAMA.* 1998; 280(18):1569-1575.
4. National Health statistic report number 18, July 30, 2009.

5. MacPherson H, Thomas K, Walters S, Fitter M. A prospective survey of adverse events and treatment reactions following 34,000 consultations with professional acupuncturists. *Acupunct Med.* 2001;19(2):93-102.
6. Melchart D, Weidenhammer W, Streng A, et al. Prospective investigation of adverse effects of acupuncture in 97 733 patients. *Arch Intern Med.* 2004;164(1):104-105.
7. World Health Organization. Acupuncture: review and analysis of reports on controlled clinical trials. 2002. http://apps.who.int/medicinedocs/pdf/s4926e/s4926e.pdf
8. Berman BM, Langevin HM, Witt CM, Dubner R. Acupuncture for chronic low back pain. *N Engl J Med.* 2010;363(5):454-461.
9. Leibing E, Leonhardt U, Koster G, et al. Acupuncture treatment of chronic low-back pain—a randomized, blinded, placebo-controlled trial with 9-month follow-up. *Pain.* 2002;96(1-2):189-196.
10. Molsberger AF, Mau J, Pawelec DB, Winkler J. Does acupuncture improve the orthopedic management of chronic low back pain—a randomized, blinded, controlled trial with 3 months follow up. *Pain.* 2002;99(3):579-587.
11. Witt CM, Jena S, Selim D, et al. Pragmatic randomized trial evaluating the clinical and economic effectiveness of acupuncture for chronic low back pain. *Am J Epidemiol.* 2006;164(5):487-496.
12. Chou R, Huffman LH; American Pain Society, American College of Physicians. Nonpharmacologic therapies for acute and chronic low back pain: a review of the evidence for an American pain Society/American college of physicians clinical practice guideline. *Ann Intern Med.* 2007;147(7):492-504.
13. Chou R, Qaseem A, Snow V, et al. Diagnosis and treatment of low back pain: a joint clinical practice guideline from the American college of physicians and the American pain society. *Ann Intern Med.* 2007;147(7):478-491.
14. He D, Veiersted KB, Hostmark AT, Medbo JI. Effect of acupuncture treatment on chronic neck and shoulder pain in sedentary female workers: a 6-month and 3-year follow-up study. *Pain.* 2004;109(3):299-307.
15. He D, Hostmark AT, Veiersted KB, Medbo JI. Effect of intensive acupuncture on pain-related social and psychological variables for women with chronic neck and shoulder pain—an RCT with six month and three year follow up. *Acupunct Med.* 2005;23(2):52-61.
16. Franca DL, Senna-Fernandes V, Cortez CM, Jackson MN, Bernardo-Filho M, Guimaraes MA. Tension neck syndrome treated by acupuncture combined with physiotherapy: a comparative clinical trial (pilot study). *Complement Ther Med.* 2008;16(5):268-277.
17. Liang ZH, Yang YH, Yu P, et al. Logistic regression analysis on therapeutic effect of acupuncture on neck pain caused by cervical spondylosis and factors influencing therapeutic effect. *Zhongguo Zhen Jiu.* 2009;29(3):173-176.
18. Witt CM, Jena S, Brinkhaus B, Liecker B, Wegscheider K, Willich SN. Acupuncture for patients with chronic neck pain. *Pain.* 2006;125(1-2):98-106.
19. Fu LM, Li JT, Wu WS. Randomized controlled trials of acupuncture for neck pain: Systematic review and meta-analysis. *J Altern Complement Med.* 2009;15(2):133-145.
20. Trinh K, Graham N, Gross A, et al. Acupuncture for neck disorders. *Spine (Phila Pa 1976).* 2007;32(2):236-243.
21. Linde K, Streng A, Hoppe A, et al. Treatment in a randomized multicenter trial of acupuncture for migraine (ART migraine). *Forsch Komplementmed.* 2006;13(2):101-108.
22. Coeytaux RR, Kaufman JS, Kaptchuk TJ, et al. A randomized, controlled trial of acupuncture for chronic daily headache. *Headache.* 2005;45(9):1113-1123.
23. Ebneshahidi NS, Heshmatipour M, Moghaddami A, Eghtesadi-Araghi P. The effects of laser acupuncture on chronic tension headache—a randomised controlled trial. *Acupunct Med.* 2005;23(1):13-18.
24. Endres HG, Bowing G, Diener HC, et al. Acupuncture for tension-type headache: a multicentre, sham-controlled, patient-and observer-blinded, randomised trial. *J Headache Pain.* 2007;8(5):306-314.
25. Endres HG, Diener HC, Molsberger A. Role of acupuncture in the treatment of migraine. *Expert Rev Neurother.* 2007;7(9):1121-1134.
26. Facco E, Liguori A, Petti F, et al. Traditional acupuncture in migraine: a controlled, randomized study. *Headache.* 2008;48(3):398-407.
27. Melchart D, Streng A, Hoppe A, et al. Acupuncture in patients with tension-type headache: randomised controlled trial. *BMJ.* 2005;331(7513):376-382.

28. Melchart D, Thormaehlen J, Hager S, Liao J, Linde K, Weidenhammer W. Acupuncture versus placebo versus sumatriptan for early treatment of migraine attacks: a randomized controlled trial. *J Intern Med.* 2003;253(2):181-188.
29. Streng A, Linde K, Hoppe A, et al. Effectiveness and tolerability of acupuncture compared with metoprolol in migraine prophylaxis. *Headache.* 2006;46(10):1492-1502.
30. Wang K, Svensson P, Arendt-Nielsen L. Effect of acupuncture-like electrical stimulation on chronic tension-type headache: a randomized, double-blinded, placebo-controlled trial. *Clin J Pain.* 2007;23(4):316-322.
31. Melchart D, Weidenhammer W, Streng A, Hoppe A, Pfaffenrath V, Linde K. Acupuncture for chronic headaches—an epidemiological study. *Headache.* 2006;46(4):632-641.
32. Linde K, Allais G, Brinkhaus B, Manheimer E, Vickers A, White AR. Acupuncture for migraine prophylaxis. *Cochrane Database Syst Rev.* 2009;(1):CD001218.
33. Linde K, Allais G, Brinkhaus B, Manheimer E, Vickers A, White AR. Acupuncture for tension-type headache. *Cochrane Database Syst Rev.* 2009;(1):CD007587.
34. Manias P, Tagaris G, Karageorgiou K. Acupuncture in headache: a critical review. *Clin J Pain.* 2000;16(4):334-339.
35. Gottschling S, Meyer S, Gribova I, et al. Laser acupuncture in children with headache: a double-blind, randomized, bicenter, placebo-controlled trial. *Pain.* 2008;137(2):405-412.
36. Witt CM, Reinhold T, Jena S, Brinkhaus B, Willich SN. Cost-effectiveness of acupuncture treatment in patients with headache. *Cephalalgia.* 2008;28(4):334-345.
37. Ramnero A, Hanson U, Kihlgren M. Acupuncture treatment during labour—a randomised controlled trial. *BJOG.* 2002;109(6):637-644.
38. Skilnand E, Fossen D, Heiberg E. Acupuncture in the management of pain in labor. *Acta Obstet Gynecol Scand.* 2002;81(10):943-948.
39. Kotani N, Hashimoto H, Sato Y, et al. Preoperative intradermal acupuncture reduces postoperative pain, nausea and vomiting, analgesic requirement, and sympathoadrenal responses. *Anesthesiology.* 2001;95(2):349-356.
40. Lin JG, Lo MW, Wen YR, Hsieh CL, Tsai SK, Sun WZ. The effect of high and low frequency electroacupuncture in pain after lower abdominal surgery. *Pain.* 2002;99(3):509-514.
41. Sim CK, Xu PC, Pua HL, Zhang G, Lee TL. Effects of electroacupuncture on intraoperative and postoperative analgesic requirement. *Acupunct Med.* 2002;20(2-3):56-65.
42. Wang SM, Kain ZN. P6 acupoint injections are as effective as droperidol in controlling early postoperative nausea and vomiting in children. *Anesthesiology.* 2002;97(2):359-366.
43. Berman BM, Lao L, Langenberg P, Lee WL, Gilpin AM, Hochberg MC. Effectiveness of acupuncture as adjunctive therapy in osteoarthritis of the knee: a randomized, controlled trial. *Ann Intern Med.* 2004;141(12):901-910.
44. Berman BM, Swyers JP, Ezzo J. The evidence for acupuncture as a treatment for rheumatologic conditions. *Rheum Dis Clin North Am.* 2000;26(1):103-15, ix-x.
45. Tsui P, Leung MC. Comparison of the effectiveness between manual acupuncture and electro-acupuncture on patients with tennis elbow. *Acupunct Electrother Res.* 2002;27(2):107-117.
46. Fink M, Wolkenstein E, Luennemann M, Gutenbrunner C, Gehrke A, Karst M. Chronic epicondylitis: effects of real and sham acupuncture treatment: a randomised controlled patient- and examiner-blinded long-term trial. *Forsch Komplementarmed Klass Naturheilkd.* 2002;9(4):210-215.
47. Alkaissi A, Evertsson K, Johnsson VA, Ofenbartl L, Kalman S. P6 acupressure may relieve nausea and vomiting after gynecological surgery: an effectiveness study in 410 women. *Can J Anaesth.* 2002;49(10):1034-1039.
48. Allen DL, Kitching AJ, Nagle C. P6 acupressure and nausea and vomiting after gynaecological surgery. *Anaesth Intensive Care.* 1994;22(6):691-693.
49. Belluomini J, Litt RC, Lee KA, Katz M. Acupressure for nausea and vomiting of pregnancy: a randomized, blinded study. *Obstet Gynecol.* 1994;84(2):245-248.
50. Butkovic D, Toljan S, Matolic M, Kralik S, Radesic L. Comparison of laser acupuncture and metoclopramide in PONV prevention in children. *Paediatr Anaesth.* 2005;15(1):37-40.

51. Ezzo J, Streitberger K, Schneider A. Cochrane systematic reviews examine P6 acupuncture-point stimulation for nausea and vomiting. *J Altern Complement Med.* 2006;12(5):489-495.
52. Frey UH, Scharmann P, Lohlein C, Peters J. P6 acustimulation effectively decreases postoperative nausea and vomiting in high-risk patients. *Br J Anaesth.* 2009;102(5):620-625.
53. Gan TJ, Jiao KR, Zenn M, Georgiade G. A randomized controlled comparison of electro-acupoint stimulation or ondansetron versus placebo for the prevention of postoperative nausea and vomiting. *Anesth Analg.* 2004;99(4):1070-1075, table of contents.
54. Ashenden R, Silagy CA, Lodge M, Fowler G. A meta-analysis of the effectiveness of acupuncture in smoking cessation. *Drug Alcohol Rev.* 1997;16(1):33-40.
55. Balk J, Day R, Rosenzweig M, Beriwal S. Pilot, randomized, modified, double-blind, placebo-controlled trial of acupuncture for cancer-related fatigue. *J Soc Integr Oncol.* 2009;7(1):4-11.
56. Avis NE, Legault C, Coeytaux RR, et al. A randomized, controlled pilot study of acupuncture treatment for menopausal hot flashes. *Menopause.* 2008;15(6):1070-1078.
57. Brinkhaus B, Witt CM, Ortiz M, et al. Acupuncture in seasonal allergic rhinitis (ACUSAR)—design and protocol of a randomised controlled multi-centre trial. *Forsch Komplementmed.* 2010;17(2):95-102.
58. Biernacki W, Peake MD. Acupuncture in treatment of stable asthma. *Respir Med.* 1998;92(9):1143-1145.
59. Bullock ML, Kiresuk TJ, Pheley AM, Culliton PD, Lenz SK. Auricular acupuncture in the treatment of cocaine abuse. A study of efficacy and dosing. *J Subst Abuse Treat.* 1999;16(1):31-38.
60. Cao H, Pan X, Li H, Liu J. Acupuncture for treatment of insomnia: a systematic review of randomized controlled trials. *J Altern Complement Med.* 2009;15(11):1171-1186.
61. Chae Y, Kang OS, Lee HJ, et al. Effect of acupuncture on selective attention for smoking-related visual cues in smokers. *Neurol Res.* 2010;32(suppl 1):27-30.
62. Chen HY, Shi Y, Ng CS, Chan SM, Yung KK, Zhang QL. Auricular acupuncture treatment for insomnia: a systematic review. *J Altern Complement Med.* 2007;13(6):669-676.
63. Cheuk DK, Yeung WF, Chung KF, Wong V. Acupuncture for insomnia. *Cochrane Database Syst Rev.* 2007;(3):CD005472.
64. Cheong YC, Hung Yu Ng E, Ledger WL. Acupuncture and assisted conception. *Cochrane Database Syst Rev.* 2008;(4):CD006920.
65. El-Toukhy T, Sunkara SK, Khairy M, Dyer R, Khalaf Y, Coomarasamy A. A systematic review and meta-analysis of acupuncture in vitro fertilisation. *BJOG.* 2008;115(10):1203-1213.
66. Ernst E. Acupuncture for persistent allergic rhinitis: a randomised, sham-controlled trial. *Med J Aust.* 2008;188(1):64; author reply 64.
67. Huang W, Kutner N, Bliwise DL. A systematic review of the effects of acupuncture in treating insomnia. *Sleep Med Rev.* 2009;13(1):73-104.
68. Fung KP, Chow OK, So SY. Attenuation of exercise-induced asthma by acupuncture. *Lancet.* 1986;2(8521-8522):1419-1422.
69. Kokkotou E, Conboy LA, Ziogas DC, et al. Serum correlates of the placebo effect in irritable bowel syndrome. *Neurogastroenterol Motil.* 2010;22(3):285-e81.
70. Lee MS, Shin BC, Ernst E. Acupuncture for treating menopausal hot flushes: a systematic review. *Climacteric.* 2009;12(1):16-25.
71. Mora B, Iannuzzi M, Lang T, et al. Auricular acupressure as a treatment for anxiety before extracorporeal shock wave lithotripsy in the elderly. *J Urol.* 2007;178(1):160-164; discussion 164.
72. Nir Y, Huang MI, Schnyer R, Chen B, Manber R. Acupuncture for postmenopausal hot flashes. *Maturitas.* 2007;56(4):383-395.
73. Smith CA, Hay PP. Acupuncture for depression. *Cochrane Database Syst Rev.* 2005;(2):CD004046.
74. Smith CA, Hay PP, Macpherson H. Acupuncture for depression. *Cochrane Database Syst Rev.* 2010;(1):CD004046.
75. Wang SM, Kain ZN. Auricular acupuncture: a potential treatment for anxiety. *Anesth Analg.* 2001;92(2):548-553.
76. Nayak S, Shiflett SC, Schoenberger NE, et al. Is acupuncture effective in treating chronic pain after spinal cord injury? *Arch Phys Med Rehabil.* 2001;82(11):1578-1586.

SECTION VI

Acute Pain

30 Adult Postoperative Pain

David A. Edwards

I. INTRODUCTION

Postoperative pain is a combination of a patient's preoperative pain in addition to that caused by the surgical insult and modified by a given patient's psychological state. To treat postoperative pain, an individualized preoperative evaluation and pre-emptive plan for pain control should be created. A treatment plan should consist of proposed pre-emptive and postoperative analgesic medications, psychological intervention, regional anesthetic, and nonmedication treatments whenever possible. Perioperative pain control may reduce the likelihood of developing persistent postsurgical pain, so an efficient individualized plan for patients undergoing surgery can have lasting implications.

II. PRINCIPLES OF POSTOPERATIVE PAIN MANAGEMENT

A. Preoperative Planning and Setting Expectations

Patients who are prepared and know what to expect on the day of surgery will have less anxiety and a better understanding of what options for pain control are available. Empowering a patient in this way enables them to feel more in control. In those patients who are prone to catastrophizing—prone to irrational thoughts that something is far worse than it actually is—having a well thought out plan will lead them to catastrophize less. An introduction to options for postoperative pain control should take place in the surgeon's office when planning the operation or in the preoperative anesthesia clinic when a description of the anesthetic plan is delivered. Less ideal is the delivery of the analgesic plan on the morning of surgery.

1. Physical Prehabilitation

The concept of prehabilitation is the physical and psychological optimization of a patient prior to surgery in order to enhance recovery afterward. Physical and psychological therapy can be formal or informal. Physical prehabilitation ensures that the patient has reached a level of function that will optimize the physiological response to surgery and enhance physical recovery.

2. *Psychological Prehabilitation*

Patients who have never had surgery before should be told what to expect. They should be aware that some degree of postoperative pain is inevitable and that their doctors and nurses will work with them to treat any pain that does occur. Patients should also be familiar with the chosen pain assessment method and the need to assess pain on a regular basis. Preparing patients psychologically in this way will optimize chances for recognizing and treating pain promptly and has been associated with lower pain scores after many types of surgery.

a. Pain Assessment. In clinical practice, pain intensity is most commonly assessed by asking a patient their pain level on a scale of 0-10, called the numerical rating scale (NRS), or pain score. This is done at regular intervals to understand each patient's subjective pain intensity and to assess efficacy of treatment. To better understand a patient's pain, it is advisable to assess the pain score preoperatively and then compare this to postoperative pain at rest, with activity, and after treatment with analgesics. Simply relying on a single, static pain report at rest will miss the inevitable increase in pain that occurs with activity and may well lead to undertreatment.

b. Pre-emptive Analgesia. Acute pain is an adaptive response to injury that prompts an organism to protect itself and allow for appropriate time to heal. Chronic pain is the pathological extension of acute pain. Pre-emptive analgesia attempts to minimize the magnitude of postoperative acute pain and lessen the potential for transition to chronic pain. Preoperative analgesics that target different aspects of pain sensation, transmission, transduction, and perception are all employed and show varying efficacy.

III. METHODS OF POSTOPERATIVE ANALGESIA

A. Pharmacology

Medications targeting pain, anxiety, muscle spasm, and sleep are all tools used to enhance the postoperative experience of patients with pain. Often pain is tolerable if a patient can sleep well, move from their bed to a chair, and distract their thoughts. A multimodal regimen using a few medications at low doses may prevent the need for a single agent at a high dose with greater risk of side effects. In recent years, multimodal regimens have been used to reduce the overall doses of opioid required to produce adequate pain control.

1. *Opioids*

Morphine is a simple agonist at μ, κ, and δ opioid receptors. Its effects and side effects are well known and understood. Other opioids are used when patients express a preference for another drug, when they are either allergic to or report significant side effects from morphine, or when morphine does not appear to be effective. Hydromorphone is a useful alternative to morphine and may be associated with less dizziness, nausea, and lightheadedness in some patients.

The side effects of opioid drugs limit their use. Respiratory depression is the most feared risk, and patients receiving opioids should be closely monitored for respiratory depression, especially at the start of treatment. Monitoring for adequacy of ventilation includes observing the patients' state of arousal and respiratory rate, including depth and pattern of breathing, as well as color (skin and mucous membranes). Pulse oximeters and respiratory monitors are critical, especially during periods of high risk, for example, during early recovery or while titrating to increased doses. A drop in oxygen saturation as measured by pulse oximetry is a relatively late indication of opioid-related respiratory depression and signals the need for immediate intervention. A drop in the respiratory rate and minute ventilation occurs somewhat before respiratory depression is severe enough to be life-threatening, and new and emerging monitoring devices are incorporating innovative ways to automatically detect early signs of respiratory depression using some of these measurements.

Severe respiratory depression should be treated with small intravenous (IV) boluses of the μ-opioid antagonist naloxone (Narcan). If naloxone is given too quickly, severe agitation and, in extreme cases, flash pulmonary edema secondary to aggressive respiratory effort may result. The ampule of naloxone (0.4 mg) can be diluted in saline in a 10-mL syringe, and then 2-3 mL can be given every minute as needed. After naloxone reversal, patients should continue to be closely monitored because naloxone's duration of action is short (~20 minutes), and the effects of the opioid may outlast those of a single dose of naloxone, leading to "renarcotization." Naloxone will reverse opioid effects quite rapidly; so if the patient does not respond, one should consider alternative causes of the respiratory compromise.

Systemic opioid therapy (either oral or parenteral) remains the primary treatment used for patients experiencing moderate to severe acute pain. No new treatment has entirely replaced opioids, yet newer accelerated recovery protocols demand an alternative to opioids as the sole analgesic because opioid side effects (nausea, sedation, reduced bowel mobility) interfere with the goal of rapid resumption of normal physiologic functions (eating, drinking, urinating, defecating, walking, coughing). Today's standard is to use multimodal analgesia, opioids being an important component, whereas the regimen also aims to minimize opioid use.

Most postoperative patients receive bolus administration of opioids, which allows for ready titration of dose according to need. Continuous IV or subcutaneous therapy is sometimes useful—for example, in patients requiring mechanical ventilation. Oral administration is resumed as soon as oral intake is re-established.

There are several options for delivery of opioids, including by mouth (PO), IV, transdermal (TD), in the epidural (EPI) or intrathecal (IT) space, and rarely as intramuscular (IM) or subcutaneous (SQ) injections (Table 30.1).

a. Patient-Controlled Analgesia. In many institutions, including MGH, patient-controlled analgesia (PCA) is a common, although less frequently needed, therapy for postoperative pain. PCA is the self-administration of analgesics (usually via the IV route) by patients instructed in the use of a microprocessor controlled device specifically designed for this purpose. The goal of PCA is to provide doses of analgesic immediately based on the demand of the patient.

The use of portable microcomputer-controlled infusion pumps allows this dosing to be achieved quickly and easily (literally at the touch of a button); therefore small, frequent doses can be given. This approach avoids the extreme swings in plasma levels and in efficacy and side effects associated with the larger, less frequent doses used during standard nurse-administered therapy.

Other advantages of PCA are the inherent safety of using small doses and the fact that obtunded patients will not press the on-demand button for additional doses; PCA is the preference of most patients for techniques

TABLE 30.1 Delivery of Opioids

Opioid	Common Routes	Common Starting Doses
Morphine	PO, IV, EPI, IT	0.5 mg IV, 5-10 mg PO q4h
Hydromorphone	PO, IV, EPI	0.2 mg IV, 2 mg PO q4-6h
Oxycodone	PO	5-20 mg PO q4-6h
Fentanyl	IV, TD	25 mcg IV, 25 mcg/h TD
Methadone	PO	2.5-5 mg PO q8h

Option	Description
Oral	As effective as parenteral in appropriate doses. Use as soon as oral medication is tolerated
IM	Has been the standard parenteral route, but injections are painful and absorption unreliable. Avoid this route when possible
SQ	Preferable to IM for low-volume continuous infusion. Injections painful and absorption unreliable. Avoid this route for long-term repeated dosing
IV	Parenteral route of choice after major surgery. Suitable for titrated bolus or continuous administration, including patient-controlled analgesia (PCA), but requires monitoring. Significant risk of respiratory depression with inappropriate dosing
PCA	Good, steady level of analgesia. Popular with patients but requires special infusion pumps and staff education. Same cautions as for IV opioids
Epidural and intrathecal	When suitable, provides good analgesia. Expensive if infusion pumps used. Significant risk of respiratory depression, sometimes delayed in onset. Requires careful monitoring

that offer a sense of control. An exception to the general safety of PCA is its use by older and confused individuals, who, despite early obtundation (or maybe because of it), will sometimes overdose themselves. Studies show that patients vary widely in their physical need for opioids and PCA accommodates a wide range of analgesic needs. With standard PCA orders, patients can receive anywhere between 0 and 10 mg of IV morphine each hour.

Nurse-controlled boluses may be needed at the start of treatment, because patients are often sedated by residual anesthesia and incapable of using PCA properly. The small, spaced doses of PCA are also inadequate to gain rapid control of severe pain; thus nurse-administered bolus doses should be given to rapidly gain control of pain before the PCA is started. It is tempting to think that once patients are connected to PCA pumps, they do not need further pain assessment or treatment, but if pain is neglected in the early postoperative period, it may be more difficult to treat later.

Individualizing the PCA settings and frequently assessing patients' analgesia levels are critical during the first 24 hours following surgery.

The success of PCA depends first and foremost on patient selection. Patients who are too old, too confused, too young, or unable to control the button or who do not want the treatment are not suitable candidates. Ideally, patients should be educated before surgery about PCA and the concept of self-dosing.

Teaching points include expectations for pain relief, informing patients of their active role in pain management (both in pain reports and medication management), elimination of fears and misconceptions about opioids, and fear of overmedication (Table 30.2).

2. Nonsteroidal Anti-inflammatory Drugs

Nonselective nonsteroidal anti-inflammatory drugs (NSAIDs) (those that inhibit both cyclooxygenase-1 and cyclooxygenase-2 or COX-1 and COX-2) are useful as sole analgesics for mild to moderate pain and useful alternatives or adjuncts to opioid therapy and regional analgesia. Because they act by a unique mechanism, mostly in the periphery (not in the CNS), their action complements that of other analgesic therapies. Their analgesic effect is secondary to their anti-inflammatory effect, which in turn is due to inhibition of prostaglandin synthesis. Prostaglandin inhibition is also responsible for their chief side effects—gastritis/gastric ulceration, platelet dysfunction, and renal damage. Renal injury is particularly common in patients with contracted intravascular volume (eg, hypovolemic patients after trauma or patients with congestive heart failure on chronic diuretics), as maintenance of renal perfusion is mediated through prostaglandin-dependent dilation of the afferent renal arterioles. NSAIDs are contraindicated in patients with a history of peptic ulcer disease, gastritis, or NSAID intolerance, with renal dysfunction (creatinine > 1.5) and with bleeding diatheses.

Many surgeons prefer not to use NSAIDs in the immediate postoperative period for patients who have undergone renal or liver surgery, grafts, muscle flap procedures, or bone fusions, since they may increase bleeding or impede healing. The cyclooxygenase-2 or COX-2 selective NSAIDs do not interfere with platelet function or protection of the gastric mucosa but share the renal effects with the nonselective NSAIDs. The COX-2 inhibitors produce similar pain relief to the nonselective agents. The exact role of the COX-2 inhibitors in the management of acute pain is still being evaluated, but many multimodal regimens have included a preoperative dose of oral celecoxib.

Ketorolac is a potent NSAID with a chief indication for acute pain. It is the only NSAID analgesic available for parenteral use in the United States.

TABLE 30.2 Patient-Controlled Analgesia (PCA): Common Adult Dosing

Drug	Demand	Demand Range	Lockout Interval (min)	1-Hour Limit	Infusion
Morphine	1 mg	0.5-3 mg	5-20	10 mg	0-10 mg/h
Hydromorphone	0.2 mg	0.1-0.5 mg	5-15	1.5 mg	0-0.5 mg/h
Fentanyl	15 mcg	10-50 mcg	3-10	100 mcg	0-100 mcg/h

TABLE 30.3 Delivery of NSAIDs

NSAID	Common Routes	Common Starting Doses
Ibuprofen	PO	200-800 mg PO q6h
Ketorolac	IV	15-30 mg IV q6-8h
Celecoxib	PO	100-200 PO q12h
Naproxen	PO	250-500 PO q12h
Acetaminophen[a]	PO, IV	500-1000 mg PO/IV q8h

[a]Acetaminophen is not anti-inflammatory but is efficacious in acute pain.

It is expensive (~20 times costlier than morphine), and because its potency extends to its side effects, its use is restricted to 5 days (manufacturer's recommendation). Ketorolac can also be used to supplement epidural analgesia, particularly when the epidural does not cover the whole surgical area, for example, after thoracotomy (Table 30.3).

3. Anticonvulsants

Anticonvulsants are most commonly used in the treatment of chronic neuropathic pain; however, evidence has shown their efficacy in reducing pain scores and improving sleep in patients with acute pain after surgery while reducing the doses of opioid required to achieve pain control. Side effects include sleepiness, confusion, bloating, leukopenia, and thrombocytopenia (Table 30.4).

4. Antidepressants

Antidepressants (tricyclic antidepressants [TCAs] and serotonin-norepinephrine reuptake inhibitors [SNRIs]) are also used commonly in the treatment of chronic pain. Many patients are on these prior to surgery. As part of a multimodal treatment strategy, patients on these medications can have their dose titrated up to higher doses over several days, particularly where severe or prolonged pain is expected after surgery. Side effects of TCAs include sleepiness, dry mouth, increase heart rate, blurred vision, urinary retention, and constipation. Side effects of duloxetine include nausea, dry mouth, and sleepiness (Table 30.5).

5. N-Methyl-D-Aspartate (NMDA) Receptor Antagonists

NMDA receptor antagonists reduce central sensitization, hyperalgesia, and opioid tolerance. The attraction of NMDA receptor antagonist treatment for acute pain is obvious—they may well reduce postoperative and postsurgical chronic pain by reducing central sensitization, and they can reduce opioid requirements and tolerance. Intraoperative ketamine results in prolonged analgesia into the postoperative period, even when administered as a single bolus dose at the start of surgery. Continuation of subanesthetic

TABLE 30.4 Delivery of Anticonvulsants

Anticonvulsant	Common Routes	Common Starting Doses
Gabapentin	PO	100-300 mg PO tid, titrate up
Pregabalin	PO	25-75 mg PO tid, titrate up

TABLE 30.5 Delivery of Antidepressants

Antidepressant	Common Routes	Common Starting Doses
Amitriptyline (TCA)	PO	25 mg PO qhs, titrate up
Nortriptyline (TCA)	PO	25 mg PO qhs, titrate up
Duloxetine (SNRI)	PO	30 mg PO qday, titrate up

doses of ketamine for analgesia into the postoperative period is limited by side effects, yet can still be very efficacious. The most common and limiting side effects of ketamine for postoperative pain are hallucinations and increased secretions. To reduce the likelihood of these side effects, it is recommended that infusions be started at the lowest dose and slowly titrated upward. The use of benzodiazepines prior to initiation may reduce the likelihood of disturbing hallucinations, and glycopyrrolate will reduce secretions (Table 30.6). However, neither adjunct is typically needed when small, subanesthetic doses are employed after surgery.

6. α2 Agonists

Although the perioperative use of systemic α2 agonists (oral or transdermal) has been advocated for blood pressure control and for analgesia, the analgesic effect has not proven satisfactory. However, neuraxial clonidine is effective, and is used as an adjunct to neuraxial local anesthetics (LAs) and opioids. Clonidine and dexmedetomidine can be useful as anxiolytics and as adjunctive analgesics in intubated patients to reduce opioid requirement and facilitate extubation. Tizanidine is a muscle relaxant that can be used to treat postoperative muscle spasm. Its common side effects include sleepiness, dizziness, dry mouth, bradycardia, hypotension, anxiety, and rarely elevation of liver enzymes. So it is recommended to trial the medication at a low dose and then to titrate upward as tolerated (Table 30.7).

7. Local Anesthetics

LAs are the most effective analgesics. They are used to prevent pain during procedures as minor as placing an IV catheter, up to use as the primary analgesics for operative procedures as with regional anesthesia techniques. LAs for acute postoperative pain have several limitations, primarily their limited duration of action and their indiscriminate interruption of motor function as well as sensory blockade. LAs are delivered via three routes:

a. **Intravenous**—as intraoperative and postoperative infusions, lidocaine has been shown to reduce pain and opioid requirement in enhanced recovery protocols.
b. **Subcutaneous**—as targeted injection or regional infiltration (ie, into surgical wound site), LAs can control postoperative pain for the duration of their action, which is typically 2-12 hours postoperatively.

TABLE 30.6 Delivery of NMDA Antagonist

NMDA Antagonist	Common Routes	Common Starting Doses
Ketamine	IV	0.5-2 mcg/kg/min when awake, 5-10 mcg/kg/min under anesthesia

TABLE 30.7 Delivery of α2 Agonists

α2 Agonist	Common Routes	Common Starting Doses
Clonidine	PO, TD, EPI	0.1-0.4 mg PO, 0.1 mg TD, 30-40 mcg/h EPI
Dexmedetomidine	IV	0.5-1 mcg/kg loading, 0.2-1 mcg/kg/h maintenance
Tizanidine	PO	2-4 mg qhs-tid, titrate up

c. **Perineural**—regional anesthesia is the targeted delivery of LAs to specific nerves that innervate the region of pain. Local anesthetic is used to provide surgical anesthesia and analgesia or postoperative analgesia (Table 30.8). Often adjuncts (clonidine, dexamethasone) are added to prolong the effect. Regional anesthesia includes neuraxial (epidural or spinal) and peripheral nerve blocks (ie, interscalene, femoral nerve).

B. Regional Anesthesia

Regional anesthesia involves control of pain principally by delivery of local anesthetic to the specific nerves innervating the surgical or otherwise painful site. This includes epidural, intrathecal, paravertebral, intercostal, transversus abdominis plane (TAP) blocks (collectively known as axial blocks), and the peripheral blocks that include the interscalene, supraclavicular, infraclavicular (upper extremity) and femoral, sciatic, popliteal, and saphenous, being the most common lower extremity blocks. The specific nerve blocks used are tailored to assure adequate block of all nerves innervating the surgical site. Regional anesthesia can be delivered as a single perineural bolus of local anesthetic or incorporate small perineural catheters to continuously deliver local anesthetic for more prolonged periods after surgery.

1. Epidural Analgesia

For certain well-chosen indications, a functioning epidural produces superior pain relief and is known to improve surgical outcome (Table 30.9). However, a considerable degree of technical expertise is needed to place epidural catheters, and, even in the best hands, this treatment can fail. Because it involves meticulously and blindly locating the epidural space (Fig. 30.1), epidural placement and management is time-consuming and labor-intensive. Nevertheless, both surgeons and anesthesiologists at MGH are sufficiently convinced of the positive benefits of epidural analgesia to offer the treatment to all our patients in whom it is indicated, being careful to explain both its risks and its benefits (Table 30.10).

2. Postoperative Pain Indications

Epidurals are recommended for treatment of postoperative pain (can be placed before or after surgery) primarily for the following indications:

a. Patients having thoracic or abdominal surgery
b. Patients having lower limb surgery in whom early mobilization is important (early active or passive mobilization)
c. Patients having lower body vascular procedures in whom a sympathetic block is desirable

TABLE 30.8 Delivery of Local Anesthetics

			Plain		With Epinephrine	
Local Anesthetic	Usual Concentration	Usual Onset (min)[a]	Maximum Dose (mg/kg)	Duration (min)	Maximum Dose (mg/kg)	Duration (min)
Lidocaine	1%, 2%	5-20	4.2	60-120	7	120-180
Ropivacaine	0.2%, 0.5%	15-30	2.8 mg	180-360	3.5	240-420
Bupivacaine	0.25%, 0.5%, 0.75%	15-30	2.5 mg	120-360	3.2	240-420
Mepivacaine	1%, 2%	5-20	4.2 mg	45-90	7 mg	120
Chloroprocaine	2%, 3%	5-20	11 mg	15-30	13 mg	30

[a]Dose- and concentration-dependent.

TABLE 30.9 Known Benefits of Postoperative Epidural Analgesia

- Superior analgesia
- Improved pulmonary function
- Better graft survival after lower limb vascular procedures
- Increased bowel mobility, associated with shorter hospital stay
- Fewer cardiac ischemic events
- Shorter recuperation after joint surgery, associated with early aggressive mobilization

3. Management Principles

The management of epidural catheters should always be under the direct supervision of anesthesiologists. Patients should be seen daily to ensure that catheters and medications are working effectively. Pain reports should be satisfactory, and side effects such as pruritus, sedation, and changes in sensation or motor function should be carefully evaluated. Catheters and their insertion sites should be inspected for migration, integrity of the dressings and inflammation or back tenderness. Anesthesia personnel should make changes to the analgesic regimen and administer specific medications as necessary. At the end of treatment, the anesthesia team should be responsible for removing the catheter and ensuring that it is removed intact. Nurses should be properly educated

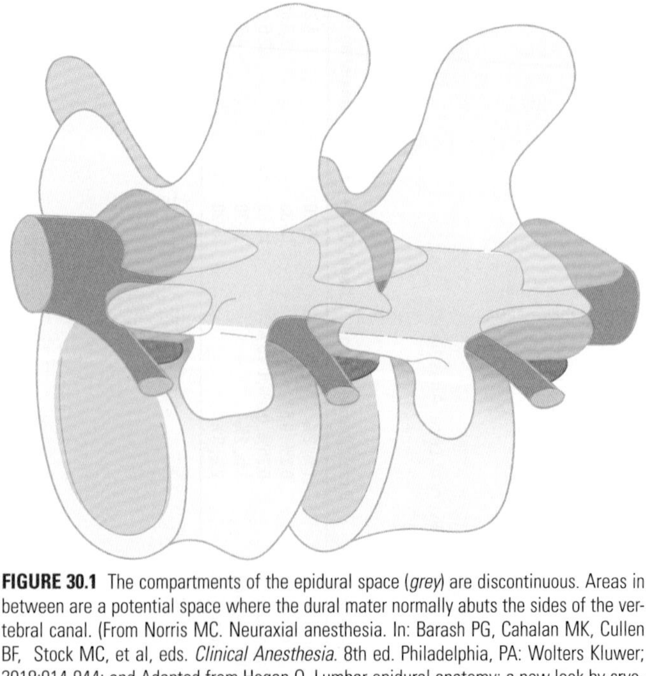

FIGURE 30.1 The compartments of the epidural space (*grey*) are discontinuous. Areas in between are a potential space where the dural mater normally abuts the sides of the vertebral canal. (From Norris MC. Neuraxial anesthesia. In: Barash PG, Cahalan MK, Cullen BF, Stock MC, et al, eds. *Clinical Anesthesia*. 8th ed. Philadelphia, PA: Wolters Kluwer; 2018:914-944; and Adapted from Hogan Q. Lumbar epidural anatomy: a new look by cryomicrotome section. *Anesthesiology*. 1991;75:767-775.)

TABLE 30.10 Contraindications to Epidural Placement

- Patient refusal
- Coagulopathy
- Concurrent or planned treatment with low-molecular-weight heparin, potent antiplatelet agents, warfarin, or newer oral anticoagulants
- Bacteremia
- Local infection at epidural insertion site
- Spine pathology (relative contraindication)

before they care for patients with epidural catheters. Important teaching points include typical medication doses and concentrations, anticoagulation issues, assessment parameters, the normal appearance of the catheter and catheter site, operation of the infusion pumps, treatment of common medication side effects, and side effects requiring a call to the physician in charge.

4. Drug Choices

The standard infusion for postoperative epidural therapy at the MGH is a mixture of 0.1% bupivacaine with 20 µg/mL of hydromorphone. A synergistic effect occurs when one combines local anesthetic with opioid, so that the mixture optimizes analgesia. However, there may be reasons to remove one or other components (eg, local anesthetic causing hypotension, or opioid causing pruritus, over sedation in elderly patients, or insufficient systemic analgesia in opioid-tolerant individuals), in which case, dose adjustments need to be made to the remaining drug. In the case of sole local anesthetic treatment, it may be necessary to add a systemic analgesic (opioid or NSAID).

Continuous epidural infusions vary between 4 and 12 mL/h depending on the catheter location, with possible infusion rates up to 20 mL/h. Fentanyl is our second choice of epidural opioid and is reserved for patients who are sensitive to opioid effects (ie, the very young and the very old). Because of its lipophilicity, fentanyl tends to bind locally to spinal cord receptors, rather than spread with cerebrospinal fluid (CSF) movement. Conventional wisdom holds that the analgesic effect of fentanyl localizes to the level of epidural insertion, whereas hydromorphone and morphine (the least lipophilic of the opioids) produce better spread but a greater risk of delayed respiratory depression secondary to the spread of drug to higher centers in the CNS. In practical use, all three of these opioids produce excellent analgesia when used epidurally in combination with low-dose local anesthetic and significant sedation, and respiratory depression is uncommon.

a. Standard epidural orders include:
  i. Infusion dose ranges for nurse-directed titration based on the patient's needs
  ii. Orders for alternative treatments should the epidural fail
  iii. Orders for the treatment of common adverse effects

The addition of clonidine to the local anesthetic and opioid has been found to significantly improve the quality and duration of neuraxial analgesia. The effect is mediated by descending modulatory pathways to the spinal dorsal horn. Despite neuraxial administration, systemic side effects (hypotension, bradycardia, and sedation) can occur. Dose-finding studies are still underway, and the therapeutic window for useful analgesia without side effects seems to be narrow. A reasonable regime uses a 1-2 μg/kg bolus followed by 0.4 μg/kg/h.

5. Management of Inadequate Analgesia

The best way to ensure that an epidural catheter is well positioned is to establish an anesthetic level using local anesthetic. Testing can be attempted at any stage, but it should be remembered that:

a. Responses are less reliable in a patient who is in the early stages of recovery after anesthesia.
b. A bolus injection can produce hypotension, and so it is necessary to closely monitor blood pressure for at least 20 minutes after bolus administration (time to the peak pharmacologic effect of an epidural local anesthetic bolus) and be prepared to treat hypotension.

First, test the dermatomes that should be covered by the epidural infusion with cold pack/ice. The patient should feel less cold in the region that should also be the level of pain. If there is no apparent coverage of this area, then a local anesthetic test dose can be given. Let the team members know you will be testing the epidural, so that all members can anticipate problems, such as hypotension, if they occur. If the catheter is well positioned, analgesia should be noticeably improved by the injection and can be confirmed with ice again.

Once good catheter function is established, several approaches to improve analgesia can be taken:

a. A bolus injection can be given (as described earlier), if it has not already been given.
b. The infusion rate can be titrated upward.
c. Systemic analgesics can be given.
d. NSAIDs can be given and serve as useful adjuncts to epidural analgesia, especially when the epidural level does not cover the area of surgical pain, as when the incision is high or when pain is referred outside the epidural area (as in shoulder pain associated with chest tubes and diaphragmatic irritation).
e. Systemic opioids (including PCA) can also be added; in this case, it is our practice to remove the opioid from the epidural mix to avoid possible overdose stemming from the synergistic effects of intrathecal and systemic opioid administered simultaneously.

6. Patient-Controlled Epidural Analgesia

Patient-controlled epidural analgesia (PCEA) has become standard in many institutions around the country. Allowing patients to gain control is one great advantage to PCEA. One must consider the lipophilicity of the opioid used, the onset of action, and the duration of pain relief when prescribing demand doses and lockout intervals. The PCEA dosing for the standard MGH epidural mix (0.1% bupivacaine with 20 μg/mL hydromorphone) is 2 mL bolus every 20 minutes (lockout), with basal infusion 4-6 mL/h.

7. Side Effects

Most side effects (see Table 30.11) are alleviated by either lowering the infusion rate or by changing the drug or dose. Pruritus is a common side effect of neuraxial opioid and usually responds well to antihistamine treatment. The mixed agonist/antagonist nalbuphine (Nubain) (5-10 mg IV, 4-6 hourly) also works well, as does low-dose naloxone infusion. Contrary to popular belief, nausea rarely occurs because opioid doses are low. Gut mobility is improved by epidural therapy. Urinary retention may occur, especially

TABLE 30.11 Common Side Effects of Epidural Analgesia

Side Effect	Treatment
Pruritus	Nalbuphine 5-10 mg IM, IV
Hypotension	Fluids, phenylephrine, ephedrine, etc.
Sedation	Naloxone 40-80 mcg IV, repeated PRN
Mild sensory/motor changes	Exam to ensure no complications
Dizziness	Evaluate for hypotension, opioid effect
Urinary retention	Consider reducing rate, concentration

when lumbar catheters are used, so we tend to continue indwelling bladder catheters until the epidural is discontinued.

Unilateral lower extremity numbness with occasional weakness or motor block is a side effect of the local anesthetic. This usually occurs when the epidural catheter tip has migrated along a nerve root and the local anesthetic is concentrated in one area. Pulling the catheter back, or lowering the infusion rate, often rectifies the problem. However, one should always remain vigilant and continue to watch for more serious complications.

8. Complications

The most common complications of epidural analgesia are failed block/analgesia and post–dural puncture headache (PDPH) (see Table 30.12). Both are considered benign, although they may be disturbing to patients who have committed to an epidural in order to optimize their surgical experience. The incidence of these common complications is difficult to establish because reports vary and the occurrences likely vary according to reporting and practice habits. Failed block/analgesia rate was 15% in one recent MGH survey, whereas PDPH may occur in up to 86% patients after accidental dural puncture (with the incidence of dural puncture at just 0.16%-1.3%). The incidence of other self-limiting neurologic complications such as radicular pain and peripheral nerve lesions is difficult to determine, because these occurrences are rarely reported.

Of far greater concern is permanent neurologic injury, including paraplegia, which may be caused by epidural hematoma or abscess, even when these are diagnosed and treated in a timely manner. A rash of reports of epidural hematoma occurring after neuraxial interventions in patients receiving low-molecular-weight heparin (LMWH) alerted us to the dangers of breaching the

TABLE 30.12 Epidural Complications

Common
- Failed block/analgesia
- Post–dural puncture headache (PDPH)

Rare
- Skin infection
- Epidural hematoma or abscess

Extremely rare
- Anterior spinal artery syndrome
- Transverse myelitis
- Meningitis

epidural space in patients receiving highly effective deep venous thrombosis prophylaxis. More problems followed when chronic treatment with potent and long-acting antiplatelet agents, such as clopidogrel, became more widespread. The use of activated protein C for severe sepsis also precludes the use of neuraxial blockade. Given the rapidity with which new anticoagulants enter practice, and the lag time before the extent of a problem can be assessed, we are left with a great deal of uncertainty about the safety of neuraxial procedures. International guidelines regarding the use of neuraxial anesthesia in patients on various anticoagulants are now widely available (see further discussion below). To make the judgment even more difficult, one of the major reasons that older studies showed a benefit to spinals and epidurals in terms of serious morbidity was their ability to reduce thromboembolism. This benefit may no longer apply in an era of improved pharmacologic thromboprophylaxis.

Epidural abscess occurs less often than epidural hematoma but may be equally catastrophic and can cause permanent and serious neurologic injury, even death. The mortality of spinal abscess can be as high as 18%. The incidence of epidural abscess secondary to neuraxial blockade is estimated at 1 in 250 000 in healthy patients but 1 in 2000 in diabetic or immunocompromised patients.

Other serious complications such as anterior spinal artery syndrome, transverse myelitis, and meningitis have been reported but are extremely rare. PDPH is thought to be the result of a small CSF leak secondary to accidental dural puncture. Typically, there is a delay in onset of the headache (~24 hours), so that the complication tends to manifest itself on the first postoperative day.

a. Characteristics of PDPH include:
  - **i.** Worsens on sitting up, and particularly on walking, and improves on lying down, so it may not present itself until the patients get out of bed for the first time after surgery.
  - **ii.** Headache that tends to occur at the back of the head (occiput) and neck and produces a tight, pulling, and throbbing sensation.

b. Treatment of PDPH:
  - **i.** Conservative management consists of bed rest (up to bathroom only), plenty of fluids (IV or oral), and headache medication (NSAIDs, acetaminophen, caffeine, and theophylline have all been used effectively).
  - **ii.** If there is no resolution, or if conservative measures are contraindicated, a blood patch is recommended. This consists of an epidural injection of 10-20 mL of the patient's own blood (drawn under sterile conditions) and is thought to close the dural puncture. The exact mechanism by which an epidural blood patch works is uncertain, but there is likely some element of pressure effect exerted by the blood placed in the epidural space that reduces the degree of intracranial hypotension immediately. The epidural clot itself likely induces a fibrotic reaction that ultimately seals the dural puncture site.

c. Epidural hematoma and abscess can have a variable presentation, but the cardinal signs of impending spinal cord compression are:
  - **i.** Sensory and motor changes in the lower extremity (often bilateral) and pain in the back.
  - **ii.** In the case of lesions in the sacral canal, cardinal signs are changes in bladder and bowel function and absence of pain.

The signs and symptoms typically appear more rapidly over a period of hours in those with an expanding epidural hematoma. Epidural abscess formation can be delayed for days to weeks after epidural removal, and the onset of signs and symptoms can be insidious, requiring a high index of suspicion to catch before the appearance of irreversible neurologic injury. If there is any reason for concern, the first response should be to discontinue the epidural infusion and possibly remove the epidural catheter, especially if there is evidence of infection at the skin (if there are coagulation issues, it may be better to leave the catheter until they are resolved; see in subsequent text). Although minimal sensory changes are common and may be benign, prolonged motor changes that do not resolve on discontinuing the epidural infusion are always worrying, as is back pain. If there is no resolution after simple measures, magnetic resonance imaging (MRI) of the appropriate level should be ordered and the involvement of neurology and neurosurgery sought. Early intervention is key to preventing permanent neurologic injury, and early surgical decompression usually results in complete resolution. Without these measures, spinal cord compression and paraplegia may develop.

9. Anticoagulation and Epidurals

The incidence of epidural hematoma after neuraxial injection, catheter placement, or catheter removal has been estimated to be 1:190 000, with many of the reported cases being associated with anticoagulant use. Unfortunately, the literature has little information about the risk of epidural hematoma and specific anticoagulants, especially the latest generation of anticoagulants and antiplatelet drugs. Published guidelines are based on the known pharmacology of the drugs, as well as clinical evidence from case reports (anecdotal and published). Epidural bleeding is known to occur secondary to single-shot neuraxial techniques as well as neuraxial catheter insertion and removal, so that recommendations are needed for the start and end of neuraxial therapy, as well as for starting anticoagulant therapy after neuraxial instrumentation or catheter removal.

The American Society of Regional Anesthesia and Pain Medicine (ASRA) periodically issues consensus guidelines on the use of neuraxial interventions in patients receiving thromboprophylaxis. ASRA also publishes the *ASRA Coags* app where guidelines are continuously updated for the many anticoagulant medications to consider. MGH guidelines are based on ASRA's recommendations, and the most common anticoagulants are summarized in Table 30.13.

The NSAIDs and low-dose subcutaneous standard heparin are not considered a risk. High-dose infusions of standard (unfractionated) heparin are relatively easy to handle because their effects are predictable. The partial thromboplastin time (PTT) usually returns to within satisfactory range of normal 2-3 hours after discontinuation, at which point epidurals can be placed or removed.

There is no practical test of LMWH activity (the anti-Xa level is not a reliable predictor of the risk of bleeding, and is available only on a limited basis); prothrombin time (PT), INR, and PTT values do not reflect LMWH activity.

Clopidogrel (Plavix) use is associated with a high incidence of surgical bleeding and epidural hematoma (anecdotal reports). These problems were particularly obvious when this drug was first used and the effect on bleeding, and slow reversal of this effect, was not appreciated. The current recommendation is that regional anesthesia is contraindicated for 7 days after termination of treatment with clopidogrel (14 days after ticlopidine [Ticlid]). The newer antiplatelet drugs seem less prone to increase surgical bleeding, but, as already mentioned, we rely on anecdotal evidence for perioperative events, and sometimes anecdotal evidence is misleading.

TABLE 30.13 Guidelines for Epidural Placement and Removal During Most Common Anticoagulant Therapy

Drug	Time After Last Dose Before Placing or Removing Catheter	Time After Placing or Removing Catheter Before Restarting Medication
Warfarin (Coumadin)	4-5 d and normal INR (<1.5)	No delay; remove catheter with INR <1.5
NSAID (ASA)	No restrictions when used alone	No restrictions when used alone
Heparin		
• (SQ bid)	Hold for 4 h (check plts if on > 4 d)	No delay
• (SQ tid)	Hold for 4 h (check plts if on > 4 d)	No delay
• (IV)	2-4 h (check coags, PTT < 35)	1 h
Enoxaparin (Lovenox)		
• (ppx dose qday)	10-12 h	12 h (catheter removed before initiation)
• (ppx dose bid)	10-12 h	12 h
• (treatment dose: 1 mg/kg q12h or 1.5 mg/kg daily)	24 h	No recommendation
Clopidogrel (Plavix)	7 d	Avoid with catheter present, no recommendation after removal

For up-to-date guidelines on many anticoagulants, refer to the ASRA Coags app or go to https://www.asra.com/advisory-guidelines, accessed January 13, 2019.
INR, international normalized ratio; NSAID, nonsteroidal anti-inflammatory drug; ASA, acetylsalicylic acid; IV, intravenous; PTT, partial thromboplastin time; plts, platelets; ppx, prophylactic.

10. Single-Shot Neuraxial Morphine

Neuraxial morphine is safe provided dosing is reasonable and patients are appropriately monitored. A single shot of morphine into the epidural space (1-4 mg) or intrathecal space (0.1-0.4 mg) can provide prolonged analgesia (up to 24 hours) but carries a risk of delayed respiratory depression. Morphine is poorly lipophilic, tends to stay in CSF once there, and is subject to CSF flow with passage to higher centers including the respiratory center. At the same time, the fact that morphine tends to remain in CSF is the reason that it produces excellent selective spinal analgesia (ie, good spread to spinal cord receptors). Single-shot neuraxial morphine is an excellent means of providing analgesia when there is no epidural catheter. Patients should be monitored in the same way as those receiving epidural opioid infusions for at least 18-24 hours after administration. PCA can be used to provide supplementary analgesia, but, for safety, only demand doses are used rather than continuous infusions.

11. Peripheral Nerve Blockade

a. Single-shot peripheral blocks

(See earlier discussion in this chapter.)

b. Continuous catheter peripheral blockade

Neural blockade can be prolonged by using continuous infusions via perineural catheters. Continuous analgesic/anesthetic infusions can be administered at various sites, offer a safer alternative to neuraxial techniques, and are particularly useful when active mobilization is needed. It is useful to infuse analgesics into the brachial plexus after shoulder or hand surgery and into the femoral sheath after knee surgery. It may also be helpful to infuse them into joints after joint surgery as well as into wounds.

Infusions of LAs via brachial and lumbar plexus catheters have established efficacy. Patients must be hospitalized, at least while the treatment is stabilized. Bupivacaine or ropivacaine 0.1% at 10-20 mL/h is used initially. If that is not effective, a higher concentration (0.25%) can be used, and/or a bolus injection of 0.25%-0.375% bupivacaine or ropivacaine can be tried. Patients may also use supplemental systemic analgesics. When a well-designed system of aftercare has been put in place, many patients can be allowed to go home with a perineural or wound infiltration catheter, either with a home pump or reserving the catheter for injection before physical therapy sessions.

12. Intraoperative Neural Blockade

Nerve blocks performed before or during surgery provide excellent pain control during the early postoperative period. Infiltration of wounds with LAs by surgeons can also contribute significantly to the control of early postoperative pain. Intraoperative neural blockade can reduce postoperative analgesic requirements and, in some cases, eliminate the need for postoperative analgesia. Intraoperative nerve blocks are particularly useful in children, who tolerate analgesics poorly and in whom pain is particularly distressing. The risk-benefit analysis for the placement of neuraxial blocks under general anesthesia favors this approach in children, where awake placement may be difficult or impossible, but argues against this approach in adults, where safe placement in a cooperative patient is easily achieved. The concern is that general anesthesia removes any chance that the patient will report needle contact with neural structures that might lead to injury during placement.

C. Nonpharmacologic Treatments

1. Education

Educating patients to the expected course of recovery and communication about the times of potential increased discomfort (dressing changes, physical therapy, analgesic taper, etc.) empowers patients to take as needed medications in anticipation of increased discomfort and improves satisfaction with care.

2. Behavioral Therapy

The goal of behavioral therapy is to provide patients with a sense of control over their pain. All patients benefit from being well prepared psychologically for the experience of surgery and postoperative pain. Simple relaxation strategies and imagery can help those patients who find such interventions appealing and do not need to be complex to be effective. Simple strategies, such as brief jaw relaxation, music-assisted relaxation, and recall of peaceful images, can reduce anxiety and analgesic requirements. Behavioral treatments take only a few minutes to teach, although they may require continual practice and reinforcement.

3. Physical Therapy

Immobility, especially out of fear of pain, can worsen pain and slow recovery with increased risks including hospital-acquired pneumonia and venous embolism. Patients should have sufficient analgesia to facilitate mobility, when appropriate. In turn, increased mobility will ensure recovery and reduce pain as strength returns.

IV. SPECIAL SUBPOPULATIONS

A. The Elderly

Elderly patients are both at increased risk for oversedation with pain medications and undertreatment with possibility of suffering. The best approach to treating elderly patients with acute pain is to keep things simple. Opioids specifically are more sedating and metabolized less efficiently, resulting in potential for overdose. Start with a low dose of a single medication and titrate upward to pain control while including nonsedating agents as adjuncts (acetaminophen and NSAIDs).

For severe pain, small, intermittent doses of IV morphine (1-5 mg every 4 hours) or the equivalent should be used. Epidural therapy with or without opioid or regional anesthesia can be particularly helpful at controlling pain while sparing need for systemic opioids.

B. The Mentally and Physically Disabled

These patients present a challenge because they may be unable to communicate the status of their pain clearly. As with the very young, effective pain management with the very old may require time and patience to be spent learning what patients are experiencing and how best to help them. Vital signs, behavioral cues, positioning, muscle guarding, and grimacing may be the only guiding factors at first. Seeking input from those who normally care for these patients is indispensable, as they will be alert to subtle changes in behavior that might signal ongoing pain. Although drugs are metabolized normally in most of these patients, individuals with baseline breathing difficulties may be more sensitive to the respiratory depressant effects of opioids.

C. Substance Use Disorder

Patients with a history of past or present substance use disorder may be difficult to manage during an acute pain episode. The behavioral factors that make inpatient management difficult are compounded because opioids do not work well in patients who have become opioid-tolerant. It is often difficult to determine whether opioid-seeking behavior is due to inadequate pain control or to addictive behavior. The medical staff may become exasperated, thereby compromising patient care.

These patients should be given the benefit of optimal control of acute pain, while detoxification should be postponed until the acute pain has resolved. It is helpful to work closely with addiction specialists, including psychiatrists and social workers, to prepare the patients for discharge and possible rehabilitation.

It is important to obtain a history of "recreational drug use," both past and present. The information may be unreliable but should at least be sought. It should be ascertained whether the patient is in withdrawal, and if so, the withdrawal should be treated. Large doses of opioids may be needed to avoid withdrawal and treat pain. Even patients who misuse substances such as alcohol, cocaine, and marijuana may exhibit some degree of cross-tolerance with opioids, thus requiring higher than normal opioid doses.

Patients on methadone or buprenorphine maintenance should continue their preadmission dose, or this should be converted to an alternative opioid or mode of delivery, and additional opioid prescribed as needed. PCA is an effective modality for those with substance use disorder, because it provides an element of control and lessens the anxiety associated with trying to obtain additional medication.

Opioid analgesia can usefully be supplemented with nonopioid treatments such as NSAIDs, regional anesthesia, and anxiolytics. Alpha-agonists such as clonidine may be useful because they provide analgesia and reverse symptoms of withdrawal. Other treatments for withdrawal include benzodiazepines and neuroleptics, in addition to supportive measures.

D. Intensive Care Patients

Patients admitted to intensive care form a special population because, in many cases, they are unable to communicate, either because of severe illness or because they are ventilated, sedated, and sometimes even paralyzed. When impossible to assess pain, as in heavily sedated or unconscious patients, it is reasonable to assess analgesic requirements on the basis of the amount of surgical or other trauma the patient has undergone, guided by patient vital signs.

Patients on mechanical ventilation can be treated with higher than normal doses of opioids (if desired) because there is no risk of respiratory depression. Continuous infusion is the most frequently chosen mode of delivery. Fentanyl or hydromorphone may be preferred to morphine in patients with renal insufficiency who tend to accumulate the active morphine metabolite morphine-6-glucuronide. Methadone may also be useful for prolonged intensive care unit (ICU) stays because there may be less risk of developing tolerance than with other opioids. It has recently been found beneficial to use the $\alpha 2$ agonist dexmedetomidine for ICU sedation, not only because of its hypnotic effects but also because of its analgesic synergy with opioids (opioid sparing). It may also help minimize withdrawal symptoms during weaning from opioids.

Alert patients or those who are breathing on their own can be treated for pain like patients in other units, with the proviso that severely ill patients may handle drugs inefficiently, resulting in more profound and prolonged drug effects. Epidurals are useful even in patients on a ventilator, and they ease weaning from ventilation.

E. Patients With Chronic Pain

Patients that live with chronic pain may have lower thresholds for pain sensation through central sensitization. Many of these patients are on chronic, long-acting opioids, including methadone that may result in opioid-induced hyperalgesia (OIH). As a result, it is even more important for this group of patients to be seen prior to the day of surgery, so that an appropriate plan of care can be established.

This group should have analgesia in excess of their baseline requirement or they will suffer in the immediate postsurgical period. They also benefit more from the use of multimodal analgesia both intraoperatively and postoperatively (ie, ketamine, lidocaine infusions) and regional anesthesia.

Care should be taken when deciding to use methadone in patients on high-dose opioids as conversion is not simple between methadone and other opioids, and the multiple receptor targets of methadone (NMDA, opioid, serotonin, norepinephrine) may sensitize the opioid-tolerant patient and more easily result in overdose. Chronic pain service consultation is recommended in those unfamiliar with methadone use.

V. CONCLUSION

Postoperative pain has often been inadequately treated in the past, in part because of complacency, and in part because of fear of analgesic side effects. Effective postoperative pain management involves adherence to certain basic principles. First and foremost, pain must be assessed regularly and systematically so that pain treatment can be modified according to need.

Pain scores and function should be documented so that the pain course is apparent to all caregivers. Pain that is treated preemptively or controlled early is easier to manage than established or severe pain. Treatment during the intraoperative and early postoperative periods is essential.

Patients should be involved in their treatment and be educated about their surgery and the options available for treating postoperative pain.

Selected Readings

Chou R, Gordon DB, de Leon-Casasola OA, et al. Management of Postoperative Pain: a Clinical Practice Guideline From the American Pain Society, the American Society of Regional Anesthesia and Pain Medicine, and the American Society of Anesthesiologists' Committee on Regional Anesthesia, Executive Committee, and Administrative Council. *J Pain.* 2016;17:131-157.

Horlocker TT, Vandermeuelen E, Kopp SL, Gogarten W, Leffert LR, Benzon HT. Regional Anesthesia in the Patient Receiving Antithrombotic or Thrombolytic Therapy: American Society of Regional Anesthesia and Pain Medicine Evidence-Based Guidelines (Fourth Edition). *Reg Anesth Pain Med.* 2018;43:263-309.

Mao J. Opioid-induced abnormal pain sensitivity. *Curr Pain Headache Rep.* 2006;10:67-70.

Masic D, Liang E, Long C, Sterk EJ, Barbas B, Rech MA. Intravenous lidocaine for acute pain: a systematic review. *Pharmacotherapy.* 2018;38(12):1250-1259.

Salicath JH, Yeoh EC, Bennett MH. Epidural analgesia versus patient-controlled intravenous analgesia for pain following intra-abdominal surgery in adults. *Cochrane Database Syst Rev.* 2018;(8):CD010434.

Schwenk ES, Viscusi ER, Buvanendran A, et al. Consensus Guidelines on the Use of Intravenous Ketamine Infusions for Acute Pain Management From the American Society of Regional Anesthesia and Pain Medicine, the American Academy of Pain Medicine, and the American Society of Anesthesiologists. *Reg Anesth Pain Med.* 2018;43:456-466.

31 Postoperative Pain in Children

Lane C. Crawford, Alexandra R. Adler, and Pascal Scemama de Gialluly

I. HISTORY

Historically, the field of pediatric acute pain management has lagged behind its adult counterpart. However, recent years have seen significant advances in our understanding of the prevalence and significance of pediatric pain. We have also made strides in our ability to assess and treat acute pain in children, with multimodal analgesia and regional techniques emerging as increasingly important strategies (Table 31.1). Contrary to previous belief, even the youngest of neonates is capable of feeling pain, as demonstrated by observable physiologic and behavioral responses. Furthermore, recent research has shown that pain in infancy and childhood can result in long-term, potentially deleterious changes in future pain responses, not only through behavioral or psychological mechanisms but also through sensitization of pain pathways in the developing central nervous system.

The phenomenon of chronic postsurgical pain, though better described in adults, has been observed in children as well, and it has been hypothesized that aggressive pain control in the perioperative period might reduce the risk of transition to chronic pain. By optimizing analgesia in this particularly vulnerable population, we have the opportunity to make

TABLE 31.1 Behavioral and Physiological Indicators of Pain in Children

- Crying, screaming, moaning, whimpering
- Facial expression (eg, grimacing, furrowed brow)
- Posture, tone, guarding, thrashing, touching painful area
- Palmar sweating
- Sleep pattern
- Respiratory rate and pattern
- Heart rate and blood pressure

a difference not only in the acute setting but potentially for the long term as well.

There are many differences between adults and children that make pain management in children a particular challenge and subsequently place children at higher risk for inadequate analgesia:

- It is not as easy to assess pain in children as it is in adults.
- The emotional and psychological aspects of pain can be more pronounced in children than in adults.
- Children, particularly neonates and infants, metabolize drugs differently than do adults.
- Epidural catheters are technically more difficult to place and more difficult to maintain in children.
- The sight of a child in pain is particularly distressing, especially to parents.

This chapter discusses general issues about postoperative pain management in children.

II. PLANNING FOR POSTOPERATIVE ANALGESIA

A plan for intraoperative and postoperative anesthesia and analgesia should be made before surgery. A multimodal perioperative pain therapy plan should be put together. Such a plan should be easy to implement and include safeguards regarding the occurrence of possible side effects.

A. Multimodal Pain Therapy

Multimodal pain therapy plans should include the following:

1. Use of regional anesthesia when appropriate
2. Nonopioid analgesics
3. Opioids
4. Coanalgesics

B. Communication

1. Children and their parents should be told honestly what to expect and be reassured that everything will be done to alleviate any pain or discomfort. It is often helpful to find out how the child copes with pain and distress, how he or she communicates pain (eg, "boo-boo," "hurt," "sore"), and whether the child relies on special blankets, toys, or other means for comfort and reassurance.
2. If the child has had surgery before, then the following questions apply:
   a. What was the past pain experience of the child?
   b. What medications were used in the past, and did they work well?

c. Were nonpharmacologic techniques used and did they work well?
d. What coping techniques were beneficial?

3. If patient-controlled analgesia (PCA) is used, it is helpful to teach the child and the parents the principles of PCA or to explain regional anesthetic techniques if they are chosen. The parents and child should be intimately involved in the evaluation, management, and decision-making whenever possible.

III. ASSESSING ACUTE PAIN IN INFANTS AND CHILDREN

Pain assessment is the key to effective pain management. Consistent assessment must occur regularly, and the same scale and format must be used for each assessment so as not to confuse the child or parents. In neonates and infants, clinical judgment alone is often used, whereas simple assessment tools are useful in older children. Broadly, there are three stages of a child's development, each of which requires a different means of pain assessment.

A. Neonates, Infants, and Children Aged 4 Years and Younger

Infants and neonates clearly cannot report their pain. However, children as young as 18 months can indicate their pain and give a location, although they cannot specify pain intensity before about 3 years of age. At the age of 3 years, they can give a gross indication, such as "no pain," "a little pain," or "a lot of pain," but their reports are not always reliable. The parents' impression is often the best indicator in these very young patients. Nurses and doctors need to listen to the parents, as well as use objective measures of pain. Behavioral and physiologic responses can be used as a measure of pain in young children, particularly those who are noncommunicating, although the signs may not be specific to pain.

Several systematic and validated measurement tools could be used to quantify pain in children, such as CRIES (developed by Krechel and Bildner in 1995), that utilize various combinations of physiological and behavioral indicators of pain, although their use is not often warranted in cases of acute pain. The principles of pain assessment in very young children and issues of the nervous system and cognitive development are described in Chapter 45.

B. Children Aged 4-8 Years

Assuming that the young children (from 4 to 8 years) have normal development, they can provide reliable self-reports of pain using assessment tools designed for young children, such as the FACES pain-rating scale (see Chapter 5, Fig. 5.1), by communicating through their parents or through direct communication with doctors and nurses. Simple numeric scales using age-appropriate language may be helpful at the upper end of this age range.

C. Children Older Than 7 Years

Children older than 7 years who understand the concept of numeric order can use verbal numeric scales or visual analog scales such as those used in adults (see Chapter 5).

D. Children With Cognitive Impairment

For children with cognitive impairment, chronological age is not a good indicator of which type of pain assessment tool to use. Input from the parents or caretakers is essential as they can help elucidate behaviors associated with pain. For this population, the revised FLACC scale (Face, Legs, Activity, Cry, Consolability) has been validated.

E. New Emerging Techniques to Assess for Pain

Pain assessment in children remains a challenge. Recent research on new and more objective techniques to assess for pain is being conducted. Preliminary results are encouraging for using EEG or pupillometry to assess for pain in infants and children.

IV. TREATMENT CHOICES

Treatment options for both procedural and postoperative pain in children should be part of a multimodal pain plan that maximizes the use of regional anesthesia, nonopioid analgesics, and coanalgesics where appropriate. Opioids should then be added in sufficient quantity and regularity to provide effective pain relief. The benefit of this multimodal approach is to minimize the side effects of opioids such as postoperative nausea and vomiting (PONV) and constipation, which are often distressing to children but also may delay their discharge, and to reduce the risk of serious complications from opioids such as respiratory depression. In addition, there has been an increased focus on other side effects of opioids especially in children (ie, opioid-induced hyperalgesia, immune suppression, suppression of the HPA axis, and decreased wound healing).

When choosing treatment options for both procedural and postoperative pain for children, the following physiological considerations should be kept in mind:

- Drug conjugation in the liver is the predominant method of metabolism for most analgesics. Neonates have an immature cytochrome P450 system and will conjugate drugs slowly.
- Renal clearance of drugs and their metabolites is usually adequate at 2 weeks after birth. Before this, the clearance of many drugs may be delayed, necessitating an increase in dosing intervals.
- Because of the increase in total body water concentration in neonates, water-soluble drugs have a larger volume of distribution.
- Neonates have less plasma protein binding, resulting in increased free drug concentration.

In general, these pharmacokinetic factors mean that lower per-kilogram doses are needed in neonates and infants, but sometimes at increased dosing intervals. However, the effects of immaturity are complex and some drugs may actually be needed in larger doses because of differences in drug sensitivity and distribution. There is no substitute for using pediatric drug tables when prescribing drugs for young children.

A. Acetaminophen and Nonsteroidal Anti-inflammatory Drugs

Acetaminophen and nonsteroidal anti-inflammatory drugs (NSAIDs) are effective as single agents for mild to moderate pain and are important components of multimodal and opioid-sparing analgesic strategies. Such drugs offer the advantages of not being associated with respiratory depression and being relatively free of side effects such as nausea and constipation. Pediatric dosing for these drugs is presented in Table 31.2.

1. **Acetaminophen.** Acetaminophen has only minimal anti-inflammatory effects because its effects are mainly in the central nervous system. In patients who have a history of asthma or an increased risk of gastrointestinal (GI) mucosal insult or renal insufficiency, acetaminophen is

TABLE 31.2 Pediatric Dosing of Commonly Used Nonsteroidal Anti-inflammatory Drugs (NSAIDs) and Acetaminophen for Children Older Than 3 Months

Drug	Dose	Comments
Acetaminophen (PO and PR)	10-15 mg/kg q4h	Doses up to 30-40 mg/kg can be given PO or PR for severe pain; maximum daily dose is 90 mg/kg. For term neonates, maximum daily dose is 60 mg/kg and interval is increased to 6-8 h.
Acetaminophen (IV)	12.5 mg/kg q4h or 15 mg/kg q6h	Maximum daily dose 60 mg/kg or 3750 mg. Reduce dose to 7.5-10 mg/kg for children under 2 years old. For term neonates, the maximum daily dose is 30 mg/kg.
Aspirin	10-15 mg/kg q4h	Limited usage in children because of its association with Reye syndrome.
Ibuprofen	4-10 mg/kg q6-8h	Maximum daily dose 40 mg/kg.
Naproxen	5 mg/kg q12h	Also available as oral liquid.
Ketorolac (IV)	0.5 mg/kg q6-8h	Potent and injectable; usage limited by side effects; should not be used for more than 5 d.

Note: Doses are for oral use unless otherwise stated.
PO, by mouth; PR, by way of the rectum; NSAIDs, nonsteroidal anti-inflammatory drugs; IV, intravenous.

favored over NSAIDs. Acetaminophen is available in many formulations, including tablets, capsules, syrups, suspensions, and suppositories. It is also included in many compound analgesics (Tylenol No. 3, Percocet, Vicodin, Ultracet, etc.). Rapid absorption without first-pass liver metabolism makes the rectal route useful in children; however, absorption can be variable and time to peak effect can be up to 3 hours. Intravenous (IV) acetaminophen is relatively new to U.S. markets, though it has been in use in other countries since 2000. Its time to onset is 5-15 minutes, and peak effect is at 1 hour. It results in peak plasma levels up to 70% higher than oral and rectal forms. IV acetaminophen is approved in the United States for use in patients 2 years of age and older. Studies have shown it to be well tolerated in younger patients as well, though dose reductions may be advisable given theoretical concerns for hepatotoxicity in infants and neonates. Acetaminophen is contraindicated in patients with severe liver disease.

2. **Nonsteroidal Anti-inflammatory Drugs.** The analgesic effect of NSAIDs results from their inhibition of cyclooxygenases involved in prostaglandin synthesis. This mechanism is also responsible for the well-recognized side effects of NSAIDs including gastric ulceration, platelet dysfunction, and renal dysfunction. These side effects may limit their use after certain surgeries (ie, when significant hemorrhage or difficult hemostasis is a concern) and in certain patients (eg, those with renal disease or coagulopathies).
3. **Aspirin.** Aspirin (acetylsalicylic acid) currently has very limited use in children and in infants because of its recognized association with Reye syndrome. The most widely used NSAID is ibuprofen, available in a number of formulations including an oral suspension and chewable tablets

appropriate for use in children and infants. An IV formulation is commercially available, but infrequently used. Ketorolac, on the other hand, is most frequently administered parenterally, making it an extremely useful opioid-sparing or adjunct agent when the oral route cannot be used. Renal and GI side effects can be avoided by adhering to recommended dosages and limiting use to 5 days.

Numerous studies have examined ketorolac's effect on surgical bleeding in children with conflicting results. As such, in the postoperative setting, its analgesic benefits must be carefully weighed against the risk of hemorrhage on a case-by-case basis. Other NSAIDs used in the treatment of children include naproxen, indomethacin, tolmetin, diclofenac, and ketoprofen. IV indomethacin is used to treat patent ductus arteriosus but has virtually no application in the treatment of pain. Indomethacin suppositories may be useful occasionally. Selective cyclooxygenase-2 (COX-2) inhibitors such as celecoxib, valdecoxib, and etoricoxib are less likely than other NSAIDs to cause GI side effects because they selectively inhibit the inducible COX-2, sparing the constitutive enzyme (COX-1), particularly in the GI tract. They may be useful as an alternative to nonselective NSAIDs when there is concern about GI irritation. Although data regarding the perioperative use of these drugs in children and infants are lacking, celecoxib has been shown to be effective and well-tolerated by children over 2 years of age in the outpatient setting at doses of 3-6 mg/kg bid.

B. Opioids

Although opioids can be effectively used in infants and children for pain relief in the perioperative period or in palliative settings, current practice favors first optimizing nonopioid medications, such as acetaminophen and NSAIDs, as well as adjuvant drugs, which are discussed at the end of this section. Opioids are described fully in Chapter 11.

Prescription opioid misuse and abuse poses a serious public health concern among children and adolescents in the United States. Prescribing rates among young adults have nearly doubled since the mid-1990s, and the number of opioid-related drug overdoses and deaths has increased. Opioids prescribed to adults, but found in the home, also pose a serious risk to children. Therefore, judicious use and prescription of these medications is essential. Providers should aim to prescribe the lowest effective opioid dose and only the quantity needed for the expected duration of pain. The prescription should include instructions for discontinuing and discarding the medication. Short-acting opioids (morphine or oxycodone) are preferred over long-acting opioids (oxycontin, fentanyl patches, methadone) for the management of acute noncancer pain. Finally, for many pain conditions, either nonopioid analgesics or adjuvant analgesics may provide comparable relief with less risk for harm than opioids.

1. **Pharmacokinetics.** Opioids are metabolized differently in children at different ages. In newborns and infants, pharmacokinetic factors indicate that lower per-kilogram doses are needed than in older children, although the larger volume of distribution of these drugs may mean that a relatively large loading dose (given under controlled conditions) may be needed. The half-life of morphine in neonates is 6-8 hours and about 10 hours in premature infants (compared to 2 hours in adults), necessitating markedly lower infusion rates than in older individuals. As children grow, morphine clearance rapidly approaches the adult level, and in adolescents, it is actually greater than that in adults.

2. **Side effects.** Neonates and premature infants are extremely sensitive to the respiratory depressant effects of opioids, and respiratory depression may occur at subanalgesic doses. Infants are also at an increased risk of apnea following a rapid bolus dose because of the rapid peak dose in the brain. Other important side effects include nausea, emesis, bradycardia, tolerance, withdrawal, dysregulation of the hypothalamic pituitary axis, and adverse effects on wound healing. Opioid-induced hyperalgesia, which manifests as an increased postoperative analgesic requirement, is poorly understood in children but has been demonstrated in adolescents undergoing scoliosis surgery and is therefore a consideration when prescribing opioids to children.
3. **Choice of opioids.** Morphine is commonly the drug of choice in infants and in children. Because of the associated histamine release with morphine, hydromorphone or fentanyl may be used in patients with asthma. Nalbuphine, a semisynthetic opioid analgesic that acts as an agonist at the k-receptor and an antagonist at the μ-receptor, has a potency comparable to that of morphine and a ceiling effect that limits respiratory depression. Oxycodone and hydrocodone are the opioids most commonly chosen for oral administration in children. Oral codeine has been removed from the MGH inpatient formulary; the FDA added a boxed warning to the label of all codeine-containing products about the risks of codeine in postoperative pain management in children following tonsillectomy and/or adenoidectomy. Children who are ultrarapid metabolizers of codeine due to a cytochrome P450 2D6 (CYP2D6) polymorphism may be particularly sensitive to the respiratory depressant effects of codeine. Routine CYP2D6 testing is not currently recommended in children.
4. **Route of administration.** Opioids can be given parenterally, orally, rectally, intranasally, transdermally, transmucosally, or neuraxially. In the immediate postoperative period, the IV route is most commonly chosen. If there is no IV in place, the rectal route may be useful.
   a. **Parenteral.** The IV route is the parenteral route of choice. Drugs can be given either intermittently or through a continuous infusion. Intermittent boluses are used if pain gets out of control or when there is a need for analgesia for anticipating noxious stimulation such as dressing changes. PCA is used when children are old enough to use this technique. Nurse-controlled analgesia (NCA) via a PCA pump is also an option.
      i. **Continuous IV infusion.** Continuous IV infusions are used in young children (<6 years of age or developmentally delayed) with moderate to severe pain, when they are not able to use PCA, in order to maintain steady plasma drug levels and stable analgesia. A loading dose of the drug is commonly given to reach a steady state before the infusion. Careful monitoring of vital signs and special monitors are sometimes necessary to prevent excessive sedation and respiratory depression. This precaution is particularly important in neonates and in all spontaneously breathing children. If pain cannot be controlled with infusion, the rate of infusion may be increased. However, the rate of infusion should not be repeatedly and rapidly increased; accelerating the infusion rate is a common misstep that frequently causes potentially dangerous respiratory depression.

         Morphine is the most commonly used opioid for continuous infusions. Analgesic levels are usually obtained after a loading dose of 10-100 mcg/kg of morphine, and an infusion at 0.01-0.03

TABLE 31.3 Guidelines for Continuous Intravenous Infusion of Opioids in Children

Drug	Rate
Morphine	≤40 kg: 0.01-0.03 mg/kg/h >40 kg: 1.5 mg/h
Hydromorphone	≤40 kg: 0.003-0.005 mg/kg/h >40 kg: 0.3 mg/h
Fentanyl	0.5-1 mcg/kg/h

Adapted from the Massachusetts General Hospital for Children: Pediatric Analgesic Dose Guide. With permission.

mg/kg/h is then started. Hydromorphone may also be used. Recommended infusion rates are listed in Table 31.3.

ii. **Patient-controlled analgesia.** PCA is used in older children (≥6 years of age) at MGH when they understand how to use it. The principles of PCA can be found in the chapter entitled "Acute Pain in Adults." It is sometimes appropriate to allow parents or nurses to operate the infusion pump or other delivery device for the child, but caution should be exercised. Before allowing parents to participate, the prescribing physician should be absolutely certain that the parents understand the principles of PCA, and, in particular, that they should not press the button unless the child is awake and is requesting analgesia for pain. Standard MGH PCA orders are shown in Chapter 30 Table 31.4 presents a PCA dosing guideline for morphine, hydromorphone, and fentanyl.

b. **Oral.** The oral route is used when the pain is mild to moderate. Oxycodone, morphine elixir, and oxycodone with acetaminophen (Percocet) are all useful in children. Recommended doses can be found in Table 31.5. Morphine and hydromorphone are available as suppositories and may be useful when the oral and IV routes are not available. Rectal doses are the same as oral doses.

c. **Transdermal.** A transdermal fentanyl patch is available for the treatment of moderate to severe pain, but this has limited application in infants and children. The lowest available dose is 25 mcg/h; therefore, the patch is not suitable for children weighing <25 kg or for those requiring a low dose (ie, those who have not yet developed a tolerance to opioids). The patch has a long onset time and a long elimination half-life, and therefore, it is not suitable when rapid titration is needed. Occasionally, the patch is useful in children undergoing surgery who have already become opioid tolerant because of preexisting cancer or chronic pain. The efficacy of the buprenorphine patch has been reported in one study of pediatric patients suffering from chronic cancer pain, but its safety and efficacy has not yet been formally established in the pediatric population.

d. **Transmucosal.** Transmucosal administration of fentanyl has been used in adults for acute pain relief. The fentanyl buccal tablet ("Fentora") is absorbed through the buccal mucosa. It is usually absorbed into the systemic circulation in 10-20 minutes, and it is more effective than oral/gastric intestinal administration because it bypasses the first-pass hepatic metabolism. There are currently no randomized controlled trials for fentanyl transmucosal delivery systems in children and they are not currently FDA approved in patients under the age of 18.

TABLE 31.4 Guidelines for Patient-Controlled Analgesia (PCA) Dosing (≥6 Years of Age)

Drug	Start Dose[a]	Dose Range	Lockout	Continuous Rate (Optional)	1 Hour Limit
Fentanyl 10 mcg/mL	0.25 mcg/kg/dose	0.1-0.3 mcg/kg/dose	6 min	Not recommended on general care units	2 mcg/kg/h
Hydromorphone 0.5 mg/mL	0.004 mg/kg/dose	0.003-0.005 mg/kg/dose	10 min	0-0.004 mg/kg/h[b]	0.015-0.02 mg/kg/h
Morphine 1 mg/mL	0.02 mg/kg/dose	0.01-0.03 mg/kg/dose	6 min	0-0.03 mg/kg/h[b]	0.1-0.15 mg/kg/h

[a]No parent- or nurse-controlled analgesia.

[b]Low-dose continuous rate in addition to PCA demand dose may improve postoperative pain management and quality of sleep but has been associated with episodic hypoxemia. Monitor for nighttime hypoxemia. Continuous rate may be required for patients with acute pain associated with chronic illness, sickle cell, or cancer.

Adapted from the Massachusetts. General Hospital for Children: Pediatric Analgesic Dose Guide. With permission.

TABLE 31.5 Recommended Starting Doses for Opioids in Children Weighing ≤40 kg

Drug	Oral	Parenteral
Morphine	0.3 mg/kg q3-4h	0.1 mg/kg q3-4h
Hydromorphone	0.04-0.08 mg/kg q3-4h	0.02 mg/kg q2-4h
Oxycodone	0.1-0.2 mg/kg q4-6h	Not available
Hydrocodone	0.1-0.2 mg/kg q4-6h	Not available
Methadone	0.1-0.2 mg/kg q6-12h	0.1 mg/kg q6-12h
Fentanyl		0.5-1 mcg/kg q3-6h

e. **Neuraxial.** Opioids given intrathecally or epidurally provide analgesia that is both effective and relatively free of side effects because much smaller doses are used. Hydromorphone and fentanyl are used at MGH. Differences among opioids when administered neuraxially are described in a previous chapter. As a general principle, an epidural dose is 1/10th of an IV dose, whereas an intrathecal (spinal) dose is 1/100th of an IV dose.

f. **Novel routes of administration.** Recently, several alternative routes have been described for children. For example, intranasal administration of fentanyl, sufentanil, and butorphanol has been used for relieving postoperative pain after myringotomy. Intranasal clonidine has been used for procedural sedation. Unfortunately, there are few studies supporting novel opioid delivery systems in children.

C. Emerging Coanalgesic Therapies

1. **Multimodal treatment.** Acute peri- and postoperative pain in infants and children is often undertreated, and multimodal pain therapy represents one way to better treat pain in children while minimizing exposure to opioids.

a. **Ketamine.** Ketamine is an *N*-methyl-D-aspartate (NMDA) antagonist that provides both anesthesia and sedation and can be administered by a variety of routes: IV, intramuscular (IM), intranasal (IN), oral (PO), and rectal. The pharmacokinetics of IV and IM ketamine are best understood: onset is within 1-2 minutes after IV use and 5 minutes after IM use, and the duration of action is around 45 minutes. Typical doses in children are 0.1-0.5 mg/kg as a bolus dose (maximum of 35 mg per dose) and 1.65-5 mcg/kg/min as a continuous infusion. The stable cardiorespiratory side effect profile of ketamine makes it desirable in children with cardiac disease, especially cyanotic subtypes.

Although ketamine has been shown to decrease postoperative pain and opioid requirements in adults, its opioid-sparing effect is less clear in children: a large meta-analysis demonstrated that systemic ketamine decreased postoperative pain intensity and analgesic requirement in the PACU but did not have a postoperative opioid-sparing effect. However, both peritonsillar and systemic use of ketamine decreased posttonsillectomy pain without adverse effects such as nausea, vomiting, sedation, or hallucinations. There is limited literature on the role of ketamine in hyperalgesia in children; there are currently no data to support the use of low-dose ketamine in children with opioid-induced hyperalgesia. Intranasal ketamine is used in the emergency department for procedural sedation—the doses used in studies vary (0.5-9 mg/kg), and while it does produce sedation and anxiolysis, it is not superior to existing therapies (such as midazolam). Ketamine can also be added to caudal injections and has been shown to significantly prolong the duration of single-shot injections at a dose of 0.5 mg/kg. Contraindications to ketamine include significantly elevated blood pressure, recent head trauma, post intracranial surgery, intracranial mass or bleed, uncontrolled seizure of psychotic disorder, known hypersensitivity to ketamine, and patients under 2 years of age or <10 kg.

b. **Dextromethorphan.** Dextromethorphan is a weak NMDA receptor antagonist and can be administered IV or PO (as a syrup) at a dose of 1 mg/kg. Similar to studies with ketamine, there is evidence for reduced early postoperative opioid use (during the first 6 hours after surgery) in patients undergoing tonsillectomy and/or adenoidectomy. Dextromethorphan lacks undesirable opioid side effects, namely, respiratory depression, nausea, and vomiting.

c. **Clonidine.** Clonidine is an α2-adrenoreceptor agonist with analgesic and sedative actions. As an IV or PO supplement to opioids at a dose of 1-3 mg/kg, it can reduce the need for these agents. It can also be used intranasally for sedation.

d. **Gabapentin.** Gabapentin is an anticonvulsant that is used in the management of chronic pain. Its opioid-sparing effects in the early postoperative period have been demonstrated in adults, and there is evidence to suggest that it may reduce postoperative morphine consumption in children at a dose of 15 mg/kg.

e. **Lidocaine.** Currently, lidocaine has only been investigated in children in reducing the laryngeal reflex response to tracheal intubation and the pain associated with propofol injection. However, coadministration of low-dose IV lidocaine (1-2 mg/kg/h) is an intriguing idea to reduce postoperative pain requirements in children.

f. **Dexamethasone.** High-dose dexamethasone (>0.2 mg/kg) has been shown to have opioid-sparing effects and to decrease pain scores in adults and is a promising potential future therapy in children.

g. **Tramadol and tapentadol.** Tramadol is a synthetic analog of codeine. It has both a mild opioid effect (via the u receptor) and also inhibits neuronal uptake of serotonin and norepinephrine. It is available as an oral form (the IV formulation is not currently available in the United States) and has been used for postoperative pain control in children undergoing ambulatory surgery at a dose of 1-2 mg/kg orally. Tramadol is not currently FDA approved for use in children. Tapentadol is a novel central-acting analgesic that also acts both via the μ-opioid receptor and norepinephrine reuptake inhibition. It has no active metabolites. Its safety and efficacy has not yet been established in patients under the age of 18.

D. Neuraxial and Regional Anesthesia and Analgesia

Neuraxial and regional techniques are often used in children and provide the advantages of prolonged analgesia extending into the postoperative period with reduced distress and opioid requirement. Catheters may be utilized to even further extend the duration of analgesia. Conveniently, infants and young children are relatively resistant to the hemodynamic and respiratory effects of epidural or spinal blockade and are also less prone to post–dural puncture headache than adults. While neuraxial and peripheral blocks in adults are performed with the patient awake to allow for reporting of paresthesia or symptoms of local anesthetic toxicity, children are less able to communicate these symptoms and moreover are simply unable to tolerate these procedures awake. The risk of injury in an uncooperative or moving patient dictates that most pediatric blocks be performed under general anesthesia. Current literature supports the safety of this practice, with no difference in the incidence of adverse events between blocks performed on anesthetized children vs awake or sedated children.

1. **Epidural analgesia.** The most commonly used regional technique in children is epidural analgesia, often via a caudal approach. For a description of epidural analgesia in adults, see Chapter 30. Many of the principles in adults also apply to children and are not repeated here. Compared to adults, thoracic and lumbar epidural catheters may be technically more difficult to place in small children due to their smaller interspaces, whereas caudal placement is easier because their sacral bones are not yet fused. Catheters are more difficult to maintain in children. Challenges include preventing catheter migration or disconnection caused by movement, protecting the catheter from diaper contamination, and maintaining catheter patency when small catheters are used. Hence, single-shot epidurals, especially caudals, are used more frequently in children than in adults and provide excellent analgesia during the early postoperative phase.
2. **Indications.** Postoperative epidural analgesia is typically reserved for children undergoing thoracic, abdominal, or lower-limb procedures that are expected to produce severe pain such as thoracotomy, laparotomy, and amputation. Single-shot techniques provide useful analgesia for less painful surgical procedures of the torso, pelvis, and lower limbs, including hernia repair, circumcision, tendon lengthening, and clubfoot release. The caudal route is most commonly selected for single-shot epidural injections.
3. **Contraindications**
   a. Patient or parent refusal
   b. Coagulopathy
   c. Bacteremia
   d. Local infection at the epidural insertion site
   e. Congenital or acquired spine pathology, neurologic deficit, and raised intracranial pressure (relative contraindications)
4. **Benefits**
   a. Superior analgesia, which facilitates mobilization and pulmonary toilet
   b. Opioid sparing and decreased risk of respiratory depression
   c. Increased bowel motility
   d. Decreased bladder spasm after urologic surgery
5. **Disadvantages and risks**
   a. This technique poses the risk of local anesthetic toxicity.
   b. If opioids are used, respiratory depression can occur.
   c. Urinary retention is common. Pruritus may be a problem in up to 30% of patients. Nausea occurs rarely in this population.
   d. Catheter migration may occur, resulting in intrathecal, intravascular, or extradural placement. Indications of catheter migration include sudden increase in block density, blood in catheter, or failure to provide analgesia.
   e. Although rare, epidural hematoma and abscess may occur. Particular caution should be used when a child has a history of coagulopathy or is receiving anticoagulant therapy. Practitioners should be familiar with the guidelines for neuraxial analgesia from the American Society of Regional Anesthesia and Pain Medicine (ASRA) (see Appendix II for Web site address). Careful monitoring of neurologic function and patient status is imperative to detect early signs of adverse events.

TABLE 31.6 Differences in Spinal Cord Anatomy by Age

Age	Dural Sac Ending	Spinal Cord Ending
Full-term neonate	S3-S4	L4
6 mo	S2	L2-L3
1 y	S1	L1

E. Epidural Placement in Children

1. **Anatomic differences.** In infants, the level of the spinal cord and dural sac are continuously changing up to 1 year of age (see Table 31.6). The relation of the line between iliac crests to the spinal cord level changes as follows: in the neonate, the line is at spinal cord level L5-S1, in an older child at L5, and in an adult at L4-L5. It is also useful to know the depth of the epidural space in children, especially because the ligaments are less dense than in adults and provide a different feel. A useful formula to approximate depth (in mm) of the epidural space from the skin in children is as follows:
   a. Infant: depth (mm) = 1.5 × weight (kg)
   b. Child: depth (mm) = 1 × weight (kg)
2. **Techniques.** Placement of thoracic or lumbar epidural is similar in children as in adults. The ligamentum flavum may be soft and therefore not provide the same tactile feedback as in adults. For caudal epidural injections, a 20- to 22-gauge needle is inserted at a 60-degree angle to the skin between the sacral cornuae at the base of the sacrum, advanced through sacrococcygeal ligament, dropped to a 30-degree angle, and advanced through the sacral hiatus into the caudal space. A catheter can be threaded through the caudal canal to the lumbar or thoracic epidural space, if desired. Because most pediatric epidural catheter placement is performed under general anesthesia, it is common practice to place epidurals at the caudal or lumbar (not thoracic) level so as to avoid spinal cord injury. Fluoroscopy can be useful both to facilitate catheter insertion and to confirm positioning of the catheter tip at the desired level.

F. Single-Shot Epidural and Caudal Analgesia

When bolusing thoracic or lumbar epidurals for single-shot injection or prior to starting continuous infusion, the following is acceptable practice: 0.05 mL/kg/spinal segment using 1% lidocaine or 0.125%-0.25% bupivacaine or ropivacaine, not to exceed a dose of 5 mg/kg of lidocaine or 2.5 mg/kg of bupivacaine or ropivacaine. For single-shot caudal injection, we commonly give 0.5, 1.0, or 1.5 mL/kg of 0.2% ropivacaine or 0.25% bupivacaine to achieve anesthesia to the level of the groin, umbilicus, and chest, respectively. Clonidine 2-4 mcg/kg added to the local anesthetic prolongs duration of analgesia with minimal risk of hypotension. Addition of fentanyl 1 mcg/kg can augment analgesia but may contribute to respiratory depression in vulnerable patients.

G. Managing Epidural Infusions

1. **Choice of medication.** Dosing for common epidural infusion solutions is summarized in Table 31.7. Epidural opioids should be avoided or used with caution in infants and children at risk (eg, those with pulmonary dysfunction, developmental delay, high risk of respiratory depression or apnea, or prematurity).

TABLE 31.7 Epidural Infusion Solution Options and Dosing

Drug	Recommended Weight (Age) Group	Dosing
Ropivacaine 0.1%	0-5 kg (<6 mo)	0.1-0.2 mg/kg/h
	6-10 kg (>6 mo)	0.1-0.3 mg/kg/h
Bupivacaine 0.1%	>5 kg (>6 mo)	0.1-0.3 mg/kg/h
Bupivacaine 0.1% with fentanyl 2 mcg/mL	>5 kg (>6 mo)	0.1-0.3 mg/kg/h
Bupivacaine 0.1% with hydromorphone 3-20 mcg/mL	>5 kg (>6 mo)	0.1-0.3 mg/kg/h
Bupivacaine 0.1% with clonidine 0.5 mcg/mL	>5 kg (>6 mo)	0.1-0.3 mg/kg/h

2. **General care.** The standard of care when providing postoperative epidural analgesia for children is similar to that for adults. This protocol consists of the following:
   - **a.** 24-hour pain service coverage for patients receiving epidural analgesia.
   - **b.** Ventilatory status monitored and recorded hourly.
   - **c.** Vital signs monitored and recorded every 4 hours.
   - **d.** Daily pain service evaluation for pain control satisfaction, side effects, and neurologic status.
   - **e.** Daily examination of the catheter site for signs of inflammation or infection.
   - **f.** Children younger than 6 months should be considered at risk of respiratory depression and a low threshold should be set for more intensive monitoring.
   - **g.** Heels should be padded to prevent pressure sores.
   - **h.** No systemic opioids should be given while the patient is receiving epidural opioids. If there is a need to treat pain in an area that the epidural does not cover, the opioid can be removed from the epidural infusion solution and be given intravenously.

H. Treatment of Side Effects and Complications

The abnormal neurologic examination, that is, motor or sensory block outside the epidural's expected coverage, should be promptly investigated. Potential causes include a too-high infusion rate, catheter migration to the intrathecal or subdural space, or the rare but more sinister possibility of developing epidural hematoma or abscess. These symptoms should always prompt the decrease or discontinuation of epidural infusion, close neurologic monitoring, and possible investigation with CT or MRI if suspicion for hematoma or abscess is high (eg, concurrent back pain, progression or persistence of deficits despite discontinuation of treatment). Should hematoma or abscess be discovered, timely surgical decompression is crucial to avoid permanent neurologic damage.

Local anesthetic toxicity is rare in the postoperative setting. If it occurs, it should be treated as described in Chapter 46. The pediatric dose for Intralipid is 2-5 mL/kg, with repeated doses as needed up to a total of 10 mL/kg.

Side effects from epidural opioid include pruritus, nausea and vomiting, urinary retention, and respiratory depression. Treatment is summarized

TABLE 31.8 Treating Side Effects of Epidural Opioid in Pediatric Patients

Drug	Indication	Dose
Naloxone	Respiratory depression	2 mcg/kg
Naloxone	Pruritus	0.5-1 mcg/kg
Diphenhydramine	Pruritus	0.5 mg/kg
Nalbuphine	Pruritus	10-20 mcg/kg
Ondansetron	Nausea	0.1 mg/kg
Metoclopramide	Nausea	0.1-0.2 mg/kg

in Table 31.8. Respiratory depression is the most serious of these complications. Treatment involves administering oxygen; providing ventilatory support, if necessary; stopping the epidural infusion; and administering naloxone (2 mcg/kg, IV). Rarely, respiratory depression can be due to catheter migration into the intrathecal space, resulting in a high or total spinal. Because children are relatively resistant to the hemodynamic effects of sympathectomy, respiratory depression can be the first manifestation of this complication.

I. Spinals

Spinal anesthesia and analgesia are most commonly used in neonates when avoidance of a general anesthetic is desirable for operations up to 120 minutes in duration. The L4-L5 space is typically chosen. For infants, the doses of local anesthetics used are relatively higher than those for an older child or an adult. The duration of action is also shorter in children than in older patients. Hyperbaric bupivacaine, ropivacaine, and tetracaine are the most commonly used agents. Common dosing regimens are listed in Table 31.9. Intrathecal opioid (most commonly preservative-free morphine sulfate [Duramorph] 2-10 mcg/kg), either alone or in combination with local anesthetic, provides prolonged analgesia (12-24 hours or more), but is reserved for children older than 5 years old. Because delayed respiratory depression may occur, close monitoring of the respiratory status is required for 24-36 hours after administration.

J. Peripheral Nerve Blocks

Peripheral nerve blocks (PNBs) of the upper and lower extremities, head and neck, and trunk are a safe and effective means of providing postoperative analgesia in children. Some blocks are also useful for treating pain after trauma. As with neuraxial blocks, both single-shot and continuous catheter techniques may be employed, and most blocks are performed under general anesthesia. The use of ultrasound guidance for PNB has become

TABLE 31.9 Dosing for Pediatric Spinal

Weight	0.5% Bupivacaine (mg/kg)	0.5% Ropivacaine (mg/kg)	0.5% Tetracaine (mg/kg)
<5 kg	0.5-0.6	0.5-1	0.5-0.6
5-15 kg	0.4	0.5	0.4
>15 kg	0.3	0.5	0.3

widespread and is the default approach at our institution. The techniques for performing PNB in children are similar to in adults, but the volume of local anesthetic administered should be carefully determined based on weight. The maximum recommended doses of commonly used local anesthetics are as follows: bupivacaine 2.5 mg/kg, ropivacaine 2.5 mg/kg, and mepivacaine 5 mg/kg. Blocks in infants and younger children should be performed using more dilute solutions such as bupivacaine 0.25% or ropivacaine 0.2%, while blocks in older children may be performed with more concentrated solutions. If continuous infusion via a peripheral nerve catheter is desired, 0.2-0.4 mg/kg/h of ropivacaine 0.1% may be used. A list of blocks commonly used in pediatrics and the settings in which they are useful are listed in Table 31.10.

K. Topical Analgesia

EMLA cream (a eutectic mixture of local anesthetics—lidocaine and prilocaine) has been proven to be useful in children to benumb the skin before needling and even to provide postoperative pain relief (eg, after circumcision). Other topical local anesthetic preparations are occasionally useful (eg, lidocaine gel for mucous membranes). Topical preparations are capable of causing local anesthetic systemic toxicity, especially in small children.

TABLE 31.10 Common Pediatric Peripheral Nerve Blocks

Block	Indication	Dosing 0.1% Ropivacaine[a]
Brachial plexus (interscalene, supraclavicular, infraclavicular, axillary)	Surgeries and trauma of the upper extremity from shoulder to hand	0.2-0.3 mL/kg
Femoral	Surgeries on the anterior knee and thigh	0.2-0.4 mL/kg
Proximal sciatic	Surgeries on the posterior knee and thigh, lower leg, and foot	0.3-0.5 mL/kg
Sciatic in the popliteal fossa	Surgery on the ankle and foot	0.2-0.4 mL/kg
Superficial cervical plexus	Surgery on the lateral neck and clavicle	0.1 mL/kg
Occipital	Occipital craniotomy	0.1 mL/kg
Transversus abdominis plane	Appendectomy, cholecystectomy, laparoscopy, laparotomy	0.4 mL/kg per side
Rectus sheath	Umbilical hernia repair, laparoscopy with midline port	0.2 mL/kg per side
Ilioinguinal/ iliohypogastric	Inguinal hernia repair, hydrocelectomy, orchiopexy	0.2 mL/kg per side
Penile	Circumcision	0.1 mL/kg
Paravertebral	Thoracotomy, renal surgery, breast surgery, cholecystectomy, rib fractures	0.5 mL/kg per side
Lumbar plexus	Surgery on the hip and upper leg	0.3-1.0 mL/kg

[a]Not to exceed maximum recommended dose.

L. Nonpharmacologic Techniques

Nonpharmacologic techniques are adjuncts to analgesic medications to help ease a child's discomfort or anxiety level associated with pain. These techniques work best when the patient and his or her family are introduced to the particular technique and if they actively participate.

M. Cognitive Approaches

1. Education has been shown to be effective in children, especially when teaching has been conducted preoperatively.
2. Distraction may be useful in all age groups, but it needs to be age specific. Attention is focused on stimuli other than the pain sensation. The stimuli must be interesting to the patient; consistent with the developmental level, energy level, and capability of the child; and stimulating to major sensory modalities (ie, hearing, vision, touch, and movements). Some examples for specific ages are as follows:
   a. Toddler/preschooler: blowing bubbles, singing, music recordings, pop-ups, or "I Spy" games
   b. School-aged/adolescent: music or story via headset, video/computer games, singing or tapping rhythm, or conversation
3. **Relaxation.** These techniques are used to decrease anxiety and skeletal muscle tension, potentially relieving some of the mental and physical effects of pain. Techniques include breathing exercises, progressive muscle relaxation, remembering past peaceful experiences, and using pacifiers and stroking in infants and toddlers.
4. **Hypnosis and guided imagery.** Hypnosis is an altered state of consciousness characterized by increased suggestibility, narrowing of attention, and relaxation. In hypnotherapy, therapeutic suggestions made by a therapist or through self-hypnosis are used to modify sensation and perception with the goal of reducing anxiety and alleviating the subjective experience of pain. Guided imagery is a related technique in which a patient imagines sensory images to make pain more acceptable or to change pain into a different sensation. Examples are throwing pain away like a snowball, blowing pain away, or imagining pain medication traveling through the body to relieve the pain.

N. Cutaneous Stimulation

Massage or rubbing the skin may be very soothing but is generally not recommended for premature and full-term neonates. The application of heat or cold is often useful in localized pain. Transcutaneous electric nerve stimulation (TENS) can also be used (see Chapter 27).

O. Acupuncture

Acupuncture has shown good effects for treating PONV in children. Although the utility of acupuncture for children with acute postoperative pain has not been established, recent studies of acupuncture for posttonsillectomy pain suggest that it may be of use as an adjunct to pharmacologic analgesia.

V. ANALGESIA FOR PEDIATRIC AMBULATORY SURGERY

When managing pain for children undergoing same-day surgery, the goal is to achieve satisfactory analgesia that can be maintained by the patient's caregiver in the home, while minimizing side effects that might require prolonged medical care and monitoring (ie, sedation, respiratory depression, nausea, constipation). To these ends, the use of opioid-sparing techniques is particularly valuable. Regional and local anesthesia should be used whenever possible. Continuous peripheral nerve blockade via catheters and portable infusion systems can be used in outpatients to extend regional analgesia for days. Keep in mind, however, that prolonged motor blockade that limits the mobility of a usually ambulatory child can present a challenge for caregivers. Parent/caregiver education is crucial to successful analgesia after same-day surgery. Misconceptions about how pain medicines work, ideal dosing, and the risk of addiction can lead to undertreatment of pain, while lack of a plan for tapering analgesics can lead to unnecessarily long courses. Caregivers should be instructed on which agents to administer on a standing basis (eg, acetaminophen, NSAIDs), which to give only as needed for breakthrough pain (eg, opioids), and in what order to taper various agents (eg, opioids before adjuncts). For children who receive regional anesthesia, caregivers should be shown how to protect the insensate limb.

VI. ANALGESIA FOR NEONATES

As our understanding of the effects of pain on the developing nervous system has grown, pain management in neonates has become increasingly important. Multiple tools have been developed for the assessment of pain in neonates, for example, the Face, Legs, Activity, Cry, Consolability (FLACC) scale and Premature Infant Pain Profile (PIPP). In this population, differences in pharmacokinetics and pharmacodynamics dictate caution when dosing analgesics. Neonates, especially those born preterm, are more sensitive to both the analgesic and respiratory depressant effects of opioids. Protocolized care and appropriate monitoring during opioid administration are key to patient safety. Regional and neuraxial techniques can be safely used in neonates and are an excellent option when avoidance of opioids is desired. Nonpharmacologic therapies such as oral sucrose, nonnutritive sucking, and kangaroo care can provide effective analgesia for minor procedural pain and as an adjunct to pharmacologic measures, perhaps through promotion of endogenous opioid release.

VII. CONCLUSION

Improvements in pain management in infants and children play an integral role in advancing the medical care of children. Further progress in education, research, and knowledge will allow us to apply those lessons learned in the adults to the care of young patients. It is incumbent upon all caregivers to consider pain and analgesia at every juncture in the care of sick children.

Selected Readings

American Society of Anesthesiologists Task Force on Acute Pain Management. Practice guidelines for acute pain management in the perioperative setting: an updated report by the American Society of Anesthesiologists Task Force on Acute Pain Management. *Anesthesiology.* 2012;116(2):248-273.

Chidambaran V, Sadhasivam S. Pediatric acute and surgical pain management: recent advances and future perspectives. *Int Anesthesiol Clin.* 2012;50(4):66-82.

Crawford MW, Hickey C, Zaarour C, Howard A, Naser B. Development of acute opioid tolerance during infusion of remifentanil for pediatric scoliosis surgery. *Anesth Analg.* 2006;102(6):1662-1667.

Dahmani S, Michelet D, Abback PS, et al. Ketamine for perioperative pain management in children: a meta-analysis of published studies. *Pediatr Anesth.* 2011;21(6):636-652.

Howard R. Postoperative pain management. In: McGrath PJ, Stevens BJ, Walker SM, Zempsky WT, eds. *Oxford Textbook of Paediatric Pain.* Oxford, UK: Oxford University Press; 2014.

Malviya S, Polaner DM, Berde C. Acute pain. In: Cote C, Lerman J, Todres D, eds. *A Practice of Anesthesia for Infants and Children.* Philadelphia, PA: Saunders, Elsevier; 2009.

McCabe SE. Medical and nonmedical use of prescription opioids among high school seniors in the United States. *Arch Pediatr Adolesc Med.* 2012;166(9):797. http://doi.org/10.1001/archpediatrics.2012.85

Russell P, von Ungern-Sternberg BS, Schug SA. Perioperative analgesia in pediatric surgery. *Curr Opin Anaesthesiol.* 2013;26(4):420-427.

Shah RD, Suresh S. Applications of regional anaesthesia in paediatrics. *Br J Anaesth.* 2013;111(suppl 1):i114-i124.

Suresh S, Giorgio I. Regional anesthesia in pediatric patients. In: Hadzic A, ed. *Textbook of Regional Anesthesia and Acute Pain Management.* New York, NY: McGraw-Hill; 2007.

Verghese ST, Hannallah RS. Acute pain management in children. *J Pain Res.* 2010;3:105-123.

Walker SM. Neonatal pain. *Paediatr Anaesth.* 2014;24(1):39-48.

32 Care of Burn Patients

Amir Mian and Jingping Wang

I. EPIDEMIOLOGY

A burn is defined as a type of injury to flesh or skin caused by heat, electricity, chemicals, friction, or radiation. Burn injuries are associated with a high level of morbidity. In the United States, ~486 000 people visited emergency rooms in 2011 for burns as the primary diagnosis including 40 000 hospitalizations and 3400 deaths. A significant source of suffering in these patients is pain associated with the burn injury.

To better understand the multimodal approach to treating these patients, it is helpful to review the anatomy and physiology underlying burn pain.

II. ANATOMY AND PHYSIOLOGY

A. Classification

Burns are characterized by destruction of tissues and subsequent alteration of the normal physiology. Traditionally, burns have been classified according to the depth of tissue destruction.

1. **First-degree burns.** Superficial burns where damage is confined to the epidermis
2. **Second-degree burns.** Partial-thickness burns involving the epidermis and a portion of the dermis
3. **Third-degree burns.** Full-thickness burns where the entire dermis is destroyed
4. **Fourth-degree burns.** Full-thickness burns involving the entire dermis where injury extends to underlying tissue (ie, muscle, bone, etc.)

The physiologic alterations caused by the injury vary depending on the depth, extent, and location of the tissue destruction. However, what is constant is the presence of an inflammatory reaction in response to the burn. This is both localized and systemic, the major characteristic being the release of the chemical mediators of inflammation that play a crucial role in the phenomena of burn pain and its morbidity.

B. Mechanism of Burn Pain

Burns can produce pain through a variety of mechanisms. Simplistically, a cutaneous (first-degree) burn stimulates nociceptors and mechanoreceptors, which send signals through their associated unmyelinated C and myelinated A delta fibers. These fibers synapse in the dorsal horn of the spinal cord and transmit to second-order neurons that ascend through the anterolateral spinothalamic tracts. Pain signals are modulated by descending inhibitory fibers (ie, endogenous opioid system). The ascending tracts terminate in the thalamus where signals are relayed to many areas of the central nervous system, including the somatosensory cortex.

The depth of the burn is thought to play a part in the severity of pain experienced; deeper burns in which nerve endings are completely destroyed are less painful than those in which they are spared. However, because most burns cause a spectrum of tissue damage, the importance of this fact is questionable, and all burn patients can be assumed to have pain. Moreover, nerve destruction may lead to disorderly nerve regeneration and resultant neuropathic pain.

Along with the acute pain caused by the immediate neural response, burn injury also causes release of the chemical mediators of the inflammatory response. These mediators in turn modify the subacute and chronic phases of the neural response to the burn.

1. **Primary hyperalgesia** is the increased sensitivity of the wounded area caused by sensitization of the remaining pain receptors caused by chemical mediators.
2. **Secondary hyperalgesia** refers to the increased sensitivity of surrounding unburned areas and is thought to be due to neuronal changes in the anterolateral tracts of the spinal cord.

The inflammatory response also increases the patient's metabolic rate with subsequent increased clearance of medications, which may also impact analgesia.

III. CLINICAL FEATURES

A. Patterns of Burn Pain

Different patterns of pain have been observed in burn patients and necessitate a tailored approach to the treatment of pain. Four specific patterns have been described:

1. **Background pain.** Pain experienced by the patient at rest
2. **Breakthrough pain.** Intermittent episodes of increased pain
3. **Procedural pain.** Pain associated with procedures including dressing changes, debridement, etc.
4. **Chronic pain.** Pain far outlasting any painful stimulus (occurs in about 52% of burn patients)

IV. MANAGEMENT

The focus of burn pain management must be multimodal to increase effectiveness and decrease adverse effects from any single modality.

A. Pharmacologic

1. Opioids

The opioids constitute the cornerstone of pharmacologic analgesia for all phases of burn pain. The wide variety of available agents with different characteristics allows treatment to be tailored to the patient's needs.

For example, IV patient-controlled analgesia (PCA) has been shown to be effective for managing burn pain in the inpatient setting. PCA allows medications with well-known profiles (ie, morphine, hydromorphone) to be administered as continuous infusions with patient-controlled boluses for breakthrough pain. In addition, most pumps allow for larger provider-administered boluses for procedural pain.

Outpatients may be treated as in other pain conditions with a long-acting opioid for background pain if needed and a short-acting medication as needed for breakthrough pain. Various well-known medications are available for this indication, although none have shown any superiority for treatment of burn pain.

Procedural pain is amenable to treatment with potent short-acting opioids (eg, fentanyl analogues) with or without anesthesia (general or regional).

Among the well-known adverse effects of opioids, pruritus may be the most significant in those with burns, as scratching can dramatically interfere with wound healing. Management has proven to be difficult although NSAIDs and antihistamines may offer some relief.

2. NSAIDs and Acetaminophen

Anti-inflammatory drugs are used in combination with opioids for synergistic effect and to decrease the adverse effects associated with opioids by lowering the doses necessary to provide analgesia. Anti-inflammatory medications decrease the inflammatory response triggered by burn injury through their actions on the arachidonic acid pathway. This mechanism is also responsible for their familiar adverse effects. In this regard, the most desirable are selective COX-2 inhibitors and acetaminophen. A well-known side effect of NSAIDs which may be especially troublesome in the burn setting is gastric ulceration. Stress (Curling) ulcers occur commonly in those with significant burn injuries, and prophylaxis with histamine-2 antagonists or proton pump inhibitors is recommended for all burn patients.

3. Anticonvulsants

The anticonvulsants or AEDs (antiepileptic drugs) are a useful group of drugs when it comes to treating the neuropathic component of burn pain. The mechanism of action varies with the specific medication; however, they all decrease neuronal excitability and impulses from damaged nerves. As such, they are useful adjuncts in the long-term management of persistent pain after burn injury.

4. Antidepressants

The antidepressants are another class of medications which may be used as adjuncts in the treatment of burn pain. Most of these agents work by inhibiting the reuptake of norepinephrine and/or serotonin at the presynaptic nerve terminal thereby modifying transmission of pain signals. Although unstudied for this indication, their effects on mood and sleep can also be used to benefit this patient population.

5. Alpha-2 Receptor Agonists

Alpha-2 receptor agonists such as clonidine and dexmedetomidine bind to presynaptic receptors thereby decreasing release of norepinephrine. This action decreases the afferent sympathetic impulses from the burn area thereby modulating the sympathetically mediated component of the patient's pain. An especially pertinent side effect of these drugs in this setting is hypotension; thus caution must be in the acutely injured patient, where hypovolemia is common.

V. ANESTHETICS

General or regional anesthesia may be required for invasive procedures including extensive dressing changes or debridement. Alternatively, IV anesthetics can be used for less invasive bedside procedures.

A. Ketamine

Ketamine, an NMDA receptor antagonist, has a long history of use for dressing changes because of its potent analgesic action with relative paucity of respiratory depressant effects.

B. Propofol

Short-acting anesthetics such as propofol are also useful when there is a recurring need for sedation such as for dressing changes, debridement, and grafting.

C. Regional Anesthesia

Regional anesthesia techniques, that is, brachial plexus blocks, femoral nerve blocks, and epidural, can be used to provide analgesia to anatomically limited burn areas (for extended periods of time, catheters can be placed and continuous infusions used).

VI. NONPHARMACOLOGIC

Nonpharmacological techniques such as cognitive behavioral therapy and hypnosis have a limited but proven role in the management of burn pain. Their utility lies in changing the patient's perception of the pain, thereby decreasing reliance on medications. This may serve them well in the long run, as prolonged pain affects mood and coping.

The treatment of pain associated with burns presents a challenge which draws upon the varied skills of the pain physician.

Selected Readings

Burn Incidence and Treatment in the United States: 2016. American Burn Association; 2012. http://ameriburn.org/who-we-are/media/burn-incidence-fact-sheet/. Accessed May 31, 2020.

Castro R, Leal P, Sakata R. Pain management in burn patients. *Rev Bras Anestesiol.* 2012;63(1):149-158.

Norman A, Judkins K. Pain in the patient with burns. *Contin Educ Anaesth Crit Care Pain.* 2004;4(2):57-61.

33 Pain Management for Sickle Cell Disease

Qing Yang and Shiqian Shen

I. INTRODUCTION

Sickle cell disease (SCD) is the most common inherited disorder in the United States, accruing $2.4 billion in health care costs each year. The majority of those affected are of African American and Hispanic origins. Acute pain associated with vaso-occlusive crisis is the hallmark presentation of SCD and the main reason for emergency room visits and hospitalizations. Inadequate treatment of pain and lack of follow-up result in high readmission rates. Treatment goals for acute pain episodes are to alleviate pain, prevent readmissions, and prevent long-term complications. Prompt administration of IV analgesia is crucial. Opioids (fentanyl, morphine, hydromorphone) are typically used. Patient-controlled analgesia (PCA) is an effective and efficient way to stabilize acute pain, followed by transition to a multimodal oral regimen. Chronic pain is associated with degenerative complications such as leg ulcers, disc disease, and avascular necrosis and managed with pharmacological and functional therapies. Chronic opioid therapy in SCD is controversial given that side effects, tolerance, and dependence are inevitable. Hydroxyurea increases fetal hemoglobin levels, prevents sickling, decreases frequency of pain episodes, and prevents organ damage and thus is recommended as a standard daily therapy. Emotional and social impacts of SCD create bias and mistrust between patients and health care providers. Respect, objectivity, and accurate assessment of patient needs are important in delivering satisfactory pain management for SCD patients.

II. OVERVIEW

A. Epidemiology

1. SCD affects 70 000-100 000 people in the United States. Another 3.5 million people are heterozygote carriers of the hemoglobin S (HbS) gene (have the "sickle cell trait"). The majority of the patients are of African descent. Smaller fractions are Hispanic, Middle Eastern, Mediterranean, or Asian Indian. Roughly 1 in 365 African Americans are born with the disease, and 1 in 13 are carriers.

2. Several subtypes of sickle cell disease exist, based on genetic composition and associated clinical severity (see Table 33.1). The most prevalent form is SS, where the patient has two copies of the HbS allele. Sβ-thalassemia patients have only one functional β-globin gene, which produces HbS, resulting in disease as severe as HbSS.
3. Average life expectancy is 42 years in men and 48 years in women. Median survival to age 18 is 94%.

B. Pathophysiology

1. Normal adult hemoglobin (HbA_1) is composed of two α-globin and two β-globin peptides. In SCD, a missense mutation from A to T converts the codon coding for amino acid 6 in the β-globin chain from glutamic acid (GAG) to valine (GTG), producing HbS.
2. When deoxygenated, HbS forms polymers through hydrophobic interactions, deforming the red cell membrane, producing the characteristic sickled shape. Sickled RBCs increase blood viscosity and activate endothelial cells that attract adhesion of both white and red blood cells, leading to formation of heterocellular aggregates and vaso-occlusion. Local hypoxia further fuels the cycle of sickling, inflammation, free radical formation, and reperfusion injury. Hb normally plays a role in nitric oxide (NO) transport, binding and releasing NO to peripheral tissues. HbS leads to functional NO deficiency, further contributing to vasoconstriction and hypoxia.
3. Fetal hemoglobin (HbF) prevents sickling. Higher HbF level is predictive of less severe disease. HbF concentration >20% is associated with decreased risk of painful crises and complications.

C. Complications and Organ Systems Affected

1. Hematologic

Fragility of sickled RBCs predisposes them to hemolysis and sequestration by the spleen. SCD patients are chronically anemic, with baseline Hb levels between 6 and 9 g/dL. Precipitous drop in Hb may develop during splenic sequestration (splenic enlargement, circulatory collapse), aplastic crisis (associated with parvovirus B19 infection), or overwhelming hemolysis, necessitating transfusion. The bone marrow has a high turnover rate and requires nutritional supplementation of iron and folic acid. Spleen autoinfarction occurs by late childhood, making patients vulnerable to infection by encapsulated organisms including meningitis, pneumonia, cholecystitis, osteomyelitis, and sepsis.

2. Neurologic

Tissue damage from vaso-occlusion and hypoxia can occur at multiple foci, leading to multisystem complications. Stroke occurs in 11% of patients by age 20. Silent small cerebrovascular infarcts are much more common, resulting in developmental delays and cognitive impairment. Routine screening of children by transcranial Doppler is recommended. Transfusion of those with increased Doppler velocities to keep HbS concentration below 30% has been shown to reduce the risk of stroke to <1%. Proliferative retinopathy results from occlusion of peripheral retinal vasculature and affects up to 70% of SCD patients.

3. Cardiopulmonary

SCD patients are at increased risk of venous thromboembolism and pulmonary embolism due to increased blood viscosity, endothelial dysfunction, and stasis. Patients with a history of acute chest syndrome (ACS) are prone to

TABLE 33.1 Genetic Variations of Sickle Cell Disease

Sickle Cell Disease Type	Prevalence (% of SCD Patients)	Common Ethnicity	Hemoglobin Composition in Adults %					Hemoglobin Level (g/dL)	Clinical Severity
			HbS	HbA_1	HbA_2	HbF	Other		
SS	65%	African	>90	0	2	<10		6-9	Severe
$S\beta^0$-thalassemia	2%	African, Mediterranean	>80	0	5	<20		7-9	Severe
$S\beta^+$-thalassemia	8%	African, Mediterranean	>60	10-30	4	<20		9-12	Mild to moderate
SC	25%	African, Hispanic	50	0	2	≤1	C: 45	9-14	Moderate
SD	Rare	South Asian, European	50	0	2-3	≤1	D: 47	7-9	Moderate to severe
SE	Rare	Southeast Asian	60	0	2	1-5	E: 33	10-12	Mild
SO	Rare	Middle East, Balkan	50	0	2	<10	O: 40	6-9	Severe
Sickle cell trait AS	—	African, Caribbean	≤40	>60	2	≤1		Normal	No disease
Normal AA	—	—	0	96	2-3	<2		Normal	No disease

Adapted from Yawn BP, et al. Management of sickle cell disease: summary of the 2014 evidence-based report by expert panel members. *JAMA*. 2014;312(10):1033-1048; CDC. Sickle Cell Disease: Data and Statistics. August 31, 2016; Lovett PB, Sule HP, Lopez BL. Sickle cell disease in the emergency department. *Emerg Med Clin North Am*. 2014;32(3):629-647; Zimmerman SA, et al. Hemoglobin S/O(Arab): thirteen new cases and review of the literature. *Am J Hematol*. 1999;60(4):279-284.

develop chronic restrictive lung diseases. Pulmonary hypertension is increasingly recognized as a chronic complication, leading to exercise intolerance, fatigue, and heart failure. Echocardiographic abnormalities have been reported in over 75% of SCD patients, most commonly enlarged left atrium and left ventricle, and tricuspid regurgitation.

4. Gastrointestinal and Renal

Chronic kidney disease occurs in 4%-18% of SCD patients due to renal medulla ischemia. Cholestasis and cholelithiasis develop over time as the result of hemolysis and increased bilirubin turnover. Priapism occurs as the result of low flow, stasis, and hypoxia and presents a urological emergency. Prolonged priapism may be preceded by stuttering priapism or short, self-limited episodes.

5. Musculoskeletal

Avascular necrosis develops in 10%-30% of patients. Bone, most commonly the femoral head, dies because of compromised vascular supply. This can cause severe chronic pain and limited mobility. Another form of vascular complications and source of chronic pain is persistent, nonhealing leg ulcers, which can coexist with osteomyelitis.

III. ACUTE PAIN

A. Vaso-occlusive Crisis (VOC)

1. Overview

Vaso-occlusive crisis is the most common presentation of SCD, responsible for 82% of emergency room visits and 76% of hospitalizations among adult sickle cell patients.

a. On average, HbSS patients have 1 VOC episode per year. The incidence is lower for other subtypes. Less than 40% of patients experience no painful episodes in any given year. About 5%-6% of patients have more than three episodes per year, and 1% has more than six episodes, accounting for significant medical resource utilization. One-month readmission rate after crisis discharge ranges from 33% to 63% in various studies. Young adults aged 18-30 exhibit the highest rates of readmission.

b. Microvascular occlusion from sickling leads to ischemia, tissue damage, inflammation, and activation of nociceptors. Triggers of VOC include increased blood viscosity, hypoxia, dehydration, vascular stasis, infection, fever, hypothermia, cardiopulmonary impairments, and acidosis. Other associated conditions include concurrent α-thalassemia, ambient weather and humidity changes, altitude change, and psychological stress. Low HbF level is an independent risk factor, and high HbF level protects against the development of acute pain episodes.

c. Extensive infarction of vascular beds due to occlusive crisis can lead to bone marrow necrosis, presenting as sharp, severe pain of the long bones or vertebra. Necrotic particles from the bone marrow may provoke ACS or fat embolism, which can be life threatening.

d. Acute painful crisis is associated with serious complications including ACS, organ infarction, and sudden death.

2. Assessment of Pain

a. Acute pain associated with SCD is often described as unbearable, agonizing, and constant, with a deep somatic quality (crushing, squeezing, pounding, throbbing). The pain experience is unique to each patient, who may be able to tell if the current episode is typical for him or her, aiding in the diagnosis.

b. Progression of VOC pain has been described in four phases:

i. Prodromal—in the few days preceding an episode, the patient may feel fluctuating aches, numbness, or paresthesia in areas that subsequently become painful.

ii. Initial—characterized by increasingly intense pain.

iii. Established—pain of maximal intensity with signs of inflammation such as joint effusion.

iv. Resolving—after a period of hours to days or even weeks, pain subsides, and the requirement for analgesia decreases. Inflammation may persist during the resolving phase, and patients are at risk for readmission.

c. Classically VOC pain is located in the back and extremities. Pain may be migratory. Most commonly affected bones are the humerus, sternum, ribs, tibia, and femur. In infants and children, VOC may affect the hands and feet, presenting as dactylitis.

d. Routine laboratory evaluation is not required for patients presenting with classical VOC pain. In fact, excessive laboratory or imaging studies may delay analgesic administration and thus are not recommended unless other etiologies are suspected, the patient appears systematically unwell, or there is worsening anemia or jaundice.

Providers should rule out other causes of pain, including infection; ACS; acute abdominal pathology such as gallstones, pancreatitis, appendicitis, and peptic ulcer disease; infarction of visceral vessels (ischemic colitis); and splenic sequestration. Providers must also be mindful of other concurrent conditions that are not painful and may be overlooked due to preoccupation with pain.

B. Treatment

1. Prompt triage and analgesic administration constitute the hallmark of treatment for patients with sickle cell crisis. As there is no reliable objective measure of pain severity, analgesia should be titrated to the patient's report. Goals of treatment are to alleviate pain, prevent readmission, and prevent long-term complications.

2. Prompt opioid administration

a. IV opioid is the fastest way to achieve analgesia for painful emergencies. Morphine (0.1 mg/kg), fentanyl (1 μg/kg), and hydromorphone (0.015 mg/kg) are routinely used. It is recommended that a potent and rapid-acting opioid be given within 30 minutes of arrival to the emergency room.

b. Transmucosal fentanyl (buccal effervescent tablet, lozenge, or sublingual tablet) offers rapid onset and has been reported to be effective for acute sickle cell pain in the absence of IV access.

c. Diamorphine (heroin) has been successfully used for VOC in the United Kingdom.

d. Meperidine and codeine are no longer preferred due to concerns for side effects (especially seizures with higher doses of meperidine), variable metabolism, and drug interactions.

e. Dosing can be guided by each patient's outpatient pain regimen and the typical dose and type of opioid that is required to relieve pain for that particular patient.

3. PCA is an efficacious alternative to frequent boluses of IV opioid during the established phase of pain. Fentanyl, morphine, and hydromorphone are commonly used for PCA.

4. Pain scores, respiratory rate, and sedation score should be checked and documented in 30-minute to 1-hour intervals initially, then every 3-6 hours during the acute pain presentation. The goal is to achieve pain scores close to the patient's baseline and maintain respiratory rate above the lower limit for age and mental status of alert to mild sedation.

5. Once pain is stabilized and the total opioid requirement is established, the patient may be transitioned to maintenance analgesia. Oral long- and short-acting morphine or oxycodone may be used in combination with around-the-clock acetaminophen and NSAIDs. Transdermal fentanyl and methadone at equal analgesic doses of total opioid requirement have also been successfully used.
6. Careful monitoring and treatment of side effects should be included as part of the management strategy. Patients should receive antiemetics for nausea and vomiting and scheduled bowel regimen for constipation.
7. Indications for fluids and transfusion
   a. Previously, hydration has been the mainstay of VOC management because of the thought that RBC dehydration contributes to sickling. Aggressive fluid therapy is no longer recommended as studies demonstrated no clear benefits and fluid overload increases the risk of pulmonary edema and ACS. IV fluid boluses should be reserved for hypovolemia.
   b. Transfusion is indicated for urgent management for acute anemia, ACS, stroke, circulatory collapse associated with splenic or hepatic sequestration or aplastic crisis, multiorgan failure, and perioperative situations. It is not indicated for routine treatment of uncomplicated VOC, priapism, or asymptomatic anemia. Transfusion is associated with risks of immune reactions, circulatory overload, iron toxicity, and increased blood viscosity and thus may worsen existing disease.
   c. In the perioperative setting, exchange transfusion to decrease HbS concentration to $<30\%$ or simple transfusion to increase total Hb to ≥ 10 g/dL may be employed. The two protocols showed no difference in mortality or major complications such as frequency of VOC, ACS, or infection.
8. Adjuncts and alternative therapies
   a. Invasive regional or neuroaxial analgesia is rarely performed in SCD patients, except for special circumstances such as in a laboring woman with concurrent pain crisis.
   b. Steroid use for acute pain in SCD is not recommended. Although some trials have shown that high doses of methylprednisolone decreased the duration of the pain, it is associated with increased length of stay, rebound pain after discontinuation, long-term toxicity, and readmission.
   c. Low-dose infusions of ketamine and dexmedetomidine (0.2-1 μg/kg/h) may be useful as adjuvant therapy, especially in patients who have persistent pain despite escalating opioid doses and/or who experience significant opioid-related side effects such as respiratory depression. Decrease in subjective pain scores and opioid requirements have been reported following 3-7 days of infusion. Weaning of dexmedetomidine should be done gradually in a controlled fashion to avoid withdrawal and rebound hypertension and may be facilitated by transitioning to a clonidine patch.
   d. NO availability has been implicated in SCD pathogenesis. Preliminary studies suggest inhaled NO promotes vasodilation and reduces the tendency of HbS to polymerize and thus may be beneficial for VOC, although large-scale trials have been inconclusive.
   e. More than 70%-90% of sickle cell patients report engaging in alternative and complementary therapy to manage their pain, including prayer, relaxation, biofeedback, acupuncture, hypnosis, herbal medicine,

and massage. Female gender, higher education, and higher household income are associated with alternative therapy utilization. Current evidence for the efficacy of these modalities is limited by poor study design, high risk of bias, and statistically nonsignificant outcomes. Providers should be aware of these behaviors and patients' belief in the potential benefits.

9. Lack of follow-up with hematologist, asthma comorbidity, pain, and treatment with steroids constitute main risk factors for readmission after discharge from a VOC episode. Thus, smooth transition of care and plan for adequate outpatient pain control are crucial.

C. Acute Chest Syndrome

1. ACS, defined as new pulmonary infiltrates (often bilateral) on chest x-ray, accompanied by fever and respiratory symptoms such as cough and rales, is a serious complication and part of the differential diagnosis during acute pain crisis admissions. Up to 3% of patients with ACS die. Mechanism of ACS encompasses hypoxia and inflammation-induced occlusion of pulmonary vasculature; hypoventilation, which may be pain or opioid related; infection; and fat embolism.
2. Management of ACS includes empirical antibiotics, supplemental oxygen if hypoxemic, and exchange transfusion for severe cases.

D. Preventive Therapy

1. Hydroxyurea is a cytotoxic nucleotide analog that induces HbF production in the bone marrow through a state of stress erythropoiesis. HbF inhibits HbS polymerization and sickling. Whether hydroxyurea also directly affect endothelial function, blood rheology, and inflammation is still under investigation. Large-scale randomized controlled trials demonstrates that long-term daily hydroxyurea leads to 40%-50% reduction in the incidence of acute pain episodes, ACS, need for transfusions, and splenic autoinfarction, as well as mortality benefit and improved quality of life. Since approved by the FDA in 1998, it has now become a standard therapy for SCD.
2. Hydroxyurea should be initiated in adult patients with ≥3 pain crises in 1 year, history of severe or recurrent ACS, or chronic pain that interferes with daily activities and quality of life and in infants or children older than 9 months of age regardless of the presence of symptoms or clinical severity in order to prevent complications. Starting dosage is typically 15 mg/kg/d for adults and 20 mg/kg/d for children. CBC with differential and reticulocyte count is monitored. Dose may be escalated to achieve mild myelosuppression (absolute neutrophil count 2000-4000/μL). Clinical response may take several months, and there is significant individual variation. An increase in HbF level to 8%-18% above baseline is expected. Hydroxyurea should be continued during episodes of acute illness and hospitalizations. Hydroxyurea is contraindicated in pregnant and lactating women. Dosage should be reduced for renal impairment.

IV. CHRONIC PAIN

A. Types of Chronic Pain in SCD

1. Chronic pain is defined as pain lasting longer than 6 months with negative effects on the patient's life. On average, sickle cell patients report having pain for half of their days at home. A third of patients report pain on 95% of the days. Over 90% of patients take pain medications on a daily basis. In SCD, the main type of chronic pain is related to degenerative complications such as leg ulcers, avascular necrosis of joints, and chronic

osteomyelitis. Patients may also have persistent pain between acute pain episodes, with central sensitization, alterations in pain pathways, and opioid-induced hyperalgesia as proposed mechanisms.

2. Neuropathic pain has been reported in sickle cell patients. This type of pain is initiated by primary dysfunction of the nervous system resulting from chronic inflammation, nerve damage, and neuronal sensitization. In studies examining patient-reported symptoms, up to 40% of patients gave descriptors characteristic of neuropathic pain, such as burning, cold, numb, and radiating. Studies have demonstrated increased temperature sensitivity (thermal hyperalgesia) and decreased neural conduction threshold in SCD patients, pointing to peripheral and central sensitization as mechanisms for the observed neuropathic pain. Clinical trials of neuropathic analgesics, for example, gabapentin, in SCD are under way.

B. Management

1. Management of chronic pain focuses the reduction of the impact of persistent pain and calls for a multidisciplinary approach. Pharmacological control mainly involves a combination of PO long-acting or controlled-release opioids and nonopioid therapy.

   a. NSAIDs

   NSAIDs have anti-inflammatory, analgesic, and antipyretic effects. Acetaminophen is a centrally acting analgesic and antipyretic. As with other types of chronic pain, general healthy habits, education, and coping skills training help manage expectations and improve function.

   b. Opioids

   Opioid use for chronic SCD, apart from acute pain crises, remains controversial. One study showed that 75% of SCD patients are prescribed opioids as part of their home regimen. Although the median opioid dosage was significantly lower in SCD compared to other chronic pain syndromes, up to 15% of patients took more than 50 mg oral morphine equivalent daily. Risk factors for high chronic opioid use include a history of avascular necrosis, low vitamin D level, and low bilirubin level. Prolonged opioid use is associated with undesirable side effects such as constipation, tolerance, and physical and psychological addiction. Prudence is needed when prescribing opioids as part of the patient's long-term management.

   c. Addiction and pseudoaddiction

   Providers need to differentiate addiction from pseudoaddiction. Drug abuse and addiction to the nonanalgesic effects of opioids have been reported in SCD patients, but the rate is no higher than the general patient population. Pseudoaddiction describes the behavior of requesting stronger analgesic because of persistent pain. The drug-seeking behavior ceases once pain is adequately controlled. The use of the term psuedoaddiction has fallen out of favor, as it is difficult to differentiate those seeking higher drug doses for abuse and diversion from those who legitimately require larger doses of opioid to control their pain.

   d. Cognitive behavioral therapy (CBT)

   CBT has the most empirical support as a nonpharmacological intervention for SCD pain. Half of the clinical trials to date have shown positive outcomes. Cognitive coping skills and education to alter pain perception may help lower pain scores and reduce the length and frequency of painful episodes.

2. Functional and surgical corrections should be considered when appropriate to the etiology of pain. For example, leg ulcers necessitate input from wound care centers. Large, persistent, gangrenous ulcers may require

amputation, which has been reported to provide pain relief and improve the quality of life. Avascular necrosis should be evaluated by orthopedics for joint replacement, as well as by physical therapy and rheumatology.

C. Curative Therapy

1. Stem Cell Transplant

Allogeneic hematopoietic stem cell transplant is the only known curative therapy for SCD. Typically patients undergo myeloablative conditioning with chemotherapy medications, followed by stem cell transplant from HLA-matched siblings, with a 5-year disease-free survival rate of 85%. The procedure not only alleviates the symptoms of SCD but also stabilizes or reverses the associated organ damage. Unrelated umbilical cord blood has also been used as an alternative source of stem cells, but the rate of graft failure is high. Currently only high-risk, severe SCD patients are candidates for stem cell transplant. Indications include history of stroke, abnormal transcranial Doppler studies, recurrent VOC and ACS, and failure, noncompliance, or contraindication for hydroxyurea.

2. Gene Therapy

Gene therapy using viral vectors and autologous stem cell transplant following *in vitro* gene correction are under investigation.

V. PSYCHOSOCIAL CONSIDERATIONS

A. The impact of pain reaches broad aspects of the sickle cell patient's life, including education, employment, independence, and social relationships. Patients often feel trapped by the intensity, frequency, and constant presence of pain, experiencing various negative emotions such as fear, uselessness, and helplessness. Depression and anxiety have been reported in 10%-27% of patients. In the United States and other Western countries, the sickle cell patient population mainly consists of minorities from socioeconomically disadvantaged backgrounds. Frequent hospitalizations for painful crisis since young age result in missed opportunities for meeting social, educational, and vocational milestones, further hindering their success and advancement in society. Children often exhibit low achievement, poor academic performance, and deficit in interpersonal skills as a result of social and cognitive deprivation. Adolescents and adults continue to have trouble building substantive relationships, gaining and keeping employment, and developing active coping strategies. These psychosocial comorbidities must be considered when treating SCD patients.

B. It is widely documented that medical providers have cognitive biases toward sickle cell patients. Providers may question the genuineness of painful crises in patients with frequent episodes and hospital visits. They may apply labels such as "drug seeking," "addicted," "demanding," and "difficult" to these patients, leading to delayed and suboptimal treatment of pain. Perceived health care injustice evokes in the patients negative emotions and maladaptive behaviors such as catastrophizing and isolation, increasing pain levels and psychological distress. Conversely, sense of justice and therapeutic alliance with providers leads to effective coping strategies and positive pain outcomes. In order to promote trust and respect, patients and their caretakers should be regarded as experts in their condition, and their views and concerns should be discussed when formulating treatment plans. As in other chronic pain conditions, social support and self-empowerment are important aspects of care.

Selected Readings

Ballas SK, Gupta K, Adams-Graves P. Sickle cell pain: a critical reappraisal. *Blood.* 2012;120(18):3647-3656.

Brandow AM, Farley RA, Panepinto JA. Early insights into the neurobiology of pain in sickle cell disease: a systematic review of the literature. *Pediatr Blood Cancer.* 2015;62(9):1501-1511.

Brown SE, et al. Sickle cell disease patients with and without extremely high hospital use: pain, opioids, and coping. *J Pain Symptom Manage.* 2015;49(3):539-547.

Campbell CM, et al. An evaluation of central sensitization in patients with sickle cell disease. *J Pain.* 2016;17(5):617-627.

CDC. *Sickle Cell Disease: Data and Statistics.* August 31, 2016. http://www.cdc.gov/ncbddd/sicklecell/data.html

Charache S, et al. Effect of hydroxyurea on the frequency of painful crises in sickle cell anemia. Investigators of the Multicenter Study of Hydroxyurea in Sickle Cell Anemia. *N Engl J Med.* 1995;332(20):1317-1322.

Chou ST, Fasano RM. Management of patients with sickle cell disease using transfusion therapy: guidelines and complications. *Hematol Oncol Clin North Am.* 2016;30(3):591-608.

Coleman B, et al. How sickle cell disease patients experience, understand and explain their pain: an Interpretative Phenomenological Analysis study. *Br J Health Psychol.* 2016;21(1):190-203.

De Franceschi L, et al. Fentanyl buccal tablet: a new breakthrough pain medication in early management of severe vaso-occlusive crisis in sickle cell disease. *Pain Pract.* 2016;16(6):680-687.

Edwards CL, et al. A brief review of the pathophysiology, associated pain, and psychosocial issues in sickle cell disease. *Int J Behav Med.* 2005;12(3):171-179.

Enninful-Eghan H, et al. Transcranial Doppler ultrasonography and prophylactic transfusion program is effective in preventing overt stroke in children with sickle cell disease. *J Pediatr.* 2010;157(3):479-484.

Estcourt LJ, et al. Preoperative blood transfusions for sickle cell disease. *Cochrane Database Syst Rev.* 2016;4:CD003149.

Ezenwa MO, et al. Coping with pain in the face of healthcare injustice in patients with sickle cell disease. *J Immigr Minor Health.* 2017;19(6):1449-1456.

Field JJ, Knight-Perry JE, Debaun MR. Acute pain in children and adults with sickle cell disease: management in the absence of evidence-based guidelines. *Curr Opin Hematol.* 2009;16(3):173-178.

Freed J, et al. Allogeneic cellular and autologous stem cell therapy for sickle cell disease: 'whom, when and how'. *Bone Marrow Transplant.* 2012;47(12):1489-1498.

Gillis VL, et al. Management of an acute painful sickle cell episode in hospital: summary of NICE guidance. *BMJ.* 2012;344:e4063.

Gladwin MT, Crawford JH, Patel RP. The biochemistry of nitric oxide, nitrite, and hemoglobin: role in blood flow regulation. *Free Radic Biol Med.* 2004;36(6):707-717.

Gladwin MT, et al. Nitric oxide for inhalation in the acute treatment of sickle cell pain crisis: a randomized controlled trial. *JAMA.* 2011;305(9):893-902.

Green NS, Barral S. Emerging science of hydroxyurea therapy for pediatric sickle cell disease. *Pediatr Res.* 2014;75(1-2):196-204.

Han J, et al. Patterns of opioid use in sickle cell disease. *Am J Hematol.* 2016;91(11):1102-1106.

Head CA, et al. Beneficial effects of nitric oxide breathing in adult patients with sickle cell crisis. *Am J Hematol.* 2010;85(10):800-802.

Inoue S, et al. Pain management trend of vaso-occlusive crisis (VOC) at a community hospital emergency department (ED) for patients with sickle cell disease. *Ann Hematol.* 2016;95(2):221-225.

Jordan L, et al. Multicenter COMPACT study of COMplications in patients with sickle cell disease and utilization of iron chelation therapy. *Curr Med Res Opin.* 2015;31(3):513-523.

Lanzkron S, Carroll CP, Haywood C Jr. The burden of emergency department use for sickle-cell disease: an analysis of the national emergency department sample database. *Am J Hematol.* 2010;85(10):797-799.

Lovett PB, Sule HP, Lopez BL. Sickle cell disease in the emergency department. *Emerg Med Clin North Am.* 2014;32(3):629-647.

Lutz B, et al. Updated mechanisms of sickle cell disease-associated chronic pain. *Transl Perioper Pain Med.* 2015;2(2):8-17.
Maioli MC, et al. Relationship between pulmonary and cardiac abnormalities in sickle cell disease: implications for the management of patients. *Rev Bras Hematol Hemoter.* 2016;38(1):21-27.
Maximo C, et al. Amputations in sickle cell disease: case series and literature review. *Hemoglobin.* 2016;40(3):150-155.
Niscola P, et al. Pain syndromes in sickle cell disease: an update. *Pain Med.* 2009;10(3): 470-480.
Pizzo E, et al. A retrospective analysis of the cost of hospitalizations for sickle cell disease with crisis in England, 2010/11. *J Public Health (Oxf).* 2015;37(3):529-539.
Powars DR, Chan L, Schroeder WA. The influence of fetal hemoglobin on the clinical expression of sickle cell anemia. *Ann N Y Acad Sci.* 1989;565:262-278.
Sheehy KA, et al. Dexmedetomidine as an adjuvant to analgesic strategy during vaso-occlusive episodes in adolescents with sickle-cell disease. *Pain Pract.* 2015;15(8): E90-E97.
Telfer P, et al. Management of the acute painful crisis in sickle cell disease—a re-evaluation of the use of opioids in adult patients. *Br J Haematol.* 2014;166(2): 157-164.
Thompson WE, Eriator I. Pain control in sickle cell disease patients: use of complementary and alternative medicine. *Pain Med.* 2014;15(2):241-246.
Uprety D, Baber A, Foy M. Ketamine infusion for sickle cell pain crisis refractory to opioids: a case report and review of literature. *Ann Hematol.* 2014;93(5):769-771.
Vichinsky EP, et al. Acute chest syndrome in sickle cell disease: clinical presentation and course. Cooperative Study of Sickle Cell Disease. *Blood.* 1997;89(5): 1787-1792.
Weiner DL, et al. Preliminary assessment of inhaled nitric oxide for acute vaso-occlusive crisis in pediatric patients with sickle cell disease. *JAMA.* 2003;289(9):1136-1142.
Williams H, Tanabe P. Sickle cell disease: a review of nonpharmacological approaches for pain. *J Pain Symptom Manage.* 2016;51(2):163-177.
Yawn BP, et al. Management of sickle cell disease: summary of the 2014 evidence-based report by expert panel members. *JAMA.* 2014;312(10):1033-1048.
Zimmerman SA, et al. Hemoglobin S/O(Arab): thirteen new cases and review of the literature. *Am J Hematol.* 1999;60(4):279-284.

34 Pain Management in the Trauma Patient

Saad Mohammad and David A. Edwards

I. INTRODUCTION

Trauma is a major source of morbidity and mortality and is the leading cause of death in those <44 years of age. The evaluation and management of trauma injury is a field supported by decades of practice and research in battlefield medicine and applied in austere environments and on the front lines by emergency medical services in urban and rural environments.

II. MECHANISM OF PAIN IN TRAUMA

Traumatic injury can result in acute severe pain. The mechanism of injury often results in damage of multiple tissue types so pain involves all modalities:

A. Nociceptive Pain (Somatic or Visceral)

This is pain that results from activation of nociceptors. Examples include pain that results from movement of limbs against fractured bones or peristalsis of viscera against an ulceration or perforation.

B. Inflammatory Pain

This is pain that is caused by injuries that result in inflammation and the release of inflammatory mediators that lower the threshold for nerve firing and trigger transmission of pain, that is, burn, abrasion, penetrating injury, contusion, fracture, and ischemia.

C. Neuropathic Pain

This is pain that is caused by injuries that result in nerve transection, crush, stretch, or other direct damage, that is, concussive sheer injury, limb crush, and burn.

The body location injured and the mechanism of injury more specifically define the tissues involved and the degree of injury expected. Some modifying factors include the timing of presentation to a practitioner for treatment, the environment (battlefield, sports arena, highway collision), and preexisting patient features including coexisting disease and psychosomatic state (catastrophizing).

III. CONSIDERATIONS

The circumstances of trauma and the individual patient state can modify the perception of pain. In high-intensity situations, sympathetic stimulation can reduce the perception of pain but is often specific to the individual. While much still needs to be learned about the mechanisms behind chronification of pain, the severity of acute pain is a predictor of chronic pain. So, it is prudent to either prevent or rapidly treat acute severe pain.

A. Austere Settings

Traumatic injury can occur anywhere so treatment will depend on available supplies. First responders, while providing rescue, also stabilize and treat pain during transport to care centers. It is extremely important to have trained personnel respond not only to safety and survival but also, once stabilized, to attend to pain control to limit suffering and the long-term sequelae of severe pain.

Multimodal analgesia should be used in austere setting to reduce the likelihood of side effects from any one modality. For example, treat acute pain with available low-risk analgesics such as acetaminophen, nonsteroidal anti-inflammatory drugs (NSAIDs) where appropriate, and ketamine in order to limit the overall dose of opioids and their risks.

A strong understanding of anatomy is crucial for regional anesthesia done by landmark technique or with a nerve stimulator. Mobile ultrasound has reduced the need for purely anatomical-based regional techniques in many austere settings.

B. Chronicity of Trauma Pain

Crush injury, blast injury, amputation, and other traumatic injuries that occur in high emotional states may result in chronic pain. Rapid treatment and control of pain lessens severe suffering and may also reduce the likelihood of developing chronic pain. Chronic pain and chronic psychological disorders (posttraumatic stress disorder) often coexist and should be treated concurrently.

C. Surgery as Trauma

Surgery is itself a controlled trauma to tissue. Setting patient expectation for surgery and empowering patients with proper education lessens the emotional impact and perception of pain.

IV. THERAPEUTIC OPTIONS

Acute severe pain is often not treated depending on the geographical location of the trauma and availability of supplies. In these instances, limb positioning, bracing, and immobilization can be used to limit nociceptive pain and ischemic pain from poor perfusion. Where medications are available, opioids are relatively inexpensive and potent analgesics but must be used by those who know how to manage the potential side effects of depressed mental state, slowed breathing and even apnea, and muscle rigidity.

A. Medications

Useful analgesics for acute pain are discussed in Chapter 30 (Adult Postoperative Pain) on postoperative acute pain. The options may be limited depending on regional availability. Some additional points regarding the use of these medications are mentioned here:

1. **Acetaminophen**—this central-acting cyclooxygenase (COX) antagonist provides analgesia through a different mechanism than other COX antagonists, such as typical NSAIDs, and therefore can be a safe adjunct for acute pain. Adjustment must be made for patients with liver disease.
2. **Ketorolac and other NSAIDs**—treatment of inflammatory pain with NSAIDs can be especially effective. Intravenous NSAIDs are as effective as low-dose opioids and can be lifesaving in scenarios where opioid sedation can further put the patient at risk (ie, rib fractures in patients at risk of aspiration, respiratory decline).
3. **Ketamine**—in controlled situations and in the hands of emergency responders or other skilled clinicians, ketamine is an extremely useful potent analgesic. The side effects of increased secretions and hallucinations must be understood and able to be managed by the clinician. Ketamine as an adjunct or alone can be used to limit the need for opioids and reduce their risks.
4. **Opioids**—the type of opioid available depends on the country. It is important for clinicians working in austere settings to know the available analgesics in their location. Opioids are some of the most potent analgesics, but they also have some high-risk side effects such as sedation and respiratory depression. Opioids are indispensable at this time, for acute severe pain unable to be controlled by regional anesthesia.

B. Regional Anesthesia

Traumatic injury that results in peripheral limb or trunk injury is often able to be treated with regional anesthetic techniques. There is a high learning curve to be able to perform regional anesthesia safely. Some risks include direct nerve injury, vascular puncture, pneumothorax, respiratory depression (ie, if multiple intercostal nerves or the phrenic nerve are blocked), infection (ie, with bowel perforation or blocks done in unsterile conditions), or paralysis (spinal cord injury). An expert understanding of external and internal anatomy, and sonographic anatomy when using ultrasound, is a prerequisite. Moreover, knowledge of weight-based maximal allowable doses for the local anesthetics is crucial to prevent local anesthetic systemic toxicity (LAST) (see Chapter 30: Adult Postoperative Pain).

1. **Rib and sternal fractures**—falls, tractor rollovers, car accidents, etc. can result in multiple rib fractures and flail chest, making it painful to breath. Proper analgesia can decrease chest wall splinting and alveolar collapse and improves deep breathing and secretion clearing, all of which can help the patient avoid pneumonia. Regional anesthesia techniques include continuous thoracic epidural infusion, paravertebral block, intrapleural infusions, and intercostal nerve blocks. Epidural and paravertebral blocks can help to control the pain without the need for high doses of opioids and prevent need for intubation. Often pneumothorax or hemothorax with contusions co-occur with rib fractures. Without adequate pain control, patients (especially elderly) may decompensate and require intubation.

   Assessment involves interviewing the patient and viewing signs of pending respiratory failure, such as inability to inspire (use an incentive spirometer to track patient ability to breathe deeply), declining oxygenation on pulse oximetry. Computed tomography or plain films should be viewed to identify the number and location of fractures. If regional anesthesia is requested for pain control, images can also be used to assess potential trajectory of epidural placement to ensure there are no free bony fragments in the way, preexisting epidural hematoma, or evidence of spinal cord injury.

Treatment of mild to moderate pain from rib fractures can be escalated if a patient's respiratory status declines. One strategy would be to start with NSAIDs and low-dose opioids, titrating to sufficient analgesia. Then, if needed, epidural or paravertebral catheter placement can provide great benefit and potentially prevent the need for intubation. Contraindication to epidural placement would include a patient on anticoagulant medications, spinal cord injury where epidural infusion may mask progressing neurological deficits, epidural hematoma, free bony fragments in the path of epidural placement, and a patient who does not consent.

For patients already intubated, epidural analgesia can facilitate in weaning a patient off the ventilator to enable extubation.

a. **Intrapleural infusion**—this involves placement of local anesthetics directly into the intrapleural space, usually by the surgeon at time of thoracostomy tube placement. Trials have failed to find a clear benefit or improved analgesia compared to epidural technique, and this technique is rarely used.
b. **Intercostal nerve blockade**—this technique can be used to achieve analgesia but is limited due to the multiple injections needed, duration of block, and the need to repeat multiple injections.
c. **Paravertebral block**—this block can be used on unilateral fractures; catheters can be placed allowing continual infusion of local anesthetic. As long as the coverage needed is limited to only a few dermatomes, this technique can be equivalent to epidural analgesia with less risk of hypotension.
d. **Epidural analgesia**—widely used to infuse local anesthetics and opioids. Data show decreased length of mechanical ventilation as well as decreased rate of nosocomial pneumonia when epidural anesthesia is used. There is better pain control and pulmonary function for patients with epidural analgesia compared to intravenous narcotics. Care should be taken in patients with spine fractures and with possible coagulopathy, and standard monitoring should be used.

2. **Limb injury or amputation**—sudden limb amputation can result in severe pain. Coupled with the strong emotional state, risk of chronic pain is high. Rapid treatment of pain with multimodal analgesia to treat all pain modalities is crucial. Sympathectomy from regional anesthesia is particularly useful to maintain limb perfusion until surgical repair can reestablish normal blood flow or to facilitate limb survival in reattachment surgery. Communication with the surgeon is important before using regional anesthesia techniques in patients who may be at risk of compartment syndrome. Although the ischemic pain from compartment syndrome will likely break through low-concentration local anesthetic block, missed diagnosis of compartment syndrome is devastating, and so regional anesthesia should be used cautiously in these patients.

V. SPECIAL POPULATIONS

A. Chronic Pain Patient

1. Opioid Dependence

Analgesia in patients with chronic pain and opioid dependence who are acutely injured can be a challenge to manage due to high rates of tolerance and unpredictable drug effects. Usually these patients are kept on their home level of opioid therapy with increased dosages used to treat increased pain while in the hospital. Multimodal strategies should be employed whenever possible including use of acetaminophen, NSAIDs, ketamine and lidocaine infusions, and regional anesthetics.

2. Methadone

Patients on chronic methadone therapy, either for chronic pain or for substance use disorder, are at risk of suffering more with pain if treatment for acute pain is not adequately managed. The usual oral dose of methadone should be given at the earliest possible time, or if not possible, half the oral dose can be given IV. Another strategy is to take the 24-hour total oral dose and convert that to an hourly dose, and then give half that dose intravenously as an hourly infusion.

3. Buprenorphine

Patients on buprenorphine (Suboxone) can be a challenge due to the high affinity (1000 times that of morphine) of the drug at mu-opioid receptors where it acts as a partial agonist and also as an antagonist at kappa-opioid receptors. The mean half-life is 37 hours. The effects on respiratory drive have a "ceiling effect."

It is recommended to discontinue buprenorphine in the setting of acute pain so that full opioid agonists can be used to control severe pain. Careful titration of the full agonist must be done under monitoring for the first 3 days as buprenorphine is cleared. During the first hours, larger than usual doses of opioid are likely to be needed for pain control. Once the buprenorphine is cleared, and there is less competitive antagonism at the mu-opioid receptor, the doses of opioid needed to control pain may fall significantly. In those with mild to moderate pain, continuation of buprenorphine with or without small supplemental doses of a pure mu-opioid agonist, or even just a slight temporary increase in buprenorphine is often sufficient to provide adequate pain control. Once the patient no longer needs opioids for pain control, buprenorphine monotherapy at the original dose be resumed. Multimodal analgesia including regional anesthesia can be helpful in controlling pain in this at-risk population.

VI. CONCLUSION

Injury during traumatic accident is a broad topic that includes scenarios as diverse as automobile accidents to battlefield blast injury. A common feature is the likelihood of severe pain as a result of multiple tissue–type injury. In this setting, multimodal analgesia is particularly important to mitigate the risks of any one therapy.

Selected Readings

Carrier FM, Turgeon AF, Nicole PC, et al. Effect of epidural analgesia in patients with traumatic rib fractures: a systematic review and meta-analysis of randomized controlled trials. *Can J Anaesth.* 2009;56:230.

Heit HA, Gourlay DL. Buprenorphine: new tricks with an old molecule for pain management. *Clin J Pain.* 2008;24:93.

Ho AM, Karmakar MK, Critchley LA. Acute pain management of patients with multiple fractured ribs: a focus on regional techniques. *Curr Opin Crit Care.* 2011;17:323.

Kelly DJ, Ahmad M, Brull SJ. Preemptive analgesia I: physiological pathways and pharmacological modalities. *Can J Anaesth.* 2001;48:1000.

McNicol ED, Schumann R, Haroutounian S. A systematic review and meta-analysis of ketamine for the prevention of persistent post-surgical pain. *Acta Anaesthesiol Scand.* 2014;58:1199.

Mohta M, Verma P, Saxena AK, et al. Prospective, randomized comparison of continuous thoracic epidural and thoracic paravertebral infusion in patients with unilateral multiple fractured ribs—a pilot study. *J Trauma.* 2009;66:1096.

Quibell R, Prommer EE, Mihalyo M, et al. Ketamine. *J Pain Symptom Manage.* 2011;41:640.

Weibel S, Jokinen J, Pace NL, et al. Efficacy and safety of intravenous lidocaine for postoperative analgesia and recovery after surgery: a systematic review with trial sequential analysis. *Br J Anaesth.* 2016;116:770.

Young A, Buvanendran A. Recent advances in multimodal analgesia. *Anesthesiol Clin.* 2012;30:91.

SECTION VII

Chronic Pain

35 Neuropathic Pain Syndromes

Andrew C. Young and Brian J. Wainger

Neuropathic pain is defined by the International Association for the Study of Pain (IASP) as pain caused by a lesion or disease of the somatosensory nervous system. Nerve injury to the nociceptive afferent tracts of the peripheral or central nervous system can result in pathologic peripheral and central sensitization thereby leading to chronic neuropathic pain. Clinically, neuropathic pain can present with spontaneous (stimulus independent) symptoms of lancinating, burning, electrical, shooting, and tingling sensations as well as evoked (stimulus dependent) features such as allodynia, pain in response to nonnociceptive stimuli, and hyperalgesia, increased pain response to ordinarily noxious stimuli. A common clinical picture of neuropathic pain includes a constellation of these aforementioned positive pain symptoms colocalized with reduced sensory function in the area innervated by injured nerves. Other neurologic symptoms, such as motor or autonomic disturbances, are also common but may go unrecognized.

Neuropathic pain can result from a wide range of etiologies—trauma, infection, ischemia, autoimmune, toxic-metabolic, and mono- or oligogenetic processes—that occur anywhere along the pain sensory transduction pathways. The development of persistent neuropathic pain involves changes in the peripheral and even more so central nervous systems that yield feed-forward amplification of pain signaling modalities. These changes occur in afferent sensory tracts as well as descending tracts that normally suppress pain transmission to the brain. Finally, alterations in the spatial and network representation of pain in the brain serve to augment pain.

Diagnosis and treatment for neuropathic pain remains challenging. While lesions to the thalamus, spinal cord, nerve roots, and large fiber somatic nerves are often more readily identified on clinical examination, nerve injury that results in neuropathic pain can occur with subtle or even no findings on neurological examination. Often, this "invisible pain" creates a psychological burden because family members and medical providers cannot localize the lesion or diagnose a specific disease using traditional lab tests or imaging. Mutual trust and communication between patient and caregivers must be established for effective care.

I. CLINICAL MANIFESTATIONS

The clinical spectrum of neuropathic pain ranges from barely noticeable to severely disabling. One or more of the following symptoms are present in neuropathic pain patients regardless of etiology, mechanism, and location of neural injury.

Evoked (or stimulus dependent) neuropathic pain is a result of hypersensitization of the somatosensory nervous system and is clinically described as allodynia and hyperalgesia. Allodynia is a pain response due to a normally innocuous stimulus. Hyperalgesia is an amplified pain response to an ordinarily noxious stimulus. Stimuli are typically classified as mechanical or temperature related (heat/cold). A patient with mechanical allodynia from postherpetic neuralgia may be so exquisitely sensitive to touch that he goes to extreme lengths to avoid contact with clothing, a bedsheet, or even by a breeze. Temporal summation or wind-up—increasing pain intensity to repetitive noxious stimuli—is a phenomenon also seen in evoked neuropathic pain. See Figure 35.1 for graphical representation of allodynia and hyperalgesia.

Neuropathic pain also presents with spontaneous (or stimulus independent) sensations without exogenous stimuli. Symptoms can be continuous or episodic. Paresthesias are abnormal sensations, typically described as "pins-and-needles" and skin crawling sensations, and dysesthesias refer to painful paresthesias. Patients may also describe pressure, squeezing, and superficial burning pain. Brief, spontaneous, lancinating, electric shock-like pain is also classical for neuropathic pain.

Neuropathic pain syndromes often include other sensory disturbances. In addition to paresthesias, patients may experience hypoesthesia, loss of sensory function, which is experienced as numbness. Hypoesthesia may involve multiple types of sensory modalities including mechanical stimuli, vibratory stimuli, and temperature stimuli, depending on the affected

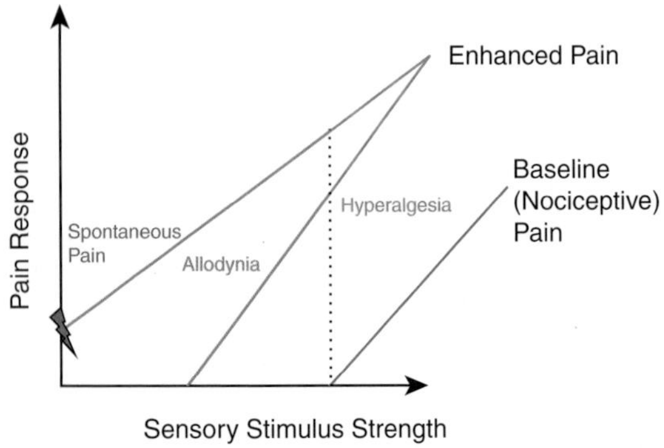

FIGURE 35.1 Graphic representation of perturbations of somatosensory function associated with pathologic pain states.

fiber types. Finally, hyperesthesia refers to an increased response to both nonnociceptive and nociceptive stimuli.

II. SPECIFIC NEUROPATHIC PAIN SYNDROMES

A. Trigeminal Neuralgia

Trigeminal neuralgia presents with paroxysmal unilateral lancinating facial pain. Episodes are brief, lasting less than fraction of a second to 2 minutes. Symptoms can be precipitated by light mechanical stimuli—chewing, speaking, or a light breeze. Spatial and temporal summation of stimuli can also trigger symptoms. Symptoms predominantly occur in the maxillary (V2) and mandibular (V3) distribution and usually spare the ophthalmic (V1) region. Classic trigeminal neuralgia is attributed to vascular compression of the trigeminal nerve. Secondary causes of trigeminal neuralgia are attributed to mass lesions (cerebellopontine angle tumors) and demyelinating disorders (multiple sclerosis). In idiopathic trigeminal neuralgia, neither of the prior two etiological criteria sets are met. Trigeminal neuralgia is almost always unilateral, except occasionally in multiple sclerosis, in which the disease can be caused by lesions of the central myelin between the root entry zone and the trigeminal nuclei, and rarely in familial neuropathies. Initial pharmacologic treatment is carbamazepine or the more recently developed agent, oxcarbazepine. Gabapentin, baclofen, and phenytoin have also been shown to have benefit. Other medications for which there is preliminary evidence of benefit include pregabalin, lamotrigine, valproic acid, and botulinum toxin. If pharmacologic treatment is ineffective, interventions include percutaneous ablative procedures directed toward Gasserian ganglion (thermal, mechanical, or chemical disruption), microvascular decompression of the trigeminal root, and Gamma Knife XRT to trigeminal root.

B. Glossopharyngeal Neuralgia

Glossopharyngeal neuralgia, due to lesions of the somatosensory component of the ninth cranial nerve, presents with neuropathic pain in the back of the throat or behind the angle of the jaw. Pain is unilateral, lasting a few seconds to minutes, severe, with electric shock-like or shooting quality. Pain can be precipitated by activities such as coughing, yawning, and swallowing. Etiologies are similar to those of trigeminal neuralgia and include vascular compression, demyelinating disease, and irritation from local infection or mass-occupying lesion. Eagle syndrome, calcification of the stylohyoid ligament, can also produce compression of the glossopharyngeal nerve.

C. Occipital Neuralgia

Occipital neuralgia presents with pain in the distribution of the greater and lesser occipital nerves, namely the suboccipital, occipital, and posterior parietal regions. Pain is described as deep, burning pain, with brief paroxysmal shock-like pains. There may be associated allodynia, hyperalgesia, paresthesia, and numbness present over the scalp. The greater occipital nerve arises from medial branch of the dorsal ramus of the C2 spinal nerve and innervates the medial occiput. The lesser occipital nerve arises from the ventral ramus of C2 and C3 spinal nerves and innervates the lateral head behind the ear. The third occipital nerve arises from the medial branch of the dorsal ramus of the C3 spinal nerve and passes along the C2-C3 facet joint to innervate the semispinalis capitis and the parasagittal region below the superior nuchal line. Injury or entrapment of the greater, lesser, or third occipital nerves is thought to cause occipital neuralgia. Diagnostically, painful symptoms should be alleviated with an occipital nerve block.

D. Brachial Plexus Syndromes

Brachial plexus syndromes are typically unilateral and present with severe pain in the shoulder, neck, and periscapular area with associated sensory and motor and changes in the affected arm. Injury can occur with trauma, inflammation, ischemia, tumors, and radiation.

1. **Traumatic brachial plexus** lesions present acutely with severe pain accompanied by weakness and numbness. Recovery may be limited depending on the severity of the trauma and concomitant nerve root avulsions that may be present.
2. **Idiopathic brachial plexitis**, known as Parsonage-Turner syndrome, is an immune-mediated disease of the brachial plexus. The classic presentation is severe shoulder and arm pain that is followed by numbness and weakness in the next few weeks. Recovery can take several months to several years.
3. **Neoplastic and postradiation** etiologies present with a less acute and more insidious progressive onset. Horner syndrome in combination with shoulder pain and arm weakness and numbness is suggestive of a mass lesion, commonly at the apex of the lung. Brachial plexopathy following radiation treatment can occur months after treatment but can also appear many years later.

E. Radiculopathy

Radiculopathy clinically presents with pain, paresthesias, or muscle weakness of the associated nerve root. The most common etiologies of radiculopathy are primarily structural insults resulting from degenerative disc herniation and spondylosis but also include acute trauma, infection, inflammation, and malignancy may lead to nerve root compression or disease. Cervical and lumbar radiculopathy are more common than thoracic radiculopathy due to greater biomechanical stresses at the neck and low back. Sensory symptoms consistent with neuropathic pain are dermatomally confined to the associated nerve root. Physical examination may be notable for weakness in the associated myotome with depressed muscle stretch reflexes. Exam maneuvers such as Spurling sign, ipsilateral straight leg raise, and contralateral straight leg raise can help support a diagnosis of radiculopathy. Electrodiagnostic testing (NCS/EMG) may be useful in subacute to chronic radiculopathy, particularly in cases for which the diagnosis is unclear. Such diagnostic uncertainty may result either due to an exam limited by pain/patient effort or if a peripheral diagnosis suspected but requires greater spatial refinement (plexopathy, mononeuropathy). MRI is an appropriate noninvasive test to evaluate for anatomical and structural contributions to radiculopathy. Treatment is based on the underlying etiology of the radiculopathy, for example antiviral treatment for HIV-associated polyradiculopathy. For radiculopathy related to disc herniation and neural foraminal stenosis, initial conservative management is recommended with nonopioid analgesics. There is insufficient evidence for physical therapy, but this is typically recommended for mild to moderate radiculopathy. Epidural steroid injections are indicated for refractory and severe radicular symptoms. Surgical management is indicated in the presence of progressive neurological deficits and should also be considered if symptoms remain severe and functionally disabling despite conservative treatment.

F. Postherpetic Neuralgia

Patients with postherpetic neuralgia, also known as zoster/shingles, experience burning, stinging, and stabbing pain in the dermatomal distribution of prior acute herpetic neuritis. Other sensory perturbations include allodynia and hyperalgesia to multiple modalities—mechanical, thermal, vibration—in the affected dermatomes. The natural history is as follows: varicella zoster virus (VZV) lies dormant in the dorsal root ganglia after acute infection and upon reactivation can cause acute herpetic neuralgia with pain associated with vesicular rash. Five to twenty percent of patients develop postherpetic neuralgia, pain that persists beyond 4 months after resolution of the rash. Risk factors for post herpetic neuralgia include age, severe rash (>50 skin lesions), and severe pain during acute herpetic neuralgia. Acute treatment with antivirals within 72 hours reduces the length of the vesicular rash and acute pain. However, the conclusions from the most recent studies are that antivirals are not effective in reducing the risk of developing postherpetic neuralgia. The same is true for early pain treatment intervention. Cranial variants of VZV include herpes zoster ophthalmicus (CN V1), which presents with headache, malaise, fever with unilateral eye pain with possible potential of vision loss. Herpes zoster auricularis (Ramsay-Hunt syndrome) presents with rash in the external ear, ear pain, and ipsilateral facial weakness. Reactivation of VZV is localized to the genicular ganglion of CN VII, the facial nerve, and commonly spreads to CN VIII. Other associated symptoms can also include hearing loss, tinnitus, and vertigo.

G. Meralgia Parethetica

Meralgia paresthetica is an isolated entrapment of the lateral femoral cutaneous nerve. It presents with pain, burning, and numbness over the anterolateral thigh without focal weakness. Prolonged standing or hip extension can provoke or amplify symptoms due to potential stretch or compression of the lateral femoral cutaneous nerve. The lateral femoral cutaneous nerve originates from the L2 and L3 nerve roots and branches off the lumbar plexus to travel underneath the inguinal ligament. The inguinal ligament is the suspected site of compression in most cases. Risk factors for impingement include obesity, diabetes, belts, and tight clothing.

H. Postamputation Stump Pain and Phantom Limb Pain

The development of postamputation stump pain and phantom limb pain is highly prevalent in amputees. Stump pain can be due to nerve injury, tissue trauma, infection, or vascular insufficiency. Chronic stump pain is frequently associated with painful neuromas; the transected nerve endings can form tangles of disorganized regenerative axonal sprouts and scar tissue. Symptomatic neuromas were initially treated by repeat excision and implantation of the nerves into muscle, bone, or veins. Unfortunately, the neuromas may then redevelop in these new locations. Restoration of function to the previously transected nerve potentially reduces recurrent neuroma formation. Thus, newer strategies include targeted muscle reinnervation where the proximal nerve stump is connected to a separate motor nerve thus providing function for the transected nerve. Phantom pain and sensation, in contrast to stump symptoms, are perceived distal to the site of the amputation. Mechanisms underlying this phenomenon remain unclear. Hyperactivity of the peripheral nervous system may contribute to spontaneous symptom generation. Neurons in the somatosensory cortex that are deprived of their normal afferent input may undergo cortical reorganization and cortical-motor sensory dissociation. Treatment options are similar to those for other neuropathic pain syndromes but are often less successful.

I. Complex Regional Pain Syndrome

Complex Regional Pain Syndrome (CRPS) is described as persistent severe regional pain that is disproportionate to the inciting event with associated sensory, vasomotor, sudomotor, and motor/trophic changes. The distribution of pain is not isolated to a specific nerve or dermatome. CRPS is subcategorized as type I (formerly known as reflex sympathetic dystrophy) where tissue injury occurs without clear evidence of peripheral nerve injury. Type II (formerly known as causalgia) refers to cases in which there is evidence of peripheral nerve injury. The Budapest criteria for CRPS requires associated symptoms in three of four categories: sensory (hyperesthesia, allodynia), vasomotor (temperature, skin color changes), and sudomotor (edema, sweating changes), motor/trophic (weakness, tremor, dystonia/nail or skin thickness, shiny, scaly discolored skin, loss of hair). For further discussion of CRPS diagnosis, evaluation, and management, please refer to Chapter 37.

J. Painful Diabetic Neuropathy

Painful diabetic neuropathy presents with tingling, shooting, and burning pain in the distal extremities with or without associated numbness, and often with concomitant autonomic symptoms. Approximately, one-third of all patients with diabetes experience neuropathic pain symptoms, and it is estimated that 50% of diabetic patients will develop peripheral neuropathy. Prolonged metabolic derangement in the setting of hyperglycemia damages axons of the small and large sensory, motor, and autonomic fibers. Classically, patients will describe a stocking and glove distribution of symptoms that ascends with progressive disease. Unlike small fiber neuropathy, diabetic neuropathy presents with a mix of small (C- and A-delta) and large (A-beta and A-alpha) fiber pathology. Loss of sensory nerves leads to impaired proprioception and hypoesthesia to multiple sensory modalities: vibration, pressure, pinprick, and temperature. More severe cases can have motor involvement as well, and weakness typically follows sensory changes and is usually observed first with intrinsic foot muscles. Autonomic symptoms are broad and affect cardiovascular, gastrointestinal, urogenital, and sudomotor systems. Treatment for painful diabetic neuropathy relies on glycemic control to limit disease progression and neuropathic agents for symptom management. A separate less common condition is known as treatment-induced diabetic neuropathy, also called **insulin neuritis**, and presents with intense neuropathic pain and dysautonomia following rapid glycemic control. The underlying etiology is not well understood, but small thinly myelinated and unmyelinated nerves are implicated in the pathophysiology as the cardinal features include orthostasis, syncope, nausea, diarrhea, erectile dysfunction, and severe neuropathic pain. Patients with insulin neuritis generally improve within months to years.

K. Diabetic Amyotrophy

Diabetic amyotrophy or diabetic lumbosacral radiculoplexus neuropathy presents with unilateral deep pain in the pelvis and hip for 4-6 weeks followed by proximal leg weakness, weight loss, and autonomic dysfunction. Clinical weakness primarily involves the obturator and femoral nerve–innervated muscles and manifests in hip flexion weakness, hip adduction weakness, and knee extension weakness, although the affected regions can be quite broad and variable. The patellar reflex is usually reduced or absent. Etiology of this condition is attributed to microvascular ischemic injury to upper lumbar plexus and nerve roots as opposed to the distal nerves in diabetic polyneuropathy. Functional recovery may take months to years. Therefore, symptomatic management of pain as well as physical therapy (and orthotics if needed) to support motor function are recommended. Incomplete recovery with residual weakness occurs in some cases.

L. Small Fiber Neuropathy

Small fiber neuropathy results in neuropathic pain and dysautonomia secondary to injury to the unmyelinated (C fibers) and thinly myelinated (A-δ) nerve fibers. Pain qualities include electric shock, shooting, and burning pain with allodynia, hyperalgesia, dysesthesias, as well as stimulus-independent pain. Injury to the small autonomic fibers can produce varied symptoms encompassing multiple systems: cardiovascular (orthostasis, syncope), gastrointestinal (constipation, diarrhea, gastroparesis), urogenital (urinary hesitancy or incontinence), and sudomotor systems (abnormal sweating). Diagnostically, expert clinical recognition remains the diagnostic standard although efforts are underway to develop objective classification. The following diagnostics tests help provide evidence for small fiber neuropathy: Distal leg skin biopsies evaluating intraepidermal nerve fiber density, autonomic function testing, and quantitative sudomotor axon reflex testing.

Small fiber neuropathy is associated with wide range of diagnosis including diabetes, celiac disease, Ehlers-Danlos Syndrome, infections, autoimmune (Sjögren's, sarcoidosis), genetic (Fabry), paraneoplastic syndromes, amyloid, toxins, and vitamin deficiencies. Interestingly, genetic mutations in ion channels that control nociceptor excitability, such as SCN9A (NaV1.7), SCN10A (NaV1.8), and SCN11A (NaV1.9), can all be associated with small fiber neuropathy. Treatment is twofold: addressing the underlying etiology and symptomatic management. In specific cases, identifying the etiology leads to straight-forward method to mitigate the disease and symptoms. However, in most cases, a unifying diagnosis remains elusive, and treatments are initiated empirically. Symptomatic management typically involves neuropathic pain medications (tricyclic antidepressants [TCAs], serotonin-norepinephrine reuptake inhibitors [SNRIs], anticonvulsants, topical agents) and in the right context—mexiletine and opioids.

M. Erythromelalgia

Erythromelalgia is a rare clinical syndrome with intermittent erythema, swelling, and burning pain in the distal extremities. Symptomatic episodes may last minutes to hours. Patients self-treat with cooling techniques—ice water immersion, ice packs, and cooling fans. Inherited erythromelalgia is most commonly from dominant activating mutations of the SCN9A gene, which encodes the NaV1.7 voltage-gated sodium channel on chromosome 2q24. The mutation results in increased entry of sodium into first-order nociceptor neurons, thus conferring a hyperexcitable state in peripheral nociceptor neurons.

N. Central Post-stroke Pain

Central post-stroke pain (CPSP) is a neuropathic pain syndrome caused by a cerebrovascular lesion in the pain pathways. The first cases were described by Déjerine and Roussy in 1906 in their paper "Le syndrome thalamique," where they reported thalamic strokes leading to severe, persistent, and paroxysmal pain associated with hemiplegic weakness. In addition to thalamic lesions, infarctions of the cerebral cortex and lateral medulla are also associated with the development of CPSP. The clinical syndrome can present days to years after the stroke. The prevalence of CPSP in stroke is estimated to be between 1% and 12%. Painful symptoms include spontaneous dysesthesias described as aching, squeezing, burning, and pricking sensations, as well as episodic lancinating and shooting pain. Evoked sensory changes of allodynia and hyperalgesia are also present in CPSP. These sensory changes are confined to areas of the body that correlate with the cerebrovascular lesion.

O. Spinal Cord Injury

Spinal cord injury (SCI) can lead to visceral pain and neuropathic pain. Neuropathic pain related to SCI is categorized as at-level and below-level symptoms. At-level SCI refers to segmental pain at the level of the lesion and within three dermatomes below the level of injury, the additional levels on account of ascent of afferent nociceptor fibers within Lissauer's tracts before projecting to the dorsal horn. Below-level SCI neuropathic pain refers to symptoms that are perceived more than three dermatomal levels below the level of injury. Etiology of SCI includes trauma, ischemia, and mass compression. Epidemiology studies demonstrate neuropathic pain is present in 40%-53% of the population with SCI and significantly impacts quality of life. Persistent neuropathic pain may occur at the time of acute injury or develop in the months afterward. Patients can experience burning, tingling, aching, squeezing, shooting, and shock-like pains. Sensory deficits or hypersensitivity phenomenon including allodynia and hyperalgesia may colocalize to the areas of pain.

P. Syringomyelia and Syringobulbia

Syringomyelia and syringobulbia are cavities that develop within the spinal cord or lower brainstem. They can be congenital or a consequence of trauma or tumor within the spinal cord. These cavities typically produce bilateral neuropathic symptoms. These symptoms primarily affect the body segments innervated by the damaged area of the cord because incoming pain axons cross close to the central canal (anterior commissure) near the level where they enter the cord. Ascending or descending tracts carrying information from other body areas travel in more peripheral regions of the cord and are less affected by these centrally located cavities. Pain is typically the earliest symptom of these syndromes.

III. TREATMENT OF NEUROPATHIC PAIN

Medications are typically the first-line therapy for neuropathic pain. Multiple drugs have proven effective against neuropathic pain in randomized placebo-controlled clinical trials, although often with modest benefits and a large NNT (number of subjects needed to treat to obtain benefit of a prespecified amount in a single subject). Because neuropathic pain constitutes a range of heterogeneous conditions and the interactions of individual genetic background and use of specific drugs are poorly understood, finding the best treatment for an individual patient is largely empiric, with the possible exception of carbamazepine and oxcarbazepine for trigeminal neuralgia. Not surprisingly, it is often necessary to try several different medications before identifying the optimal agent and dose. This sequential process should be explained to patients to ensure that their expectations for the extent and timing of relief are realistic. In general, the initial medication should be introduced, titrated to a reasonable dose, and monitored for efficacy and side effects. It is a common mistake to declare a medication ineffective without having titrated to a therapeutic dose.

The four major classes of medications for treating neuropathic pain syndromes are antidepressants—including TCAs and SNRIs, anticonvulsants, opioid analgesics, and topical agents. A systemic meta-analysis of neuropathic pain treatments demonstrated the following NNT:

3.6—TCAs
4.3—strong opioids—defined as oxycodone (10-120 mg/day) or morphine (90-240 mg/day)
4.7—tramadol (up to 400 mg daily)
6.4—serotonin-noradrenaline reuptake inhibitors (mainly duloxetine)
7.2—gabapentin
7.7—pregabalin
10.6—capsaicin patches 8% patches

Factoring in tolerability and safety profile of these treatments, the authors recommend first-line use of TCAs, SNRIs, pregabalin, and gabapentin. Second-line treatments include lidocaine patches, capsaicin patches, and tramadol. Strong opioids are a third-line recommendation and should be considered with care due to the known associated risks and paucity of high-quality outcome data. A more complete description of dosing, side effects, and mechanisms of medications used in the treatment of pain can be found in Chapters 10, 11, and 12, and Appendix IV. Specific considerations for the use of opioids in chronic nonterminal pain are discussed in Chapter 43.

Adjunctive treatments can improve function and reduce the pain and disability caused by chronic neuropathic pain. Physical and occupational therapies may be indicated to address loss of strength, decreased range of motion, and abnormal muscle tone. Physical and occupational therapies maximize functional gains and minimize secondary problems from disuse. Cognitive behavioral therapy fosters thoughts, emotions, and behaviors related to chronic pain that are less negative and self-defeating. The overall goal is to the address psychosocial burdens and functional impact of living with chronic pain.

Interventional approaches to neuropathic pain include local anesthetic and steroid nerve blocks, radiofrequency ablation, spinal cord stimulation, peripheral nerve stimulation, intrathecal analgesic delivery, and decompressive surgery. These topics are discussed elsewhere in this Handbook.

IV. CONCLUSION

Whereas neuropathic pain was considered a distinct entity associated with specific pain conditions, it is better understood as a heterogeneous clinical manifestation of the diverse and incompletely understood mechanisms that are responsible for many chronic pain syndromes. Neuropathic pain results from pathological structural and functional changes in the nervous system that promote pain sensitization, initiation, and amplification. It is perhaps the most challenging type of pain we treat in the pain clinic. Not surprisingly, neuropathic pain remains prominent focus of attention for clinicians and neuroscience researchers who together are attempting to unravel its mechanisms and improve treatments. For physicians, neuropathic pain is an integral target of the practice of pain management and worthy of an intensive effort to help the unfortunate effected individuals.

Selected Readings

Abbott CA, Malik RA, Van Ross ER, Kulkarni J, Boulton AJ. Prevalence and characteristics of painful diabetic neuropathy in a large community-based diabetic population in the U.K. *Diabetes Care.* 2011;34(10):2220-2224. doi: 10.2337/dc11-1108.

Baron R, Binder A, Wasner G. Neuropathic pain: diagnosis, pathophysiological mechanisms, and treatment. *Lancet Neurol.* 2010;9(8):807-819. doi: 10.1016/S1474-4422(10)70143-5.

Bryce TN, Biering-Sørensen F, Finnerup NB, et al. International spinal cord injury pain classification: part I. Background and description. *Spinal Cord.* 2012;50(6):413-417. doi: 10.1038/sc.2011.156.

Burke D, Fullen BM, Stokes D, Lennon O. Neuropathic pain prevalence following spinal cord injury: a systematic review and meta-analysis. *Eur J Pain.* 2017;21(1):29-44. doi: 10.1002/ejp.905.

Chen N, Li Q, Yang J, Zhou M, Zhou D, He L. Antiviral treatment for preventing postherpetic neuralgia. *Cochrane Database Syst Rev.* 2014;2014(2):CD006866. doi: 10.1002/14651858.CD006866.pub3.

Dejerine J, Roussy G. Le syndrome thalamique. *Rev Neurol.* 1906;14:521-532.

Dib-Hajj SD, Yang Y, Waxman SG. Chapter 4: genetics and molecular pathophysiology of Nav1.7-related pain syndromes. *Adv Genet.* 2008;63:85-110. doi: 10.1016/S0065-2660(08)01004-3.

Dworkin RH, O'Connor AB, Kent J, et al. Interventional management of neuropathic pain: NeuPSIG recommendations. *Pain.* 2013;154(11):2249-2261. doi: 10.1016/j.pain.2013.06.004.

Dyck PJ, Windebank AJ. Diabetic and nondiabetic lumbosacral radiculoplexus neuropathies: new insights into pathophysiology and treatment. *Muscle Nerve.* 2002;25(4):477-491. doi: 10.1002/mus.10080.

Eberlin KR, Ducic I. Surgical algorithm for neuroma management: a changing treatment paradigm. *Plast Reconstr Surg Glob Open.* 2018;6(10):e1952. doi:10.1097/GOX.0000000000001952

Ellenberg MR, Honet JC, Treanor WJ. Cervical radiculopathy. *Arch Phys Med Rehabil.* 1994;75(3):342-352. doi: 10.1016/0003-9993(94)90040-X.

Ephraim PL, Wegener ST, MacKenzie EJ, Dillingham TR, Pezzin LE. Phantom pain, residual limb pain, and back pain in amputees: results of a national survey. *Arch Phys Med Rehabil.* 2005;86(10):1910-1919. doi: 10.1016/j.apmr.2005.03.031.

Farhad K. Current diagnosis and treatment of painful small fiber neuropathy. *Curr Neurol Neurosci Rep.* 2019;19(12):103. doi: 10.1007/s11910-019-1020-1.

Finnerup NB, Attal N, Haroutounian S, et al. Pharmacotherapy for neuropathic pain in adults: a systematic review and meta-analysis. *Lancet Neurol.* 2015;14:162-173. doi: 10.1016/S1474-4422(14)70251-0.

Flor H, Elbert T, Knecht S, et al. Phantom-limb pain as a perceptual correlate of cortical reorganization following arm amputation. *Nature.* 1995;375(6531):482-484. doi: 10.1038/375482a0.

Gibbons CH, Freeman R. Treatment-induced diabetic neuropathy: a reversible painful autonomic neuropathy. *Ann Neurol.* 2010;67(4):534-541. doi: 10.1002/ana.21952.

Harden RN, Bruehl S, Perez RS, et al. Validation of proposed diagnostic criteria (the "budapest Criteria") for Complex Regional Pain Syndrome. *Pain.* 2010;150(2):268-274. doi: 10.1016/j.pain.2010.04.030.

Harney D, Patijn J. Meralgia paresthetica: diagnosis and management strategies. *Pain Med.* 2007;8(8):669-677. doi: 10.1111/j.1526-4637.2006.00227.x.

Hatem SM, Attal N, Ducreux D, et al. Clinical, functional and structural determinants of central pain in syringomyelia. *Brain.* 2010;133(11):3409-3422. doi: 10.1093/brain/awq244.

Jensen MP, Chodroff MJ, Dworkin RH. The impact of neuropathic pain on health-related quality of life: review and implications. *Neurology.* 2007;68(15):1178-1182. doi: 10.1212/01.wnl.0000259085.61898.9e.

Klit H, Finnerup NB, Jensen TS. Central post-stroke pain: clinical characteristics, pathophysiology, and management. *Lancet Neurol.* 2009;8(9):857-868. doi: 10.1016/S1474-4422(09)70176-0.

Levine TD. Small fiber neuropathy: disease classification beyond pain and burning. *J Cent Nerv Syst Dis.* 2018;10:117957351877170. doi: 10.1177/1179573518771703.

Oaklander AL, Nolano M. Scientific advances in and clinical approaches to small-fiber polyneuropathy: a review. *JAMA Neurol.* 2019;76(10):1240-1251. doi: 10.1001/jamaneurol.2019.2917.
Olesen J. The International classification of headache disorders, 3rd edition. *Cephalalgia.* 2018;38(1):5. doi: 10.1177/0333102417738202.
Peltier A, Goutman SA, Callaghan BC. Painful diabetic neuropathy. *BMJ.* 2014;348:g1799. doi: 10.1136/bmj.g1799.
Sampathkumar P, Drage LA, Martin DP. Herpes zoster (Shingles) and postherpetic neuralgia. *Mayo Clin Proc.* 2009;84(3):274-280. doi: 10.4065/84.3.274.
Sengupta DK, Herkowitz HN. Lumbar spinal stenosis: treatment strategies and indications for surgery. *Orthop Clin North Am.* 2003;34(2):281-295. doi: 10.1016/S0030-5898(02)00069-X.
Subedi B, Grossberg GT. Phantom limb pain: mechanisms and treatment approaches. *Pain Res Treat.* 2011;2011:864605. doi: 10.1155/2011/864605.
Tsairis P, Dyck PJ, Mulder DW. Natural history of brachial plexus neuropathy. *Arch Neurol.* 1972;27(2):109. doi: 10.1001/archneur.1972.00490140013004.

36 Low Back Pain: Evaluation and Management

Moises A. Sidransky and Boris Spektor

I. LOW BACK PAIN OVERVIEW

A. Location of Pain: Definitions

1. **Axial lumbosacral back pain** comprises pain in the lumbar (L1-L5 vertebral region) and sacral spine (S1 to sacrococcygeal junction).
2. **Radicular** leg pain travels into an extremity along a dermatomal distribution secondary to nerve or dorsal root ganglion irritation.
3. **Referred** pain spreads to a region remote from its source but along a nondermatomal trajectory.

B. Epidemiology

1. Low back pain (LBP) is very common in the United States and worldwide—the fourth most common reason for visiting a U.S. physician.
2. Approximately 25% of U.S. adults experienced LBP of at least 24 hours' duration in the last 3 months.
3. Lifetime prevalence is 65%-80% in the general U.S. adult population with an annual prevalence of 10%-30%.
4. Total health care costs attributable to pain in the United States were estimated at over $500 billion in 2011, and LBP is a major contributor.
5. The 2010 Global Burden of Disease study identified LBP as the leading contributor to disability and work days lost.

C. Acute (<6 weeks) and Subacute (6-12 weeks) Low Back Pain

1. Majority of acute LBP is self-limited to 6 weeks or less.
2. 10%-40% of patients develop symptoms lasting >6 weeks.
3. Assess for red flags to screen patients for more serious etiology and need for further evaluation (see Section II.A.2, Fig. 36.1).

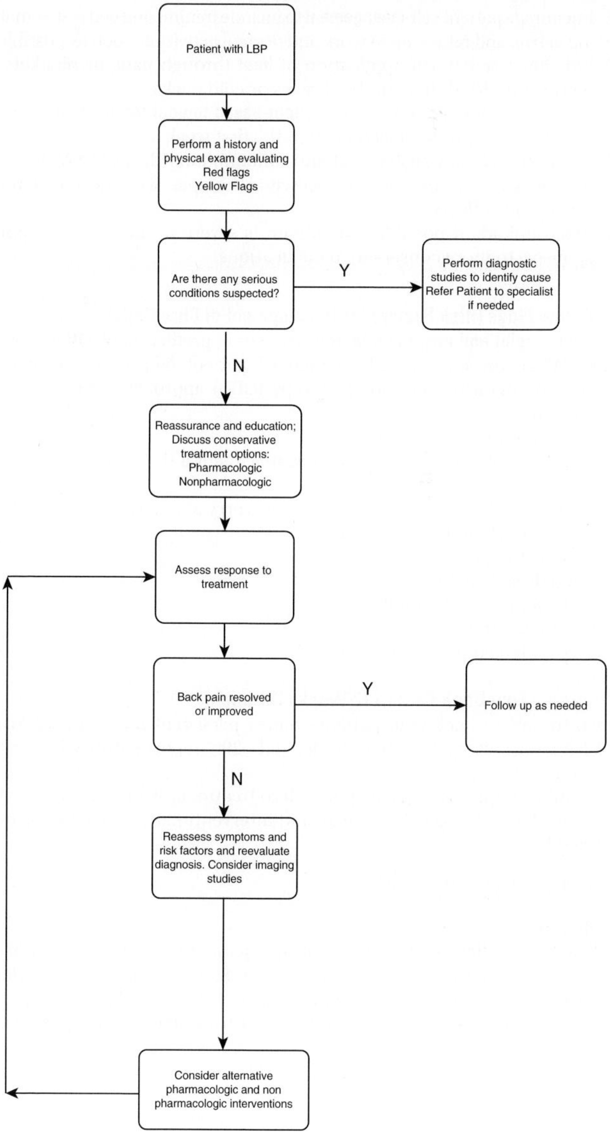

FIGURE 36.1 Low back pain assessment and management.

4. If no red flags, provide **patient education** about generally nonspecific etiology, favorable prognosis, likelihood of similar recurrences in most people, and **reassurance** to expect a favorable course.
5. Reevaluate those patients with persistent pain beyond 1 month.

6. Encourage patient **self-management** to include minimizing bed rest, remaining active, and returning to work and normal activity as soon as possible.
7. Judicious short-term application of **heat** through pads or blankets is better supported than lumbar braces or cold packs.
8. Short-term application of a **capsaicin-based topical formulation** showed analgesia relative to placebo within the first week of use.
9. Acetaminophen, nonsteroidal anti-inflammatory drugs (NSAIDs), and muscle relaxants are first-line medicinal therapies with the aim of minimizing side effects.
10. Avoid opioids if possible unless pain is severe in intensity and unresponsive to more conservative medications.

D. Yellow Flags (Risk Factors for Development of Chronicity)

1. **Psychosocial and emotional factors** are strong predictors of LBP chronicity. When present, consider enhanced patient education and earlier focused cognitive behavioral therapy (CBT) approaches to target the following:
   a. Anxiety and depression
   b. Catastrophizing (exaggerated negative mental thinking regarding the painful experience)
   c. Fear avoidance behavior (significant worry about aggravating LBP by engaging in normal activities)
   d. Passive coping strategies
   e. Job dissatisfaction
   f. Higher levels of disability
   g. Somatization
   h. Disputed compensation claims

E. Chronic Low Back Pain (>12 Weeks Duration)

1. Up to 33% of back pain patients report persistent moderate-intensity LBP 1 year after an acute episode, and ~20% report substantial limitation in activity.
2. A multidisciplinary logical approach to treatment is most effective with medical, psychological, physical, and interventional approaches as outlined below.

II. PATIENT ASSESSMENT

A. History

1. **Nonspecific Etiology:** When evaluating a patient with LBP it may not be possible to define a precise cause—up to 85% of patients will be diagnosed with *nonspecific* LBP upon primary evaluation. However, look for evidence of specific serious etiologies of back pain by elucidating the following:
   a. **Duration:** Symptom duration stratifies the patient into acute, subacute, or chronic LBP to help guide decision-making.
   b. **Location:** Ascertain pain location and radiation to clarify axial vs radicular vs referred LBP
   c. **Severity:** Use a specific pain severity scale (eg, Visual Analog Scale or Numerical Rating Scale). Determine current, average, worst, and best scores.
   d. **Pain character:** Can help differentiate neuropathic from nociceptive somatic pain. Neuropathic pain is often described as burning, shooting, electric, or pins-and-needle pain. Nociceptive pain is often described as dull, sharp, aching, and focal.

e. **Inciting event:** Circumstances that initiated the pain such as a motor vehicle accident should be noted, including whether patient was a driver or passenger, airbag deployment, site of impact, speed and damage to vehicle, and type of vehicles involved. Additional important information includes whether or not the patient was evaluated in urgent care or an emergency room, what workup was performed, and whether the patient was admitted.
f. **Alleviating and provoking factors** such as pain change with sitting, standing, walking, and lying down help clarify differential diagnosis.
g. **Previous history:** Prior similar episodes of lower back pain should be documented to clarify intermittent recurrent nature of symptoms.
h. **Prior evaluation and management:** Noting previous diagnostic studies and interventions is helpful in guiding further management.
i. **Progression of symptoms:** Note temporal changes in presentation to assess symptom progress.
j. **Function:** Determine how pain is affecting work and activities of daily living.

2. **Red flags:** The initial evaluation should include screening questions to rule out concerning constitutional symptoms that point to a **serious progressive or unstable cause** for pain such as cancer, infection, trauma, and neurologic compromise (see Possible Etiologies for Low Back Pain, Table 36.1). Among patients who present with LBP, <1% will have a serious systemic etiology. However, the posttest probability has been estimated at 33% for emergency room presentation for LBP in people with a prior history of cancer.
   a. **History of cancer** (excluding nonmelanoma skin cancers) is the strongest risk factor for back pain from bone metastasis. **Common bone metastasizing cancers include breast, lung, renal cell, thyroid, GI adenocarcinomas, and prostate.** Less predictive risk factors include **recent weight loss, worsening pain at night, and inability to attain relief at rest or in the supine position.**
   b. **History of recent fever, malaise, spinal injection, IV drug use, immunosuppression, and other concurrent infections.** These are risk factors for vertebral infection including discitis, epidural abscess, or osteomyelitis.
   c. **History of recent or substantial trauma.** Ascertain mechanism of traumatic injury and potential for ligamentous instability or fracture.
   d. **Neurologic compromise** such as **numbness, saddle anesthesia, gait instability, weakness in the legs,** or **bowel and bladder control changes** are concerning for severe spinal cord or cauda equina compression. For cauda equina syndrome, urinary retention and overflow incontinence are the main features, giving both ≥90% sensitivity and specificity.
3. **Psychosocial factors:** Evaluate patients for social or psychological distress as these are stronger predictors of LBP outcome than physical examination or pain characteristics (see Section I.D. Yellow Flags).

B. Physical Exam

1. **General physical examination** should be performed including **vital signs, ambulation status** (assistive devices, mobility, and gait), **appearance, signs of distress, mood and affect,** and **multisystem evaluation.**
2. **Neurological examination** is critically important to rule out neurologic compromise and consists of **motor strength, sensation, deep tendon reflex testing,** and **upper motor neuron reflexes (ankle clonus, Babinski).**
3. **Spine examination:**
   a. **Inspection:** Evaluating the thoracolumbar spine will provide information on posture and alignment. Abnormal kyphosis, lordosis, or

TABLE 36.1 Possible Etiologies of Low Back Pain and Evaluation

Possible Etiologies	Key Positives on History and Physical Examination	Imaging	Supplemental Tests
Cancer	History of cancer with acute or progressively worsening LBP	MRI +/− contrast	ESR, CRP
	Unintentional weight loss, failure to improve with conservative therapy after 4 wk, age > 50	Lumbar x-ray	ESR, CRP
	Multiple risk factors and high clinical cancer suspicion	MRI +/− contrast	ESR, CRP
Spinal infection	Fever, IV drug use, malaise, recent spinal intervention, immunosuppression, other infections	MRI +/− contrast	ESR, CRP, CBC
Cauda equina syndrome	New bowel or bladder incontinence, saddle anesthesia, significant motor deficits not localized to a single nerve root	MRI without contrast	None
Vertebral compression Fracture	History of osteoporosis, older age, corticosteroid use, recent trauma	Lumbar X-ray; MRI for acuity, malignant vs benign fracture	None
Ankylosing spondylitis	Gradual onset, morning stiffness, improves with exercise, nocturnal back or buttock pain, age < 40	Pelvic/SI joint x-ray	ESR, CRP, HLA-B27
Herniated disk	Radicular back pain to L4-S1 dermatomes of leg; Positive straight leg raise test	None	None
	No improvement after 4-6 wk of conservative therapy, worsening symptoms, or neurologic deficits	MRI without contrast	Confirmatory EMG/NCV if neurologic deficits
Spinal stenosis	Neurogenic claudication with ambulation or extension, older age; improved with sitting	None	None
	No improvement after 4-6 wk of conservative therapy, worsening symptoms, neurologic deficits	MRI without contrast	None

scoliosis should be noted. Skin evaluation should focus on rashes, scars, erythema, swelling, and signs of trauma.

b. **Palpation** over the spinous processes can reveal localized tenderness. Light palpation will help detect allodynia (pain to nonnoxious stimuli), which often indicates presence of neuropathic pain.

c. **Range of motion:** Assess range of motion with regard to flexion, extension, lateral bending, and rotation (with the pelvis stabilized). While nonspecific, pain that is provoked by lateral bending and back extension is suggestive of facet arthropathy. Pain that is provoked by forward flexion is suggestive of discogenic pain because flexion of the lumbar spine causes axial loading.

4. **Selected tests for specific etiologies:**
   a. **Patrick/FABER Test:** Evaluates **hip and sacroiliac pathology**, which are both associated with lower back pain. With the patient in supine position, the examiner passively **f**lexes, **ab**ducts, and **e**xternally **r**otates the hip (FABER). Pain in the groin area suggests hip pathology, while pain in the back suggests sacroiliac joint pathology.
   b. **Straight leg raise:** With the patient in a supine position, the examiner slowly lifts the patient's leg at the heel while the knee is straight. This produces tension in the **lower lumbar nerve roots (L4-S1)**. A positive straight leg raise reproduces radicular pain experienced by the patient radiating from his lower back or buttock down to his ankle in a radicular pattern. If pain remains localized to the posterior thigh area, it is most likely secondary to tension on the hamstring muscles.
   c. **Gaenslen test:** With the patient in the supine position, the hip joint is flexed maximally on one side and the opposite hip joint is extended beyond the edge of the examination table. Buttock pain reproduction is suggestive of **sacroiliac joint** pathology.

C. Diagnostic Testing

1. **Laboratory studies—rarely indicated.** For patients with suspected malignancy or infection, ESR, CRP, and CBC are helpful (see Table 36.1: Possible Etiologies of Low Back Pain and Workup)
2. **Electrodiagnostic testing: Electromyography (EMG) and nerve conduction testing** may be indicated if objective neurologic signs are found on examination. These tests can help **differentiate acute from chronic radiculopathy as well as help localize the pathologic lesion** to confirm clinical suspicion.
3. **Imaging:** Most acute LBP patients **do not require imaging. Imaging should only be performed when neurologic deficits are present or when serious etiology is suspected (ie, red flags).** Additionally, patients with signs and symptoms of spinal stenosis or radiculopathy should receive imaging for **planning of surgery or minimally invasive interventions.**
   a. **X-rays:** When indicated, obtain **weight-bearing AP/lateral radiographs of the lumbar spine.** Of note, lumbar radiography affected management in only 1%-2% of patients receiving it. The average radiation exposure from lumbar x-Ray is 75 times higher than for chest radiography.
   b. **Lumbar MRI:** Indicated when there is substantial clinical suspicion for an underlying systemic disease (See Table 36.1). **MRI *with and without contrast* is indicated in patients suspected of cancer or infection or in the setting of prior lumbar surgery where enhancement can help differentiate scar from disk. Noncontrast lumbar MRI** is optimal for spinal stenosis or radiculopathy assessment.
   c. In patients who require advanced imaging but **cannot have an MRI (eg, pacemaker)**, a **lumbar CT** scan is an alternative though with inferior resolution of soft tissue and nerves.

III. ETIOLOGY OF LOWER BACK PAIN

a. **Myofascial pain** refers to a focal muscle region of palpable tightness and tenderness (ie, **trigger point**) characterized by limited passive muscle stretching and a typical pattern of **referred pain on palpation.** Myofascial pain often develops secondary to **underlying mechanical factors** such as postural abnormalities or spondylosis as well as chronic anxiety. These regions exhibit biochemical changes including inflammatory mediators and neuropeptides that chronically are **associated with central sensitization.** Stretching, massage, and topical analgesics are first-line therapy followed by possible trigger point injection, though evidence is limited.

b. **Facet-mediated pain:** Lumbar facet joint degeneration is a multifactorial process that is associated with degeneration of the intervertebral disks. Pain can be caused by osteoarthritis of the facet joint or stress of the facet joint capsule. Pain is often **described as deep and aching, unilateral or bilateral, with occasional radiation to one or both buttocks and thighs, stopping generally above the knee.** Physical examination, though nonspecific, will often show **pain on extension, rotation, lateral bending (ie, facet loading), and paraspinal palpation.** Imaging studies are nonspecific.

c. **Discogenic pain**: Approximately 40% of lower back pain can be attributed to the intervertebral disk. Patients often report **pain in the center of the low back with limited radiation typically to the buttocks or thighs.** Pain generally **improves with standing and worsens with sitting, lumbar flexion, Valsalva maneuver, and coughing (ie, axial loading).** Disk degeneration occurs secondary to diminished vascular supply (atherosclerosis, smoking), genetic factors affecting collagen, and inflammatory mediators that can subsequently promote **nerve ingrowth of nociceptors** deeper into the annulus fibrosis causing pain. Importantly, **degenerated desiccated (low T2 signal) disks are often asymptomatic**; pain is more often associated with **disk extrusions, significantly decreased disk height, high-intensity zones** (bright T2 signal at the posterior annulus), and **Type I Modic endplate changes** (dark on T1, bright on T2). The use of provocative diskography for identifying painful disks is controversial.

d. **Lumbar post-laminectomy syndrome:** This is a multidimensional postoperative condition of **persistent low back pain with or without radicular symptoms after one or more spine surgeries.** Its incidence has been reported as between 10% and 40% after spine surgery. Etiology is related to multiple factors: **preoperative factors** include patient history of anxiety, depression, poor coping strategies, litigation, and compensation secondary gains; **intraoperative factors** include poor technique and inability to achieve the goal of surgery; **postoperative** factors include progression of disease, epidural fibrosis, surgical complications, new instability, and the development of associated myofascial pain and central sensitization.

e. **Spinal stenosis:** A condition caused by decreased space available for nerves and vasculature in the vertebral canal resulting in **neural ischemia and compression.** The condition is most often secondary to degeneration and hypertrophy of the disk, facet joints, and ligamentum flavum at **L3-L4 and L4-L5** in patients **above 65** years of age. Clinical presentation includes **gluteal and lower extremity pain with or without associated lower back pain.** Pain classically **worsens with standing and walking and improves with sitting and lumbar flexion (ie, neuroclaudication).** Imaging with MRI or CT confirms the diagnosis: absolute lumbar spinal stenosis is radiologically defined as **cross-sectional canal area <75 mm^2 or AP diameter of <10 mm.**

f. Sacroiliac (SI) joint pain: The sacroiliac joint is a diarthrodial synovial joint with both ventral and dorsal sacral innervation. SI joint pain **typically overlies the low back and buttock with possible referred pain into the leg usually above the knee level.** Patients with **spondyloarthropathy** and **prior lumbar fusion** are at higher risk for sacroiliac arthropathy. Multiple positive provocative tests are more suggestive for SI pain including **posterior superior iliac spine (PSIS) tenderness, Patrick (FABER) and Gaenslen tests** (see Section II.B.4).

IV. TREATMENT FOR LOW BACK PAIN (TABLE 36.2)

A. Multidisciplinary Approach to Treatment

1. Not all patients respond to the same treatment approach, and no single intervention is generally completely effective for all patients.
2. Limited trials of one or more interventions guided by evidence and effectiveness are utilized to decrease overall costs.

B. Pharmacologic Treatment

1. Acetaminophen

a. For *acute* LBP, there is no clear difference in analgesia between acetaminophen at dosages up to 4 g/day and NSAIDs.

b. For *chronic* LBP, acetaminophen is slightly inferior to NSAIDs for pain relief.

c. Generally favorable safety profile and low cost; uncertain clinical significance of generally asymptomatic aminotransferase elevations above 3 g/day; caution with other acetaminophen-containing drugs

TABLE 36.2 Interventions for Acute and Chronic Low Back Pain

	Acute LBP	Chronic LBP
Pharmacologic Treatments		
Acetaminophen	X	X
NSAIDs	X	X
Muscle relaxants	X	X
Tramadol	X	Mixed
Potent opioids	X	X
TCA		X
SNRI		X
Antiepileptic		X
Psychological Treatments		
Education and reassurance	X	
CBT	X (if yellow flags)	X
Progressive relaxation		X
Biofeedback		Mixed
Physical and Rehab Treatments		
Maintain normal activities	X	
Exercise program		X
Multidisciplinary rehab		X
Complementary/Alternative		
Acupuncture		X
Manual manipulation	X	X
Medium-firm mattress		X

2. *NSAIDs*
   a. For *acute* and *chronic* LBP, nonselective and COX-2 selective NSAIDs are superior to placebo with no clear difference in efficacy between NSAIDs.
   b. Use NSAIDs with caution in patients with chronic kidney disease, cardiovascular pathology, bleeding risk, and history of GERD/peptic ulcer disease. Use lowest effective dose for shortest duration possible.

3. *Skeletal Muscle Relaxants*
   a. For *acute* LBP, short-term studies (2 weeks' duration) show analgesia superiority to placebo, with no clear difference between specific muscle relaxants.
   b. Primary associated side effect is CNS sedation and risk for falls.
   c. Particular caution with carisoprodol, which is metabolized to the sedating and potentially addictive barbiturate meprobamate.

4. *Tramadol and More Potent Opioids*
   a. Consider judiciously for severe, disabling acute and chronic pain uncontrolled with other therapeutic options. Use time-limited course with reevaluation of **A**nalgesic efficacy, improved **A**ctivity, **A**dverse effects, and **A**berrant behavior (4A's).
   b. Caution should be exercised in patients at **risk for addiction** or aberrant behavior (eg, personal or family history of addiction, poorly controlled psychological comorbidity, sexual abuse history, young age <45).
   c. While tramadol has shown limited analgesia with mild functional improvement for *chronic* LBP, potent opioids have shown significant analgesia and improved function at 3 and 6 months' duration in randomized trials.

5. *Tricyclic Antidepressants (TCAs)*
   a. RCT efficacy established for *chronic* LBP.
   b. Exert analgesia primarily through serotonin and norepinephrine reuptake inhibition, sodium channel blockade, and NMDA antagonism.
   c. Most common side effects include dry mouth/constipation (anticholinergic) and dizziness/drowsiness (antihistaminergic).

6. *Serotonin Norepinephrine Reuptake Inhibitors (SNRIs)*
   a. RCT efficacy of duloxetine and venlafaxine established for *chronic* LBP, with duloxetine being better tolerated.
   b. Analgesic mechanism via serotonin and norepinephrine reuptake inhibition important for descending pain inhibition.
   c. Most common side effects include dry mouth, self-limited nausea, dizziness, headache, and insomnia.

7. *Antiepileptics*
   a. While gabapentin has shown analgesic efficacy for chronic LBP with radiculopathy, only topiramate has been studied for chronic axial LBP with evidence of analgesia and improved quality of life.
   b. Topiramate has the advantageous side effect of weight loss but is also associated with dizziness, somnolence, and rare nephrolithiasis.

C. Psychological Treatments

1. Psychological interventions have been most studied for *chronic* LBP, though application to *acute* LBP patients with multiple yellow flags (see Section I.D) is prudent to prevent chronicity of pain.

2. Addressing psychosocial and motivational factors is important within a multidisciplinary framework for analgesic efficacy and reducing disability.
3. **Cognitive behavioral therapy (CBT)**
   a. Goal-oriented approach that targets maladaptive thinking and coping strategies to change behavior and improve mood
   b. RCT evidence for short-term improvement in pain intensity and disability
4. **Progressive relaxation**
   a. Muscle tension-reducing technique involving systematic flexing and relaxing of specific muscles with the aim of achieving profound relaxation.
   b. Provides short-term improvement in pain and function.
5. **Biofeedback**
   a. Relaxation approach that utilizes auditory and visual feedback from muscle activity to reduce muscle tension
   b. Mixed data for pain intensity reduction

D. Physical and Rehabilitation Treatments

1. Exercise Therapy

a. Defined as a series of specific movements with the goal of training the body to promote good physical health
b. Short-term reduction in pain intensity and disability in *chronic* LBP relative to usual care
c. Stretching exercises most associated with pain reduction; strengthening yields greatest functional gains

2. Multidisciplinary Functional Rehabilitation Programs

a. Defined as multidisciplinary biopsychosocial rehabilitation with at least one physical dimension (exercise, physical modalities) and one other dimension (psychological or social or occupational)
b. Effective for pain relief, disability reduction and improved mood

3. Other PT/Rehab Modalities Lacking RCT Support for Chronic LBP

a. No RCT studies assessing effectiveness of **lumbar support**.
b. Inadequate data to support **massage** therapy, **back schools**, **traction**, **superficial heat/cold** application.
c. **TENS** is not supported compared to placebo for chronic LBP.

E. Complementary and Alternative Medicine Approaches

1. Acupuncture

a. Intervention that utilizes specific anatomical points along classic meridians typically with the use of small needles that are either manipulated or electrically stimulated to achieve effect.
b. Meta-analysis of RCTs focusing on *chronic* LBP reveals reduced pain intensity and improved function immediately postintervention compared to sham, NSAIDs, or muscle relaxants.

2. Manual Medicine/Manipulation

a. Through osteopathic or chiropractic treatment, manipulation of the spine involves the goal of restoring spinal alignment and optimal range of motion.
b. Meta-analysis reveals equal effectiveness to general practitioner care, analgesics, physical therapy, and exercise therapy.

3. *Sleep Support*
   a. **Medium-firm mattress** reduced pain levels during the day, during the night, and with rising from bed relative to firm mattress.

F. Interventional Minimally Invasive Percutaneous Approaches for Axial Low Back Pain

1. *General Principles*
   a. In cases when pain remains refractory to conservative multidisciplinary treatment, minimally invasive interventional approaches are rationally considered with the goal of improving function, relieving pain, and reducing side effects from medical management.
   b. **Predictors of poor outcome** to interventional procedures:
      i. Poorly controlled psychiatric disorder
      ii. Catastrophizing and fear avoidance behavior
      iii. Coexisting chronic pain complaints
      iv. High baseline pain scores and disability
      v. Previous treatment failures
      vi. Chronic escalating opioid use
      vii. Secondary gain
      viii. Previous spine surgery

2. *Lumbar Facet (Zygapophyseal) Joint Interventions*
   a. Lumbar facet joints are innervated by the **medial branches** of the dorsal rami, with anatomical studies documenting nerve endings within the facet joints.
   b. Facet joint pain has been targeted by intra-articular injections, medial branch nerve blocks, and radiofrequency neurotomy of the medial branch nerves.
   c. **Intra-articular facet joint steroid injections** have limited or negative RCT evidence for benefit and are not recommended.
   d. If **diagnostic lumbar medial branch nerve blocks** (single or preferably comparative to decrease placebo response) provide substantial temporary relief, neuroablation via radiofrequency neurotomy is considered for longer-term benefit.
   e. **Lumbar medial branch radiofrequency neurotomy** has good RCT evidence for improved pain and function lasting 6-12 months.
   f. **Complications** from facet joint interventions are rare and are primarily limited to pain or swelling at needle insertion site and temporary flare of pain postneurotomy.

3. *Sacroiliac Joint Interventions*
   a. Sacroiliac joints are known to be a significant source of pain in patients with spondyloarthropathies as well as with advanced age and post–lumbar fusion.
   b. **Intra-articular sacroiliac joint steroid injections** have been studied in one small RCT in patients with ankylosing spondyloarthropathy with analgesia and decreased NSAID use. No RCTs explore this intervention for nonrheumatologic sacroiliac joint pain.
   c. The sacroiliac joints are innervated by both ventral and dorsal sacral rami. The posterior sacroiliac joint and ligaments (**posterior sacroiliac complex**) are innervated by the **lateral branches** of the sacral dorsal rami.
   d. **Sacral lateral branch radiofrequency neurotomy** targeting the posterior sacroiliac complex has been studied in two small RCTs utilizing cooled as well as unipolar radiofrequency lesioning techniques.

Diagnostic blocks were performed either with sacroiliac joint intra-articular injections or with L5 dorsal ramus plus S1-S3 lateral branch blocks. Analgesia postneurotomy was significant for ~3-6 months with improved function.

4. Lumbar Radicular Pain and Spinal Stenosis Treatment with Epidural Steroid Injections (ESI)

a. Epidural injections of steroid provide significant though temporary (<3 month) analgesia with best supportive RCT evidence in patients with **acute radicular pain** concordant with site of lumbar disk herniation rather than axial lumbar pain.

b. Epidural steroid injection for neurogenic claudication secondary to spinal stenosis has been studied with RCT evidence revealing equivalent reduction in pain and improved function for both the steroid and local anesthetic groups, but no sham injection group was included. Local anesthetic alone can provide analgesia by increasing blood flow to ischemic nerve roots, suppressing nociceptive transmission, and washing out inflammatory mediators.

5. Lumbar Postlaminectomy Syndrome and Spinal Cord Stimulation (SCS)

a. Spinal cord stimulation delivers electrical pulses via epidural electrodes at vertebral levels associated with pain, either overlapping the pain with masking paresthesia (traditional low-frequency SCS devices) or through the use of high-frequency (10 kHz) nonparesthesia neuromodulation. The latter is thought to provide better analgesia for axial LBP.

b. RCT studies have shown significantly improved analgesia, function, and patient satisfaction with use of SCS compared to conventional medical management or repeat spine surgery in patients with lumbar postlaminectomy syndrome up to 2 years postimplantation.

c. High-frequency neuromodulation has shown RCT superiority to low-frequency SCS for both axial and radicular analgesia at 2-year follow-up.

Selected Readings

Abrahm JL. Assessment and treatment of patients with malignant spinal cord compression. *J Support Oncol.* 2004;2:88-91.

Chou R. In the clinic. Low back pain. *Ann Intern Med.* 2014;160:ITC6.

Chou R, et al. Diagnosis and treatment of low back pain: a joint clinical practice guideline from the American College of Physicians and the American Pain Society. *Ann Intern Med.* 2007;147:478-491.

Chou R, et al. Nonsurgical interventional therapies for low back pain: a review of the evidence for an American Pain Society clinical practice guideline. *Spine.* 2009;34(10):1078-1093.

Chou R, et al. Diagnostic imaging for low back pain: advice for high-value health care from the American College of Physicians. *Ann Intern Med.* 2011;154:181-189.

Chou R, Huffman LH. Medications for acute and chronic low back pain: a review of the evidence for an American Pain Society/American College of Physicians clinical practice guideline. *Ann Intern Med.* 2007;47:505-514.

Chou R, Huffman LH. Nonpharmacologic therapies for acute and chronic low back pain: a review of the evidence for an American Pain Society/American College of Physicians clinical practice guideline. *Ann Intern Med.* 2007;147:492-504.

Chung JWY, et al. Drug therapy for the treatment of chronic nonspecific low back pain: systematic review and meta-analysis. *Pain Physician.* 2013;16:E685-E704.

Cohen SP, et al. Epidural steroids: a comprehensive, evidence-based review. *Reg Anesth Pain Med.* 2013;38:175-200.

Dagenais S, et al. Synthesis of recommendations for the assessment and management of low back pain from recent clinical practice guidelines. *Spine J.* 2010;10:514-529.

Downie A, Williams CM, Henschke N, et al. Red flags to screen for malignancy and fracture in patients with low back pain: systematic review. *BMJ.* 2013;347:f7095.

Falco FJE, et al. An update of the effectiveness of therapeutic lumbar facet joint interventions. *Pain Physician.* 2012;15:E909-E953.

Hartvigsen J, et al. What low back pain is and why we need to pay attention. *Lancet.* 2018;391:2356-2367.

Koes BW, et al. An updated overview of clinical guidelines for the management of non-specific low back pain in primary care. *Eur Spine J.* 2010;19:2075-2094.

Lam ML, et al. Effectiveness of acupuncture for nonspecific chronic low back pain. *Spine.* 2013;38:2124-2138.

Middelkoop M, et al. A systematic review on the effectiveness of physical and rehabilitation interventions for chronic non-specific low back pain. *Eur Spine J.* 2011;20:19-39.

Shaheed CA, et al. Interventions available over the counter and advice for acute low back pain: systematic review and meta-analysis. *J Pain.* 2014;15(1):2-15.

Wellington J. Noninvasive and alternative management of chronic low back pain (efficacy and outcomes). *Neuromodulation.* 2014;17:24-30.

37 Complex Regional Pain Syndrome

Eugenia-Daniela Hord

Complex regional pain syndrome I (CRPS I) and complex regional pain syndrome II (CRPS II) are a relatively new terminology used to rename two classic neuropathic pain syndromes previously known as **reflex sympathetic dystrophy** and **causalgia.** These syndromes remain among the most fascinating and enigmatic of the pain syndromes.

I. HISTORY

The clinical syndrome we refer to as CRPS was scarcely mentioned in the medical literature before 1864 when Weir Mitchell, an American Civil War physician, described a syndrome consisting of burning pain, hyperesthesia, and trophic changes following nerve injury in the limbs of the soldiers. He named this pain syndrome **causalgia**.

Similar pain states were later documented in postsurgical patients, as well as in those with no clearly inciting cause. In the 1920s, Leriche, a French surgeon, established a link between the sympathetic nervous system and causalgia by demonstrating that sympathetic blockade or sympathectomy relieved the symptoms of many of his patients. Patients with no clear-cut peripheral nerve injury, or those with pain in more than one peripheral nerve distribution, had what became known as reflex sympathetic dystrophy, which is now called CRPS I.

In 1946, Evans devised the term **reflex sympathetic dystrophy** to describe a similar syndrome in patients with no obvious nerve damage. Since then, numerous attempts have been made to explain the pathophysiology behind these clinical features, and a host of different names have been used to describe them.

In 1995, the International Association for the Study of Pain introduced the name CRPS. CRPS I and CRPS II are new names for two classic neuropathic pain syndromes previously known as **reflex sympathetic dystrophy** and **causalgia.** The new terminology was suggested to avoid the misleading term "sympathetic" and to create uniform diagnostic criteria. Although there was some dissention, the new terminology is now largely accepted. CRPS I occurs without evidence of major nerve damage, whereas CRPS II follows an identifiable major nerve lesion. Based on the presence or absence of the sympathetic component of pain, both types of CRPS can be divided further into sympathetically maintained pain (SMP) and sympathetically independent pain (SIP). A diagnostic sympathetic blockade can help distinguish SMP from SIP. In 2003, a consortium of CRPS experts met in Budapest Hungry to review the IASP diagnosis criteria and published the results of that workshop in 2007, yielding greater accuracy in the diagnosis of CRPS.

II. BASIC MECHANISMS

Numerous theories have been offered to explain the pathophysiology of CRPS, but the exact mechanisms remain unclear. While many theories postulate that sympathetic dysfunction plays a significant role in the development and maintenance of the syndromes, there are CRPS syndromes in which part or all the pain appears to be SIP.

CRPS most likely involves both peripheral and central mechanisms. Peripherally, one observes events after nerve injury that herald long-term changes in neural processing. In animal models, persistent afferent small-fiber activity begins days to weeks after peripheral nerve ligation or section and can be measured at the site of a developing neuroma as well as in the dorsal root ganglia. The neural sprouts at these sites have growth cones, which have mechanical and chemical sensitivities not possessed by the original neurons. These neural sprouts also may have increased numbers of sodium channels, leading to increased ionic conductance and hence increased spontaneous activity. There is also evidence of an abnormal coupling between sympathetic efferent and nociceptive afferent neurons (C-fibers and/or afferent somata within the dorsal root ganglia). It is hypothesized that a partial nerve lesion induces an upregulation of functional α_2 adrenoceptors at the plasma membrane of nociceptive fibers. These mechanisms could be the pathologic pathway of SMP. Additionally, more recent evidence supports the involvement of neurogenic inflammation, as well as, axonal damage to small sensory fibers in the pathogenesis of edema, vasodilation, and sweating in CRPS.

Centrally, changes in the morphology of the spinal dorsal horn ipsilateral to a peripheral nerve injury may be secondary to intrinsic mechanisms arising in response to a chronic barrage of impulses, or in response to retrograde transport of chemical factors from the area of the lesion. Increased spontaneous activity in the primary afferent neuron may be a factor leading to spinal cord glutamate release. The activated peripheral nociceptors transmit messages to the spinal cord through lightly myelinated A-delta fibers and unmyelinated C fibers. This process leads to the release of excitatory amino acids like glutamate and asparagine. The excitatory amino acids act on *N*-methyl-D-aspartic acid (NMDA) receptors causing the release of substance P which subsequently lowers the threshold for synaptic excitability in normally silent second-order spinal synapses. The role of glutamate release in the spinal cord after peripheral nerve injury is being evaluated with growing interest. In addition to the functional changes described, there is some suggestion that the brains of patients with CRPS could have structural changes consisting of decreased thickness of the gray matter in areas related to pain, or decreased thickness of prefrontal cortices, or enlargement of choroid plexus. The observation that some patients appear to have hemineglect further supports also some involvement of the cortex in the pathogenesis of CRPS.

III. CLINICAL PRESENTATION

The initial signs and symptoms of CRPS may begin at the time of injury or may be delayed for weeks. Sometimes, the traumatic event cannot be identified. CRPS I occurs without evidence of major nerve damage, whereas CRPS II consists of the same signs and symptoms following an identifiable major nerve lesion. Because CRPS I and II have identical diagnostic criteria, it seems likely that the cause of CRPS I is also nerve injury but that the nerve injuries go undetected because they are partial, fascicular, or involve primarily small unmyelinated axons. These specific types of nerve lesions are notoriously difficult to diagnose by examination or electrodiagnostic studies.

CRPSs are characterized by pain, changes in cutaneous sensitivity, autonomic dysfunction, trophic changes, and motor dysfunction. Untreated CRPS was characterized by three stages: acute, dystrophic, and atrophic. However, the sequential progression is hard to identify now that most patients are treated and do not display the later stages of disease progression.

Spontaneous pain is present in most of the patients. It can be burning, sharp stabbing, electric shocklike aching, and the quality can vary in time. The pain appears disproportionate to the inciting event. Sensory changes are common CRPS and include allodynia and hyperalgesia. Sensory deficits also can be present.

Autonomic dysfunction manifests as edema, changes in sweating (hypo- or hyperhidrosis), skin color changes (red or pale), and skin temperature differences. These signs can vary from time to time and may be reported despite not being obvious at the time of the examination.

Trophic changes are largely the result of disuse. They include changes in nail growth and aspect, skin changes (can be thin and shiny or thick), hair loss, or hypertrichosis (see Fig. 37.1). Bones are osteoporotic, and joints may ankylose (see Fig. 37.2).

The motor dysfunction includes weakness and later atrophy. Dystonia and tremor are also described.

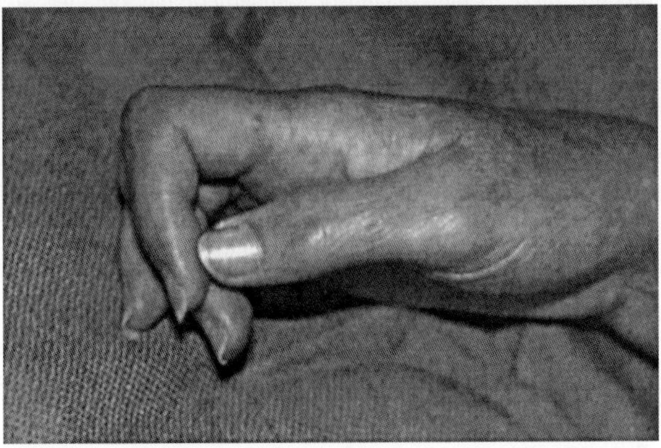

FIGURE 37.1 The appearance of the hand in CRPS. The skin is smooth, glossy, tight, and cool, the overlying hair has fallen out, and the nails are severely brittle. The digits are thin and tapered. The joints are ankylosed.

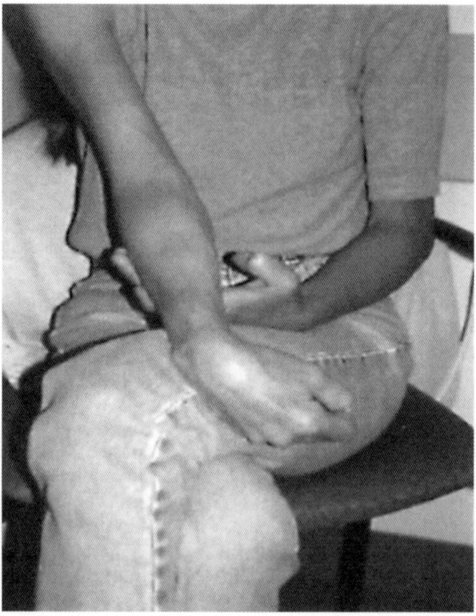

FIGURE 37.2 Woman with severely affected right arm. Muscle wasting is pronounced, and there are flexion contractures.

IV. DIAGNOSIS

Pain is the cardinal feature of CRPS, but there are also sensory changes, autonomic dysfunction, trophic changes, motor impairment, and psychological changes. The diagnosis is based on the overall clinical picture, with additional information from carefully performed and interpreted confirmatory tests to ascertain the presence or absence of SMP and autonomic dysfunction. These include diagnostic sympathetic blockade (eg, stellate ganglion block, lumbar sympathetic block) and tests such as the quantitative pseudomotor axon reflex test, which allows a continuous hygrometric assessment of pseudomotor activity and is considered a good indicator of C-fiber function.

The diagnosis of CRPS requires the exclusion of confounding medical problems, as well as the evaluation of diagnostic criteria. The IASP continues to clarify and refine the diagnostic criteria for CRPS, and hopefully, this will help eliminate diagnostic and therapeutic dilemmas.

Based on IASP-revised CRPS clinical diagnostic criteria, a diagnosis of CRPS can be made when the following criteria are met:

A. Continuing pain that is disproportionate to any inciting event
B. At least one symptom reported in at least three of the following categories
1. **Sensory:** Hyperesthesia or allodynia
2. **Vasomotor:** Temperature asymmetry, skin color changes, skin color asymmetry
3. **Sudomotor:** Edema, sweating changes, or sweating asymmetry
4. **Motor/trophic:** Decreased range of motion, motor dysfunction, or trophic changes

C. At least one sign at the time of evaluation in at least two of the following categories:

1. **Sensory:** Evidence of hyperesthesia to pinprick or allodynia to light touch, temperature sensation, deep somatic pressure of joint movement
2. **Vasomotor:** Evidence of temperature asymmetry (>1°C), skin color changes, skin color asymmetry
3. **Sudomotor:** Evidence of edema, sweating changes, or sweating asymmetry
4. **Motor/trophic:** Decreased range of motion, motor dysfunction, or trophic changes

V. TREATMENT

Progress has been slow in refining treatment of CRPS. Because the condition is complex and incompletely understood, the treatment has been varied and formulated to address presumed pathophysiologic causes and to ameliorate specific symptoms. The common goal is functional restoration. Pharmacologic therapy as well as regional anesthetics and surgical interventions should be used in conjunction with physical therapy (PT). CRPS prognosis in adults is more guarded than in children. Most children with recent-onset CRPS will improve spontaneously and should be treated conservatively.

A. Physical Therapy

PT should be started as soon as a diagnosis is made, even a presumptive diagnosis. In cases in which PT has already been started (eg, after surgery on the hand or foot, or after casting for a fracture), the pain may worsen as CRPS develops, but discontinuing PT will only make matters worse. PT should continue, but the approach may be altered. The major role of PT seems to be to treat the secondary complications such as decreased joint and tendon range of motion and subsequent atrophy. One randomized controlled study demonstrated that physical and, to a lesser extent, occupational therapies reduced pain and improved active mobility in recent-onset CRPS I. Mobilization of the affected limb is of paramount importance. Elevation, massage, and contrast bath also have been used. Often, the pain must be aggressively treated (as in subsequent text) to accomplish this. A gentle approach using heat, massage, vibration, and other mild stimuli will help to restore more normal sensory processing. Isometric strengthening should be followed by progressive stress loading as tolerated. One must be careful when using medication or, in particular, regional anesthesia in conjunction with PT to avoid aggressive range of motion exercises and heavy loading of the affected limb. (Chapter 27 contains a full description of PT for patients with CRPS.)

B. Pharmacologic Treatments

Research into treatments has been gravely hindered by the loose definitions used, and there have been almost no multicenter, randomized, placebo-controlled trials. There are currently no medications approved by the U.S. Food and Drug Administration (FDA) for the treatment of CRPS.

In 2018, Duong and colleagues reviewed the controlled clinical trials for CRPS concluding that the current evidence from RCTs supports use of bisphosphonates and short courses of oral steroids in the setting of CRPS. They also found emerging evidence suggesting a therapeutic role for ketamine, memantine, intravenous immunoglobulin, epidural clonidine, intrathecal clonidine/baclofen/adenosine, aerobic exercise, mirror therapy, and dorsal root ganglion stimulation. Evidence from RCTs also suggest efficacy of spinal cord stimulation (SCS) for management of CRPS pain and associated symptoms. Despite the posited role of the sympathetic nervous system in the pathophysiology of CRPS, an update of a Cochrane review (O'Connell et al., 2016) found that there is inadequate evidence to support or refute efficacy of local anesthetic sympathetic blockade. Here, we describe medications proven effective for neuropathic pain, even if not specifically tested in multicenter randomized trials on patients with CRPS.

1. Neuropathic Pain Medications

a. Tricyclic Antidepressants. TCAs are effective in treating neuropathic pain syndromes, including postherpetic neuralgia, diabetic neuropathy, and CRPS. These agents have independent analgesic effects but also can facilitate the treatment of pain by improving mood, sleep, and anxiety states. Few patients experience total relief, and usage is often limited by side effects. This should be considered when prescribing these drugs, particularly in the elderly. Refer to Chapter 10 for a full description of these drugs.

b. Anticonvulsants. The anticonvulsants are a heterogeneous group of drugs, some of which have known efficacy for the treatment of neuropathic pain. Several anticonvulsants have been used successfully for CRPS, including phenytoin, carbamazepine, vaproic acid, and gabapentin. Gabapentin has advantages over older agents such as carbamazepine and phenytoin because of its better side effect profile. Case reports and small series support the efficacy of gabapentin in adult and pediatric CRPS. Newer antiepileptic medications also may be effective, but randomized placebo-controlled clinical trials are lacking. The anticonvulsant drugs and their use in pain management are described in Chapter 10.

c. Local Anesthetics. Mexiletine, a sodium channel blocker, originally was developed as an anticonvulsant, but until recently, it has been used almost solely as a Class Ib antiarrhythmic. It is structurally similar to lidocaine and has been demonstrated to be useful in treating neuropathic pain states. Although few studies exist, it has been felt that mexiletine may be useful in the treatment of CRPS though its use is limited by safety concerns.

Recently, transdermal lidocaine patches have been used successfully in areas of localized neuropathic pain with allodynia and hyperalgesia in postherpetic neuralgia. EMLA (eutectic mixture of local anesthetic) cream is a topical preparation containing both lidocaine and prilocaine. These topical lidocaine preparations appear to be useful in the treatment of localized areas of hyperesthesia associated with CRPS, but this efficacy has not been confirmed by trials (see Chapters 10 and 21).

2. Nonsteroidal Anti-inflammatory Drugs

Nonsteriodal anti-inflammatory drugs (NSAIDs) are not useful as sole pharmacologic therapy in CRPS because pain relief is generally inadequate, although they may be helpful during the early stages of the disease. They may occasionally be useful as adjunctive therapy, especially when there is joint and tendon involvement. The risks, benefits, and desirability of NSAIDs are discussed in Chapter 12.

3. Opioids

For many reasons, the use of opioids in neuropathic pain states is controversial. Formerly, neuropathic pain was believed to be unresponsive to opioids, although currently opioid responsiveness with a rightward shift of the dose-response curve (indicating efficacy but at higher doses) is accepted. Although there are no well-controlled trials of opioid therapy in patients with CRPS, it appears that in certain patients, opioid treatment can usefully improve pain. Therefore, for refractory pain, a trial of opioids may be warranted. Opioids should only be used as adjuncts to other treatments, and great care should be taken when prescribing for patients with a history of substance abuse or obvious risk factors for abuse (see Chapter 11).

4. Inhibitors of Osteoclast Activity

Some patients with CRPS have abnormalities of bone metabolism, including excess bone resorption in the affected area, although this is likely a secondary consequence of reduced mobility and/or loss of innervation to the bone. For this reason, inhibitors of osteoclast activity (eg, bisphosphonates or regulators of bone metabolism like calcitonin) have been evaluated as treatments for recent-onset CRPS. There is also evidence of direct antihyperalgesic effects of some of these compounds. The mechanisms by which calcitonin and bisphosphonates control pain in early CRPS are unclear: bisphosphonates hinder the synthesis of prostaglandin E2, proteolytic enzymes, lactic acid, and pro-inflammatory cytokines; calcitonin inhibits the synthesis of proteolytic enzymes and lactic acid. None of these agents can be given orally; calcitonin is available as a nasal spray, and bisphosphonates usually are administered intravenously.

5. Corticosteroids

Corticosteroids have been advocated for use in the early stages of CRPS. There is evidence that by decreasing inflammation, they relieve pain and minimize ectopic electrical activity after nerve injury. Recent studies suggest that there is a marked inflammatory component in the early stages of CRPS. Thus, if a patient has pain secondary to joint movement and trophic changes, a trial of corticosteroids with a reasonably rapid taper is recommended. Using this approach, one may avoid many of the undesirable side effects of steroids when evaluating and treating the inflammatory component of CRPS early in the disease.

6. Others

a. **Lioresal (Baclofen)** is a γ-aminobutyric acid-receptor (type B) agonist that increases the function of dorsal-horn interneurons that inhibit the output of projection neurons, including those transmitting pain signals via the spinothalamic tracts. For some time, it has been used successfully both orally and intrathecally for treatment of spasticity. Some patients with CRPS develop dystonia. Short-term efficacy of intrathecal baclofen for relieving CRPS spasticity was demonstrated in one recent study. Oral and intrathecal baclofen as a treatment of neuropathic pain independent of spasticity have been evaluated in preclinical and clinical studies. There is some evidence for efficacy in treating CRPS pain, even in patients without dystonia. However, further studies are necessary.

b. **Phentolamine,** an α-adrenergic blocker, is used by intravenous infusion to test the susceptibility of CRPS to sympathetic blockade. It is reported that ~30% of patients with sympathetically mediated pain will respond positively to an intravenous infusion test. In these patients, intravenous regional sympathetic blockade may subsequently prove useful. Oral α-blockers have not been found useful because side effects, most importantly hypotension and tachycardia, preclude anything but the smallest doses, which severely limits their utility as analgesics.

c. Clonidine, an α_2 agonist, has been shown to have significant analgesic properties. It can be administered systemically or neuraxially and has proven effective for both nociceptive and neuropathic pain. Intravenous regional blockade using 1 μg/kg clonidine can provide marked pain relief in patients with sympathetically mediated pain. Likewise, transdermal clonidine is believed to be useful, particularly when applied to discreet areas of hyperalgesia. Clonidine has both central and peripheral actions and may be a useful adjunct in the treatment of CRPS. Clonidine is described in more detail in Chapter 10.

d. Ketamine is a NMDA antagonist administered as an infusion for neuropathic pain including CRPS. In CRPS, there is an increase in glutamate release from first-order afferents which in turn stimulates the NMDA receptors on second-order neurons from the spinal cord causing windup and central sensitization. The reported efficacy is between 50% and 100% improvement in pain control, but it is also depending on the other endpoint measures of efficacy and duration of patient posttreatment follow-up. Of note, these studies are generally of low quality (eg, open label). There is also high variability in the published protocols for ketamine infusion regarding dosing, duration, frequency, and timing of the ketamine infusions. More commonly, one low-dose ketamine infusion of 1-4 hours is administered followed by a longer infusion at higher doses in next few weeks if there was some degree of improvement. Many patients will require periodic infusions, but some will not require additional treatments. Other options include inpatient 4-5 day infusions, or outpatient 5-10 daily infusions. There are CNS side effects including dysphoria, hallucinations, agitation, and night terrors, which can be treated with benzodiazepines. It can cause liver dysfunction.

C. Regional Anesthesia

Several regional anesthetic modalities have been used in the treatment of CRPS. The primary indication is as an adjunct to PT in the process of functional restoration. Regional sympatholysis in patients with SMP can be both diagnostic and therapeutic (in conjunction with PT). The regional anesthetic techniques are described in detail in Chapters 16 and 30.

1. Sympathetic Blockade

a. Temporary sympatholysis of the upper extremity can be accomplished by a stellate ganglion block or a cervical sympathetic block. A lumbar sympathetic block will provide sympathetic blockade in the lower extremities. In addition to providing temporary pain relief, sympathetic blocks can be helpful in determining the extent of the sympathetic component of a patient's pain, thereby predicting potential benefit from pharmacologic therapy and from SCS. However, one must keep in mind that some degree of somatic blockade is almost certain to occur in conjunction with these blocks; therefore, the test is not entirely clean. It cannot be overemphasized that the aim of temporary sympatholysis in CRPS is to achieve sufficient pain relief to allow functional restoration during a course of PT. The endpoint for the combined therapy is either adequate functional restoration, or the point at which the patient is no longer able to increase his or her endurance and workload after sympathetic blockade. A series of blocks may be necessary, in conjunction with the PT sessions.

b. Sympathetic neurolysis has been advocated in the past but is no longer recommended. Chemical neurolysis lasts only 3-6 months, and patients may then suffer a recurrence, or even worsening, of their original pain.

There is also a risk of spread of the neurolytic agent to the sensorimotor fibers in close proximity to the targeted nerves (eg, phrenic nerve, lumbar plexus). In addition, there is a high risk of deafferentation pain, which is worse and harder to treat than the initial pain. More recently, **percutaneous radiofrequency lesioning of the sympathetic trunk** and **endoscopic sympathectomy** have been used in selected patients with clearly demonstrable SMP. Long-term evaluation of these treatments has not yet been completed. However, current experience suggests that there may be a similar risk of deafferentation pain.

2. Intravenous Regional Blockade

Intravenous regional blockade has been attempted using several different medications, with varying reports of success. Several of the medications previously used for IV regional blockade are no longer available in the United States. If a patient has failed conservative treatment, an IV regional trial may be warranted. However, it is now clearly established that this intervention does not provide long-lasting pain relief. Bretylium and guanethidine can provide up to 3 weeks of relief. Local anesthetic and clonidine often are used in combination. Some practitioners advocate adding ketorolac if the patient is in the acute stage of CRPS when there is a significant inflammatory component. Again, the main purpose of treatment should be pain relief to facilitate PT. Many patients are unable to tolerate the procedure because of severe pain with limb exsanguination and tourniquet placement.

3. Epidural Blockade

Lumbar epidural blockade and, less frequently, cervical epidural blockade have been used for extended periods of time to treat cases of CRPS that have been unresponsive to less invasive therapies. Lumbar epidural catheters can be used to provide continuous lumbar plexus blockade for patients who have inadequate pain relief and have been unable to participate in PT. A low concentration of local anesthetic is used, as high concentrations tend to produce sensory and motor blockade, which hamper functional restoration. Often an opioid or clonidine is used in combination with the local anesthetic to augment pain relief. Temporary epidural catheters have been left in place for up to 6 weeks, allowing successful functional restoration. Obviously, there are risks associated with long-term epidural catheters, and sometimes, the external infusion system can interfere with the exercise regime. Implanted epidural infusion systems are more secure and less intrusive, but the risks of the surgical procedure are probably not warranted other than in the most refractory cases.

4. Brachial Plexus Blockade

Continuous brachial plexus blockade for patients with CRPS of the upper extremity is sometimes used. This can be accomplished with an axillary, infraclavicular, or supraclavicular catheter. The advantage, as with epidural catheters, is that the prolongation of neural blockade enables patients to make relatively rapid progress in their PT. Under neural blockade, care should be taken to avoid overextending the passive and active range of motion exercises. As with any catheter treatment, there are risks of dislodgement and infection. A relatively high infusion rate of local anesthetic is needed for successful brachial plexus catheter treatment, which limits the utility of these catheter treatments in outpatients. The treatment is best suited to patients who have been unresponsive to pharmacologic therapy but are likely to have a good and rapid response to PT with adequate sensorimotor blockade.

D. Neuromodulation

1. Spinal Cord Stimulation

SCS has been shown to be effective in patients with refractory CRPS in several clinical trials. A preliminary report suggests that short-term efficacy of sympathetic blockade may predict a positive response to SCS in patients with CRPS. Stimulation is conducted at the C5-C7 level for the upper extremities and the T8-T10 level for the lower extremities. It seems critical to have good overlap between the induced paresthesias and the painful area. Approximately 50% of preselected patients with CRPS will have a positive response to stimulation during the period of a trial. Approximately 70% of these patients will have good-to-excellent long-term benefit. A goal of pain relief is reasonable in view of the refractory nature of the pain in patients selected for this expensive therapy, although if treatment is started early, one could hope that functional restoration may be achieved. The is literature suggesting utility for earlier use of SCS in patients with CRPS, although an exact recommendation on timing has yet to be determined. See Chapter 13 for a more complete description of SCS.

2. Peripheral Nerve Stimulation

Peripheral nerve stimulation has been advocated for use in patients with CRPS II, with symptoms entirely or mainly in the distribution of a single major peripheral nerve, who have been unresponsive to other therapeutic modalities. It is not considered an option for patients with CRPS involving an entire limb or further extension to the trunk or other extremities. Peripheral nerve stimulators present a special problem in that they generally cross several mobile joints and therefore may be dislodged with movement. In select patients, however, early small studies suggest this might be successful treatment for patients with CRPS II who have been unresponsive to other therapies.

E. Psychotherapy

Because of the discrepancy between the subjective complaints of pain made by patients with CRPS and the limited objective evidence of underlying pathology, it may be suggested that psychiatric factors are a major cause of CRPS. Many patients with CRPS become depressed during their illness. There has been a great deal of discussion on whether a premorbid tendency to depression predisposes patients to CRPS or whether CRPS causes depression or uncovers a preexisting condition, and no consensus has been reached. Early in the illness, only ~10%-15% of patients with CRPS report being depressed; this is similar to the incidence of depression in the general population. Furthermore, when psychological tests are conducted at this stage, the results are similar to those in the general population. As CRPS progresses, anxiety and depression play more of a role. This is confirmed by psychological testing. Clinicians should be aware of the high rate of secondary psychiatric problems in CRPS and refer patients for counseling and medical treatment as needed. A psychiatrist, psychologist, or social worker familiar with CRPS should be involved in caring for patients if possible at this juncture. Biofeedback for relaxation and reduction of muscle tension is a useful adjunct to pharmacologic therapy, PT, and psychotherapy.

VI. CONCLUSION

Most CRPS patients are best managed with a combination of skilled physical therapist with medication(s) and interventional pain modalities. The aim is always to start treatment early and to optimize function. Use of appropriate medications in conjunction with neuromodulation techniques—and in some cases, also sympathetic blocks—is sufficient therapy in all but the most refractory cases. With a team approach to the treatment of patients with CRPS, a successful outcome is most likely.

Selected Readings

Baron R, Binder A. Complex regional pain syndromes. In: Pappagallo M, ed. *The Neurological Basis of Pain.* New York, NY: McGraw-Hill; 2005:359-378.

Becker WJ, Ablett DP, Harris CJ, et al. Long term treatment of intractable reflex sympathetic dystrophy with intrathecal morphine. *Can J Neurol Sci.* 1995;22:153-159.

Blumberg H, Janig W. Clinical manifestations of reflex sympathetic dystrophy and sympathetically maintained pain. In: Wall PD, Melzack R, eds. *Textbook of Pain.* 3rd ed. Edinburgh, UK: Churchill Livingstone; 1994:685-698.

Bossut DF, Perl ER. Effects of nerve injury on sympathetic excitation of A-delta mechanical nociceptors. *J Neurophysiol.* 1995;73:1721-1723.

Bruehl S, Harden RN, Galer B, et al. External validation of IASP diagnostic criteria for complex regional pain syndrome and proposed research diagnostic criteria. *Pain.* 1999;81:147-154.

Cepeda MS, Lau J, Carr DB. Defining the therapeutic role of local anesthetic sympathetic blockade in complex regional pain syndrome: a narrative and systematic review. *Clin J Pain.* 2002;18:216-233.

Devor M, Wall P, Catalan N. Systemic lidocaine silences ectopic neuroma and DRG discharge without blocking nerve conduction. *Pain.* 1992;48:261-268.

Duong S, Bravo D, Todd KJ, Finlayson RJ, Tran Q. Treatment of complex regional pain syndrome: an updated systematic review and narrative synthesis. *Can J Anaesth.* 2018;65(6):658-684.

Eisenach J, DeKock M, Klimscha W. Alpha 2 adrenergic agonists for regional anesthesia: a clinical review of clonidine (1984-1995). *Anesthesiology.* 1996;85:655-674.

Galer BS, Bruehl S, Harden RN. IASP diagnostic criteria for complex regional pain syndrome: a preliminary empirical validation study. *Clin J Pain.* 1998;14:48-54.

Harden RN, Bruehl S, Galer BS, et al. Complex regional pain syndrome: are the IASP diagnostic criteria valid and sufficiently comprehensive? *Pain.* 1999;83:211-219.

Harden RN, Bruehl S, Stanton-Hicks M, et al. Proposed new diagnostic criteria for complex regional pain syndrome. *Pain Med.* 2007;6(4):326-331.

Hord ED, Cohen S, Ahmed S, et al. The predictive value of sympathetic block for the success of spinal cord stimulation. *Neurosurgery.* 2003;53(3):626-633.

Hord ED, Oaklander AL. Complex regional pain syndrome: a review of evidence-supported treatment options. *Curr Pain Headache Rep.* 2003;7:188-196.

Janig W, Stanton-Hicks M, eds. *Reflex Sympathetic Dystrophy: A Reappraisal.* Seattle, WA: IASP Press; 1996.

Kamibayashi T, Maze M. Clinical uses of alpha 2-adrenergic agonists. *Anesthesiology.* 2000;93:1345-1349.

Kingery WS. A critical review of controlled trials for peripheral neuropathic pain and complex regional pain syndromes. *Pain.* 1997;73:123-139.

Kumar K, Toth C, Nath RK, et al. Epidural spinal cord stimulation for treatment of chronic pain—some predictors of success. A 15-year experience. *Surg Neurol.* 1998;50:110-120.

Lee DH, Lee KJ, Cho KI, et al. Brain alterations and neurocognitive dysfunction in patients with complex regional pain syndrome. *J Pain.* 2015;16(6):580-586.

Mellick GA, Mellicy LB, Mellick LB. Gabapentin in the management of reflex sympathetic dystrophy. *J Pain Symptom Manage.* 1995;10:265-266.

Merskey H, Bogduk N, eds. Classification of chronic pain. In: *Description of Chronic Pain Syndromes and Definition of Pain Terms.* 2nd ed. Seattle, WA: IASP Press; 1994.

Mitchell SW. *Injuries of Nerves and Their Consequences.* Philadelphia, PA: JB Lippincott Co; 1872; Reprinted in *Clinical Orthopedics and Related Research* 1982;163:2-7.

Mitchell SW, Morehouse GR, Keen WW, et al. *Gunshot Wounds and Other Injuries of Nerves.* Philadelphia, PA: JB Lippincott Co; 1864.

O'Connell NE, Wand BM, Gibson W, Carr DB, Birklein F, Stanton TR. Local anaesthetic sympathetic blockade for complex regional pain syndrome. *Cochrane Database Syst Rev.* 2016;7:CD004598.

Perez RS, Kwakkel G, Zurmond WW, et al. Treatment of reflex sympathetic dystrophy (CRPS type 1): a research synthesis of 21 randomized clinical trials. *J Pain Symptom Manage.* 2001;21(6):511-526.

Rockett M. Diagnosis, mechanisms and treatment of complex regional pain syndrome. *Curr Opin Anaesthesiol.* 2014;27(5):494-500.

Stanton-Hicks M, Baron R, Boas R, et al. Consensus report. Complex regional pain syndromes: guidelines for therapy. *Clin J Pain.* 1998;14:155-166.

Van Hilten BJ, van de Beek WJ, Hoff JI, et al. Intrathecal baclofen for the treatment of dystonia in patients with reflex sympathetic dystrophy. *N Engl J Med.* 2000;343:625-630.

Visnjevac O, Costandi S, Patel BA, et al. A comprehensive outcome-specific review of the use of spinal cord stimulation for complex regional pain syndrome. *Pain Pract.* 2017;17(4):533-545.

Wheeler AH, Murrey DB. Spinal pain: pathogenesis, evolutionary mechanisms and management. In: Pappagallo M, ed. *The Neurological Basis of Pain.* New York, NY: McGraw-Hill; 2005:421-452.

Wheeler DS, Vaux KK, Tam DA. Use of gabapentin in the treatment of childhood reflex sympathetic dystrophy. *Pediatr Neurol.* 2000;22:220-221.

Woolf CJ, Mannion RJ. Neuropathic pain: aetiology, symptoms, mechanisms, and management. *Lancet.* 1999;353:1959-1964.

Zhou G, Hotta J, Lehtinen MK, et al. Enlargement of choroid plexus in complex regional pain syndrome. *Sci Rep.* 2015;5:14329.

Zollinger PE, Tuinebreijer WE, Kreis RW, et al. Effect of vitamin C on frequency of reflex sympathetic dystrophy in wrist fractures: a randomised trial. *Lancet.* 1999;354:2025-2028.

38 Headache

Nathaniel M. Schuster and
Brian J. Wainger

Headache is the third leading cause of disability worldwide according to the Global Burden of Disease.[1–5] Given its high prevalence, pain medicine practitioners interested in headache can receive many referrals for headache consultation. Also, given the association between headache disorders and chronic pain and chronic widespread musculoskeletal pain, pain medicine providers encounter many patients with headache disorders for other pain-related reasons.[6] Having a good understanding of headache diagnoses and management enables pain medicine providers to reduce polypharmacy by choosing medications proven to have both headache and pain benefits and to avoid medications likely to cause medication overuse headache (rebound headache).

I. EPIDEMIOLOGY

Migraine is the primary headache disorder for which people most often seek medical care. Forty-three percent of women and eighteen percent of men will experience a migraine during their lives.[7] Migraine has a one-year prevalence of 17.1% in women and 5.6% in men.[8] About 1% of people have chronic migraine, or migraines more than 8 days a month and headaches more than 15 days a month.[9] Migraine is the seventh leading cause of disability worldwide according to the Global Burden of Disease.[1–5]

Tension-type headache is more common than migraine, but given that tension-type headaches are less severe and less disabling than migraines, they are often merely a nuisance to people and are a less common reason for presentation for medical care. The one-year prevalence in a Danish study was 79% in 1989 and 87% in 2001.[10] However, other studies have found a lower prevalence. The male-female ratio in the Danish study in 1989 was 1:1.4 and in 2001 was 1:1.1.[10]

Cluster headache is estimated to have a prevalence of 0.1%-0.4%.[11-14] It causes pain so severe that patients often contemplate suicide.[15] Unlike many other pain disorders, it has a male predominance, estimated at about 3:1.

II. HEADACHE HISTORY

A. Red Flags for Secondary Causes of Headache

While most headaches are due to primary headache disorders (such a migraine or tension-type headache), the first task in the evaluation of a new patient is excluding secondary headache disorders (such as vascular, infectious, and neoplastic causes), several of which warrant urgent or emergent treatment.

At initial visit, a thorough history and physical examination including neurologic examination should be performed. The mnemonic SNOOP can be used to remember red flags for secondary headache disorders (Table 38.1).

While it is standard to ask patients presenting with headache whether they have a prior personal history of migraines, motion sickness, or infantile colic and to ask whether they have a family history of migraine, an affirmative answer to any of these questions should not cause providers to overlook red flag signs and symptoms which may be present.

B. Distinguishing Primary Headache Disorders

In the absence of red flag signs and symptoms, the headache history focuses on headache timing and duration and the presence of migrainous features (photophobia, phonophobia, nausea, and vomiting), autonomic features (ptosis, conjunctival injection, lacrimation, nasal congestion), and associated features such as visual aura.

Location and quality are also asked, but it is important to know the pitfalls and where these may be misleading. Most notably, "squeezing"

TABLE 38.1 SNOOP Mnemonic of Red Flags for Secondary Headache

S	Systemic Signs or Symptoms	Such as fever, chills, or unexplained weight loss
	Secondary Risk Factors	Especially history of cancer or immunosuppression
N	Neurologic Signs or Symptoms	Particularly new focal neurological features
O	Onset	Thunderclap headache, or severe headache of maximal severity within 1 minute of onset
O	Older	New-onset headache starting at age > 50 (some say 40)
P	Positional Headache	High-pressure headache if present upon awakening and improving with standing up. Low-pressure headache if present when standing and remitting with lying down
	Prior Headache	Change in quality from prior headache
	Papilledema	Critical assessment as it results in divergent diagnostic and treatment algorithms
	Pregnancy	Increased risk associated with hypercoagulability, hypertension, and vascular permeability

bifrontal headaches with migrainous features may be misdiagnosed as tension-type headache rather than migraine, and "stabbing" unilateral retroorbital headaches with migrainous features and timing and duration consistent with migraine may be misdiagnosed as cluster headache. In many cases, these conclusions are influenced by consideration of Bayesian pretest probability: undiagnosed migraine are particularly common.

1. **Triggers.** Triggers to ask about include:
   a. Cough or valsalva
   b. Exertion
   c. Sex
   d. Sleep (or "alarm-clock" headaches awakening from sleep at same time nightly)
   e. Cutaneous triggers in face or mouth

   These triggers are to help distinguish primary headache disorders from one another and are distinct from the common migraine triggers to be asked once a diagnosis of migraine has been made.
2. **Algorithm.** Bigal and Lipton provide an excellent algorithm for classifying primary headache disorders.[16] Duration of untreated headache should be distinguished as short duration headaches (<4 hours) and long duration headaches (≥4 hours). Headache frequency should be categorized by low frequency (<15 days a month) or high frequency (more than 15 days per month). If patients have multiple headaches per day, the range of daily headaches should be recorded (Figs. 38.1-38.3).

III. HEADACHE PHYSICAL EXAMINATION

In addition to complete neurologic examination, the headache examination should include funduscopic examination to evaluate for papilledema, temporomandibular joint examination to assess temporomandibular joint dysfunction, body habitus, neck circumference, Mallampati scoring of posterior oropharynx examination to assist with screening for obstructive sleep apnea, and examination of the nuchal region and cervical spine to exclude nuchal rigidity and to evaluate for possible occipital neuralgia and cervicogenic component of headaches.

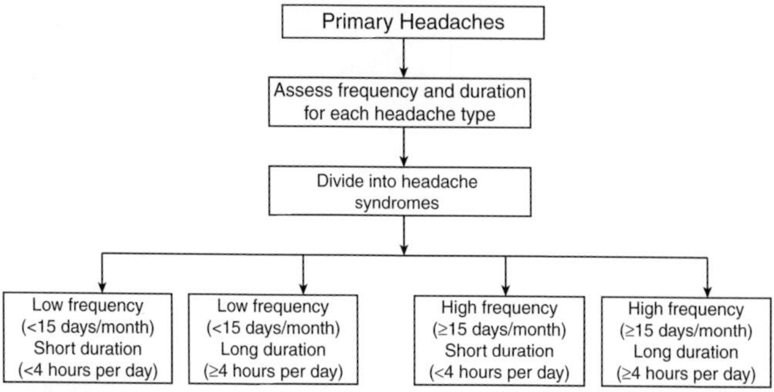

FIGURE 38.1 Dividing primary headache disorders by duration and frequency. (Reprinted by permission of Springer: Bigal ME, Lipton RB. The differential diagnosis of chronic daily headaches: an algorithm-based approach. *J Headache Pain*. 2007;8(5):263-272. doi: 10.1007/s10194-007-0418-3.)

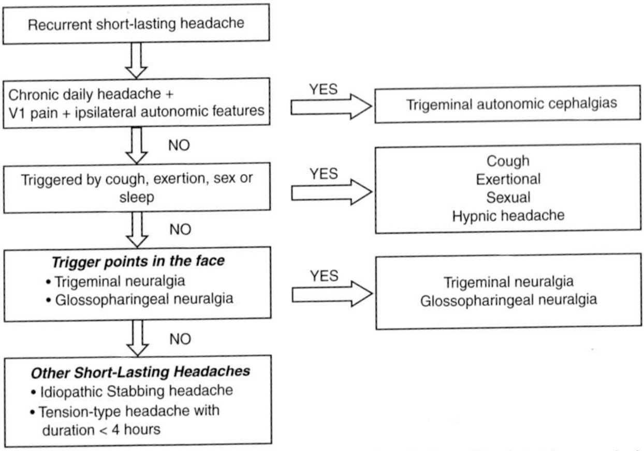

FIGURE 38.2 Algorithm of recurrent short-lasting headaches. (Reprinted by permission of Springer: Bigal ME, Lipton RB. The differential diagnosis of chronic daily headaches: an algorithm-based approach. *J Headache Pain*. 2007;8(5):263-272. doi: 10.1007/s10194-007-0418-3.)

IV. HEADACHE LABORATORY TESTING AND IMAGING

Laboratory testing is not routinely warranted. In patients age > 50 with headache and other concerning symptoms including episodes of vision loss, jaw claudication and/or proximal pain and stiffness, giant cell arteritis, and temporal arteritis must be excluded. Immediate evaluation should

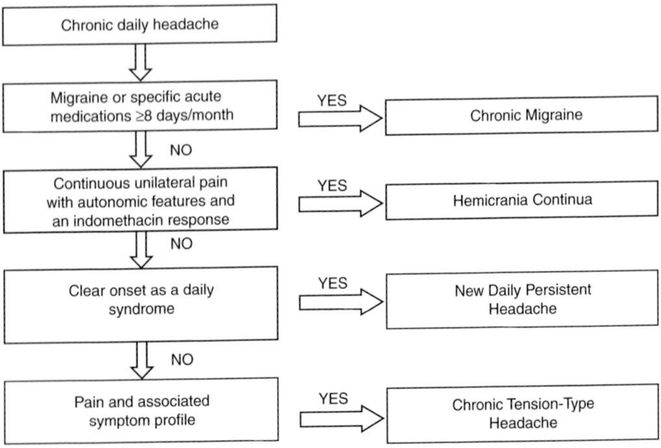

FIGURE 38.3 Algorithm of high-frequency, long-duration headaches. (Reprinted by permission of Springer: Bigal ME, Lipton RB. The differential diagnosis of chronic daily headaches: an algorithm-based approach. *J Headache Pain*. 2007;8(5):263-272. doi: 10.1007/s10194-007-0418-3.)

begin with ordering erythrocyte sedimentation rate (ESR) and C-reactive protein (CRP). High-dose steroid treatment is not delayed for arterial biopsy if suspicion is strong.

Imaging should only be ordered if secondary headache is suspected based on the presence of red flags (Table 38.1). The American Headache Society recommends against imaging patients with stable migraine.[17] Brain MRIs are more helpful than CTs for excluding most causes of secondary headache, and MRIs should be ordered unless in emergency department situations if MRI is not readily available.[17]

The most common, and important, exception to the recommendation of ordering an MRI is if subarachnoid hemorrhage (SAH) is suspected. Clinicians should consider SAH if patients report the worst headache of their life and "thunderclap headache" (severe headache of maximal intensity within 1 minute of onset, although usually the peak severity is reached within seconds). Onset with exertion and associated nausea and neck stiffness are common but not always present in SAH. SAH is a medical emergency and when suspected, an emergent noncontrast CT should be performed. If the noncontrast CT is nondiagnostic and high clinical suspicion of SAH remains, it is controversial whether the next step should be CT with CT angiogram, MRI, or lumbar puncture.

While migraine and tension-type headache do not require imaging in the absence of red flag symptoms, TACs and exertional headaches require imaging (MRI brain preferred) to exclude pituitary and posterior fossa pathology. If trigeminal neuralgia or glossopharyngeal neuralgia are suspected, MRI with and without contrast with CISS or FIESTA sequence should be performed to evaluate for vascular loops overlying the pertinent cranial nerves as well as dorsal root entry zone demyelination which may herald a new diagnosis of multiple sclerosis.

V. DIFFERENTIAL DIAGNOSIS

A. Secondary Headache Disorders

The differential diagnosis for headache with red flags should include causes listed in Table 38.2.

Patients with migraine may believe that they have an ocular problem or sinus pathology and may seek treatment from ophthalmology or ENT prior to receiving a migraine diagnosis. Most self-reported sinus headache

TABLE 38.2 A List of Secondary Headache Causes

Subarachnoid, Epidural, Subdural, or Intraparenchymal Hemorrhage
Pituitary Apoplexy
Cerebral Venous Thrombosis
Hypertensive Disorders including Posterior Reversible Encephalopathy Syndrome (PRES)
Cervical (Carotid or Vertebral) Dissection
Meningitis or Encephalitis
Temporal Arteritis and Giant Cell Arteritis
Primary (Benign or Malignant) or Secondary (Metastatic) Brain Tumor
Intracranial Hypertension (Idiopathic Intracranial Hypertension, previously known as pseudotumor cerebri, or Communicating or Noncommunicating Hydrocephalus)
Intracranial Hypotension (Spontaneous or Iatrogenic CSF Leak)

is actually migraine, as supported by a 2006 ENT, neurology, allergy, and primary care consensus statement.[18]

If secondary headache disorder is suspected, clinical judgment should be used to decide whether referral to the emergency department, to a neurologist, or to other specialties is indicated. The broad range of consequence between severe but minimally threatening migraine and life-threatening SAH, for which more than half of patients present with headache alone, make the accurate assessment of headache critical.

B. Primary Headache Disorders

The definitive reference for headache disorders is the *International Classification of Headache Disorders 3*, which can be found at ichd-3.org.[19] An excellent algorithm for considering primary headache disorders based on frequency and duration can be found in an article by Bigal and Lipton[16] (Figs. 38.1-38.3).

Most common are long-duration (≥4 hour) headaches, especially migraine, which should be ≥4 hours in duration if untreated, although with treatment with analgesics, triptans, or other acute medications, the headache may last <4 hours. Other long-duration headaches are hemicrania continua (a side-locked headache with ipsilateral autonomic features), tension-type headache (which can be 30 minutes to 7 days in duration), and new daily persistent headache (a headache which is continuous from onset for >3 months and can be migrainous or nonmigrainous).

1. The short-duration headaches include the TACs:
   a. Cluster headache
   b. Paroxysmal hemicrania
   c. Short-lasting unilateral neuralgiform headache with conjunctival injection and tearing (SUNCT)
   d. Short-lasting unilateral neuralgiform headache with autonomic symptoms (SUNA).
2. They also include the exertional headaches:
   a. Primary cough headache
   b. Primary exercise headache
   c. Primary headache associated with sexual activity.
3. Primary thunderclap headache is another primary headache disorder which is a diagnosis of exclusion; "thunderclap headache" is a red flag symptom for which subarachnoid hemorrhage, and reversible cerebral vasoconstriction syndrome are on the differential.
4. The two short-duration headaches that patients often report awaken them in the middle of the night "like an alarm clock" are:
   a. Cluster headache (unilateral headache with ipsilateral autonomic features)
   b. Hypnic headache (pain is usually bilateral and mild to moderate and without autonomic features).

C. Selected Headache Disorders In-Depth

Among primary headache disorders encountered in pain medicine and primary care clinics, the most common is migraine. Migraine is defined as a headache lasting 4-72 hours, often unilateral, throbbing/pulsating, moderate/severe, and worsened by routine activity, associated with photophobia and photophobia and nausea and vomiting.

A common pitfall is misdiagnosing patients with tension-type headache based on headache location and/or quality alone; migraines can be bilateral and may be described as "squeezing" in quality. Differentiating migraine from tension-type headache is crucial since many of the

TABLE 38.3 The ID Migraine Screener

During the last 3 months, did you have any of the following with your headaches?		
P	Photophobia	Light bothered you (a lot more than when you do not have headaches)?
I	Incapacitating	Your headaches limited your ability to work, study, or do what you needed to do for at least 1 day?
N	Nausea	You felt nauseated or sick to your stomach when you had a headache?
An affirmative answer to 2 of those 3 questions conveys 81% sensitivity and 75% specificity for a diagnosis of migraine.		

Reprinted with permission from Lipton RB, Dodick D, Sadovsky R, et al. A self-administered screener for migraine in primary care: the ID Migraine validation study. *Neurology.* 2003;61(3):375-382, Ref. [21]

most effective treatments for migraine (such as triptans, topiramate, and onabotulinumtoxinA) are ineffective in patients with pure tension-type headache. In patients who experience both migraine and tension-type headache, triptans and onabotulinumtoxinA can benefit both types of headaches.[20]

Use of the ID Migraine screener (mnemonic "PIN") can help to avoid missing a diagnosis of migraine (Table 38.3).

Identifying subtypes of migraine is important as they may warrant differences in treatment (Table 38.4).

Tension-type headache, while likely more prevalent than migraine, is less often encountered in pain and neurology clinics than is migraine due to its mild/moderate severity and should be considered only after inquiring about migrainous features and excluding migraine. Tension-type headaches are "featureless" headaches (lacking photophobia, phonophobia, nausea, or autonomic symptoms) and are typically bilateral, nonpulsating, and mild/moderate in severity, lasting 30 minutes to 7 days in duration. Migraine can also be bilateral and described as "tightening" in quality but is associated with photophobia and phonophobia or nausea and is more severe and disabling.

The trigeminal autonomic cephalgias (TACs) are unilateral, side-locked headaches with ipsilateral autonomic features. These autonomic features may include ptosis, lacrimation, conjunctival injection, and nasal congestion and should be strictly unilateral, in comparison to in migraine, where bilateral autonomic symptoms may be present. Distinguishing the TACs from one another is crucial since they respond to different medications. The most common, and well-known, TAC is cluster headache. It differs from the others (hemicrania continua, paroxysmal hemicrania, SUNCT, and SUNA) in duration and frequency of attacks (Table 38.5).

There are also other uncommon primary headache conditions. Hypnic headache is a featureless "alarm clock" headache that awakens patients from sleep at a fixed time of night; effective treatments include caffeine before bedtime. Primary cough headache, primary exertional headache, and primary headache associated with sexual activity are diagnoses of exclusion that can be made after excluding structural causes with MRI brain; indomethacin 25-50 mg 30-60 minutes before exercise or intercourse is effective for many patients and could be dosed three times daily for primary cough headache. Additional recommendations about indomethacin are provided later in this chapter.

TABLE 38.4 Subtypes of Migraine and Clinical Considerations

Name	Definition	Clinical Considerations
Migraine with Aura	Visual aura affects only one side of vision, lasts 5-60 minutes, starts before or during headache, develops gradually, causes partial loss of vision or blind spot in vision (scotoma), often with a zig-zag line or shimmering leading edge (fortification spectrum). Sensory and motor auras are less common.	Conveys slightly increased risk of ischemic stroke. Counsel women who both use tobacco and are on estrogen-containing oral contraceptives about increased stroke risk and encourage to stop tobacco.
Episodic Migraine	Migraines <8 days a month or headaches <15 days a month.	Consider preventive treatment if patient is having 4 or more migraine days a month.
Chronic Migraine	Migraines more than 8 days a month and headaches more than 15 days a month.	Consider botulinum toxin or CGRP inhibitors if patient has not responded to treatment with 2-3 oral migraine preventives (from antihypertensive, antiepileptic, and antidepressant classes).
Medication Overuse	Using simple analgesics more than 3 days a week or using combination analgesics, triptans, butalbital-containing compounds, or opioids more than 2 days a week.	Chronic migraine and medication overuse headache frequently cooccur. May revert to episodic migraine with decreasing use of offending medication.
Pure Menstrual Migraine	Migraines exclusively with menstrual periods on headache calendar.	Consider miniprophylaxis with a long-duration NSAID or triptan twice a day for 5 days starting 2 days before menstrual period.
Hemiplegic Migraine	Migraines associated with hemibody weakness; may also have aphasia, usually together with right hemibody weakness. May be familiar or sporadic.	Triptans and ergot derivatives are contraindicated.
Migraine with Brainstem Aura	Previously called basilar migraine.	Triptans and ergot derivatives are contraindicated.
Typical Migraine Aura without Headache	Previously called acephalgic migraine.	
Status Migrainosus	Migraine lasting longer than 72 hours.	May require rescue treatments such as IM/IV ketorolac, IV dopamine antagonists, and/or IV dihydroergotamine

TABLE 38.5 Trigeminal Autonomic Cephalalgias

	Cluster Headache	Paroxysmal Hemicrania	SUNCT/SUNA
Sex ratio	3 Males to 1 female	Males = females	1.5 Males to 1 female
Pain			
Quality	Sharp/stab/throb	Sharp/stab/throb	Sharp/stab/throb
Severity	Very severe	Very severe	Severe
Distribution	V1>C2>V2>V3	V1>C2>V2>V3	V1>C2>V2>V3
Attacks			
Frequency (per day)	1-8	11	100
Length (minutes)	30-180	2-30	1-10
Triggers			
Alcohol	+++	+	–
Nitroglycerin	+++	+	–
Cutaneous	+	–	+++
Agitation/restlessness	90%	80%	65%
Episodic versus chronic	90:10	35:65	10:90
Circadian/circannual periodicity	Present	Absent	Absent
Treatment effects			
Oxygen	70%	No effect	No effect
Sumatriptan (6 mg)	90%	20%	<10%
Indomethacin	No effect	100%	No effect
Migraine features with attacks			
Nausea	50%	40%	25%
Photophobia/phonophobia	65%	65%	25%

SUNCT/SUNA, short-lasting unilateral neuralgiform headache attacks with conjunctival injection and tearing/short-lasting unilateral neuralgiform headache attacks with cranial autonomic features; C, cervical; V, trigeminal.

Goadsby PJ. Trigeminal autonomic cephalalgias. *Continuum (Minneap Minn)*. 2012;18(4):883–895. doi: 10.1212/01.CON.0000418649.54902.0b.

Pseudotumor cerebri syndrome (PCS), also known as idiopathic intracranial hypertension (IIH), is not truly a headache disorder, but rather a neuro-ophthalmologic disorder often presenting with headache and diagnosed based on the presence of papilledema, cranial nerve abnormalities, opening pressure on lumbar puncture, and MRI findings such as empty sella, flattening of posterior aspect of the globe, distention of perioptic subarachnoid space, and transverse venous sinus stenosis.[22] Providers likely over-test for PCS/IIH based on body habitus, as migraine is much more common than PCS/IIH even in the typical PCS/IIH population of obese, reproductive-age women. If patients do not meet the other diagnostic criteria of IIH/PCS, IIH/PCS is unlikely and lumbar puncture is not indicated.[23] If IIH/PCS is suspected, we advise ophthalmology evaluation (neuro-ophthalmology, if available) for expert funduscopic examination and Humphrey Visual Fields prior to subjecting patients to lumbar puncture. Reduction in visual fields should be the key clinical finding that motivates aggressive treatment such as shunting.

Intracranial hypotension causes orthostatic headaches (provoked with rising and palliated by lying flat) often associated with neck pain, changes in hearing (which may include tinnitus), photophobia, and nausea. Intracranial hypotension is most often iatrogenic in the setting of recent prior dural puncture, whether deliberate in the setting of a lumbar puncture, or inadvertent in the setting of a "wet tap" while performing procedures such as epidural injection or catheter placement. Dural tear may also occur during spine surgery. Spontaneous CSF leaks may also occur, most often in the setting of connective tissue disorders or Tarlov cysts. Postdural puncture headache (PDPH) is most common in young women; risk can be decreased by orienting the needle bevel parallel with the longitudinal dural fibers, by using a higher gauge (smaller bore) spinal needle, and by reinserting the stylet prior to withdrawing the needle. Instructing patient to lay supine after dural puncture has not been found to reduce likelihood of developing PDPH. Following iatrogenic dural puncture, imaging is unnecessary unless neurologic examination raises concern for impending herniation. However, if clinical suspicion for intracranial hypotension in the absence of known iatrogenic cause, MRI brain may show signs of intracranial hypotension including smooth pachymeningeal enhancement, sagging of the brainstem, and dilated cerebral venous sinuses. CT or MRI myelography may be helpful to find the location of the CSF leak and to guide intervention. Treatment should begin with conservative measures such as laying supine, hydration, simple analgesics, and caffeine. If these are ineffective, blood patch may be pursued. If two blood patches are ineffective, could consider fibrin patch or surgical closure. The role of blood patch is less clear in spontaneous CSF leaks than it is in PDPH.

VI. TREATMENTS

Treatments that can be provided by pain medicine physicians include acute (or abortive), preventive (or prophylactic), and rescue pharmacologic treatments, interventional treatments, and education (including lifestyle modifications, trigger avoidance education, and medication overuse education). Figure 38.4 provides an algorithm to guide appropriate migraine treatment.

A. Lifestyle Treatments

1. Patient education of migraine patients should include:
   a. Lifestyle modifications
   b. Regular sleep times
   c. Three regular meals a day
   d. Ample hydration
   e. If patients drink caffeine, they should use a consistent amount of caffeine at the same time every morning and should limit overall caffeine use.
   f. Regular exercise
   g. Stress reduction

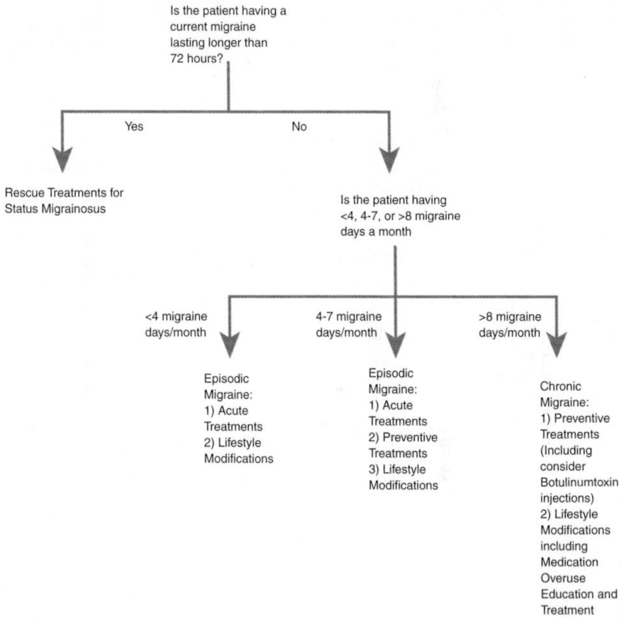

FIGURE 38.4 Algorithm for migraine treatment.

2. Trigger avoidance: Some common, avoidable triggers that patients may recognize include red wine and chocolate.
3. Medication overuse education: Using simple analgesics more than 3 days a week or using combination analgesics, triptans, butalbital-containing compounds, or opioids more than 2 days a week may cause headaches to become more frequent.

B. Preventive Migraine Treatments

Oral preventive medications include those listed in the 2012 American Academy of Neurology/American Headache Society guidelines (Table 38.6). In addition to treatments on this table, other treatments with more recent evidence to support their use include memantine, simvastatin with vitamin D, magnesium, riboflavin, and melatonin. Three monoclonal antibodies targeting the calcitonin gene-related peptide (CGRP) ligand (eptinezumab, fremanezumab, and galcanezumab) and one targeting the CGRP receptor (erenumab) are now FDA approved and are administered either monthly or once every three months.[24,25]

C. Interventional Treatments

Interventional treatments can be used for migraine prevention or for treating status migrainosus. Chemodenervation with onabotulinumtoxinA (Botox) is FDA approved for migraine prevention in patients with chronic migraine (at least 8 headache days and 15 migraine days per month). Chemodenervation with onabotulinumtoxinA was more effective than sham injections with saline with regard to reduction in headache days in the pooled data of the PREEMPT studies,[27] two randomized, controlled trials

TABLE 38.6 Classification of Migraine Preventative Therapies (Available in the United States)

Level A: Medications with Established Efficacy (≥2 Class I Trials)	Level B: Medications are Probably Effective (1 Class I or 2 Class II Studies)	Level C: Medications are Possibly Effective (1 Class II Study)	Level U: Inadequate or Conflicting Data to Support or Refute Medication Use	Other: Medications that are Established as Possibly or Probably Ineffective
Antiepileptic drugs	Antidepressants/SSRI/SSNRI/TCA	ACE inhibitors Lisinopril	Carbonic anhydrase inhibitor	Established as not effective
Divalproex sodium	Amitriptyline	Angiotensin receptor blockers	Acetazolamide	Antiepileptic drugs
Sodium valproate	Venlafaxine	Candesartan	Antithrombotics	Lamotrigine
Topiramate	β-Blockers	α-Agonists	Acenocoumarol	Probably not effective
β-Blockers	Atenolol[a]	Clonidine[a]	Coumadin	Clomipramine[a]
Metoprolol	Nadolol[a]	Guanfacine[a]	Picotamide	Possibly not effective
Propranolol	Triptans (MRM[b])	Antiepileptic drugs	Antidepressants SSRI/SSNRI	Acebutolol[a]
Timolol[a]	Naratriptan[b]	Carbamazepine[a]	Fluvoxamine[a]	Clonazepam[a]
Triptans (MRM[b])	Zolmitriptan[b]	β-Blockers	Fluoxetine	Nabumetone[a]
Frovatriptan[b]		Nebivolol	Antiepileptic drugs	Oxcarbazepine
		Pindolol[a]	Gabapentin	Telmisartan
		Antihistamines	TCAs	
		Cyproheptadine	Protriptyline[a]	
			β-Blockers	
			Bisoprolol[a]	
			Ca++ blockers	
			Nicardipine[a]	
			Nifedipine[a]	
			Nimodipine	
			Verapamil	
			Direct vascular smooth muscle relaxants	
			Cyclandelate	
CGRPsc	Erenumab	Galcanezumab	Fremanezumab	Eptinezumab

ACE, angiotensin-converting-enzyme; MRM, menstrually related migraine; SSNRI, selective serotonin–norepinephrine reuptake inhibitor; SSRI, selective serotonin reuptake inhibitor; TCA, tricyclic antidepressant; CGRP, calcitonin gene-related peptide. [a]Classification based on original guideline and new evidence not found for this report.

[b]For short-term prophylaxis of MRM. [c]Added by the authors of this chapter; FDA approved after Silberstein et al was written. Reprinted with permission from Silberstein SD, Holland S, Freitag F, Dodick DW, Argoff C, Ashman E. Evidence-based guideline update: pharmacologic treatment for episodic migraine prevention in adults report of the quality standards subcommittee of the American academy of neurology and the American headache society. *Neurology.* 2012;78(17):1337-1345. doi: 10.1212/WNL.0b013e3182535d20, Ref. [26]

in which patients with chronic migraine received injections of 5 units each in 31 protocolized sites as well as up to 40 additional units as "follow the pain" treatments, for a total of 155-195 units (see Fig. 38.5).

Pericranial peripheral nerve blocks (PPNBs) can be used either for migraine prevention or for breaking a cycle of migraines or status migrainosus. The most common PPNBs are greater occipital nerve blocks. Others include lesser occipital, supraorbital, supratrochlear, infraorbital, and auriculotemporal nerve blocks, as well as sphenopalatine ganglion blocks.

Anecdotally, trigger point injections can also break severe cycles of migraines or status migrainosus in some patients. Common locations of myofascial pain in patients with migraine include the cervical paraspinals, trapezeii, and levator scapulae. Myofascial temporomandibular disorder may be present in headache patients; for such patients, trigger point injections in the temporalis and masseters (as well as medial and lateral pterygoid muscles) may be performed. For patients with arthrogenic temporomandibular disorder, intraarticular joint injections may be performed.

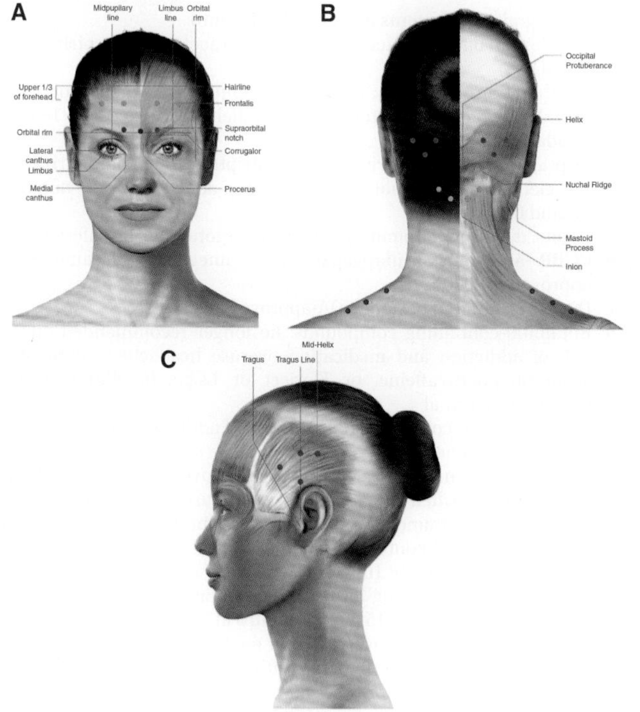

FIGURE 38.5 Fixed-site, fixed dose. PREEMPT injection site locations. (a) Corrugator, as depicted by *purples dots*; procerus, as depicted by the *red dot*; frontalis, as depicted by *orange dots*. (b) Occipitalis area, as depicted by *purple dots*; cervical paraspinal area; as depicted by *orange dots*; trapezius, as depicted by *red dots*. (c) Temporalis, as depicted by *purple dots*. (From Blumenfeld AM, Silberstein SD, Dodick DW, Aurora SK, Brin MF, Binder WJ. Insights into the functional anatomy behind the PREEMPT injection paradigm: guidance on achieving optimal outcomes. *Headache*. 2017;57(5):766-777, Ref.[28])

Cervicogenic headache is likely over diagnosed by pain medicine physicians and physiatrists. Neck pain during migraine is a common symptom of migraine due to the convergence of trigeminal and cervical sensory afferents in a part of the medulla and high cervical spinal cord known as the trigeminocervical complex.[29] If neck pain is present as part of a patient's migraine attack, it should be responsive to migraine treatments. However, if it is present between migraine attacks, treatments targeting neck pain such as trigger point injections or cervical medial branch nerve blocks and radiofrequency ablation should be considered.[30] The third occipital nerve provides the sole innervation of the C2/3 facet joint, and third occipital nerve radiofrequency ablation is a treatment for C2/3 facet arthropathy, with best evidence for its prevalence and effectiveness among patients with whiplash injuries.[31,32]

D. Acute Migraine Treatments

In 2015, the American Headache Society published an updated assessment of evidence of acute migraine treatments[33] (see Table 38.7).

1. Acute migraine treatments are often divided into:
   - **a.** Simple analgesics: acetaminophen/paracetamol, aspirin, and NSAIDs
   - **b.** Combination analgesics: aspirin/acetaminophen/caffeine, or Excedrin Migraine, and acetaminophen/caffeine, or Excedrin Tension Headache
   - **c.** Triptans: 5 fast-acting triptans—sumatriptan, zolmitriptan, rizatriptan, eletriptan, and almotriptan, and 2 long-acting triptans—naratriptanand frovatriptan.
   - **d.** Ergots: dihydroergotamine and caffeine/ergotamine, or Cafergot
   - **e.** CGRP antagonists: ubrogepant and rimegepant became FDA-approved in 2020
   - **f.** Ditans: lasmiditan became FDA-approved in 2020
   - **g.** Butalbital-containing compounds: no longer recommended due to risk of addiction and medication overuse headache[17]—butalbital/acetaminophen/caffeine, or Fioricet or Esgic, butalbital/aspirin/caffeine, or Fiorinal
   - **h.** Opioids—not recommended due to risk of addiction and medication overuse headache[17]
2. Pain physicians must be aware of medication-overuse headache. Medication overuse is when simple analgesics are used more than 3 days a week and other migraine treatments are used more than 2 days a week. Overusing butalbital-containing compounds and opioids doubles the risk of episodic migraine (migraines <8 days a month or headaches <15 days a month) turning into chronic migraine (migraines >8 days a month and headaches >15 days a month) at 1 year.[34] However, not all patients with medication overuse have medication-overuse headache; nonetheless, about 50% of patients with chronic migraine and medication overuse revert to episodic migraine after removing the inciting medication. A history of migraine frequency increasing as the frequency of the overused medication increased may help identify responders. How to treat severe headaches while patients with medication overuse headache reduce their use of acute treatments is a particularly challenging question in headache medicine. Treatment approaches being studied include adding prevention without withdrawing the overused medication, withdrawing the overused medication and afterwards adding prevention, and adding preventive therapy while weaning the overused medication.

TABLE 38.7 Acute Migraine Treatments and Strength of Evidence

Level A	Level B	Level C	Level U	Others
Analgesic Acetaminophen 1000 mg (for nonincapacitating attacks)	**Antiemetics** [a]Chlorpromazine IV 12.5 mg Droperidol IV 2.75 mg [a]Metoclopramide IV 10 mg [a]Prochlorperazine IV/IM 10 mg; PR 25 mg	**Antiepileptic** Valproate IV 400-1000 mg	**NSAIDs** Celecoxib 400 mg	**Level B negative Other** Octreotide SC 100 μg
Ergots DHE [a]Nasal spray 2 mg Pulmonary inhaler 1 mg	**Ergots** DHE[a] IV, IM, SC 1 mg [a]Ergotamine/caffeine 1/100 mg	**Ergot** [a]Ergotamine 1-2 mg	**Others** [a]Lidocaine IV [a]Hydrocortisone IV 50 mg	**Level C negative Antiemetics** [a]Chlorpromazine IM 1 mg/kg Granisetron IV 40-80 μg/kg
NSAIDs [a]Aspirin 500 mg Diclofenac 50, 100 mg Ibuprofen 200, 400 mg [a]Naproxen 500, 550 mg	[a]Flurbiprofen 100 mg Ketoprofen 100 mg Ketorolac IV/IM 30-60 mg	**NSAIDs** Phenazone 1000 mg	**NSAIDs**	**NSAIDs** Ketorolac tromethamine nasal spray
Opioids [a]Butorphanol nasal spray 1 mg	**Opioid**	**Analgesic** [a]Butorphanol IM 2 mg [a]Codeine 30 mg PO [a]Meperidine IM 75 mg [a]Methadone IM 10 mg [a]Tramadol IV 100 mg		Acetaminophen IV 1000 mg

(Continued)

TABLE 38.7 Acute Migraine Treatments and Strength of Evidence (*Continued*)

Level A	Level B	Level C	Level U	Others
Triptans Almotriptan 12.5 mg Eletriptan 20, 40, 80 mg Frovatriptan 2.5 mg [a]Naratriptan 1, 2.5 mg [a]Rizatriptan 5, 10 mg Sumatriptan [a]Oral 25, 50, 100 mg [a]Nasal spray 10, 20 mg Patch 6.5 mg [a]SC 4, 6 mg Zolmitriptan nasal spray 2.5, 5 mg [a]Oral 2.5, 5 mg	**Others** $MgSO_4$ IV (migraine with aura) 1-2 g [a]Isometheptene 65 mg	**Steroid** Dexamethasone IV 4-16 mg		
Combinations [a]Acetaminophen/aspirin/caffeine 500/500/130 mg Sumatriptan/naproxen 85/500 mg	**Combinations** [a]Codeine/acetaminophen 25/400 mg Tramadol/acetaminophen 75/650 mg	**Others** [a]Butalbital 50 mg [a]Lidocaine intranasal		

Level A	Level B	Level C	Level U	Others
		Combinations		
CGRPs		[a]Butalbital/acetaminophen/ caffeine/codeine 50/325/40/30 mg		
[b]Ubrogepant 50, 100 mg				
[b]Rimegepant 75 mg Ditans				
[b]Lasmiditan 50, 100, 200 mg		[a]Butalbital/acetaminophen/ caffeine 50/325/40 mg		

[a]Based on 2000 American Academy of Neurology evidence review.
[b]Added by the authors of this chapter, approved by the FDA after Marmura et al was written
Level A: Medications: are established as effective for acute migraine treatment based on available evidence.
Level B: Medications are probably effective for acute migraine treatment based on available evidence.
Level C: Medications are possibly effective for acute migraine treatment based on available evidence.
Level U: Evidence is conflicting or inadequate to support or refute the efficacy of the following medications for acute migraine.
Level B negative: Medication is probably ineffective for acute migraine.
Level C negative: Medication is possibly ineffective for acute migraine.
From Marmura MJ, Silberstein SD, Schwedt TJ. The acute treatment of migraine in adults: the American headache society evidence assessment of migraine pharmacotherapies. *Headache.* 2015;55(1):3-20.

3. Patients should be counseled to use their fast-acting triptan within 15-30 minutes of onset of headache pain. Triptans are less effective later during a migraine. The two long-acting triptans, naratriptan and frovatriptan, are less suited for acute migraine and better suited for short-term prevention of pure menstrual migraine (usually starting 2 days before the period and continuing twice a day for 5 days) or for treatment of status migrainosus (often used twice a day for 3-5 days). Strong vascular risk factors are contraindications for triptans and ergots due to their vasoconstrictive effects.
4. Nonoral treatments may be necessary for patients with severe nausea with or without vomiting and gastric stasis with their migraines; these includes subcutaneous sumatriptan, intranasal sumatriptan or zolmitriptan, intramuscular dihydroergotamine, and prochlorperazine rectal suppositories.
5. Lasmiditan, a novel 5HT-1F agonist, is an option for patients for whom triptans are contraindicated, ineffective, or not tolerated. The 5HT-1F receptor is not found on blood vessels, and lasmiditan does not cause vasoconstriction. It can be considered for patients with vascular risk factors. Oral CGRP antagonists ubrogepant and rimegepant are also options for acute migraine treatment.

E. Rescue Migraine Treatments

Some patients will require a rescue treatment if they have a propensity toward status migrainosus, other prolonged migraines not responding to acute migraine treatments, or emergency room presentation.[35–37] Most of the evidence is based on emergency room studies of IV treatments such as NSAIDs, D2 antagonists with or without diphenhydramine for akathisia prevention, magnesium, dexamethasone, valproic acid, or dihydroergotamine. Of note, D2 antagonists are antimigraine and not merely antiemetic; in a recent RCT, the response rate for migraine in the ED was 60% in the group treated with IV prochlorperazine 10 mg plus diphenhydramine 25 mg as compared to 31% in the group treated with IV hydromorphone 1 mg.[38] Greater occipital nerve blocks may also be effective for rescue therapy, as supported by two positive emergency department sham-controlled RCTs.

F. Treatment of Trigeminal Autonomic Cephalgias and Selected Other Primary Headache Disorders

1. Treatment of the trigeminal autonomic cephalalgias varies based on diagnosis, with first-line treatments including:
   a. Cluster headache: Injectable sumatriptan and high-flow oxygen for acute treatment, and oral steroids or occipital nerve blocks with steroids, galcanezumab, and verapamil for preventive treatment.
   b. Hemicrania continua and paroxysmal hemicrania: Indomethacin trial.
   c. SUNCT and SUNA: Lamotrigine.
2. Other indomethacin-responsive headaches include primary exertional headaches and primary stabbing headache.
3. Indomethacin trials can be performed in several ways, including a single injection of indomethacin (not available in the United States), or one of several titration schedules of indomethacin. One is starting with 25 mg three times a day for 3 days, after which can titrate to 50 mg three times a day for 3 days and then followed by 75 mg three times a day for an additional 8 days and titrating up as necessary and tolerated. We recommend taking oral indomethacin together with

sucralfate or H2B or PPI and meals. A complete response is expected to declare a positive indomethacin trial. After achieving a complete response, due to the poor long-term tolerability of indomethacin, one should taper down the indomethacin dose to a minimally effective dose. If indomethacin is not tolerated long-term, there are other options that can be tried, although none with consistent, equivalent effectiveness.[39]

VII. CONCLUSIONS AND KEY POINTS

A. SNOOP Mnemonic

The SNOOP mnemonic can help clinicians decide when to order laboratory tests or imaging and when to refer to neurology or the emergency department for evaluation of secondary headache disorders. A history of thunderclap headache may warrant immediate evaluation as it may signify a sentinel headache and risk of aneurysm rupture.

B. Migrainous and Autonomic Features

Diagnosing primary headache disorders requires asking patients about migrainous features (chiefly photophobia, phonophobia, nausea), autonomic features (ptosis, conjunctival injection, lacrimation, nasal congestion), and associated features such as visual aura.

C. Patient Education

Migraine treatment should include education about lifestyle modifications. Clinicians treating patients with migraine should be familiar with medication overuse headache. Risk of stroke is increased in women with migraine with aura who both use tobacco and use estrogen-containing oral contraceptives.

D. Preventative Medications

Migraine preventive medications are typically recommended for patients with 4 or more migraine days per month. Chemodenervation with botulinum toxin is only indicated in patients with chronic migraine (8 or more migraine days a month and 15 or more headache days a month).

E. Rescue Treatment Plans

A rescue treatment plan can help treat patients with status migrainosus and keep patients from going to the emergency room for IV therapies or opioids. This can include self-administered medications such as dexamethasone 5 mg twice daily for 3 days or injections such as intramuscular ketorolac, occipital nerve blocks, or trigger point injections.

References

1. Steiner TJ, Birbeck GL, Jensen RH, Katsarava Z, Stovner LJ, Martelletti P. Headache disorders are third cause of disability worldwide. *J Headache Pain.* 2015;16:58. doi: 10.1186/s10194-015-0544-2.
2. Steiner TJ, Stovner LJ, Birbeck GL. Migraine: the seventh disabler. *J Headache Pain.* 2013;14(1):1. doi: 10.1186/1129-2377-14-1.
3. Steiner TJ, Stovner LJ, Birbeck GL. Migraine: the seventh disabler. *Headache.* 2013;53(2):227-229. doi: 10.1111/head.12034.
4. Steiner TJ, Stovner LJ, Birbeck GL. Migraine: the seventh disabler. *Cephalalgia.* 2013;33(5):289-290. doi: 10.1177/0333102412473843.

5. Stovner L, Hagen K, Jensen R, et al. The global burden of headache: a documentation of headache prevalence and disability worldwide. *Cephalalgia.* 2007;27(3):193-210. doi: 10.1111/j.1468-2982.2007.01288.x.
6. Hagen K, Linde M, Steiner TJ, Zwart JA, Stovner LJ. The bidirectional relationship between headache and chronic musculoskeletal complaints: an 11-year follow-up in the Nord-Trøndelag Health Study (HUNT). *Eur J Neurol.* 2012;19(11):1447-1454. doi: 10.1111/j.1468-1331.2012.03725.x.
7. Stewart WF, Wood C, Reed ML, Roy J, Lipton RB. Cumulative lifetime migraine incidence in women and men. *Cephalalgia.* 2008;28(11):1170-1178. doi: 10.1111/j.1468-2982.2008.01666.x.
8. Lipton RB, Bigal ME, Diamond M, Freitag F, Reed ML, Stewart WF. Migraine prevalence, disease burden, and the need for preventive therapy. *Neurology.* 2007;68(5):343-349. doi: 10.1212/01.wnl.0000252808.97649.21.
9. Buse DC, Manack AN, Fanning KM, et al. Chronic migraine prevalence, disability, and sociodemographic factors: results from the American migraine prevalence and prevention study. *Headache.* 2012;52(10):1456-1470. doi: 10.1111/j.1526-4610.2012.02223.x.
10. Lyngberg AC, Rasmussen BK, Jørgensen T, Jensen R. Has the prevalence of migraine and tension-type headache changed over a 12-year period? A Danish population survey. *Eur J Epidemiol.* 2005;20(3):243-249. doi: 10.1007/s10654-004-6519-2.
11. Ekbom K, Svensson DA, Pedersen NL, Waldenlind E. Lifetime prevalence and concordance risk of cluster headache in the Swedish twin population. *Neurology.* 2006;67(5):798-803. doi: 10.1212/01.wnl.0000233786.72356.3e.
12. Torelli P, Beghi E, Manzoni GC. Cluster headache prevalence in the Italian general population. *Neurology.* 2005;64(3):469-474. doi: 10.1212/01.wnl.0000150901.47293.bc.
13. Sjaastad O, Bakketeig LS. Cluster headache prevalence. Vaga study of headache epidemiology. *Cephalalgia.* 2003;23(7):528-533.
14. Tonon C, Guttmann S, Volpini M, Naccarato S, Cortelli P, D'Alessandro R. Prevalence and incidence of cluster headache in the Republic of San Marino. *Neurology.* 2002;58(9):1407-1409.
15. Rozen TD, Fishman RS. Cluster headache in the United States of America: demographics, clinical characteristics, triggers, suicidality, and personal burden. *Headache.* 2012;52(1):99-113. doi: 10.1111/j.1526-4610.2011.02028.x.
16. Bigal ME, Lipton RB. The differential diagnosis of chronic daily headaches: An algorithm-based approach. *J Headache Pain.* 2007;8(5):263-272. doi: 10.1007/s10194-007-0418-3.
17. American Headache Society. *Choosing Wisely.* 2013. http://www.choosingwisely.org/societies/american-headache-society/. Accessed May 16, 2017.
18. Levine HL, Setzen M, Cady RK, et al. An otolaryngology, neurology, allergy, and primary care consensus on diagnosis and treatment of sinus headache. *Otolaryngol Head Neck Surg.* 2006;134(3):516-523. doi: 10.1016/j.otohns.2005.11.024.
19. Headache Classification Committee of the International Headache Society. The International Classification of Headache Disorders, 3rd edition (beta version). *Cephalalgia.* 2013;33(9):629-808. doi: 10.1177/0333102413485658.
20. Cady RK, Lipton RB, Hall C, Stewart WF, O'Quinn S, Gutterman D. Treatment of mild headache in disabled migraine sufferers: results of the spectrum study. *Headache.* 2000;40(10):792-797. doi: 10.1046/j.1526-4610.2000.00144.x.
21. Lipton RB, Dodick D, Sadovsky R, et al. A self-administered screener for migraine in primary care: the ID Migraine validation study. *Neurology.* 2003;61(3):375-382. http://www.ncbi.nlm.nih.gov/pubmed/12913201. Accessed May 16, 2017.
22. Friedman DI, Liu GT, Digre KB. Revised diagnostic criteria for the pseudotumor cerebri syndrome in adults and children. *Neurology.* 2013;81(13):1159-1165. doi: 10.1212/WNL.0b013e3182a55f17.
23. Fisayo A, Bruce BB, Newman NJ, Biousse V. Overdiagnosis of idiopathic intracranial hypertension. *Neurology.* 2016;86(4):341-350. doi: 10.1212/wnl.0000000000002318.
24. Silberstein SD, Dodick DW, Bigal ME, et al. Fremanezumab for the preventive treatment of chronic migraine. *N Engl J Med.* 2017;377(22):2113-2122. doi: 10.1056/NEJMoa1709038.
25. Goadsby PJ, Reuter U, Hallström Y, et al. A controlled trial of Erenumab for episodic migraine. *N Engl J Med.* 2017;377(22):2123-2132. doi: 10.1056/NEJMoa1705848.
26. Silberstein SD, Holland S, Freitag F, Dodick DW, Argoff C, Ashman E. Evidence-based guideline update: pharmacologic treatment for episodic migraine

prevention in adults report of the quality standards subcommittee of the American academy of neurology and the American headache society. *Neurology.* 2012;78(17):1337-1345. doi: 10.1212/WNL.0b013e3182535d20.
27. Dodick DW, Turkel CC, Degryse RE, et al. OnabotulinumtoxinA for treatment of chronic migraine: pooled results from the double-blind, randomized, placebo-controlled phases of the PREEMPT clinical program. *Headache.* 2010;50(6): 921-936. doi: 10.1111/j.1526-4610.2010.01678.x.
28. Blumenfeld AM, Silberstein SD, Dodick DW, Aurora SK, Brin MF, Binder WJ. Insights into the functional anatomy behind the PREEMPT injection paradigm: guidance on achieving optimal outcomes. *Headache.* 2017; 57(5):766-777.
29. Calhoun AH, Ford S, Millen C, Finkel AG, Truong Y, Nie Y. The prevalence of neck pain in migraine. *Headache.* 2010;50(8):1273-1277. doi: 10.1111/j.1526-4610.2009.01608.x.
30. Robbins MS, Kuruvilla D, Blumenfeld A, et al. Trigger point injections for headache disorders: expert consensus methodology and narrative review. *Headache.* 2014;54(9):1441-1459. doi: 10.1111/head.12442.
31. Govind J. Radiofrequency neurotomy for the treatment of third occipital headache. *J Neurol Neurosurg Psychiatry.* 2003;74(1):88-93. doi: 10.1136/jnnp.74.1.88.
32. Lord SM, Barnsley L, Wallis BJ, Bogduk N. Third occipital nerve headache: a prevalence study. *J Neurol Neurosurg Psychiatry.* 1994;57(10):1187-1190. doi: 10.1136/jnnp.57.10.1187.
33. Marmura MJ, Silberstein SD, Schwedt TJ. The acute treatment of migraine in adults: The American headache society evidence assessment of migraine pharmacotherapies. *Headache.* 2015;55(1):3-20. doi: 10.1111/head.12499.
34. Bigal ME, Serrano D, Buse D, Scher A, Stewart WF, Lipton RB. Acute migraine medications and evolution from episodic to chronic migraine: a longitudinal population-based study. *Headache.* 2008;48(8):1157-1168. doi: 10.1111/j.1526-4610.2008.01217.x.
35. Kelley NE, Tepper DE. Rescue therapy for acute migraine, part 1: triptans, dihydroergotamine, and magnesium. *Headache.* 2012;52(1):114-128. doi: 10.1111/j.1526-4610.2011.02062.x.
36. Kelley NE, Tepper DE. Rescue therapy for acute migraine, part 2: neuroleptics, antihistamines, and others. *Headache.* 2012;52(2):292-306. doi: 10.1111/j.1526-4610.2011.02070.x.
37. Kelley NE, Tepper DE. Rescue therapy for acute migraine, part 3: opioids, NSAIDs, steroids, and post-discharge medications. *Headache.* 2012;52(3):467-482. doi: 10.1111/j.1526-4610.2012.02097.x.
38. Friedman BW, Irizarry E, Solorzano C, et al. Randomized study of IV prochlorperazine plus diphenhydramine vs IV hydromorphone for migraine. *Neurology.* 2017;89(20):2075-2082. doi: 10.1212/WNL.0000000000004642.
39. Zhu S, McGeeney B. When indomethacin fails: additional treatment options for "indomethacin responsive headaches." *Curr Pain Headache Rep.* 2015;19(3):7. doi: 10.1007/s11916-015-0475-2.

39

Orofacial Pain

Steven J. Scrivani, Shehryar N. Khawaja, and David A. Keith

I. DIAGNOSTIC EVALUATION

- A. Chief Complaint
- B. History of Present Complaint
- C. Medical History
- D. Physical Examination
- E. Intraoral Examination

II. PAIN CAUSED BY PATHOLOGY OF THE HEAD, FACE, AND ORAL CAVITY

- A. Dental Pain (Table 39.1)
- B. Disorders of the Periodontium (Periodontal Disease)
- C. Oral Mucous Membrane Disorders (Table 39.2)
- D. Salivary Gland Disorders (Table 39.3)
- E. Disorders of Maxilla and Mandible
- F. Sinus Disorders
- G. Disorders of Eye and Ear
- H. Vascular Disorders
- I. Tumors

III. TEMPOROMANDIBULAR DISORDERS (TABLE 39.7)

- A. Masticatory Muscle Disorders (Table 39.8)
- B. Temporomandibular Joint Disorders (Table 39.9)

IV. NEUROPATHIC PAIN DISORDERS (TABLES 39.10 AND 39.11)

- A. Trigeminal Neuralgia
- B. Painful Posttraumatic Trigeminal Neuropathy
- C. Postherpetic Neuralgia
- D. Burning Mouth Syndrome

Facial pain syndromes are common in clinical practice. Many of these syndromes are also unique, given the complex anatomy and specialized sensory innervation of the head, face, and neck, and can pose diagnostic challenges. In general, acute pain symptoms closely correlate with other signs and symptoms of disease. However, in complex chronic pain problems in the orofacial region, the association between pain and other symptoms may not be as apparent.[1]

The common descriptive terms for craniofacial pain complaints are frequently misleading. To avoid confusion, clinicians should be familiar with the International Headache Society's Diagnostic Classification for Head, Face, and Neck Pain Disorders, the "International Classification of Headache Disorders III-Beta".[2] Clinicians need to be able to distinguish among painful conditions that arise from structural pathology of the oral and facial structures, temporomandibular joint (TMJ) disorders, myofascial pain disorders, headache syndromes, and primary cranial neuralgias.

Although nociceptive transmission in the trigeminal and spinal systems is similar, the two systems have important differences. In the perioral region, the trigeminal divisions contain afferents that subserve the dermatomes, which include the lips, teeth, gingival, anterior two-thirds of the tongue, upper pharynx, uvula, and soft palate. In addition to this cutaneous distribution, the trigeminal nerve contains afferents that provide sensory innervation to a variety of deep structures in the head, including the muscles of mastication and facial expression, the nasal and oral mucosa, the cornea, tongue, tooth pulp, TMJ, dura mater, intracranial vessels, external auditory meatus, and ear (partially, and with cranial nerves VII, IX, and X). The trigeminal system carries somatosensory information from these cutaneous and deep afferent structures as well as from specialized organs that have principally nociceptive innervation.

Most nociceptive afferents relay through the trigeminal brainstem complex, with oral and perioral structures represented more rostral than peripheral sites on the face. In addition, nociceptive afferents from the other cranial nerves and the upper cervical spinal segments (C2-C4) also are relayed through the trigeminal brainstem complex. In the subnucleus caudalis, cells relaying nociceptive signals (nociceptive-specific cells and wide dynamic-range cells) are primarily localized to analogous regions of lamina I and V in the spinal cord. Deep afferents converge on cells that also receive cutaneous nociceptive input, providing a substrate for referred pain in the head, face, and neck through the trigeminal system. Finally, the trigeminal nociceptive relay cells are strongly modulated by central pathways (descending opioidergic, noradrenergic, and serotonergic) that may dynamically modulate nociception under a variety of environmental situations and behavioral states.

Although the trigeminal dermatomes do not generally overlap those supplied by the adjacent cervical spinal nerves and other cranial nerves, dermatomes overlap extensively in the spinal afferent system. Three adjacent spinal roots must be injured to render any one region anesthetic. In the trigeminal system, under normal conditions, a section of one trigeminal division renders almost the entire dermatome anesthetic. Because the peripheral sensory nerves overlap so little with the trigeminal system, nerve lesions may result in more pronounced central somatosensory changes than those evoked by similar lesions in spinal nerves. These changes may partly underlie trigeminal neuropathic pain disorders.

Additionally, the trigeminal system may be developmentally and functionally distinct as a result of three hypothetical factors: (1) it innervates highly specialized tissues that are engaged in highly specialized functions; (2) it experiences two developmentally unique events: one programmed pain event and one programmed denervation event (eruption and exfoliation of teeth); and (3) it can be affected by dental surgery procedures performed with local anesthesia, which alters the afferent input into the system. These factors may also influence the development of chronic facial pain.

I. DIAGNOSTIC EVALUATION

A. Chief Complaint

The patient's description of the pain may provide clue to its cause. Primary neuralgias are frequently described as electric, sharp, shooting, and lancinating, secondary neuralgias have a burning nature, and muscle pain is characterized as deep dull ache, or soreness and typically aggravated by jaw function. TMJ disorders can cause pain, limitation of jaw movement, mandibular dysfunction, noises in the joint (clicking, popping and crepitus), joint tenderness and/or swelling, and potentially jaw locking and a change in the way the teeth meet in occlusion (bite).

B. History of Present Complaint

Patient should be asked about the duration, frequency, chronicity, onset, location, modifying factors, associated factors and pattern of pain. Each of these characteristics provides important information that may help to reach the differential diagnosis. Associated symptoms and signs can be ear pain, ear pressure and a clogged sensation, neck pain and stiffness, headache disorders, hyperesthesia, allodynia, and tactile evoked pain trigger areas. The pattern of the pain and associated problems are generally the most important differentiating factors in making an accurate diagnosis from the history.

C. Medical History

A careful and thorough medical history is necessary. Associated rheumatological, immunological, neurological, and other chronic pain disorders are of particular importance. Note for any trauma to the orofacial region, including surgical procedures of the teeth and other maxillofacial structures, external beam radiation therapy, and chemotherapy. Identify medications (prescription and over-the-counter) and supplements (herbal or alternative and complementary therapies) use, relevant family history, and jaw habits (such as clenching, grinding, posturing the jaw, nail biting, gum chewing) that may have an impact on the prognosis, diagnosis and management plan. A comprehensive psychosocial history is imperative for all the patients with chronic disorders. Furthermore, establish the details of any pending or planned disability claims or litigation.

D. Physical Examination

The examination should be completely systematical and not directed by a presumed diagnosis.

1. **Muscle function.** Pain in the masticatory muscles, posterior cervical region, and upper back are common causes of pain in the orofacial and the cervical region. The muscles should be palpated, trigger points noted, and the posture should be assessed. A more thorough evaluation of the masticatory muscles includes palpation for taut bands in muscle, tender or trigger points, range of motion and restrictions, measuring the maximum interincisal mouth opening, and lateral and protrusive jaw excursions. In addition, tremors, deviations, and fasciculation should also be noted.
2. **Temporomandibular joint function.** Palpate the lateral pole of the mandibular condyle for tenderness and/or swelling with the mouth in open and closed position. Joint sounds should be palpated or auscultated during range of vertical and horizontal motion. Clicking or popping should are usually indicative of intra-articular disc disorder, and crepitus is usually indicative of degenerative joint disease. Inspect for symmetrical movement of the mandible and palpate the movements of the mandibular condyles with jaw function.
3. **Neurological examination.** Gross examination of all of the cranial nerves should be carried out, in particular detailed evaluation of cranial nerves V (trigeminal) and VII (facial) IX-X complex (glossopharyngeal-vagus) and upper cervical nerves (C2-C4). During examination of trigeminal nerve, note for directional sense, light touch (nonnoxious) and sharp touch (noxious) sensations, two-point discrimination, tactile sensory perception with microfilaments (such as, "von Frey hairs"), hot and cold sensitivity, and taste acuity of the tongue.

E. Intraoral Examination

Note the dentition for any evidence of wear on the occlusal, palatal, and cervical region of the teeth, tooth decay (dental caries), or loss of dental restorations. The health of the gingival tissues around the teeth, oropharyngeal mucosa, base of the tongue, lateral and posterior pharyngeal structures, tonsillar fossa, hard and soft palate (discolorations, lesions, swellings, or masses), and oral hygiene should be recorded. Determine the moistness of the oral mucosa or pooling of saliva. Palpate the submandibular, sublingual, and parotid gland regions. Similarly, movements and appearance of the tongue and soft palpate should be assessed.

1. **Diagnostic Imaging and Laboratory Studies.** Periapical dental radiographs and panoramic radiographs offer detailed information about the teeth, jaws, maxillary sinuses, and TMJ complex. Computerized tomography (CT) can provide more detailed images of the hard structures of the jaws, TMJ, and the base of skull. Magnetic resonance imaging (MRI) is the reference standard for evaluating the soft tissue and may aid in assessment of internal structure of the TMJ, and oropharyngeal and nasopharyngeal anatomy, skull base, salivary glands, brain, and trigeminal system. Laboratory studies, such as complete blood count and erythrocyte sedimentation rate, may help to diagnose blood dyscrasias and temporal arteritis, respectively. Rheumatoid factor and Lyme titer may be helpful in evaluating TMJ articular disease.

II. PAIN CAUSED BY PATHOLOGY OF THE HEAD, FACE, AND ORAL CAVITY

A. Dental Pain (Table 39.1)

Dental pain in most cases is caused by dental disease; however, it can arise from other tissues and be referred from other sources. Tooth pulp has specialized and possibly exclusively nociceptive innervation. Dental pain is usually well localized, and the quality of the pain can range from a dull ache to severe electric shocks, depending on the specific etiology and extent of disease.[3] In general, dental pain is provoked by thermal or mechanical stimulation of the damaged tooth. Clinical and radiographic findings of dental decay, tooth fracture, or infection may corroborate the diagnosis.[4–6]

1. **Dentin Hypersensitivity**
   a. Exposure of dentin (coronal or cervical) may result in sharp pain of short duration. However, not all exposed dentin give rise to symptoms. Pain arises in response to exposure to thermal, tactile, and osmotic stimulus, and there is cessation of pain after removal of the stimulus.[7]
   b. The treatment involves alleviation of etiological factors (ie, intrinsic and extrinsic dental erosion) and use of desensitizing agents (such as, toothpaste, mouthwash or varnish containing strontium, or fluoride), or restoring (eg, restoration or crown) the exposed dentin.[4–7]
2. **Pulp Inflammation and Pain**
   a. The dental pulp may be subjected to a wide array of stimuli (eg, bacterial, thermal, chemical, or traumatic), the effects of which may result in inflammation (pulpitis). A characteristic sign of pulpitis is that the patient is unable to localize the affected tooth. Pulpitis can be reversible or irreversible; the duration of pain is commonly used as a clinical guide to determine the difference.[8]
      i. **Reversible Pulpitis:** Pain is sharp and lingers for seconds (approximately <10 seconds) after exposure to stimuli. The treatment consists of removal of the offending stimuli and placement of a sedative dressing or restoration.
      ii. **Irreversible Pulpitis:** Pain is sharp and lingers for prolong period of time (approximately >10 seconds) after exposure to stimuli. The treatment consists of extirpation of the pulpal tissues and performing formal endodontic (root canal) treatment.[8]

TABLE 39.1 Odontogenic Pain

Diagnosis	Pulpitis	Periodontal	Cracked Tooth	Dentinal
Diagnostic Features	Spontaneous and/or evoked deep/diffuse pain in compromised dental pulp. Pain may be sharp, throbbing, or dull.	Localized deep continuous pain in compromised periodontium (eg, gingiva, periodontal ligament) exacerbated by biting or chewing.	Spontaneous or evoke brief sharp pain in a tooth with a history of trauma or restorative work (eg, crown, root canal).	Brief, sharp pain evoked by different kinds of stimulus to the dentin (eg, hot or cold drinks).
Diagnostic Evaluation	Look for deep caries and recent or extensive dental work. Pain provoked/exacerbated by percussion, thermal, or electric stimulation of affected tooth. Dental x-rays helpful (periapical).	Tooth percussion over compromised periodontum provokes pain. Look for inflammation or absecess (eg, periodontitis). Apical dental x-rays are helpful (bitewings, periapical).	Presence of tooth fracture may be detectable by x-ray. Percussion should elicit pain. Dental x-rays are helpful (periapical taken from different angles).	Exposed dentin or cementum due to recession of periodontium. Possible erosion of dentinal structure. Cold stimulation reproduce pain.
Treatment	Medication: NSAIDs, nonopiate analgesics. Dentistry: remove carious lesion, tooth restoration, endodontic treatment, or tooth extraction.	Medication: NSAIDs, nonopiate analgesics, antibiotics, mouthwashes. Dentistry: drainage and débridement of periodontal pocket, scaling and root planning, periodontal surgery, endodontic treatment, or tooth extraction.	Medication: NSAIDs, nonopiate analgesics. Dentistry: depends on level of the tooth fracture restoration; treatment, or extraction of the tooth. Medication: mouthwash (fluoride), desensitizing toothpaste. Dentistry: fluoride or potassium salts, tooth restoration, endodontic treatment. Patient education, diet, tooth brushing force and frequency, proper tooth paste.	

3. Periapical Inflammation and Pain

a. Irreversible pulpitis ultimately progresses to pulpal necrosis. The periapical inflammation may not always result in pain. The pain takes place during the exacerbation phase of the inflammatory process. A characteristic clinical sign of periapical inflammation is that patient is able to precisely localize the affected tooth.[4,5,8]

b. Radiographically, it is characterized by periapical radiolucency; however, a periapical inflammation may flare up before radiographic signs are visible.

c. The treatment of periapical inflammation is similar to that of irreversible pulpitis (ie, pulpal extirpation and root canal treatment) or potentially extraction of the tooth.[3–5]

4. Cracked Tooth

a. Fracture of the tooth structure. It may be incomplete (ie, enamel, and/or dentin) or complete (ie, extending up to the pulpal chamber), or limited to crown or involve the root. It is often characterized by sharp momentary pain on biting or releasing in addition to occasional pain on exposure to cold stimulus (drink or food). There is often a history of trauma, or restorative work (eg, large dental filling, crown, root canal). Clinically, a crack may not be apparent; however, transillumination examination, removal of restoration, periapical dental radiographs, maxillofacial CT scan, and additional specific diagnostic tests may aid in diagnosis.[4,6]

b. Treatment depends on the level of the tooth fracture and includes simple restoration, temporary fixation of fractured segments, full crown restoration, or extraction of the tooth.[4]

B. Disorders of the Periodontium (Periodontal Disease)

1. Gingival Disease (Gingivitis)

a. It is the inflammation of gingival tissues. It may clinically present as gingival edema or hyperplasia, gingival erythema, or bleeding with brushing or mastication. It is not associated with alveolar bone resorption or apical migration of the gingival margins. It can be local or generalized and is associated with local (eg, plaque, calculus) or systemic (eg, endocrine, medication-induced, malnutrition) factors.

b. Treatment consists of scaling and root planning (deep cleaning, curettage, and débridement) of teeth and removal of the exacerbating factors.[9]

2. Periodontal Disease (Periodontitis)

a. Periodontitis is an immune-mediated inflammatory process that is initiated by pathogenic oral microorganisms that result in either focal or generalized of destruction of periodontal ligament and alveolar bone. It may clinically present as gingivitis, gingival apical migration, tooth mobility, or as an abscess, and radiographically, it is characterized by loss of bone support. In the presence of acute infection in the periodontal tissues, dull aching pain to palpation, erythema, bleeding, and purulent discharge from an abscess are common.

b. Treatment consists of scaling and root planning of the teeth, curettage, and débridement of the gingival pocket. An acute abscess may require incision and drainage and possibly local or systemic antibiotic therapy.[9]

C. Oral Mucous Membrane Disorders (Table 39.2)

Diseases of the oral mucosa are numerous and attributed to a variety of local (infections, traumatic and iatrogenic injuries, neoplastic, neurologic) and systemic (immune or autoimmune, nutritional and metabolic, gastro-

TABLE 39.2 Common Painful Mucosal Conditions

Infections
- Herpetic stomatitis
- Varicella zoster
- Candidiasis
- Acute necrotizing gingivostomatitis

Immune/Autoimmune
- Allergic reactions (toothpaste, mouthwashes, topical medications)
- Erosive lichen planus
- Benign mucous membrane pemphigoid
- Aphthous stomatitis and aphthous lesions
- Erythema multiform
- Graft versus host disease

Traumatic and Iatrogenic Injuries
- Factitial, accidental (burns: chemical, solar, thermal)
- Self-destructive (rituals, obsessive behaviors)
- Iatrogenic (chemotherapy, radiation)

Neoplasia
- Squamous cell carcinoma
- Mucoepidermoid carcinoma
- Adenoid cystic carcinoma
- Brain tumors

Neurological
- Burning mouth syndrome and glossodynia
- Neuralgias
- Postviral neuralgias
- Posttraumatic neuropathies
- Dyskinesias and dystonias

Nutritional and Metabolic
- Vitamin deficiencies (B-12, folate)
- Mineral deficiencies (iron)
- Diabetic neuropathy
- Malabsorption syndromes

Miscellaneous
- Xerostomia, secondary to intrinsic or extrinsic conditions
- Referred pain from esophageal or oropharyngeal malignancy
- Mucositis secondary to esophageal reflux
- Angioedema

intestinal) causes. They are characterized by pain and oral mucosal lesions (ie, vesicles, bullae, erosions, erythematous or keratotic patches). Treatment consists of local (topical or injection) and systemic antiinflammatory agents (eg, corticosteroids), newer immunosuppressive agents, and/or removal of underlying pathology.[9]

D. Salivary Gland Disorders (Table 39.3)

1. There are three major (parotid, submandibular, and sublingual) and hundreds of minor salivary gland present in the oral cavity. Disorders of

TABLE 39.3 Salivary Gland Disease

- Inflammatory
- Noninflammatory
- Infectious
- Obstructive
- Immunologic (Sjögren syndrome)
- Tumors
- Others (Red herrings)

salivary glands may result in pain as a primary or an associated symptom. Furthermore, pain may be accompanied by swelling, drainage, cervical adenopathy, or generalized symptoms of systemic infection, depending on the etiology of the disorder.

2. Disorders of the parotid gland can extend locally to produce symptoms of impairment of cranial nerve fifth, seventh, and/or ninth. Disorders of the submandibular gland may result in symptoms of impaired swallowing, or impairment of cranial nerves fifth, ninth, and/or twelfth.[10,11]
3. Treatments vary based upon the diagnosis and etiology of the salivary gland disease. This can include home care treatments, sialogogues, anti-inflammatory agents, immunosuppressive agents, antimicrobial agents, minimally invasive surgical procedures (sialendoscopy) or surgical resection, and adjunctive therapy for tumors (benign or malignant).

E. Disorders of Maxilla and Mandible

Numerous disorders of the bony structure of the jaws may present with pain. These disorders are generally classified as being of odontogenic or nonodontogenic origin. Tumors may be benign or malignant (either primary or metastatic disease). Often, additional historical or examination findings warrant further evaluation (ie, swelling, mass, discoloration, numbness, weakness, bleeding, drainage, tooth loss, or mobility). Pain can be treated symptomatically until a definitive diagnosis is established and definitive therapy is initiated.

F. Sinus Disorders

1. Sinus pain presents as unilateral or bilateral, throbbing or pressure-like pain in the frontal, malar, or glabellar region. Pain is exacerbated with forward head posture and with palpation over the affected sinus. Patients often have history of chronic allergies, frequent upper respiratory tract infections, sinusitis, headaches of various types, and multiple sinus surgeries.
2. Unilateral symptoms or associated bloody discharge may result from neoplasm and necessitates further evaluation and identification of the pain source. Immediate referral is necessary when any of the following symptoms are present: periorbital edema, a displaced globe, double vision, reduced visual acuity, or frontal swelling.
3. The American Academy of Otolaryngology-Head and Neck Surgery (AAO-HNS) recommends nasal endoscopy and CT imaging of the paranasal sinuses for definitive diagnosis of rhinosinusitis, though most cases can be diagnosed clinically.[6]
4. Treatment consists of pharmacological therapy (eg, topical and systemic decongestants, systemic antibiotics, nonopiate analgesics, topical anesthetics) and surgical intervention.[6]

G. Disorders of Eye and Ear

Numerous disorders can cause pain in and around the eye and ear. Most ophthalmologic conditions producing eye pain are associated with obvious ocular symptoms, signs, or histories that implicate the eye as the origin of pain (eg, extraocular muscle paresis, diplopia, autonomic symptoms, swelling, discharge, tinnitus, hypoacusis, pressure) (Table 39.4). Eye and ear pain warrants a thorough evaluation by either an ophthalmologist or an otolaryngologist, respectively.[12,13]

1. Eye Pain

a. A complete ocular history should include any prior visual loss, ophthalmic diseases (eg, corneal infections, uveitis, and glaucoma), use of

TABLE 39.4 Pain in or Around the Eye "Quite Eye" and Normal Examination

- Cluster headache and cluster-tic syndrome
- Paroxysmal hemicrania
- SUNCT/SUNA syndrome
- Migraine and tension-type headache
- Ice-pick HA/Ice cream HA/valsalva HA
- Trigeminal neuralgia
- Sinus disease (acute)
- Teeth, jaws (TMD)
- Carotid disease
- Temporal arteritis
- Eye pain, headache, and lung cancer

contact lenses, recent or remote ocular surgery, and ocular trauma. In addition to noting the specific features of pain when taking the history for eye pain, such as time of onset, severity, exacerbating and palliating factors, radiation, quality, duration, and frequency, ask about the specific location of pain; for example, intraocular, retrobulbar, periocular, or frontal and associated symptoms, such as tearing, loss of vision, double vision, photophobia, and discharge.

b. In some ocular causes of eye pain, the eye is superficially normal (Table 39.5).

c. There are a number of facial pain syndromes that present with prominent ophthalmologic signs and symptoms (Table 39.6).

2. Ear Pain

a. Ear pain is a common complaint that may be due to otologic or non-otologic causes. The pain, often described as dull and aching with a stopped-up sensation, may be localized to the area around the ear or may spread to involve half or all of the head. It may also refer to the vertex. Pain in the ear is as likely to be referred from other structures as it is to be stemming from the ear itself. If ear pain is not part of the orofacial pain complaint, it is highly unlikely that the ear is the pain source.

b. Primary otalgia arises from disease of the external or middle ear and is identified by inspection of the external ear and tympanic membrane. If the inspection reveals abnormal findings, ontological referral for

TABLE 39.5 Headache and Facial Pain Syndromes With Predominant Ophthalmologic Findings

- Carotid artery disease
- Orbital inflammatory pseudotumor
- Increased ICP (pseudotumor cerebri)
- Intracranial hemorrhage and stroke
- Intracranial A-V malformation
- Tolosa-Hunt syndrome
- Raeder's paratrigeminal syndrome
- Gradenigo syndrome
- Postherpetic neuralgia

TABLE 39.6 Red Flags for a Patient With Eye Pain

- New visual acuity defect, color vision defect, or visual field loss
- Relative afferent pupillary defect
- Extraocular muscle abnormality, ocular misalignment, or diplopia
- Proptosis
- Lid retraction or ptosis
- Conjunctival chemosis, injection, or redness
- Corneal opacity
- Hyphema or hypopyon
- Iris irregularity
- Nonreactive pupil
- Fundus abnormality
- Recent ocular surgery (<3 months)
- Recent ocular trauma

comprehensive diagnosis and treatment would be appropriate. In the absence of local pathology, the pain is likely referred to the ear from another structure.

c. Sensory innervation of the ear involves cranial nerves V, VII, IX, and X as well as C2 and C3. Pain referred to the ears (secondary otalgia) may originate in any structure with common innervations. Treatment of referred ear pain requires proper identification of the pain source.

H. Vascular Disorders

1. Giant Cell Arteritis

a. In giant cell arteritis (GCA), giant cells infiltrate the walls of the cranial arteries. In temporal arteritis, the superficial temporal artery is affected. Other arteries commonly affected by GCA include the maxillary, ophthalmic, and posterior ciliary arteries. It most commonly affects the elderly.

b. The involved artery may be enlarged and tender to palpation. Patients often complain of intense or deep headache that worsens upon lying flat, malaise, weakness, and weight loss. Jaw claudication is a common finding which can mimic the much more common temporomandibular disorders (TMDs). Occlusion of the optic artery may result in visual disturbances, including blindness.

c. Laboratory studies reveal elevated erythrocyte sedimentation rates and C-reactive protein. Artery biopsy may be required for definitive diagnosis.

I. Tumors

1. Numerous intra- and extra-cranial tumors can cause oral cavity, oropharyngeal, facial and head pain as a primary presenting symptom. Cancers of the upper aerodigestive tract, jaws, base of skull, and neck may all present with pain along with other associated signs and symptoms. In addition, numerous intracranial tumors and lesions (ie, vascular malformations) can present with facial pain and headache. These are primarily tumors of the cerebellopontine angle (CPA); however, various primary brain neoplasms and metastatic disease have been associated with facial pain and headache. Headache and facial pain of unknown origin should warrant a careful evaluation for an underlying occult tumor.[5,6]

2. Patients presenting with facial pain or headache should undergo a comprehensive medical history and careful physical examination with particular attention to the cranial neurological examination. Consideration should be given to obtaining appropriate imaging studies including CT, MRI, and magnetic resonance angiography (MRA).

III. TEMPOROMANDIBULAR DISORDERS (TABLE 39.7)

TMDs are a group of musculoskeletal and neuromuscular conditions that involve the TMJ, masticatory muscles, and associated head and neck tissues[5,14] (see Tables 39.8 and 39.9). The prevalence of pain-related TMDs, such as, masticatory myalgia, masticatory myofascial pain, and TMJ arthralgia, has been estimated to be between 2.5% and 10% in the general adult population, making it the second most common musculoskeletal condition, after chronic back pain, which results in pain and disability. Common manifestations of pain-related TMD consist of pain, of a persistent, recurring, or chronic nature, limitation in the range of mandibular motion, jaw dysfunction (difficulty with eating), and joint noises. The pathophysiology of pain-related TMD is poorly understood. However, multiple risk factors have been identified, such as, gender, pain during jaw function and palpation, oral parafunctions, presence of other chronic pain conditions, pain sensitivity, and psychosocial characteristics.[4–6]

A. Masticatory Muscle Disorders (Table 39.8)

The mechanisms that produce pain in skeletal muscles are poorly understood. It appears to be similar to other forms of myofascial pain disorders.

1. **Myalgia**
   a. **Masticatory Myalgia**
      i. It is a disorder characterized by regional unilateral or bilateral dull and aching pain in the masticatory muscles (masseter muscle, temporalis muscle, lateral pterygoid, or medial pterygoid) that is affected by jaw movement, function, or parafunction.[14] Pain is often associated with limited mouth opening, subjective feeling of tightness in the masticatory muscles, and pain on palpation of the masticatory muscles.[4–6]
      ii. Treatment consist of pharmacotherapy (eg, analgesics, muscle relaxants, antidepressants, anticonvulsants), physical therapy (eg, manual manipulation, massage therapy, ultrasound therapy, laser therapy, transcutaneous electric nerve stimulation therapy), orthotic jaw appliance/device therapy (eg, full-arch coverage appliance, partial coverage appliance), injection therapy (eg, local anesthetics, corticosteroid, botulinum toxin), and biobehavioral therapy (eg, cognitive behavior therapy, relaxation therapy, lifestyle coaching, biofeedback).[4–6]
   b. **Myofascial Pain With Referral**
      i. It is a unilateral muscle pain disorder characterized by presence of myofascial trigger points.[14] A myofascial trigger point is defined as a focal area of deep tenderness within a taut band of skeletal muscle located in the masticatory muscle, fascia, or tendon, stimulation of which results in characteristic referral pain and autonomic phenomena. In addition, there may be a localized twitch response during palpation or insertion of needle into the trigger point. Common referral sites include eyes, ears, teeth, and TMJs, depending on the specific muscles. Active trigger points may cause pain spontaneously or during movement. Latent trigger points are

TABLE 39.7 Temporomandibular Disorders

Diagnosis	TMJ Articular Disorders	Muscle Disorders	Myofascial Disorders
Diagnostic Features	Pain localized in the preauricular area during jaw function. Usually presence of painful click or crepitus during mouth opening. Limited opening (<35 mm), deviated or painful jaw movements.	Tenderness of the masticatory muscles. Dull, aching pain exacerbated by jaw function or palpation	Diffused dull or aching pain affecting multiple groups of muscles of the head and neck region, as well as other parts of the body
Diagnostic Evaluation	Internal derangement of the TMJ with abnormal function of the disc-condyle complex, and/or degeneration of the joint surface. Palpation is painful. Possible joint swelling in acute phases. MRI, CT, etc. of the joint may rule out tumors and advanced degenerative stages	Tenderness during palpation of the masticatory muscles and tendons. Possible limited range of jaw movement and during passive stretching examination. Can be associated with a parafunctional habit (bruxism—early morning pain).	Presence of trigger or tender points in one or more groups of muscles. Pain can radiate to distant areas with stimulation or not of the trigger points. Rule out presence of lupus erythematosus.
Treatment	Patient education and self-care Medication: NSAID, nonopiate analgesics. Physical therapy: exercise program. Occlusal splints Oral maxillofacial surgery: arthrocentesis, arthroscopic surgery, open surgery	Patient education and self-care. Medication: topical and systemic NSAIDs, nonopiate analgesics, muscle relaxants, antidepressants (usually TCAs), anxiolytics, anticonvulsants, BTX, trigger point injections, and vapocoolant spray. Physical therapy: TENS, massage, exercise program. Occlusal splints Cognitive-behavior: biofeedback, relaxation, coping skills.	***Same as muscle disorders***

TABLE 39.8 Masticatory Muscle Disorders

1. Muscle pain limited to the orofacial region
   - Myalgia
   - Tendonitis
   - Myositis
   - Spasm
2. Myofibrotic contracture
3. Hypertrophy
4. Neoplasms
5. Movement disorders—dyskinesia/dystonia
6. Masticatory muscle pain due to systemic/central disorders

nonpainful. However, result in muscle weakness and restriction in range of motion. Trigger points may become activated by sudden overloading contraction, viral infection, cold temperature, fatigue, and increased emotional stress.[5]

ii. Treatment of myofascial pain with referral consists of thermal compressions, physical therapy (eg, spraying the involved muscle with cold spray followed by stretching, myofascial release therapy, craniosacral therapy, and ischemic compression of the trigger points), isotonic and isometric exercises, dry needling or injection of local anesthetic, saline, corticosteroid, or botulinum toxin into the trigger point, and acupuncture. Other treatment options consist of pharmacotherapy (eg, analgesics, muscle relaxants) and orthotic jaw device therapy.

c. Tendonitis

i. It is a disorder characterized by dull or sharp pain of tendon origin affected by jaw movement, function, and parafunction.[14] Pain is often associated with subjective feeling of tightness, limited range of motion, and tenderness to palpation. The temporalis tendon is the most common site of tendonitis in orofacial region, and it may refer pain toward ipsilateral maxillary teeth.

ii. Treatment is similar to that of masticatory myalgia or myofascial pain with referral.[5]

B. Temporomandibular Joint Disorders (Table 39.9)

1. Joint Pain

a. Arthralgia

i. It is a disorder characterized by sharp pain of TMJ origin affected by jaw movement, function, or parafunction. Pain is often associated with limitation in movements, and joint tenderness to palpation.[14]

ii. Treatment consists of pharmacotherapy (eg, analgesics, in particular nonsteroidal anti-inflammatory medication), thermal compressions, occlusal orthotic device therapy, and physical therapy and exercises to maintain joint mobility.[5,6]

2. Disc-Condyle Complex Disorders

It is the most common TMJ arthropathy and is characterized by abnormal position of the articular disc with respect to the head of the condyle, or the temporal fossa. Commonly the articular disc is displaced either anteriorly, or anteromedially.[14] However, lateral and posterior

TABLE 39.9 Temporomandibular Joint Articular Disorders

1. Congenital or developmental
   - Aplasia
   - Hypoplasia
   - Hyperplasia
2. Joint pain
   - Arthralgia
   - Arthritis
3. Joint disorders
   - Disc-condyle complex disorders
   - Other hypomobility disorders—adhesions, ankylosis
   - Hypermobility disorders—subluxation, dislocation
4. Joint diseases
   - Degenerative joint diseases—osteoarthritis/arthrosis
   - Condylosis—ICR
   - Osteonecrosis
   - Systemic arthritides—RA, AS, Rieter's, etc.
   - Neoplasm
   - Synovial chondromatosis
5. Fractures

displacements may also occur. The etiology of disc displacement is not well established. It is postulated to be a result of impairment of lubrication of the TMJ complex, or elongated or torn collateral TMJ ligaments.[5]

a. Disc-Displacement With Reduction

i. It is a disc-condyle complex disorder in which during the closed-mouth position, articular disc is positioned anteriorly with respect to the condylar head, and during the full open-mouth position, articular disc is positioned between the condylar head and articular fossa. Clicking, popping, and/or snapping sound are often present during the mandibular range of motion. These joint sounds are eliminated during protrusive opening and closing of the mandible. Furthermore, there may be deviation (S-shaped) in the mandibular opening and closing pattern.

ii. Magnetic resonance imaging of the TMJ illustrates that the posterior band and the intermediate zone of articular disc are located anterior to the 11:30 position during the closed-mouth position. However, the intermediate zone of the articular disc is located between the condylar head and the articular eminence during the open-mouth position.[14]

iii. Displacement of disc anteriorly is considered a physiologic accommodation and does not warrant a therapy other than patient education. Disc-displacement with reduction may present with intermittent locking of the TMJ. This disorder can be managed with physical therapy (eg, joint manipulation), exercises to improve joint mobility and stabilization, and occlusal orthotic device therapy.[4–6]

b. Disc-Displacement Without Reduction (Closed Lock)

i. It is a disc-condyle complex disorder in which the articular disc is positioned anteriorly with respect to the condylar head in the closed-mouth and the full open-mouth position. Clinically, it is associated with limited mouth opening (<40 mm), ipsilateral deflection during the opening and closing movement, and limitation in the contralateral laterotrusive movement of the mandible. Patient may also complain of difficult chewing, ipsilateral joint pain during function and parafunctional movements, and changes is habitual occlusion (bite).

ii. Magnetic resonance imaging of the TMJ illustrates the posterior band of articular disc, and the intermediate zone are located anterior to the 11:30 position during the closed-mouth and the open-mouth position.[14]

iii. Primarily, the treatment is conservative and consists of an attempt to reduce the articular disc using physical therapy (eg, joint manipulation) and exercises. However, if there is limited success, minimal surgical interventions (eg, arthrocentesis and arthroscopy) can provide relief in symptoms.[4–6]

iv. Disc-displacement without reduction may not result in pain, or limitation in range of motion (>40 mm). In such cases, no treatment is necessary.

c. **Subluxation and Dislocation of TMJ (Open Lock)**

i. It is a TMJ hypermobility disorder characterized by anterior displacement of the condylar process, beyond the articular eminence. The posterior translation of the condylar process is limited, resulting in locking of the mandible in an open-mouth position.

ii. In subluxation, patient achieves the mouth closure, with a specific manipulation maneuver. If patient fails to reposition the condyle, it is called luxation. Imaging of the TMJ will illustrate condylar process positioned anterior, or anterior and superior to the articular eminence during an attempt to close the mouth.[14]

iii. Treatment consists of patient education, thermal compressions, and pharmacotherapy (eg, analgesics, and muscle relaxants). In acute cases, muscles may need to be relaxed, using local anesthetic injection, or pharmacotherapy (eg, benzodiazepines, muscle relaxants). Chronic cases can be managed using physical therapy (eg, joint manipulation), intrajoint injections using sclerosing agents (sodium morrhuate, or sodium tetradecyl sulphate) or autogenous blood, injection of botulinum toxin to the lateral pterygoid muscle. Surgical options include, striping of the lateral pterygoid muscle, eminectomy, and arthroplasty.[4–6]

3. **Degenerative Joint Disease**

a. It is defined as a degenerative condition of the TMJ characterized by deterioration and abrasion of articular tissue and concomitant remodeling of the underlying subchondral bone due to overloading of the remodeling mechanism.

b. Clinically, it may be associated with TMJ crepitus, crunching, grinding, or grating sounds during mandibular movements, TMJ stiffness, ipsilateral TMJ pain, limitation in range of motion, and alteration in occlusion (bite). However, its asymptomatic cases are also present. Radiographically, it presents as flattening, erosion, generalized sclerosing of the articular surfaces, and osteophyte formation. Degenerative joint disease can be primary (eg, idiopathic) or secondary (eg, rheumatoid arthritis, reactive arthritis, psoriatic arthritis, in response to trauma or infection) in nature.[14]

c. Treatment consists of physical therapy (eg, joint manipulation), exercises to improve joint mobility, thermal compressions, pharmacotherapy (eg, analgesics, corticosteroids, and other anti-inflammatory agents), intra-joint corticosteroid injections, orthotic jaw device therapy, and surgical interventions (eg, arthrocentesis, arthroscopy, arthroplasty or total prosthetic joint replacement).[4–6]

IV. NEUROPATHIC PAIN DISORDERS (TABLES 39.10 AND 39.11)

Neuropathic pain is defined as pain that arises from injury, disease, or dysfunction of the peripheral or the central nervous system. These disorders are particularly common in the head and neck region. This may be due to dense and specialized sensory innervation of this region. Neuropathic pain disorders can be divided, based on temporal features, into episodic or continuous. As mentioned previously, orofacial pain is mediated by afferent fibers in the trigeminal nerve, nervous intermedius, glossopharyngeal nerve, vagus nerve, and by the upper cervical roots via the occipital nerves.

A. Trigeminal Neuralgia

1. Trigeminal neuralgia is a painful disorder characterized by brief (<120 seconds) paroxysms of severe, unilateral, and electric shocklike, or lancinating pain in the trigeminal region. Maxillary and mandibular divisions are the most commonly affected. The average age of onset is ~50 years, and women are slightly more affected than men. It has an incidence of 4 per 100,000.
2. Pain can be spontaneous or precipitated by nonpainful stimuli, such as washing or lightly touching the face, shaving, talking, and brushing the

TABLE 39.10 Painful Cranial Neuropathies and Other Facial Pains

13.1 Trigeminal neuralgia
13.1.1 Classical trigeminal neuralgia
13.1.1.1 Classical trigeminal neuralgia, purely paroxysmal
13.1.1.2 Classical trigeminal neuralgia with concomitant persistent facial pain
13.1.2 Painful trigeminal neuropathy
13.1.2.1 Painful trigeminal neuropathy attributed to acute Herpes zoster
13.1.2.2 Postherpetic trigeminal neuropathy
13.1.2.3 Painful posttraumatic trigeminal neuropathy
13.1.2.4 Painful trigeminal neuropathy attributed to multiple sclerosis plaque
13.1.2.5 Painful trigeminal neuropathy attributed to space-occupying lesion
13.1.2.6 Painful trigeminal neuropathy attributed to other disorder
13.2 Glossopharyngeal neuralgia
13.3 Nervus intermedius (facial nerve) neuralgia
13.4 Occipital neuralgia
13.5 Optic neuritis
13.6 Headache attributed to ischemic ocular motor nerve palsy
13.7 Tolosa-Hunt syndrome
13.8 Paratrigeminal oculosympathetic (Raeder) syndrome
13.9 Recurrent painful ophthalmoplegic neuropathy
13.10 Burning mouth syndrome
13.11 Persistent idiopathic facial pain
13.12 Central neuropathic pain
- Central neuropathic pain attributed to multiple sclerosis
- Central poststroke pain

Pilch BZ. *Head and Neck Surgical Pathology*. Lippincott Williams & Wilkins; 2001.

TABLE 39.11 Trigeminal Neuropathic Pain Disorders

Diagnosis	Trigeminal Neuralgia	Deafferentation Pain	Acute and Postherpetic Neuralgia	Burning Mouth Syndrome
Diagnostic Features	Brief severe lancinating pain evoked by mechanical stimulation of trigger zone (pain-free between attacks). Usually unilateral, affects the V2/V3 areas (rarely V1). Possible pain remission periods (for months/years)	Spontaneous or evoked pain with prolonged after-sensation after tactile stimulation. Trigger zone due to surgery (tooth extraction) or trauma. Positive and negative descriptors (eg, burning, nagging, boring).	Pain associated with herpetic lesions, usually in the V1 dermatoma. Spontaneous pain (burning and tingling) but may present as dull and aching. Occasional lancinating evoked pain.	Constant burning pain of the mucous membranes of the tongue, mouth. Hard or soft palate, or lips. Usually affects women of age > 50 years.
Diagnostic Evaluation	MRI for evidence of tumor or vasocompression of the trigeminal tract or root (cerebellopontine angle). Rule-out MS, especially in young adults.	Etiologic factors such as trauma or surgery in the painful area. Order MRI if the area is intact to rule out peripheral or central lesions.	Small cutaneous vesicles (AHN) or scarring (PHN), usually affecting V1. Loss of normal skin color. Corneal ulceration can occur. Sensory changes in affected area (eg, hyperesthesia, dysesthesia).	Rule out salivary gland dysfunction (xerostomia) or tumor, Sjögren, candidiasis, geographic or fissured tongue, and chemical or mechanical irritations. Nutrition and menopause.
Treatment	Medication: anticonvulsionants (eg, carbamazepine, gabapentin); antidepressants (eg, amitriptyline, nortriptyline, desipramine); nonopiate analgesics, BTX. Combination of baclofen and anticonvulsants can produce good results. Surgery: microvascular decompression of trigeminal root, ablative surgeries (eg, rhizotomy, gamma knife).	Medication: anticonvulsants (eg, carbamazepine, gabapentin); antidepressants; nonopiate analgesics; topical agents (eg, lidocaine 5% patches). Surgery: ablative surgeries (eg, rhizotomy, gamma knife).	Medication: acyclovir (acute phase) anticonvulsants, antidepressants; nonopiate analgesics; topical agents (eg, lidocaine 5% patches). Surgery: ablative surgeries (eg, rhizotomy, gamma knife).	Medication: anticonvulsants, benzodiazepines, antidepressants; nonopiate analgesics; topical agents (eg, lidocaine, mouthwashes). Cognitive-behavior: biofeedback, relaxation, coping skills.

teeth. Many patients demonstrate a discrete sensory "trigger zone" in the orofacial region, tactile or thermal stimulation of this area evokes a TN pain attack. In individual patients, the attacks are stereotyped in terms of pain intensity and distribution. The findings during clinical examination are normal and show no sensory abnormality. The condition is often marked by remission periods lasting days to years during which little or no pain is noted.

3. Trigeminal neuralgia can be further classified based on temporal duration of pain and on bases of etiology.
   a. **Type I TN** is characterized by brief paroxysmal sharp lancinating or electric shocklike pain episodes.
   b. In **type II TN**, in addition to paroxysmal pain, there is presence of dull background ache.
4. In case if TN is due to compression of the dorsal root entry zone by a vascular loop, or due to an unknown etiology, it is considered **Classical (Idiopathic/Primary) TN**. However, if there is presence of an underlying pathology such as, multiple sclerosis, benign tumor (schwannoma, meningioma), cyst, or aneurysm, it is considered **Symptomatic (Secondary) TN.**[6,15,16]
5. Treatment of TN can be medical or surgical.
   a. Medical management consists majorly of pharmacotherapy using antiepileptic drugs (eg, carbamazepine, oxcarbazepine, lamotrigine, phenytoin, topiramate, gabapentin, pregabalin) and nonepileptic drugs (baclofen, tizanidine, tramadol), injection therapy, using local anesthesia, and/or botulinum toxin. Additional medical management for severe intractable attacks can include intravenous therapy (in hospital) with lidocaine, fosphenytoin (Cerebyx), and/or valproate sodium (Depacon).
   b. Surgical management consists of peripheral procedures (glycerol injections, nerve resection, cryotherapy), percutaneous rhizotomy procedures (thermal, glycerol injection, balloon compression), and central procedures (stereotactic gamma knife radiosurgery, and microvascular decompression surgery).[6,15,17,18]

B. Painful Posttraumatic Trigeminal Neuropathy

1. It is a neuropathic disorder that develops following trauma to sensory nerves in the trigeminal region. It is characterized by presence of chronic or recurrent pain in the area of the previous nerve injury, numbness, paraesthesia, dysesthesia, allodynia, hyperesthesia, and chronic burning pain. Examples of such neuropathy include postherpetic trigeminal neuropathy, inferior alveolar neuropathy following complicated tooth extraction (such as third molars), and infraorbital nerve neuropathy following maxillary trauma.
2. Treatment is similar to that of TN, consisting of medical and surgical interventions.[6,17,18] In addition, pharmacotherapy for other neuropathic pain disorders is effective along with multidisciplinary pain management care (physical medicine, biobehavioral medicine, and several complementary and alternative medicine treatments).[19]

C. Postherpetic Neuralgia

1. Postherpetic neuralgia (PHN) is a constant baseline burning and aching pain. Pain is usually spontaneous, intermittent, and lancinating with jabbing bouts. There is hyperesthesia and/or allodynia to mechanical and thermal stimuli. There are often sensory abnormalities such as itching, numbness, and tingling along with sensory deficits (such as absent or diminished thermal or tactile sensations). There are frequently skin pigmentation changes and/or scarring in the area of the acute lesions.

2. Herpes zoster (HZ) has a reported incidence of 2 to 3.4 per 1000 persons/year in the United States, mainly over age 50. The transition from HZ to PHN is immediately after the rash, or at about 1 month, 3 months, or 6 months after crusting of the skin lesions. Among all HZ patients, 9%-36 % will develop PHN. The risk factors for developing PHN include age, severity of acute pain and associated rash, and inflammation during HZ.
3. There are several forms of pharmacological therapies along with nerve blockade and topical agents. Tricyclic antidepressants, antiepileptic agents, opioids, ketamine, and other neuropathic agents remain the primary pharmacological therapy. Lidocaine has shown to be most effective among topical agents[5,6,17] (Fig. 39.1).

D. Burning Mouth Syndrome

1. It is an intraoral neuropathic pain disorder, characterized by chronic and persistent burning pain, or dysesthesia. The average age of onset is ~50 years, and women are more affected than men. It generally has a symmetric bilateral distribution, most frequently involving anterior two-thirds of tongue, the dorsum and lateral borders of tongue, the anterior hard palate, and the mucosa of the lower lip. Pain symptoms are often associated with dysgeusia (metallic taste), and xerostomia.

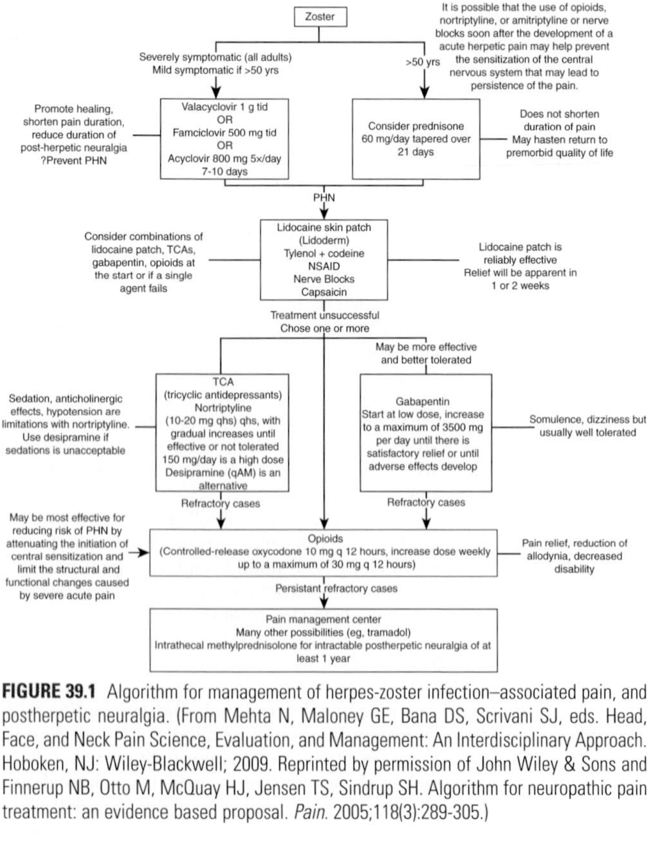

FIGURE 39.1 Algorithm for management of herpes-zoster infection–associated pain, and postherpetic neuralgia. (From Mehta N, Maloney GE, Bana DS, Scrivani SJ, eds. Head, Face, and Neck Pain Science, Evaluation, and Management: An Interdisciplinary Approach. Hoboken, NJ: Wiley-Blackwell; 2009. Reprinted by permission of John Wiley & Sons and Finnerup NB, Otto M, McQuay HJ, Jensen TS, Sindrup SH. Algorithm for neuropathic pain treatment: an evidence based proposal. *Pain.* 2005;118(3):289-305.)

2. The oral mucosa is generally of normal appearance. In **idiopathic BMS**, there is absence of local (allergic contact stomatitis, lesions, infections) and systemic (endocrine disorders, hormonal deficiencies, autoimmune disorders, medication-induced, psychogenic) causes. However, if local or systemic disease is present, it is referred to as **secondary BMS**.
3. Treatment consists of pharmacotherapy consisting of antiepileptic drugs, tricyclic anti-depressants, serotonin reuptake inhibitors, and benzodiazepines, supplements, and biobehavioral therapy, such as, cognitive behavior therapy, biofeedback, and relaxation therapy.[5,6,17,20]

References

1. Maciewicz R, Mason P, Strassman A, Potrebic S. Organization of trigeminal nociceptive pathways. *Semin Neurol.* 1988;8:255-264.
2. Headache Classification Committee of the International Headache Society. The International Classification of Headache Disorders, 3rd edition (beta version). *Cephalalgia.* 2013;33:629-808.
3. Närhi M, Jyväsjärvi E, Virtanen A, Huopaniemi T, Ngassapa D, Hirvonen T. Role of intradental A-and C-type nerve fibres in dental pain mechanisms. *Proc Finn Dental Soc.* 1991;88:507-516.
4. Okeson JP. *Bell's Orofacial Pains: The Clinical Management of Orofacial Pain.* Chicago, IL: Quintessence Publishing Company; 2005.
5. De Leeuw R, Klasser GD, eds. *Orofacial Pain: Guidelines for Assessment, Diagnosis, and Management.* Chicago: Quintessence; 2008.
6. Sharav Y. *Orofacial Pain and Headache.* Philadelphia, PA: Elsevier Health Sciences; 2008.
7. Jacobsen PL, Bruce G. Clinical dentin hypersensitivity: understanding the causes and prescribing a treatment. *J Contemp Dent Prac.* 2001;2:1-12.
8. Bender I. Pulpal pain diagnosis—a review. *J Endod.* 2000;26:175-179.
9. Newman MG, Takei H, Klokkevold PR, Carranza FA. *Carranza's Clinical Periodontology.* Philadelphia, PA: Elsevier Health Sciences; 2011.
10. Myers EN, Ferris RL. *Salivary Gland Disorders.* Pittsburgh, PA: Springer Science & Business Media; 2007.
11. Eveson J, Cawson R. Salivary gland tumours. A review of 2410 cases with particular reference to histological types, site, age and sex distribution. *J Pathol.* 1985;146: 51-58.
12. Spencer WH. *Ophthalmic Pathology: An Atlas and Textbook.* Philadelphia, PA: WB Saunders; 1985.
13. Pilch BZ. *Head and Neck Surgical Pathology.* Philadelphia, PA: Lippincott Williams & Wilkins; 2001.
14. Schiffman E, Ohrbach R, Truelove E, et al. Diagnostic Criteria for Temporomandibular Disorders (DC/TMD) for clinical and research applications: recommendations of the International RDC/TMD Consortium Network* and Orofacial Pain Special Interest Group†. *J Oral Facial Pain Headache.* 2014;28:6-27.
15. Scrivani SJ, Mathews ES, Maciewicz RJ. Trigeminal neuralgia. *Oral Surg Oral Med Oral Pathol Oral Radio Endod.* 2005;100:527-538.
16. Scrivani SJ, Mehta N, Mathews ES, Maciewicz R. Clinical criteria for trigeminal neuralgia. *Oral Surg Oral Med Oral Pathol Oral Radio Endod.* 2004;97:544; author reply 544-545.
17. Attal N, Cruccu G, Baron R, et al. EFNS guidelines on the pharmacological treatment of neuropathic pain: 2010 revision. *Eur J Neurol.* 2010;17:1113-e1188.
18. Cruccu G, Gronseth G, Alksne J, et al. AAN-EFNS guidelines on trigeminal neuralgia management. *Eur J Neurol.* 2008;15:1013-1028.
19. Finnerup N, Attal N, Haroutounian S, et al. Pharmacotherapy for neuropathic pain in adults: a systematic review and meta-analysis. *Lancet Neurol.* 2015;162-173.
20. Klasser GD, Fischer DJ, Epstein JB. Burning mouth syndrome: recognition, understanding, and management. *Oral Maxillofac Surg Clin North Am.* 2008;20:255-271.

SECTION VIII

Cancer Pain and Palliative Care

40 Pain in Adults With Cancer

Richard E. Leiter, Mark J. Stoltenberg, and Mihir M. Kamdar

I. THE INCIDENCE AND IMPACT OF CANCER PAIN

Pain is one of the most feared consequences of cancer. It can markedly affect a patient's mood, independence, and functioning and therefore reduce a patient's quality of life. It is estimated that ~30%-40% of patients with cancer will experience pain early in their illness, and in patients with advanced cancer this number rises to 70%-90%. While ~75% of this pain emanates from the cancer itself, around 25% of cancer-related pain experienced by patients is related to treatments such as chemotherapy, surgery, and radiation.

Cancer-related pain also takes a toll on the health care system. Poorly controlled pain is a common cause of urgent clinic visits, emergency room evaluations, and hospital admissions. Therefore, effective treatment of cancer pain can significantly improve a patient's quality of life while also reducing the associated impact on the health care system.

II. ASSESSMENT OF CANCER PAIN: THE IMPORTANCE OF A DIAGNOSTIC APPROACH

While it is tempting to simply titrate pain medications, clinicians should instead use a diagnostic approach to treating pain. A clinician should have a low threshold to seek additional diagnostic information when a patient presents with new or more intense pain. The diagnostic workup should have two goals: assess the possible cause of pain and determine the most effective therapies. Assessment is crucial because pain in the cancer setting is often a sign of an impending oncologic emergency. For example, a patient with known spinal metastases who reports severe back pain should be evaluated immediately for cord compression with an MRI. A patient with worsening abdominal pain and vomiting should be evaluated for an evolving small bowel obstruction. Assessment helps rule out a potentially irreversible or life-threatening complication that could be causing the pain.

This diagnostic approach also generally results in more effective therapies. For example, if a clinician correctly identifies a new vertebral compression fracture as the source of pain, radiation therapy and vertebral augmentation may become options. Reviewing a wide array of options may yield better pain control and cause fewer side effects than relying solely on pharmacologic strategies.

III. TREATMENT OF CANCER PAIN

Multiple modalities exist to treat cancer-related pain, but certain medications are more effective than others in treating specific pain syndromes. Once a clinician has determined the etiology of the pain, he or she can tailor treatment to this pathophysiological etiology. To effectively tailor pain treatment, a clinician should be aware of the general prescribing guidelines for treating pain in the cancer setting.

A. The WHO Stepladder and Modern Approach to Pain

The World Health Organization (WHO) has created an extensively researched and well-established "Pain Relief Ladder" that outlines a general approach to pain management in patients with cancer. The ladder (Fig. 40.1.) has three ascending steps that correspond to the severity of the patient's pain. Step 1 involves the use of nonopioids such as aspirin, acetaminophen, or nonsteroidal anti-inflammatory drugs (NSAIDs) such as ibuprofen or naproxen. If pain persists or increases, clinicians should move to mild opioids such as tramadol and then to stronger opioids such as morphine until the patient's pain is effectively relieved. The WHO recommends starting at Step 1 and then escalating as necessary to ensure adequate pain control without overmedication. In practice, clinicians may opt to start at a higher step for patients in severe pain who may require more potent analgesia at the outset.

B. Nonopioids

Nonopioids vary widely and fall into many therapeutic classes. Common examples of nonopioids include acetaminophen, NSAIDs, and neuropathic agents. As recommended in the WHO analgesic ladder, nonopioids should be the first step in the treatment of mild cancer-related pain. As pain increases and opioids are prescribed, nonopioids should continue to be utilized as they may provide both synergistic analgesia and opioid-sparing effects.

C. Acetaminophen/NSAIDs

Acetaminophen and NSAIDs are the most common nonopioid pain medications used in patients with cancer. Although they do not carry the risk of physiologic dependence, there is a "ceiling" beyond which drug-specific toxicities limit their effectiveness. For mild pain, acetaminophen can be prescribed on an as-needed basis; however, clinicians should be willing to start patients on a scheduled regimen (such as 1000 mg every 8 hours). This

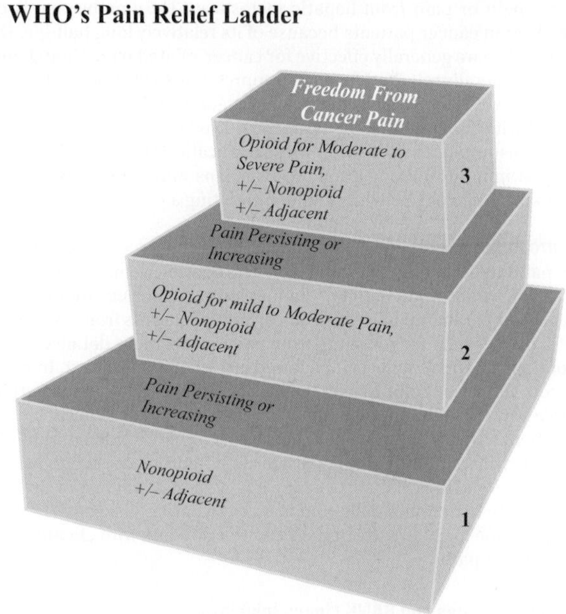

FIGURE 40.1 WHO's stepladder for cancer pain. (© 2020 World Health Organization.)

can be particularly effective in older patients, for whom clinicians worry about the cognitive side effects of opioids. The maximum daily dose of acetaminophen is 4 g, although this should ideally be limited to 3 g in chronic use. The maximum daily dose for patients with chronic liver disease or significant hepatic metastases is 2 g. Clinicians should also exercise caution, as acetaminophen is found in multiple combinations with opioids. Patients frequently do not realize that they are taking acetaminophen in multiple forms and may unintentionally exceed the maximum daily dose. Because these medications also reduce fever, acetaminophen should be minimized in patients with neutropenia.

NSAIDs can be markedly helpful for bony pain and pain from visceral capsule stretch or irritation, such as hepatic metastases or bulky lymphadenopathy. Like acetaminophen, NSAIDs can suppress fever and should be used cautiously in neutropenic patients. Because many patients with cancer are prone both to bleeding and to renal impairment, thought should be given prior to NSAID initiation. Selective COX-2 inhibitors such as celecoxib may be reasonable options in cancer patients on anticoagulation or with thrombocytopenia. Ketorolac is a parenteral nonselective COX inhibitor with opioidlike potency. It should be used for a maximum of 3-5 days due to side effects, but can be helpful in management of acute, severe cancer pain crises.

D. Corticosteroids

Corticosteroids are more potent anti-inflammatory agents than NSAIDs. High-dose corticosteroids are often used in specific cancer pain syndromes such as epidural spinal cord compression. In lower doses, they are effective for bony pain or pain from hepatic metastases. Dexamethasone is commonly used in cancer patients because of its relatively long half-life. Doses of 2-8 mg/day are generally effective for cancer-related pain, though higher doses are generally required for cord compression. Corticosteroids can also be helpful for cancer-related nausea and fatigue, but these benefits must be balanced with the potential for systemic side effects, such as immunosuppression, insomnia, and delirium. These medications may also decrease the efficacy of immunotherapy drugs, so clinicians may want to consult with the patients' oncology providers before initiating a corticosteroid regimen.

E. Neuropathic Agents

Many patients with cancer experience neuropathic pain. Neuropathy can stem from tumor-related nerve compression, treatment-induced nerve damage, and paraneoplastic syndromes. Multiple agents from various therapeutic classes help treat neuropathic pain, and a more detailed description of their pharmacology can be found elsewhere in this text. In general, clinicians should attempt to use a medication that may benefit a patient in multiple ways while avoiding a drug that that may cause side effects based on a patient's comorbidities. For example, a tricyclic antidepressant (TCA) may be very helpful for a young patient with neuropathic pain, insomnia, and depression. However, a TCA may not be a good choice in an elderly patient prone to delirium, falls, and urinary retention. Recent data suggest that duloxetine may have the best efficacy for patients with chemotherapy-induced neuropathy.

F. Bisphosphonates and RANK Ligand Inhibitors

Many patients with solid tumors (particularly prostate, breast, and lung cancer) and those with multiple myeloma will develop painful bony metastases. Bisphosphonates (such as zolendronic acid and pamidronate) and RANK ligand inhibitors (such as denosumab) work to inhibit osteoclasts. Data suggest that these agents can reduce skeletal-related events from osteoblastic solid tumors metastases and in multiple myeloma. These agents are unlikely to help with acute pain but can be a helpful long-term adjuvant in the treatment of bone pain and reduction of fracture risk.

G. Cannabinoids

Cannabinoids such as medical marijuana and its synthetic derivatives are frequently used by patients. Therefore, it is important for clinicians to understand their potential benefits and drawbacks in order to properly counsel patients. There is speculation that cannabidiol (CBD) is responsible for the primary analgesic effects found in marijuana, while tetrahydrocannabinol (THC) may mediate appetite stimulation, antiemetic properties, and CNS side effects. Unfortunately, most data involving synthetic cannabinoids have shown only mild benefit in cancer pain, and a recent international phase III study of a CBD/THC compound did not show benefit over placebo. Aside from synthetic agents, there are unfortunately few data to determine the benefits and toxicities of medical marijuana for cancer patients. Medical marijuana is now legal in multiple states, which means that use of cannabinoids will become more common. High-quality studies are needed to fully evaluate and determine their role in cancer-related pain

IV. OPIOID MANAGEMENT

Opioids are the mainstay of treatment for moderate to severe cancer pain. Though this section will focus on optimal use of opioid therapy, clinicians should continue to use nonopioids as part of a multimodal regimen tailored to each patient's pain syndrome.

A. Opioid Selection

There are many opioids available, and clinicians should consider multiple factors in selecting the most appropriate opioid for each patient. Specific considerations include available routes of delivery, renal and hepatic function, and prior patient experience. In addition, clinicians should be aware of cost and insurance factors that may limit access to certain medications. In general, clinicians should consider use of morphine as a first-line opioid, unless there are contraindications. Morphine is inexpensive and widely available throughout the world.

B. Routes of Administration

Opioids are available in oral, parenteral, subcutaneous, transdermal, sublingual, and buccal forms. In most situations, the oral route is preferred. However, many patients with advanced cancer lose the ability to take oral medications either due to direct effects of the disease or its treatment. For example, patients in the terminal phase of cancer often experience generalized debility or altered level of consciousness which affect the ability to swallow. It is important to note that hydrophilic opioids such as morphine, oxycodone, and hydromorphone have poor sublingual absorption. Alternative routes in this situation include sublingual or transbuccal (via lipophilic opioids such as fentanyl or methadone), transdermal, or parenteral delivery.

Patients with gastrostomy tubes have limited options for basal analgesia, as common extended-release oral opioids cannot be crushed and placed through a gastrostomy tube. Patients in this population who need continuous analgesia may require transdermal fentanyl or continuous infusion of parenteral opioid, either intravenously or subcutaneously. Methadone is a unique long-acting opioid that can both be crushed and comes in an elixir solution and can be used through a gastrostomy tube.

Fentanyl patches are the most widely used preparation for transdermal delivery. A patch lasts between 48 and 72 hours and, for this reason, can be logistically easier for patients to use. That said, its relatively long half-life limits rapid dose titration. Changes in the patient's body, such as fever or cachexia, can alter the rate of absorption, which may lead to overdosing or underdosing.

Parenteral delivery of opioids offers benefit for patients who cannot take oral medications, but it is also an ideal option for patients with severe pain. Patient-controlled analgesia (PCA) can be very helpful for patients with severe pain who require rapid dose titration or those with refractory incident pain. Use of PCAs is generally limited to inpatient use, though there are cases in which PCAs can be arranged in the home. Subcutaneous delivery is another parenteral option that approximates the pharmacokinetics of intravenous delivery and is commonly used in patients on home hospice.

Epidural and intrathecal drug delivery are alternate routes for opioid delivery that involve administration of opioids and other agents near drug receptors in the spine. These modes of delivery will be discussed later in the chapter.

C. Renal and Hepatic Dysfunction

Renal dysfunction is common in cancer patients, and this should be a consideration in choosing pain medications for them. Patients with renal dysfunction should avoid opioids with neurotoxic renally cleared metabolites, such as morphine, codeine, and meperidine. Conversely, fentanyl and methadone are both considered safe for patients with renal dysfunction as they do not have active renally excreted metabolites. Hydromorphone has similar metabolites to morphine, but data suggest it is safer in patients with renal insufficiency. There is a lack of data guiding the use of oxycodone in patients with renal insufficiency, and it should be used with caution given that it does have renally excreted neuroactive metabolites.

The liver is a primary site for metabolism of all opioids, which is why cautious dosing of opioids should be utilized in patients with hepatic dysfunction. Morphine, oxycodone, and hydromorphone should be prescribed initially at more conservative dosages and frequencies and then titrated to effect. While methadone does not have active metabolites, its half-life can increase in hepatic dysfunction, and its pharmacokinetics are affected by hypoalbuminemia. It should be used very cautiously in patients with hepatic dysfunction. Fentanyl may be the safest drug in hepatic failure due to its lack of active metabolites and short half-life. However, short-acting formulations of fentanyl are limited to intravenous and transmucosal agents, and transdermal fentanyl should be used cautiously given its long duration of action. The rule of thumb when using opioids in patients with hepatic dysfunction is to "start low and go slow."

D. Opioid Dosing and Titration

In general, clinicians should start treating pain with short-acting medications for patients naive to opioids. This allows clinicians to quickly find the correct dose while limiting the risk of unintentional overdose. Short-acting oral opioids (such as immediate-release morphine, oxycodone, and hydromorphone) should be dosed on an as-needed basis every 3-4 hours, unless patient-specific factors such as hepatic/renal dysfunction dictate otherwise.

If a patient requires more than three or four daily doses of a short-acting opioid, the prescribing clinician should start long-acting medications because the patient is signaling a need for more continuous pain control. Doses of long-acting opioid should equate 50%-100% of the total daily short-acting opioid dose and can then be split into divided doses. Most long-acting oral medications should be dosed every 8 or 12 hours.

All patients who take long-acting opioids should have a short-acting opioid for "breakthrough pain," or pain that is refractory to the long-acting medication. Typically, this is dosed at 10%-15% of the patient's total daily opioid dose. If a patient continues to require more than 3-4 daily doses of breakthrough medication after the long-acting medication has reached steady state, further increase of the long-acting opioid should be considered.

E. Opioid Rotation

Frequently, patients must rotate from one opioid to another. An initial opioid choice may lack efficacy, come with intolerable side effects, or be prohibitively expensive. Opioid rotation has the potential to provide patients with significant benefit. However, if done incorrectly, opioid rotation can lead to significant over- or underdosing. Therefore, clinicians must understand how to properly rotate from one opioid to another. The first step in opioid rotation is to understand opioid equianalgesic doses, which are presented in the Table 40.1.

Clinicians must also understand the important principle of *incomplete cross-tolerance.* Due to variances in the mu-opioid receptor subtypes

TABLE 40.1 Opioid Equianalgesic Doses

Drug	PO/PR (mg)	SC/IV (mg)
Morphine	30	10
Oxycodone	20	N/A
Hydrocodone	20	N/A
Hydromorphone	7.5	1.5
Oxymorphone	10	1
Fentanyl (**IV only**)	N/A	0.1 (100 μg)

that different patients express and that different opioids target, patients will be less tolerant to a new opioid than their previous opioid. The new opioid dose must be reduced by 25%-50% to account for this.

Remember that equianalgesic ratios are meant as guidelines and there may be significant variability between patients when rotating between opioids. Clinicians should use discretion as to how much to dose reduce when accounting for incomplete tolerance. For example, clinicians may choose to reduce less for a patient in severe pain. However, the clinician may prefer to be more conservative in their conversion with a medically frail patient or when rotating from one opioid to another in a patient on a high-dose regimen.

F. Methadone

Methadone is a unique opioid that can be particularly helpful in cancer pain but also requires a thorough understanding of its nuances in order to prescribe safely. Methadone is structurally distinct from the other opioids. It has unique pharmacokinetic and pharmacodynamic properties, and its half-life is extremely variable. Although its half-life lasts typically 15-60 hours, it may last >100 hours in some patients. Given this half-life, methadone is an effective long-acting pain medication. At the same time, toxicities may not develop for several days after its initiation or dose titration. There is also a disconnect between its analgesic half-life and its plasma half-life, which means it is dosed more frequently for pain than for addiction.

Methadone can be an extremely effective analgesic medication for cancer pain as it has activity not only on the mu-opioid receptors but also on the NMDA receptors. Its NMDA antagonism theoretically may provide adjuvant relief of neuropathic pain and possibly offset opioid-induced hyperalgesia (OIH).

Because of its unique and variable pharmacokinetic properties, rotation to methadone is not straightforward. Multiple methods have been published in the literature, including fixed conversion ratios and ratios that increase as the total opioid dose increases. Given this variability and the risk of significant toxicities, clinicians should seek guidance from colleagues with experience in prescribing and titrating methadone prior to initiating it. Methadone can also prolong the QT interval, and electrocardiogram monitoring should be implemented. Metabolism is also dependent on the CYP450 system, which can lead to multiple drug-drug interactions. Clinicians should also discuss the initiation of methadone with a patient's oncology provider as it may interact with other medications, including certain clinical trial agents.

G. Adverse Effects

Many patients limit their use of opioids because of side effects, which leads to inadequate pain control. It is important for clinicians to proactively manage expected side effects when initiating an opioid regimen. At subsequent visits, patients should be assessed for these side effects.

A nearly universal side effect to which patients will not develop tolerance is opioid-induced constipation (OIC). All patients who begin an opioid regimen should start a concurrent bowel regimen, generally with a stimulant such as senna, with the goal of one bowel movement every 1-2 days. Recent data demonstrate that docusate is no more effective than senna alone and should not be used. For patients who do not respond to senna, clinicians can add an osmotic agent such as polyethylene glycol. Lactulose is another alternative, but it tends to cause more discomfort from cramping. Some patients may need occasional stimulants per rectum, that is, bisacodyl, or enemas. For refractory OIC, clinicians can consider peripherally acting mu-opioid antagonists such as subcutaneous methylnaltrexone or oral naloxegol.

Another common side effect of opioid therapy is mild somnolence or mental clouding. Patients may benefit from the addition of a psychostimulant such as methylphenidate or modafinil. These medications can be taken on a regular or as-needed basis, and patients should be counseled to avoid doses after early to mid afternoon to prevent disrupting their sleep.

Patients may also experience nausea, particularly when they begin a new opioid regimen. This often improves after a period of days. Clinicians should proactively screen for OIC, as this is a common cause of nausea among patients new to opioids. Patients may benefit from the use of antiemetic that targets the chemoreceptor trigger zone such as ondansetron or haloperidol, which they should take ~30 minutes prior to each dose of opioid. For nausea that is either refractory to antiemetics, or does not improve over time, clinicians should rotate to an alternative opioid. Other less common side effects include xerostomia, pruritus, urinary retention, and myoclonus.

H. Addiction and Cancer Pain

There is currently an epidemic of opioid addiction in the United States. Patients with cancer were initially thought to be at lower risk for opioid use disorders, but recent data suggest that this is may not be the case, with some estimates of aberrant opioid-related behavior in a cancer population as high as 20%. Management of cancer patients with addiction is particularly challenging given the prevalence of pain and the need for opioid therapy to effectively treat moderate to severe cancer pain. Given the psychological overlay of pain and suffering, patients may unintentionally begin to use opioids for nonphysical pain, a phenomenon known as chemical coping.

Clinicians should treat their patients with empathy and attempt to attend to the multiple needs of the individual. Although there is no clear consensus on how to prevent opioid use disorder in patients with cancer, there is an emerging evidence base on how best to screen for, prevent, and then treat opioid use disorders. Overall, best practice for patients with concurrent cancer pain and opioid use disorder should involve the use of a harm reduction model, including use of opioid agreements, toxicology screens, and shortened refill intervals with frequent visits. At-risk patients do best when their clinicians work in collaboration with an interdisciplinary team with skills in psychiatry, addiction medicine, social work, palliative care, and pain management. Care should be taken to ensure patients have adequate control of their cancer pain and simultaneously reduce the risk of harm from opioids.

V. NONPHARMACOLOGIC THERAPIES FOR CANCER PAIN

Pharmacologic management results in adequate pain control for most cancer patients. Unfortunately, ~15%-24% of patients will not have adequately controlled pain despite adherence to WHO guidelines. Nonpharmacologic strategies can be helpful not only in alleviating opioid-refractory pain but can also decrease patient's opioid needs and associated side effects. It is important not to wait until pain becomes refractory to traditional opioid management to consider nonpharmacologic strategies.

A. Radiation and Radionuclide Therapies

Radiation therapy is a first-line treatment for direct palliation of painful malignant lesions. In fact, the majority of radiation therapy is palliative in nature. Radiation therapy can be particularly helpful for solitary, painful metastases. Remember that certain types of malignancy are more radiosensitive than others, and consultation with a radiation oncologist can be very helpful.

Radionuclide therapy can be helpful for multifocal bone pain from osteoblastic metastases, such as those arising from breast or prostate cancer. Radionuclides are isotopes that are taken up into areas of high bone turnover such as bony metastases and destroy painful cancer cells. Samarium, strontium, and radium are the best studied and most commonly used agents. The ideal use of radionuclide therapy is in a patient with multisite pain from widespread osteoblastic metastases whose pain is beyond the treatment field of traditional radiation therapy.

B. Interventional Procedures: Vertebral Augmentation, Neurolytic Blockade, Cryoablation, and Cordotomy

For patients with malignant compression fractures of the spine, vertebral augmentation can be a very helpful intervention. Vertebral augmentation refers to the injection of bone cement into a fractured vertebral body in order to stabilize its architectural integrity and reduce mechanical pain. Vertebral augmentation can be performed either via kyphoplasty or vertebroplasty. Kyphoplasty involves inflation of a balloon within the fractured vertebral body in the hopes of restoring bony architecture prior to injection of cement, while vertebroplasty involves cement injection without prior balloon inflation. Data suggest vertebral augmentation can be a safe and effective therapy for malignant compression fractures.

Neurolytic blockade involves the intentional destruction of neural pathways to alleviate pain and can be very helpful for pain transmitted by a specific nerve or nerve plexus. Celiac plexus blockade is one the most commonly performed neurolytic blocks. The celiac plexus is a network of sympathetic ganglia located near the celiac artery and transmits pain signals from a host of organs including the pancreas, liver, gallbladder, and stomach. Blockade of the celiac plexus can reduce cancer pain from various types of malignancies in the upper abdomen. Similarly, neurolysis of the superior hypogastric plexus and the ganglion impar can be helpful in alleviating pain from the lower abdomen and pelvis. Neurolytic intercostal blockade can be a useful tool to ameliorate pain from cancer involving in the chest wall.

Cryoablation is an image-guided percutaneous procedure in which probes are inserted into cancerous masses and freeze the cancerous cells, causing cell death. This is typically done under computed tomography guidance. The target of cryoablation is the interface between painful tumors and normal tissue. Data suggest that cryoablation can be particularly effective for musculoskeletal cancers that are either refractory or not amenable to radiation therapy.

Percutaneous or surgical cordotomy can be considered for refractory pain. This procedure involves direct disruption of the spinal pain pathways and can be particularly helpful for pain which affects one side of the body.

C. Neuraxial Drug Delivery: Epidural and Intrathecal Analgesia

Neuraxial drug delivery refers to the administration of analgesic medications in direct proximity to pain receptors in the spine. Examples of neuraxial analgesia include intrathecal and epidural drug delivery. By administering analgesics near spinal receptors, neuraxial drug delivery has the potential to offer more potent pain relief with significantly smaller doses of analgesics than when administered systemically. For example, 1 mg of intrathecal morphine is equianalgesic to 10 mg of epidural morphine, which is equianalgesic to 100 mg of intravenous morphine. Patients with severe pain may experience better pain control with fewer side effects than they do with systemic analgesics.

For patients with a prognosis of >3 months, intrathecal drug delivery systems (commonly known as "intrathecal pumps") are often utilized. These devices involve surgical implantation of subcutaneous drug reservoir that delivers analgesics to the intrathecal space via an internalized catheter. For patients with a prognosis of <3 months, use of a less-invasive percutaneous tunneled intrathecal or epidural catheter connected to an external drug pump can be considered. Risk of infection and catheter dislodgement is greater with this approach; however, it is much less invasive as it does not require surgical implantation of a drug reservoir.

VI. REFRACTORY CANCER PAIN

In the vast majority of patients, adequate pain control can be achieved with adherence to the WHO ladder. However, there are patients for whom usual measures do not yield adequate pain control. When a patient continues to experience pain despite optimization of both pharmacologic and nonpharmacologic therapies and common barriers to pain control have been addressed, the clinician should continue to refine their differential diagnosis. Possibilities may include the following: disease progression, OIH, aberrant opioid-taking behavior, and psychological distress.

OIH is a physiologic phenomenon in which exposure to opioids results in a lowering of the pain threshold. If clinical suspicion for OIH is high, use of nonopioid therapies should be optimized, opioid rotation to an agent with NMDA antagonism such as methadone should be employed, and additional use of more potent NMDA antagonists such as ketamine may be considered.

Lastly, patients dealing with the extreme stressors of cancer are at risk for what Dame Cicely Saunders described as "total pain." This refers to the overwhelming physical, psychological, social, spiritual, and existential challenges that patients experience while dealing with serious illness. These often-unspoken factors can significantly worsen a patient's experience of pain, making it difficult to separate physical distress from emotional pain. Clinicians should actively screen for these factors and involve assistance from mental health professionals, palliative care, social work, and chaplaincy whenever possible.

In the rare situations where all physiologic and nonphysiologic sources of refractory cancer pain have been addressed and a patient with a terminal malignancy continues to struggle with physical pain, palliative sedation may be an option to alleviate suffering. Palliative sedation is a medical intervention to alleviate intractable pain in terminally ill patients by means of continuous infusion of a sedation medication. It is considered separate from physician-assisted suicide and euthanasia and has been deemed both ethical and legal by the American Medical Association and the United Supreme Court, respectively. However, prior to considering this option, patients should consult with pain specialists and palliative care clinicians to ensure that all possible therapies have been explored. Ethics consultation is also often helpful to review the case and provide guidance prior to initiating palliative sedation. These dire situations require careful and thoughtful discussions with the patient, family, and entire treatment team. However, when deemed medically and ethically appropriate and necessary, palliative sedation can be an important therapy to alleviate intractable suffering in the dying patient.

VII. CONCLUSION

Pain is common among patients dealing with the challenges of cancer. Clinicians should utilize a diagnostic approach to cancer pain to rapidly identify potential impending oncologic emergencies and to identify targeted therapies. Pharmacologic management can be successful for the majority patients. Clinicians should also consider interventional strategies for patients who have refractory pain or side effects to systemic analgesics. An interdisciplinary approach should be employed to tend to both the physical and emotional suffering that cancer patients experience.

Selected Readings

Arcidiacono PG, Calori G, Carrara S, McNicol ED, Testoni PA. Celiac plexus block for pancreatic cancer pain in adults. *Cochrane Database Syst Rev.* 2011;(3):CD007519.

Berenson J, Pflugmacher R, Jarzem P, et al.; Cancer Patient Fracture Evaluation (CAFE) Investigators. Balloon kyphoplasty versus non-surgical fracture management for treatment of painful vertebral body compression fractures in patients with cancer: a multicentre, randomised controlled trial. *Lancet Oncol.* 2011;12(3):225-235.

Callstrom MR, Dupuy DE, Solomon SB, et al. Percutaneous image-guided cryoablation of painful metastases involving bone: multicenter trial. *Cancer.* 2013;119(5):1033-1041.

Hershman DL, Lacchetti C, Dworkin RH, et al.; American Society of Clinical Oncology. Prevention and management of chemotherapy-induced peripheral neuropathy in survivors of adult cancers: American Society of Clinical Oncology clinical practice guideline. *J Clin Oncol.* 2014;32(18):1941-1967.

Kamdar MM, Doyle KP, Sequist LV, et al. Case records of the Massachusetts General Hospital. Case 17-2015. A 44-year-old woman with intractable pain due to metastatic lung cancer. *N Engl J Med.* 2015;372(22):2137-2147.

Raslan AM. Percutaneous computed tomography-guided radiofrequency ablation of upper spinal cord pain pathways for cancer-related pain. *Neurosurgery.* 2008;62 (3 Suppl 1):226-233; discussion 233-234.

Smith TJ, Staats PS, Deer T, et al.; Implantable Drug Delivery Systems Study Group. Randomized clinical trial of an implantable drug delivery system compared with comprehensive medical management for refractory cancer pain: impact on pain, drug-related toxicity, and survival. *J Clin Oncol.* 2002;20(19):4040-4049.

Spencer K, Parrish R, Barton R, Henry A. Palliative radiotherapy. *BMJ.* 2018;360:k821.

Swarm RA, Abernethy AP, Anghelescu DL, et al.; National Comprehensive Cancer Network. Adult cancer pain. *J Natl Compr Canc Netw.* 2013;11(8):992-1022.

Tomblyn M. The role of bone-seeking radionuclides in the palliative treatment of patients with painful osteoblastic skeletal metastases. *Cancer Control.* 2012;19(2):137-144.

von Moos R, Costa L, Ripamonti CI, Niepel D, Santini D. Improving quality of life in patients with advanced cancer: targeting metastatic bone pain. *Eur J Cancer.* 2017;71:80-94.

Zech DF, Grond S, Lynch J, Hertel D, Lehmann KA. Validation of World Health Organization Guidelines for cancer pain relief: a 10-year prospective study. *Pain.* 1995;63(1):65-76.

41 Pediatric Cancer Pain

Kevin Madden and Richard D. Goldstein

I. OVERVIEW OF PEDIATRIC CANCER

A. Epidemiology

Approximately 16 000 children and adolescents are diagnosed with cancer each year in the United States. Acute lymphoblastic leukemia and acute myelogenous leukemia, the most common pediatric cancer diagnoses, represent about 25% of new diagnoses. Multidisciplinary care combining chemotherapy, radiation, and surgery has revolutionized outcomes, and the 5-year survival rate of ALL has increased from 57% in the late 1970s to nearly 90% in 2014. Nonetheless, cancer remains the second leading cause of death in children 5-14 years of age. As children live with cancer for longer periods of time, the risk for suffering has, in some ways, increased.

B. Illness Trajectory

Children whose treatment does not cure their cancer tend to follow an undulating trajectory of illness (Chapter 46), regardless of their specific cancer diagnosis. With initial treatment, the child's physical condition typically improves and symptom burden decreases. Relapse is accompanied by worsening pain, hopefully mitigated by more treatment. As the cycle of disease-treatment-remission-relapse-treatment progresses, more time is spent feeling burdened by pain and other physical symptoms. In fact, 80% of parents of children with cancer reported that their child suffered "a lot" or "a great deal" from pain in the last month of life.

II. PEDIATRIC CANCER PAIN PRESENTATION

A. General

Virtually all children with cancer will experience pain. Regardless of their prognosis, it is a priority to spare them from significant symptoms and help them live as normally as possible and participate in meaningful activities while supported by those who love them. Pain management occurs in a life-centered context that is crucial to the mission of caring for these children.

B. Myths About Pediatric Pain

Historically, there was widespread belief in the medical community that infants and young children were not able to perceive pain. Evidence supporting the idea that neonates and infants experience genuine pain was first published in 1987, yet many persistent myths about pediatric pain warrant attention.

1. **Children cannot reliably report pain location or amount.** Young children may lack the capacity to know all body parts, but the use of pictures or diagrams can be accurately used in children as young as 3 years of age to identify the location of pain. Children 5 years or older can reliably quantify their pain using the Wong-Baker FACES Pain Rating Scale.
2. **If a child is in pain, he or she will report it.** Children often do not report pain for many reasons. One of the primary reasons is from a desire to please those around them. Older children often do not want to appear "weak" by admitting to pain, especially in front of peers. Children also minimize their pain in an attempt to avoid further painful experiences or prolonging their hospital stay.
3. **A child in pain cannot sleep.** The observation that a child who is sleeping cannot be in pain is often misguided as children are often physically exhausted by chronically undertreated pain. Moreover, children with chronic pain suffer from a wide spectrum of sleep disorders that are not readily noticeable even to vigilant parents.
4. **If the child engages in activity, then the pain is well controlled.** As in adults, focused distracting activities modulate pain for children. The "job" of a child is to play, and many children endure significant pain to remain engaged in activities yet report significant pain. While a level of activity and function can be set as a goal for pain management, activity without guarding or discomfort is important.

C. Developmental Issues in the Expression of Pain

While the type of pain a child experiences is categorized no differently than in adults, the *expression* is influenced dramatically by the developmental stage of a child.

1. **Infants and toddlers.** Children at this age lack object permanence, which is the awareness that something exists without seeing, touching, or feeling it. Attachment to a parent or consistent caregiver is paramount to feeling security and comfort. Hospitalizations often interrupt this bond, leaving children with prolonged physical separation from their primary caregiver causing emotional and psychological stress that in turn amplifies their physical pain. Effective analgesia for minor, routine procedures, such as using EMLA for peripheral IV starts, must be incorporated into the treatment plan.
2. **Preschoolers.** Children in this age range are more imaginative, are developing autonomy, and are starting to experience guilt. Having a serious illness poses a significant challenge to the development of self-initiative, and so these children will often regress to more secure, familiar immature behaviors. "Magical thinking" is central to this developmental stage, and children may draw connections and inferences that affect their experience of painful conditions and procedures. For example, hospitalization and pain may be interpreted as punishment for bad behavior or

thoughts. It is important to remind children that they did not do anything to deserve their diagnosis and the painful procedures that come with it.

3. **School-aged children.** While there is still a mythical component to the internal narrative of children, they also are developing a concrete awareness of the world and their body—how it functions or how it *does not* function properly in most cases. The physical pain they endure from either the disease or the treatment of the disease challenges their drive to be a "normal" child and to be integrated into an increasingly important and dynamic social milieu. An important goal in this age group is to understand the importance of how much the child will continue going to school or be "homebound" and receive his or her education at home. Similarly, the child's desire not to disappoint may affect the disclosure of symptoms. Pain management and its side effects are an important aspect of their success. One must be prepared to listen carefully to these children's worries and anxieties while simultaneously provide age-appropriate information. Children in this age range are not easily reassured by "Don't worry about it" or "It will be OK" responses to their concerns.
4. **Teenagers and adolescents.** With the development of abstract thinking, the sense of "mystery" in life and striving to discover their place in the world, teenagers and adolescents can feel isolated even when they do not have a serious illness such as cancer. Body image is starting to occupy a central role in their identity and how they position themselves in their social sphere. They often worry that intense medical treatment will physically disfigure them while also preventing them from spending time with their friends. It is important to endorse feelings that what is often considered trivial to adults is likely central to their decision-making process.

Other than infants and the very youngest of children, it is crucial to understand that children have a basic desire to please not only their parents but most authority figures. Being mindful of the language used when communicating with children about pain can go a long way in ensuring that the child's pain is effectively managed. For example, saying "Great job, you only used two as-needed doses of morphine" implies that a "bad child" would have used more. In this context, the child will likely feel pressured to underreport his or her pain in order to continue to receive praise from their health care provider. A better way of stating the same concept would be "I'm glad to hear that you are feeling better," which allows for the child or parent to disagree and provide more information as to why a limited number of as needed doses were used.

III. ASSESSMENT OF PEDIATRIC CANCER PAIN

A. Types of Pain

Similar to adults, pain is generally divided into three main categories—nociceptive somatic, nociceptive visceral, and neuropathic. The characteristics of the different types of pain are addressed more fully in other chapters in this book.

B. Instruments to Report Pain

Given the developmental changes in capacities of children, no single standardized assessment tool is suitable to assess pain. In general, there are three major categories of the assessment tools used in pediatrics—single dimension, multiple dimension, and behavioral observational.

1. **Single dimension self-report measures** represent the vast majority of the assessment tools used in pediatrics. The Wong-Baker FACES Pain Rating Scale and, to a lesser extent, the Faces Pain Scale-Revised are both

examples of visual analog scales (VAS) and are age appropriate for children over the age of 5 years of age. The assumptions of these scales are that the child understands pain along a continuum and can comprehend proportionality; that is, they must be able to translate their experience of pain to the abstract line and anchors provided. For children over 9 years of age, verbal rating tools using Likert scales with anchor points of 1 = no pain and 5 = extreme pain have been studied but demonstrated no advantage over VAS. The major limitation of these assessment tools is that they are designed to assess only the severity of acute pain despite the fact that many confounders influence the child's experiences and interpretation of pain.

2. Because pain is attenuated by many things, including insomnia, fatigue, anxiety, depression, and spiritual distress, **multidimensional self-report symptom assessment scales** have been developed and validated for use in children as young as 7 years of age. The Memorial Symptom Assessment Scale (MSAS), originally developed for adults with cancer, has been modified and validated for use in children with cancer in two age groups, 7-12 and 10-18 years of age. These versions of the MSAS allow children to quantify many symptoms including pain severity, frequency, and distress caused by pain, as well as other sources of suffering that modify experiences of pain such as nausea, fatigue, sadness, and irritability. One of the challenges in completing these self-report measures is that the MSAS 10-18 consists of 30 questions; completing such a lengthy questionnaire on a frequent basis is difficult.
3. Children who have significant preexisting neurologic injury or are very young cannot participate in self-report measures. **Rating scales for nonverbal children** are addressed in Chapter 46.
4. Children 8 years and older have the cognitive capacity to reliably report their pain with the traditional **visual analog or verbal analog scales.**

IV. DISEASE AND TREATMENT-RELATED PAIN

A. Disease-Related Pain

Pain due to the underlying disease typically occurs at time of diagnosis or disease recurrence or when the disease becomes refractory to treatment. When disease is in remission, children often have little pain. Pain caused by disease can be either acute or chronic. Acute pain can arise as the primary tumor invades tissue, joints, or nerves or obstructs hollow viscera. Metastatic disease can cause spinal cord compression or, if in the cranial vault, increased intracranial pressure. The characteristics of pain due to bone marrow infiltration, tumor burden, metastatic disease, mucositis, and phantom limb pain are no different than what occurs in adult patients with cancer, and these are addressed more fully in other chapters in this book.

B. Treatment-Related Pain

1. **Procedure Related.** The most common source of pain for all children with cancer is the frequent invasive procedures necessary for diagnosis and treatment. The pain associated with these procedures often sets the narrative for how a child will experience pain in the future, and so it is vital that the child be adequately prepared psychologically by the parents and, with great skill, child life specialists. It is important for a plan for pain management be established beforehand. Venipuncture, accessing central venous catheters, diagnostic and therapeutic lumbar punctures, bone marrow aspirates, and biopsies all become part of the "normal" life of a child with cancer. It is now the standard of care that children undergoing invasive procedures such as a lumbar puncture or bone marrow biopsy receive anesthesia or deep sedation.

2. There are a variety of cognitive and behavioral techniques that are often beneficial to the child undergoing painful procedures as anxiety plays an integral role in child's perception and experience of pain. As mentioned earlier, child life specialists are essential for minimizing the pain and anxiety a child has with respect to painful procedures. Their role is to provide age- and developmentally appropriate information to a child undergoing any procedure, from the seemingly benign such as a CT scan to the universally painful such as surgical procedures. They also are skilled in helping children manage anxiety through perhaps the most accessible, affordable, universal, and side effect–free intervention available—distraction. From the use of virtual reality games, iPads, and storytelling in older children to bubbles, playing "peekaboo," and a pacifier with sucrose in infants, distraction is often the best intervention when the procedure will be brief such as venipuncture or accessing a central line.

V. TREATMENT OF CANCER-RELATED PAIN IN CHILDREN

A. General Strategy

The role of the parents in the treatment of their child's pain is complex. Parents may have limited experience in caring for children with life-threatening illnesses. Decisions about pain are often influenced by two countervailing ideas—a desire to minimize their child's pain and suffering and concerns related to opioids. The practitioner must be willing to devote substantial time reassuring a parent that opioids will be used in a thoughtful manner. Significant trust in the health care provider by the parents will be gained if reassurance is provided proactively that opioid therapy will be reassessed at each visit and will be weaned when the etiology of pain is better controlled.

It is important to provide patients and their families with realistic expectations of pain management. It is often helpful to counsel children and their families before significant interventions have started that the goal is twofold: to (1) minimize pain and (2) maximize functionality. Emphasis should be placed on minimizing pain and on being explicit that the intent is not to "cure" the pain. A personalized pain goal (PPG) of 0 is not realistic and will often result in unmet expectations and subsequent false hope that more interventions will lead to a complete cessation of pain. Realistic goals, as determined through collaboration with the child and family, can then be set, monitored, and assessed as time and treatment progress.

All medications for children are indexed according to the child's weight in kilograms, that is, morphine is 0.1 milligram per kilogram per dose (mg/kg/dose). Extra caution should be taken when looking up doses, as some sources will list a medication as "mg/kg/dose," while others may list as "mg/kg/day divided BID or TID." Another unique consideration in pediatric pain management is that most children cannot reliably swallow tablets or pills until 6 or 7 years of age. Most medications discussed in this chapter are available as liquid or elixir preparations. For those that are not, compounding pharmacies can often be helpful in creating suspensions of the desired medication with the exception of extended-release opioids.

B. Nonpharmacologic

The treatment of pain in children with cancer should always start with and continue to include nonpharmacologic measures. Parents are requesting these modalities with increasing frequency; at the same time, these nonpharmacologic measures are being studied and gaining more acceptance by the larger medical community. See Table 41.1 for the most commonly used strategies and techniques employed.

TABLE 41.1 Nonpharmacologic Interventions for the Treatment of Pediatric Cancer Pain

Aromatherapy	Occupational Therapy
Art therapy	Physical therapy
Hypnosis	Reiki
Massage	Vibration stimulation
Meditation	Warm/cold compresses
Music therapy	Weighted blankets

C. Nonopioids, Opioids, and Adjuvants

The medications used to treat pain in children with cancer are no different than in adults. See Table 41.2 for pediatric doses of nonopioids, opioids, and adjuvants used to manage pediatric cancer pain. There are, however, some important considerations that are specific to pediatrics that need to be considered.

Codeine is no longer used in children. Approximately 35% of children receive no analgesia due to inability to convert codeine to morphine, while some children are "ultrarapid metabolizers" who convert codeine to morphine in higher-than-normal amounts. The only long-acting opioid

TABLE 41.2 Pharmacologic Interventions for the Treatment of Pediatric Cancer Pain

Drug	Dose	Route	Frequency
Nonopioids			
Acetaminophen	15 mg/kg	PO	q4 h
	15 mg/kg	IV	q6 h
Celecoxib	1-2 mg/kg	PO	q12-24 h
Ibuprofen	10 mg/kg	PO	q6 h
Ketorolac	0.5 mg/kg	IV	q6 h (maximum 20 doses/5 d)
Opioids			
Fentanyl	0.5-2 μg/kg	IV	q1 h
Hydromorphone	0.04-0.06 mg/kg	PO	q3-4 h
	0.015 mg/kg	IV	q2-4 h
Methadone	0.1 mg/kg	PO/IV	q8-12 h
Morphine	0.2-0.3 mg/kg	PO	q3-4 h
	0.05-0.1 mg/kg	IV	q2-4 h
Oxycodone	0.1-0.2 mg/kg	PO	q3-4 h
Tramadol	1-2 mg/kg	PO	q4-6 h
Adjuvants			
Amitriptyline	0.2 mg/kg	PO	qhS
Nortriptyline	0.2 mg/kg	PO	qhS
Gabapentin	2 mg/kg (titrate to a maximum of 15 mg/kg)	PO	TID
Clonidine	0.002 mg/kg	PO	q8-24 h
Ketamine	0.25-0.5 mg/kg	PO	q8 h
Methylphenidate	0.05-0.1 mg/kg	PO	Daily to BID
Dexamethasone	0.1 mg/kg	PO/IV	q6 h

that comes in a liquid preparation is methadone, and so for many young children, this is the only extended-release opioid available to them. As such, methadone is commonly used in children with cancer pain.

D. Regional Anesthesia and Analgesia

The use of anesthesiologists and pain physicians to provide pain relief is becoming more common in the treatment of pediatric cancer pain. Skilled practitioners can provide local nerve blocks in the head/neck, upper extremity, chest, abdominal viscera, and lower extremity. These blocks are beneficial for many reasons including pain relief without increasing opioid medications and potentially suffering side effects including opioid-induced neurotoxicity, respiratory depression, and constipation. The use of nerve blocks facilitates pediatric surgical patients regaining physical functionality sooner than patients whose postoperative pain was managed only with traditional pain medication. Postoperative cancer pain management will often use epidural analgesia as well, usually managed by an anesthesia or pain team. Truly intractable pain that is not relieved by any of the modalities above may find benefit from intrathecal analgesia provided by an experienced anesthesiologist or pain medicine physician. Applications involving continuous infusions are beyond the scope of this chapter.

VI. CONCLUSION

The most common types of cancer that afflict children are different than those of adult patients. Practitioners who do not frequently treat pediatric cancer pain are often uncertain whether traditional pain medications can be safely used in children. Consulting trusted sources for the proper starting doses is essential, and for the most part, the general pharmacologic approaches to the management of pain are philosophically not very different than in adults. The utilization of nonpharmacologic measures is often of great benefit. Consultation with pediatric palliative care or pediatric pain physicians may be helpful in constructing comprehensive strategies to manage pain in children with cancer.

Selected Readings

Anand KJ, Hickey PR. Pain and its effects in the human neonate and fetus. *N Engl J Med.* 1987;317:1321-1329.

Bieri D, Reeve RA, Champion GD, Addicoat L, Ziegler JB. The Faces Pain Scale for the self-assessment of the severity of pain experienced by children: development, initial validation, and preliminary investigation for ratio scale properties. *Pain.* 1990;41:139-150.

Ciszkowski C, Madadi P, Phillips MS, Lauwers AE, Koren G. Codeine, ultrarapid-metabolism genotype, and postoperative death. *N Engl J Med.* 2009;361:827-828.

Collins JJ, Byrnes ME, Dunkel IJ, et al. The measurement of symptoms in children with cancer. *J Pain Symptom Manage.* 2000;19:363-377.

Collins JJ, Devine TD, Dick GS, et al. The measurement of symptoms in young children with cancer: the validation of the Memorial Symptom Assessment Scale in children aged 7-12. *J Pain Symptom Manage.* 2002;23:10-16.

Edwards BK, Noone AM, Mariotto AB, et al. Annual Report to the Nation on the status of cancer, 1975-2010, featuring prevalence of comorbidity and impact on survival among persons with lung, colorectal, breast, or prostate cancer. *Cancer.* 2014;120:1290-1314.

LeBaron S, Zeltzer L. Assessment of acute pain and anxiety in children and adolescents by self-reports, observer reports, and a behavior checklist. *J Consult Clin Psychol.* 1984;52:729-738.

Murphy SL, Xu J, Kochanek KD; Centers for Disease Control and Prevention, National Center for Health Statistics, National Vital Statistics System. Deaths: final data for 2010. *Natl Vital Stat Rep.* 2013;61:1-117.

Rork JF, Berde CB, Goldstein RD. Regional anesthesia approaches to pain management in pediatric palliative care: a review of current knowledge. *J Pain Symptom Manage.* 2013;46:859-873.

Savedra M, Gibbons P, Tesler M, Ward J, Wegner C. How do children describe pain? A tentative assessment. *Pain.* 1982;14:95-104.

Valrie CR, Bromberg MH, Palermo T, Schanberg LE. A systematic review of sleep in pediatric pain populations. *J Dev Behav Pediatr.* 2013;34:120-128.

Ward E, DeSantis C, Robbins A, Kohler B, Jemal A. Childhood and adolescent cancer statistics, 2014. *CA Cancer J Clin.* 2014;64:83-103.

Williams DG, Patel A, Howard RF. Pharmacogenetics of codeine metabolism in an urban population of children and its implications for analgesic reliability. *Br J Anaesth.* 2002;89:839-845.

Wolfe J, Grier HE, Klar N, et al. Symptoms and suffering at the end of life in children with cancer. *N Engl J Med.* 2000;342:326-333.

42 Palliative Medicine

Bethany-Rose Daubman, Leah B. Rosenberg, April Zehm, and Mihir M. Kamdar

I. PALLIATIVE CARE OVERVIEW

Palliative care is a medical specialty that provides relief from the symptoms and stress of a serious illness. It focuses on quality of life for the patient and family and is appropriate at any stage of serious illness. Palliative care aims to relieve all sources of suffering. In patients with serious illness, suffering may involve physical symptoms but may also pervade into emotional, cultural, and spiritual realms. Palliative care utilizes an interdisciplinary team model, often involving physicians, nurse practitioners, nurses, social workers, and chaplains, who work together with the patient and family to tend to these various elements of suffering. The palliative care team may also work to help clarify and support the patient's goals of care.

Palliative care is not an alternative to curative or life-prolonging care but is an additional measure that can be provided at any point along the time continuum of serious illness. Clinicians sometimes only involve palliative care in the very last stages of illness, feeling that palliative care is equivalent with "comfort measures only." However, palliative care is actually aggressive management of symptoms and stress at any stage of serious illness and can coexist along with curative therapy. In fact, there are data to suggest that early involvement of palliative care near the time of the diagnosis of a serious or life-threatening illness can result in better clinical outcomes than waiting until the patient is near the end of life. There may be a point in the illness where disease-prolonging therapy is no longer desired, possible, or indicated, at which point hospice becomes appropriate.

A. Palliative Care Vs Hospice

Palliative care is an umbrella term that includes hospice. Hospice is specialized medical care that focuses on comfort and end-of-life care in the last 6 months of life. However, it is important for patients and medical providers to understand that there is a difference between hospice and palliative care and that palliative care is not synonymous with just end-of-life care. Table 42.1 demonstrates some differences between hospice and palliative care.

II. CORE ELEMENTS OF PALLIATIVE CARE

A. Symptom Control

Patients with serious illness often experience severe and distressing symptoms. Often these symptoms are underrecognized and inadequately treated, thereby limiting functionality and quality of life. Though pain is a commonly recognized symptom, other important symptoms can include nausea, vomiting, dyspnea, constipation, fatigue, anorexia, depression, and anxiety. Attending to physical symptoms not only can improve physical quality of life but also allows patients and families to address nonphysical elements of suffering that come with serious illness. This can help patients better tend to the social, financial, and spiritual challenges of their illness, which can be incredibly important particularly as they near the end of life.

B. Patient-Centered Decision-Making

A key tenet of palliative care is to work with both patients and medical care teams to help with shared medical decision-making. Many patients with chronic illness face complex medical decisions that can feel overwhelming and isolating. Clinicians should not only ensure that patients have a clear sense of prognosis and treatment options but also explore their goals and values related to their health care. When clinicians have an understanding of a patient's goals and values (eg, how would a patient want to spend his or her time if he or she became sicker?), they can then align medical

TABLE 42.1 Comparing and Contrasting Palliative Care and Hospice

	Hospice	Palliative Care
Treatment	Focus is on comfort rather than on curative or disease-directed therapy	Attention to quality of life and advance care planning can occur concomitantly with disease-directed therapy
Timing	Patient has less than a 6-month prognosis if disease runs its expected course	Can occur at any stage of serious illness. Data suggest early involvement is better
Location	Mainly provided in the home and relies upon family caregiver and visiting hospice team. May also be provided in skilled nursing facilities or hospice houses for patients whose needs cannot be met at home	Often provided as inpatient or outpatient consultations. Some institutions may also have dedicated palliative care units as well as home-based palliative care teams

treatment decisions within this personalized frame. The result is that medical decision-making becomes much more patient-centered, and care is delivered that is concordant with a patient's wishes.

C. Common Misconceptions

Among both clinicians and the public, there are many misconceptions about palliative care. Many fear that palliative care is only for patients at the very end of life and erroneously equate palliative care with hospice. Patients and families may erroneously worry that palliative care is akin to "giving up" or may worry that palliative care involvement means they are near death. Patients and even clinicians may think that palliative care should only be involved when there is "nothing left to offer" and also have fears that providing comfort medications at the end of life will hasten death.

When introducing palliative care, it is important to ask patients if they have heard of palliative care and, if so, to then explore their understanding of palliative care. This is an important step in addressing any misconceptions and also an opportunity for clinicians to explain the benefits of palliative care. Palliative care involvement has been shown to improve the quality of life of both patients and families and has even been associated with patients living longer. Furthermore, early palliative care involvement in a patient's disease course has been demonstrated to have significant benefits. Hence, clinicians should avoid waiting until late in a patient's clinical course to involve palliative care. Lastly, clinicians should remember that palliative care can be provided simultaneously alongside life-prolonging care.

D. Psychosocial and Spiritual Care

No one person can meet all of the needs of a patient with complex or serious illness. Palliative care utilizes an interdisciplinary approach to tend to the multitude of psychosocial stressors that patients and families experience when dealing with a life-threatening illness. In addition to physicians and nurses, palliative care teams often include social workers, chaplains, counselors, and trained volunteers. These team members have additional expertise in counseling family members, addressing spiritual concerns, assisting with the financial burdens of serious illness, and supporting the bereaved.

III. MODES OF PALLIATIVE CARE DELIVERY

Palliative care can be provided in a wide variety of care settings. Most large hospitals in the United States offer palliative care inpatient consultations. Nearly 90% of tertiary medical centers with >300 beds have palliative care consultation services available. Over the last 10 years, there has been a significant increase in outpatient palliative care clinics and home-based programs. In addition, certain hospice agencies can also provide palliative care services to patients at health care facilities and at home. Through these programs, patients and families who may not be eligible or ready for hospice care may obtain specialist-level management of their palliative care needs.

Hospice, on the other hand, is provided in four main care settings in the United States: the patient's place of residence, a hospice inpatient facility, a residential facility such as a nursing home, or an acute-care hospital. Hospice is covered under Medicare Part A and is generally covered by private insurance.

Most patients in the United States would like to die at home if possible, and hence most hospice occurs at home. While hospice nurses will visit regularly and are on-call 24 hours a day, it is important to know that hospice at home relies on family support to provide the vast majority of nursing care. If there is not family support to meet a patient's needs at home, another venue of care should be considered.

For those patients whose care needs cannot be met at home, the remaining options are hospice care at a nursing facility or long-term care facility, free-standing dedicated hospice, or in an acute-care hospital setting. In order to meet criteria to be cared for in either a hospice house or hospice in an acute hospital setting, a patient must have acute hospice care needs that cannot be provided in a less acute setting such as the home or a residential facility.

It is also important to know that typically while on hospice, life-prolonging therapies that do not offer comfort are generally stopped. This generally includes therapies such as chemotherapy, intravenous fluids, total parenteral nutrition, and nonessential medications. There has also been a recent trend towards "open-access" hospices which allow patients to remain on life-prolonging therapies while receiving hospice care. However, these presently are limited in both scope and situation. Hospices generally provide social work and chaplaincy support to patients and families and also provide bereavement support to family members after a patient's death. The National Hospice and Palliative Care Organization (http://www.nhpco.org/) can be a very helpful resource for identifying hospice services based on a patient's geographic location.

IV. PAIN MANAGEMENT AT THE END OF LIFE

A. Overview

For an in-depth discussion of acute, chronic nonmalignant, or cancer pain management, please see the other relevant chapters of this book. This section will focus on pain management for the imminently dying patient who may only have hours to days of life remaining. It has been estimated by some authors that nearly 25% of patients with end-stage diagnoses die with moderate to severe pain. During the last hours of life, clinicians may need to quickly respond to escalating analgesic requirements and changing available routes of administration.

Given their potency and rapid onset, opioid analgesics are the mainstay of managing end-of-life pain. When evaluating a patient with pain, one should consider the routes available and the severity of pain. For example, dysphagia is common in the last hours of life, and medications may then need to be given subcutaneously or intravenously. Many clinicians are surprised to hear that subcutaneously administered opioids have similar pharmacokinetic profiles to intravenous opioids, making this a common route of use for hospice patients who may not have intravenous access. When pain is severe, we also favor using parenteral routes due to rapidity of effect over oral administration (Fig. 42.1). By convention, many clinicians will often place patients on continuous hourly infusions of opioids at the end of life, so-called morphine drips. However, this is not an effective means of controlling acute symptoms because the dose of medication is spread out over the course of an hour. Hence it will take several hours for the continuous infusion to reach steady state, and in the meantime, the patient may be in distress. As detailed in the section that follows, we recommend treating acute pain with bolus dosing.

B. Patient Case: Pain Management at the End of Life

Rita is a 65-year-old teacher with metastatic ovarian cancer who is admitted to an inpatient medical ward for uncontrolled abdominal pain. Imaging

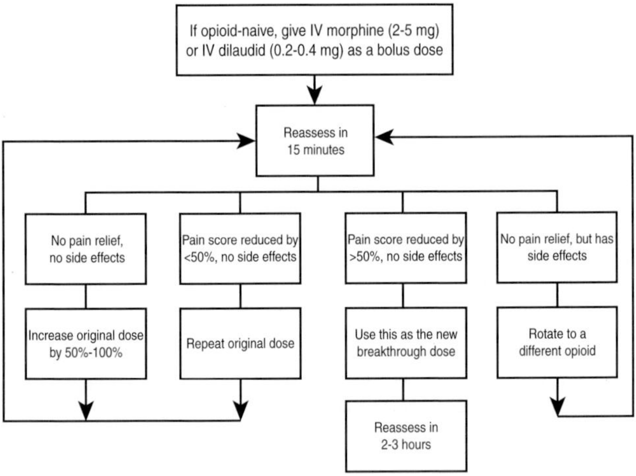

FIGURE 42.1 Managing a pain crisis.

suggests that the pain is secondary to diffuse peritoneal carcinomatosis. She has just been transferred to the unit and is complaining of "10 out of 10" abdominal pain as well as nausea.

1. **Step 1: Consider if the patient is opioid-naive or opioid-tolerant.** Rita has been taking morphine extended-release 30 mg twice daily and morphine immediate-release 7.5 mg by mouth about four times a day. She would be considered an opioid-tolerant patient.
2. **Step 2: Choose the route based on acuity of pain, patient dysphagia, and available vascular access.** Rita is too nauseated to swallow at this time. If swallowing has become unsafe, and the patient has been using an oral long-acting medication, at minimum this must converted into a continuous infusion of opioid using equianalgesic ratios. In Rita's case, her long-acting oral morphine extended-release (60 mg is the total daily dose) would correspond to 20 mg of IV morphine or a continuous infusion of 0.8 mg morphine/hour (20 mg divided by 24 hours). If Rita were opioid naive, we would not recommend initiation of a continuous infusion initially but rather bolus dosing. Once an opioid-naive patient's pain is under control with acute boluses, the clinician can then consider a continuous infusion as outlined in the section that follows.
3. **Step 3: Use bolus dosing to control the pain crisis.** Rita has been using 7.5 mg of immediate-release oral morphine for breakthrough pain with partial effect. This is equianalgesic to 2.5 mg of IV morphine. Hence reasonable starting dose for Rita would be morphine IV 2.5-3 mg with clinician reassessment after 15 minutes. If pain remains >7/10, once could increase the dose 50%-100% of the initial dose (eg, 4-6 mg). If pain decreased to 5-7/10, we would repeat the same dose, since the dose is having partial effect and it is possible that merely repeating the dose may bring the pain to a tolerable level. If her pain did not improve and she developed side effects, it would be wise to consider an opioid rotation and consideration of contacting a pain or palliative care specialist.
   a. It can be helpful to offer a range of doses (100%-150% of bolus) to enable nursing to adequately respond to pain variability. Depending on the

opioid, bolus doses can be administered as often as every 30 minutes to every 2 hours as needed based upon the level of symptoms.

b. If >4-6 doses of bolus opioid are used in a 8-hour period, it is prudent to start or increase a continuous infusion of opioid. This can be done by determining the average hourly amount of opioid used in bolus form (eg, dividing the total amount of opioid used in boluses over the past × hours by × as demonstrated below). The provider can then start or increase and opioid infusion by 50%-100% of that amount per hour. Opioid continuous infusions generally should not be increased more frequently than twice per 12-hour period. Clinicians must remember that acute periods of discomfort are best managed with repeated bolus doses prior to then initiating or starting a continuous infusion.

4. **Step 4: Reassess patient once crisis resolved.** Rita is more comfortable now, stating 2/10 pain, 10 hours later, after a total of 6 mg of IV morphine in bolus dosing (3 mg × 2 doses). She is on a continuous infusion of 0.8 mg/hour you initiated to replace her oral long-acting opioid. You divide the 6 mg/10 hours to derive an additional 0.6 mg/hour from her boluses, which you then add to the 0.8 mg/hour infusion to find a final infusion rate of morphine 1.4 mg/hour. You continue with rescue boluses of morphine 2.5-3 mg IV every 1 hour as needed in the event her pain worsens (Table 42.2).

V. NONPAIN SYMPTOM MANAGEMENT

A. Overview

Basic symptom palliation is a fundamental skill for all providers who care for patients with serious illness. In all cases, consideration of the underlying etiology and additional diagnostic testing is warranted. However, the extent of the diagnostic workup should be tailored based on the patient's underlying disease, prognosis, and goals of care. For example, if additional testing will be highly invasive or not result in therapies that will improve quality of life, purely symptomatic approaches may be appropriate in this population.

B. Depression and Anxiety

Dame Cicely Saunders, considered by many as the founder of hospice, coined the term "total pain" in reference to physical, emotional, interpersonal, and existential suffering that patients with life-threatening illness experience. Episodic sadness and anxiety are expected when adjusting to serious illness, but persistent anxiety or depression which interferes with

TABLE 42.2 Pearls of Managing an Acute Pain Crisis

- Stay at the bedside or nearby
- Consider ketorolac if no contraindication, since it may have opioid-like analgesia without causing sedation or respiratory depression
- Call for help when out of comfort range
- Look for a diagnosis (based on goals of care)
- Consider interventional options (if appropriate based on goals of care)
- Note that the same principles above for pain at the end of life can also be applied to terminal dyspnea, given that opioids are considered first-line agents for dyspnea at the end of life

daily functioning is not a normal part of serious illness or the dying process. Hence, clinicians should actively screen for mood issues in patients with life-threatening illness and treat as such. Clinicians should always assess for underlying physical causes of depressive or anxious symptoms, such as poorly controlled pain or dyspnea. While beyond the scope of this text, therapy for depression and anxiety generally entails some combination of supportive psychotherapy, cognitive therapy, and pharmacotherapy.

C. Constipation

Constipation is prevalent and multifactorial in serious illness and may result from dehydration, electrolyte disturbances, pain, immobility, neurologic dysfunction, structural gastrointestinal abnormalities, and medications.

Nonpharmacologic therapies for constipation include physical activity, scheduled toileting, and adequate fluid intake. However, adherence to these interventions may prove challenging for seriously ill patients, and pharmacologic therapy is often required. Furthermore, constipation is a nearly universal side effect of opioid use to which tolerance does not develop. Hence, a prophylactic bowel regimen should be prescribed at initiation of opioid therapy.

Both stimulants (senna glycosides, bisacodyl) and osmotic laxatives (lactulose, polyethylene glycol) have been shown to be effective for constipation and are considered first-line agents. Bulk-forming laxatives such as psyllium or methylcellulose can worsen constipation without adequate fluid intake, so we do not recommend routine use of these for palliative care patients. The stool softener docusate has not been shown to be more beneficial than placebo for constipation among terminally ill patients. Failure of escalating oral laxatives usually requires rectal-based therapies, including stimulant suppositories or enemas, or newer peripherally acting mu-opioid antagonists such as methylnaltrexone, naloxegol, and naldemedine.

D. Delirium

Delirium is an acute, acquired disturbance of attention and awareness accompanied by a change in baseline cognition that often fluctuates rapidly. It can manifest as hyperactive, hypoactive, or mixed subtypes. Hyperactive delirium is often quite noticeable, characterized by symptoms of restlessness, paranoia, hallucinations, or agitation. A more commonly missed entity is hypoactive delirium, which often manifests as lethargy, sedation, and decreased awareness. Delirium is highly prevalent among patients with serious or terminal illness and is associated with high morbidity and mortality. Underlying etiologies include medications, organ failure, metabolic abnormalities, uncontrolled pain, infection, constipation or impaction, urinary retention, hypoxemia, and central nervous system insults. Given that delirium is reversible in up to half of cases even among patients with terminal illness, management should begin with a detailed assessment for possible causes of delirium. Clinicians should perform a thorough history and examination, including a complete medication review, to identify potentially correctable causes.

Nonpharmacologic strategies for the prevention and treatment of delirium should be used for all patients with delirium, including frequent reorientation and cueing, correcting sensory deficits, normalizing sleep-wake cycles, minimizing noise or other stimulating environmental factors. While no medications are FDA approved for the treatment of delirium, antipsychotic medications are often used to treat unsafe or distressing delirium symptoms such as agitation or hallucinations. There is no evidence to support treating hypoactive delirium pharmacologically, and hence decisions to treat this subtype of delirium with medication are made on a case-by-case basis.

Haloperidol has long been considered first-line therapy for hyperactive delirium due to its efficacy, relative safety, versatility, and low cost. Chlorpromazine is an effective alternative to haloperidol, especially for severe agitation, but can have anticholinergic adverse effects. Recently, the atypical antipsychotics olanzapine and risperidone have been shown to be equally effective to haloperidol in managing delirium and carry less risk of extrapyramidal symptoms. Intramuscular delivery of neuroleptics should be avoided when possible due to erratic absorption and because painful injections can worsen agitation. Of note, antipsychotic drugs have been shown to be associated with a small increased risk of death in elderly patients with dementia, resulting in an FDA-issued black box warning for these medications in 2005. This mortality risk has not been demonstrated specifically in delirium. The use of these medications for this indication should be individualized, as the benefits of controlling agitated delirium among terminally ill patients usually outweigh the risk.

Benzodiazepines can worsen delirium and should be avoided unless specifically treating alcohol withdrawal–related delirium or if antipsychotics are contraindicated or not tolerated. Physical restraints should be only used for agitated delirium that poses a threat to the patient or staff and is unresponsive to both pharmacologic and nonpharmacologic therapies.

E. Dyspnea

Dyspnea is common in seriously ill patients, exacerbated by physical deconditioning and cachexia, and often worsens during the dying process. Dyspnea can occur in the absence of lung pathology and does not always correlate with degree of hypoxemia. Air hunger can be highly distressing, often contributing to anxiety. Anxiety can then worsen dyspnea, fueling a vicious cause-and-effect cycle. Nonpharmacologic techniques can help alleviate dyspnea, including pursed-lip breathing or the use of a bedside fan. Contrary to popular belief, there is no data supporting the use of oxygen to alleviate dyspnea in a patient who is not hypoxemic, although non-oxygenated air movement with a fan can be helpful. Opioids are the drug of choice for refractory dyspnea that is unresponsive to both treatment of the underlying cause and nonpharmacologic therapies. Fears about respiratory depression and carbon dioxide retention can be mitigated if opioids are dosed safely and appropriately, and the American College of Chest Physicians now recommends opioid titration for dyspnea management in patients with advanced cardiopulmonary disease. Benzodiazepines should be considered second-line agents for dyspnea. They can be helpful if there is significant anxiety present, but the risks of delirium and somnolence must be weighed. Specific disease-modifying agents such as diuretics, bronchodilators, and corticosteroids should be considered depending on the underlying etiology.

F. Nausea and Vomiting

The common causes of nausea in serious illness include medications (chemotherapy agents, opioids, etc.), uremia, electrolyte disturbances, infection, constipation, bowel obstruction, delayed gastric emptying, ascites, increased intracranial pressure, and anxiety. A mechanistic approach to nausea treatment based on etiology and antiemetic neuropharmacology is recommended (Table 42.3). However, in advanced disease, the etiology of nausea is often multifactorial or unidentifiable, in which case an empiric approach is acceptable. Because the most common etiologies include gastrointestinal

TABLE 42.3 Nausea Management

Medication	Dose and Frequency	Comments
Dopamine Antagonists		
Metoclopramide	5-10 mg (20 mg maximum) PO or IV or SC Q6H	Useful for opioid-induced N/V, partial malignant bowel obstruction (can worsen colicky pain if complete obstruction), impaired GI motility, N/V of unknown etiology Can cause extrapyramidal symptoms (EPS)
Prochlorperazine	5-10 mg PO or IV Q6H or 25 mg PR Q6H	Useful for opioid-induced N/V or N/V of unknown etiology Can cause EPS, sedation (especially in the elderly)
Haloperidol	0.5-5 mg PO or SC or IV Q6H	Very potent antiemetic Useful for opioid-induced N/V, malignant bowel obstruction, N/V of unknown etiology Can cause EPS
Serotonin Antagonists		
Ondansetron	4-8 mg PO or IV Q4-8H	Useful for chemotherapy or radiation-induced N/V Can cause constipation Expensive Also available in oral disintegrating tabs
Corticosteroids		
Dexamethasone	Varies. Suggest 4-16 mg PO or IV daily in divided doses	Useful for CNS tumor, malignant bowel obstruction Can cause delirium, anxiety, insomnia (avoid dosing at night)
Anxiolytics		
Lorazepam	0.5-2 mg PO or IV Q6H	Only useful if anticipatory or anxiety-related N/V Can cause sedation, confusion, delirium (especially in the elderly)
Atypical Antipsychotics		
Olanzapine	2.5-20 mg daily in divided doses	Targets multiple receptors Can cause sedation
Antihistamines		
Promethazine	12.5-25 mg PO or IV Q6H or 25 mg rectally Q6H	Dystonia, akathisia Confusion and sedation (especially in the elderly)

pathology or medications, dopamine antagonists are often recommended as first-line treatment for nausea of unknown cause. Benzodiazepines may be helpful for anticipatory nausea and vomiting that is anxiety induced but are otherwise not good antiemetics and can be sedating as well as delirium inducing, especially in the elderly. If nausea is unresponsive to optimized scheduled dosing of a single antiemetic, we recommend combination therapy using agents from different drug classes.

VI. SERIOUS ILLNESS COMMUNICATION WITH PATIENTS AND FAMILIES

Communicating effectively with seriously ill patients and their families should be an essential element of daily medical practice of all clinicians. A variety of investigations have found that patients and families benefit from clear, compassionate discussion with their providers about their illness understanding, goals, and values.

Although trained palliative care clinicians can provide these discussions to patients, it has become clear that the growing numbers of seriously ill individuals will continue to outstrip the reach of specialist palliative care workforce. It is also estimated that over the next 25 years, the palliative care needs of the US health care system will double with the aging of the baby boom population. Hence in order to meet these growing palliative care needs, every clinician will need to possess the basic palliative care competencies required to communicate effectively with patients and families about advanced care planning. For those clinicians seeking further training in honing their communication skills, we suggest exploring communication training programs such as VitalTalk or the Serious Illness Communication Guide (Web sites in Selected Readings section).

VII. PALLIATIVE SEDATION FOR REFRACTORY SYMPTOMS AT END OF LIFE

When other interventions have failed to relieve severe, intractable physical symptoms in a terminally ill patient, palliative sedation (PS) should be considered. PS involves administering proportionate doses of sedating medications to relieve otherwise refractory physical symptoms at the end of life by inducing a state of unconsciousness. The goal is relief of suffering and not to intentionally end a patient's life or hasten death, distinguishing it ethically from physician aid-in-dying or euthanasia (Table 42.4). While there is often concern about the unintended effect of hastening death, multiple studies have shown no demonstrable survival difference with this intervention. The goal is to use as little medication as needed to alleviate the distressing symptom. The most common indication for PS is refractory pain. PS may also be considered for intractable agitated terminal delirium that is refractory to maximal standard pharmacologic therapies. PS has ethical support from the American Medical Association as well as legal permissibility from the U.S. Supreme Court. Common medications used in PS include benzodiazepines, barbiturates, and propofol. Institutional protocols should be followed if available. Formal palliative care and ethics consultation is strongly recommended prior to initiating PS to provide guidance on the process and to ensure all other palliative measures have been exhausted.

VIII. CONCLUSION

Palliative care is a medical subspecialty that uses an interdisciplinary approach to tend to the multitude of stressors that patients and families dealing with serious or life-threatening illness experience. As discussed,

TABLE 42.4 Differentiation Between Interventions of Last Resort

Intervention	Cause of Death	Intention of Intervention	Legal Status
Palliative sedation	Underlying disease	Relief of intractable symptoms/ suffering	Legal in the United States
Physician aid-in-dying	Medication(s) prescribed by a physician and self-administered by the patient	Death	Legal in ten states (CA, CO, DC, HI, ME, MT, NJ, OR, VT, and WA) at the time of publication
Euthanasia	Medication(s) administered by a physician	Death	Illegal in the United States

these stressors can be both physical and emotional, and it is imperative that clinicians tend to both aspects. Another important goal of palliative care is to help foster patient-centered decision-making through effective communication. Palliative care encompasses but is not synonymous with hospice or end-of-life care and can be provided alongside life-prolonging therapies.

In the context of serious illness, palliative care provides both a framework and an extra layer of support for patients, families, and providers. Clinicians should consider involving palliative care whenever they are caring for a patient with a challenging prognosis and could use assistance in managing physical symptoms, addressing emotional needs, or clarifying goals of care.

Selected Readings

Ariadne Labs. Serious Illness Communication Guide. https://www.ariadnelabs.org/wp-content/uploads/sites/2/2015/08/Serious-Illness-Conversation-Guide-5.22.15.pdf. Accessed January 18, 2017.

Bernacki R, Hutchings M, Vick J, et al. Development of the Serious Illness Care Program: a randomised controlled trial of a palliative care communication intervention. *BMJ Open.* 2015;5:e009032.

Breitbart W, Alici Y. Agitation and delirium at the end of life: "We couldn't manage him". *JAMA.* 2008;300(24):2898-2910, E1.

Casarett D, Inouye S; American College of Physicians-American Society of Internal Medicine End-of-Life Care Consensus Panel. Diagnosis and management of delirium near the end of life. *Ann Intern Med.* 2001;135(1):32-40.

Center to Advance Palliative Care. About Palliative Care. https://www.capc.org/about/palliative-care/. Accessed December 13, 2016.

Center to Advance Palliative Care. 2015 Scorecard. https://reportcard.capc.org/. Accessed January 18, 2017.

El-Jawahri A, LeBlanc T, VanDusen H, et al. Effect of inpatient palliative care on quality of life 2 weeks after hematopoietic stem cell transplantation: a randomized clinical trial. *JAMA.* 2016;316(20):2094-2103.

Glare P, Pereira G, Kristjanson LJ, Stockler M, Tattersall M. Systematic review of the efficacy of antiemetics in the treatment of nausea in patients with far advanced cancer. *Support Care Cancer.* 2004;12(6):432-440.

Kamal A, Maguire J, Wheeler J, Currow D, Abernethy A. Dyspnea review for the palliative care professional: treatment goals and therapeutic options. *J Palliat Med.* 2012;15(1):106-114.

LeBlanc T, Tulsky J, Block SD. Addressing Goals of Care: "REMAP" (VITALtalk). http://www.vitaltalk.org/sites/default/files/REMAPforVitaltalkV1.0.pdf. Accessed February 24, 2015.

Librach S, Bouvette L, De Angelis C, et al. Consensus recommendations for the management of constipation in patients with advanced, progressive illness. *J Pain Symptom Manage.* 2010;40(5):761-773.

Lupu D. Estimate of current hospice and palliative medicine physician workforce shortage. *J Pain Symptom Manage.* 2010;40:899-911.

National Hospice and Palliative Care Organization. Facts and Figures 2012. http://www.nhpco.org/sites/default/files/public/Statistics_Research/2012_Facts_Figures.pdf. Accessed October 7, 2016.

Quill T, Lo B, Brock D, Meisel A. Last-resort options for palliative sedation. *Ann Intern Med.* 2009;151:421-424.

Schneider LS, Dagerman KS, Insel P. Risk of death with atypical antipsychotic drug treatment for dementia: metaanalysis of randomized placebo-controlled trials. *JAMA.* 2005;294:1934-1943.

Temel JS, Greer JA, Muzikansky A, et al. Early palliative care for patients with metastatic Non–Small-cell lung cancer. *N Engl J Med.* 2010;363(8):733-742.

VitalTalk. http://www.vitaltalk.org/. Accessed January 18, 2017.

Wood G, Shega J, Lynch B, Von Roenn J. Management of intractable nausea and vomiting in patients at the end of life: "I was feeling nauseous all of the time…nothing was working." *JAMA.* 2007;298(10):1196-1207.

World Health Organization. Definition of Palliative Care. http://www.who.int/cancer/palliative/definition/en/. Accessed December 13, 2016.

[illegible]

SECTION IX

Special Considerations in Pain Medicine

43

Opioids in Chronic Nonterminal Pain

Shawn G. Hughes and Rene Przkora

I. INTRODUCTION

The explosion of medical and scientific knowledge over the past century has profoundly altered the role of opioids in our lives. In present-day Western civilization, an expectation can exist that it is possible to eliminate pain through the judicious use of opioid medications. Of particular interest is the increasing use of opioids for the treatment of chronic, nonterminal pain, and the patients most commonly associated with this category include those suffering from chronic low back and/or neuropathic pain. The surge in opioid use was initially fostered by a growing concern that patients with chronic pain conditions were overwhelmingly undertreated. In the 1990s, a series of reforms resulted in the relaxing of regulations that had previously restricted the prescribing and dispensing of opioid medications. In 2001, as a means of further bolstering the recognition and treatment of pain, the Joint Commission on the Accreditation of Healthcare Organizations introduced pain as "the 5th vital sign." However, as opioid use has escalated, so too has the incidence of accidental overdose, abuse, and diversion. This trend has been especially evident in opioids to treat chronic nonterminal pain (CNTP). An initial response to this trend was to assume that opioids themselves were unsafe. In 2014, the United States Centers for Disease Control reported 18 893 overdose deaths related to opioid use. However, as this chapter will discuss, when opioids are prescribed to appropriate patients in a structured manner, the incidence of adverse events is quite low. It is therefore crucial that medical providers who choose to treat CNTP with opioids possess the understanding and tools necessary to prescribe these medications in a safe and effective manner.

II. RATIONALE FOR CHOOSING OPIOID THERAPY

There are a multitude of options available for the treatment and management of pain. Like all therapies in medicine, the decision as to what treatment is best for a given patient is highly influenced by a balance of risk vs benefit, physician experience, and the patient's preferences and cultural beliefs. The current approach, at least in the Western world, often relies heavily on medications as the most trusted and applicable of the treatment options. Opioids are the only class of pain medication offering powerful analgesia without a ceiling effect, meaning that doses can be increased until pain is overcome. This advantage makes opioids theoretically attractive options for the management of pain and the reason that many pain advocates believe that all patients with pain have a right to opioid therapy.

No one doubts that opioids are powerful and effective analgesics, and scientific evidence supports this claim. However, whether analgesic efficacy is maintained with prolonged use of opioids is less clear, and there are several areas of concern that can interfere with long-term treatment. There must be sustained and obvious benefit to justify continued use. Current guidelines suggest using opioid therapy for CNTP only when all other nonopioid strategies have been exhausted.

When making the decision to eventually begin opioid treatment of CNTP, one can usefully consider two phases—an initial phase in which opioid treatment is used as part of a multimodal and aggressive rehabilitative approach to restore function and to reduce reliance on medications, followed by a chronic phase in which opioids are used according to strict criteria. As important as deciding when to start opioid therapy is, careful consideration must also be taken in deciding when opioid therapy should be discontinued. The decision to continue or terminate opioid therapy should consider multiple factors, including the patient's level of pain, quality of life, functional status, tolerance of side effects, and signs of aberrancy or misuse.

III. AREAS OF CONCERN

A. Loss of Efficacy

Many patients receiving opioid therapy for chronic pain appear to obtain satisfactory and sustained pain relief without dose escalation. This seems counter to the belief that the development of tolerance, a pharmacologic phenomenon, is an inevitable consequence of prolonged opioid use. It is evident, nevertheless, that in many patients, tolerance "levels off," not only in the case of side effects but also in the case of analgesia, allowing these patients to derive adequate analgesia at a stable dose.

In other patients, the outcome is less favorable. Satisfactory analgesia is not sustained, and the patients request increasing doses. Tolerance develops to the analgesic and euphoric effects of opioids, as well as to their side effects (except direct bowel effects). Tolerance to opioids can be learned (associative), involving psychological factors, and linked to environmental clues, or adaptive (nonassociative), involving down-regulation and/or desensitization of opioid receptors. Mechanisms of pharmacologic tolerance to opioids have not been fully elucidated, but many mechanisms appear to be linked to the *N*-methyl-D-aspartate receptor cascade.

Opioid-induced hyperalgesia (OIH) is a phenomenon in which increasing the dosage of opioid does not decrease pain but instead results in a paradoxical increase in pain intensity and distribution beyond the initial area of injury. OIH has been described in both acute and chronic opioid users and at varying dosages. Anecdotal evidence suggests that patients on long-term, high-dose opioids are at highest risk for developing OIH. The exact prevalence is currently unknown, and there are no clearly defined criteria to differentiate OIH from tolerance. There is ongoing debate regarding the precise mechanism of OIH; the most commonly described model involves the activation of glutaminergic pathways mediated by *N*-methyl-D-aspartate receptors, resulting in central sensitization. The issue of decreasing opioid efficacy presents one of the major dilemmas prescribers will face: either to maintain the current medication and/or dosage at the expense of optimal pain management or to escalate the therapy, which will increase the risk of intolerable side effects, including OIH.

B. Unacceptable Side Effects

The side effects of opioids include sedation, respiratory depression, nausea and vomiting, slowing of bowel activity, pruritus, and dysphoria. These side effects are described in more detail in Chapter 11. As mentioned earlier, it is common for tolerance to develop to all of these side effects except bowel effects, which are peripherally mediated and to which tolerance does not develop. Patients taking opioids for longer periods should always receive bowel prophylaxis to prevent constipation, as this is an almost inevitable consequence of chronic opioid therapy. Several studies have described nausea and constipation as the most common reasons for patients with CNTP discontinuing opioid therapy. In general, when presented with intolerable side effects in the setting of CNTP, the physician should consider either reducing the opioid dosage or switching to an alternate medication.

Overdose leading to respiratory depression is the most feared complication of opioid therapy. Patients with underlying respiratory pathology such as sleep apnea and/or concomitant use of central nervous system depressants (benzodiazepines and alcohol) are at increased risk of respiratory depression when using opioids. Zedler and colleagues developed the **Risk Index for Overdose or Serious Opioid-Induced Respiratory Depression Scale** (RISORD) as an objective means to identify and quantify risk of overdose and respiratory depression in opioid users. The RISORD tool assigns values based on the presence of 15 separate variables (see Table 43.1). The sum of these variables is termed the **Risk Index Score**, which is compared to a table that assigns the probability of developing overdose or respiratory depression (Table 43.2). Although it was developed exclusively using Veterans Health Administration data, the RISORD scale is one of the few objective, evidence-based, and validated measures of opioid-induced respiratory depression. If respiratory depression is of particular concern, buprenorphine could be considered, as it is has a ceiling effect for respiratory depression.

C. Hormonal Effects

Opioids influence at least two major hormonal systems: the hypothalamic-pituitary-adrenal axis and the hypothalamic-pituitary-gonadal axis. Opioids can increase levels of prolactin and decrease levels of plasma cortisol, follicular-stimulating hormone, luteinizing hormone, testosterone, and estrogen. This can result in deleterious clinical effects, including male and female infertility, decreased libido and aggression, menstrual disorders, and galactorrhea. These opioid effects were clinically observed long before they were chemically confirmed in heroin addicts. Testosterone depletion was later demonstrated in male patients in methadone programs. Testosterone levels can be particularly low in patients receiving intrathecal opioids, to the extent that these patients often feel better and regain energy when they are treated with testosterone. The extent of hormonal changes in patients with CNTP treated with opioids, and the clinical significance of the change is unknown, but one recent study did find decrements in testosterone and cortisol in these patients. Whether hormonal replacement

TABLE 43.1 Risk Index for Overdose or Serious Opioid-Induced Respiratory Depression (RIOSORD)

Description	Y/N	Score
In the past 6 months, has the patient had a health care visit (outpatient, inpatient, or ED) involving:		
Opioid dependence?		15
Chronic hepatitis or cirrhosis?		9
Bipolar disorder or schizophrenia?		7
Chronic pulmonary disease? (eg, emphysema, chronic bronchitis, asthma, pneumoconiosis, asbestosis)		5
Chronic kidney disease with clinically significant renal impairment?		5
Active traumatic injury, excluding burns? (eg, fracture, dislocation, contusion, laceration, wound)		4
Sleep apnea?		3
Does the patient consume:		
An extended-release or long-acting (ER/LA) formulation of any prescription opioid or opioid with long and/or variable half-life? (eg, OxyContin, Oramorph SR, methadone, fentanyl patch, levorphanol)		9
Methadone? (Methadone is a long-acting opioid, so also write Y for "ER/LA formulation")		9
Oxycodone? (If it has an ER/LA formulation [eg, OxyContin], also write Y for "ER/LA formulation")		3
A prescription antidepressant? (eg, fluoxetine, citalopram, venlafaxine, amitriptyline)		7
A prescription benzodiazepine? (eg, diazepam, alprazolam)		4
Is the patient's current maximum prescribed opioid dose:		
>100 mg morphine equivalents per day?		16
50-100 mg morphine equivalents per day?		9
20-50 mg morphine equivalents per day?		5
In the past 6 months, has the patient:		
Had one or more ED visits?		11
Been hospitalized for 1 or more days?		8
Total Score		**115**

Adapted from Zedler B, Xie L, Wang L, et al. Development of a risk index for serious prescription opioid-induced respiratory depression or overdose in Veterans' Health Administration patients. *Pain Med.* 2015;16:1566-1579.

would improve the well-being of patients with CNTP who are treated with opioids remains uncertain.

D. Immune Effects

Animal and human studies have demonstrated the presence of opioid receptors on a wide range of immune cells (human leukocytes possess mu receptors) and the ability of opioids to alter the development, differentiation, and function of immune cells. Prolonged exposure to opioids appears more likely to suppress immune function than short-term exposure, and the abrupt withdrawal of opioids also seems to cause immunosuppression.

TABLE 43.2 Opioid-Induced Respiratory Depression (OIRD) Probability Based on Calculated Risk Index

Risk Index Score	OIRD Probability (%)
0-24	3
25-32	14
33-37	23
38-42	37
43-46	51
47-49	55
50-54	60
55-59	79
60-66	75
≥67	86

Adapted from Zedler B, Xie L, Wang L, et al. Development of a risk index for serious prescription opioid-induced respiratory depression or overdose in Veterans' Health Administration patients. *Pain Med.* 2015;16:1566-1579.

There is a paucity of studies assessing immune function in patients with CNTP receiving opioids, but the direct evidence that opioids impair immune function does give rise for concern. Pain itself can produce immunosuppression, so the greatest concern is likely to pertain to patients who receive high doses of opioids and yet do not experience pain relief.

E. Problematic Opioid Use

Problematic opioid use, comprising addiction, diversion, and other less serious problematic behaviors, is an inescapable consideration of opioid treatment. To deny these problems exist is to sweep aside the most challenging aspect of treating long-term pain with opioids. This in turn compromises care and denies patients appropriate treatment when problematic behavior does arise, many of which are manifestations or harbingers of substance use disorder. Problematic behaviors arise in a substantial proportion of chronic pain patients who are treated with opioids, with published reports suggesting a rate of up to 19%. Typical problematic behaviors for patients with pain who are treated with opioids are listed in the chapter addressing opioid use disorder.

The subject of substance use disorder is covered in detail in Chapter 44, but it is important to emphasize here how physical dependence differs from substance use disorder. Although the syndrome of drug addiction is often characterized in part by physical dependence—a state of adaptation manifest as a withdrawal syndrome upon cessation or reversal of the drug—addiction is a syndrome of maladaptive behavior, and maladaptive behavior must be present to diagnose addiction. Physical dependence is likely to develop in almost all patients receiving long-term opioids, but most patients do not develop an opioid use disorder without preexisting risk factors. A 2010 Cochrane review reported a 0.3% incidence of iatrogenic addiction in patients on long-term opioid therapy for noncancer pain. However, if an opioid use disorder does arise, physical dependence can be a powerful factor in maintaining the addictive state. Therefore, it is important to understand that signs of physical dependence may coincide with opioid use disorder but also to appreciate that physical dependence is not synonymous with addiction.

Diversion of opioids from their intended use, usually for profit, occasionally occurs in the pain treatment setting. This is sometimes driven by the need for the patient to obtain more drugs to satisfy the substance use disorder, but more often it is a criminal act. Occasionally, the whole treatment course is a sham when a patient fabricates pain to obtain opioids. It is not the job of the physician to monitor patients for criminal activity; nevertheless, it would be irresponsible to continue to prescribe opioids to patients who are found to be diverting. A combination of aberrant behavior and a negative drug screen may alert the physician to the possibility that the prescribed drug is being diverted. Requesting the patient present for spontaneous pill counts when there is concern for diversion may be helpful.

The medical community will likely continue to grapple with issues surrounding long-term opioid use and, in particular, finding the balance between effective pain control and the risks of problematic opioid use. How confident can clinicians be that during the course of treatment, they are treating physical pain and not life stressors? How many patients who started self-medicating with illicit opioids did so to relieve psychologic turmoil or emptiness? What is important is that physicians do not replace poorly controlled pain with poorly controlled pain plus untreated chemical coping or substance use disorder, thereby worsening the lives of their patients. Hence, it is necessary to provide long-term opioid therapy only in a highly structured and monitored setting, so the risks of substance use disorder and its attendant problems can be minimized.

F. Opioid Use in Elderly Populations

As the elderly population in the United States increases, so too has the awareness of the unique issues regarding treatment of CNTP in this group. It is reported that pain is the most common complaint among elderly patients, particularly in nursing home residents. However, cognitive impairment and altered perception of painful stimuli may result in the failure of providers to recognize and treat pain in these individuals. High-quality data regarding long-term opioid use in elderly CNTP patients is lacking. Thus it is recommended that medical providers follow general opioid prescribing guidelines (described in Section IV) in addition to considering the following caveats in this population: (1) alterations in volume of distribution and decreased hepatic and renal function may significantly alter the onset and duration of action of many medications, (2) altered or impaired cognitive function may not only be exacerbated by opioids, but may also lead to issues with compliance, and (3) polypharmacy carries significant risks of iatrogenesis in this population. In general, opioid use for CNTP in the elderly is considered safe and well tolerated by most patients when prescribed in a "start low, go slow" manner that adheres to prescribing guidelines and takes into account individual patient needs.

IV. STRUCTURED, GOAL-ORIENTED APPROACH TO LONG-TERM TREATMENT

In 2016, the United States Centers for Disease Control published guidelines for primary care providers regarding opioids for the treatment of CNTP. These 12 guidelines are described in Table 43.3. Ideally, opioids should be used for the shortest duration necessary to provide adequate pain relief. Early aggressive treatment, using a rehabilitative approach that aims to restore function and reduce reliance on medications, can be utilized when a patient first presents with debilitating pain (see Chapter 27). The structured approach suggested here should be used when the clinician and patient agree to a trial of opioid treatment for chronic pain.

TABLE 43.3

2016 CDC Guidelines for Prescribing Opioids for Chronic Pain

1. Nonpharmacologic therapy and nonopioid pharmacologic therapy are preferred for chronic pain. Clinicians should consider opioid therapy only if expected benefits for both pain and function are anticipated to outweigh risks to the patient. If opioids are used, they should be combined with nonpharmacologic therapy and nonopioid pharmacologic therapy, as appropriate.
2. Before starting opioid therapy for chronic pain, clinicians should establish treatment goals with all patients, including realistic goals for pain and function, and should consider how opioid therapy will be discontinued if benefits do not outweigh risks. Clinicians should continue opioid therapy only if there is clinically meaningful improvement in pain and function that outweighs risks to patient safety.
3. Before starting and periodically during opioid therapy, clinicians should discuss with patients known risks and realistic benefits of opioid therapy and patient and clinician responsibilities for managing therapy.
4. When starting opioid therapy for chronic pain, clinicians should prescribe immediate-release opioids instead of extended-release/long-acting (ER/LA) opioids.
5. When opioids are started, clinicians should prescribe the lowest effective dosage. Clinicians should use caution when prescribing opioids at any dosage, should carefully reassess evidence of individual benefits and risks when considering increasing dosage to ≥50 morphine milligram equivalents (MME)/day, and should avoid increasing dosage to ≥90 MME/day or carefully justify a decision to titrate dosage to ≥90 MME/day.
6. Long-term opioid use often begins with treatment of acute pain. When opioids are used for acute pain, clinicians should prescribe the lowest effective dose of immediate-release opioids and should prescribe no greater quantity than needed for the expected duration of pain severe enough to require opioids. Three days or less will often be sufficient; more than 7 days will rarely be needed.
7. Clinicians should evaluate benefits and harms with patients within 1-4 weeks of starting opioid therapy for chronic pain or of dose escalation. Clinicians should evaluate benefits and harms of continued therapy with patients every 3 months or more frequently. If benefits do not outweigh harms of continued opioid therapy, clinicians should optimize other therapies and work with patients to taper opioids to lower dosages or to taper and discontinue opioids.
8. Before starting and periodically during continuation of opioid therapy, clinicians should evaluate risk factors for opioid-related harms. Clinicians should incorporate into the management plan strategies to mitigate risk, including considering offering naloxone when factors that increase risk for opioid overdose, such as history of overdose, history of substance use disorder, higher opioid dosages (≥50 MME/day), or concurrent benzodiazepine use, are present.
9. Clinicians should review the patient's history of controlled substance prescriptions using state prescription drug monitoring program (PDMP) data to determine whether the patient is receiving opioid dosages or dangerous combinations that put him or her at high risk for overdose. Clinicians should review PDMP data when starting opioid therapy for chronic pain and periodically during opioid therapy for chronic pain, ranging from every prescription to every 3 months.
10. When prescribing opioids for chronic pain, clinicians should use urine drug testing before starting opioid therapy and consider urine drug testing at least annually to assess for prescribed medications as well as other controlled prescription drugs and illicit drugs.
11. Clinicians should avoid prescribing opioid pain medication and benzodiazepines concurrently whenever possible.
12. Clinicians should offer or arrange evidence-based treatment (usually medication-assisted treatment with buprenorphine or methadone in combination with behavioral therapies) for patients with opioid use disorder.

A. Decision Phase

The commitment to long-term opioid therapy is a serious one and should be considered as such by both patient and clinician. The need for careful review of the risks and benefits of long-term treatment is still a very necessary step even after a long-term opioid treatment phase has already been entered. The pain diagnosis must be clearly established and documented. Both clinician and patient must be satisfied that all other treatment options have been explored and have not provided adequate relief. The clinician must also be satisfied that the possible risks, particularly those of opioid use disorder or functional deterioration, do not outweigh the potential benefit of treatment. This is the single most challenging aspect of the decision phase, especially knowing that although there are established markers of risk (see Table 43.4), the presence of these markers do not necessarily mean that benefits will not outweigh risks with a carefully monitored treatment plan. The Opioid Risk Tool (ORT) and the Screener and Opioid Assessment for Patient with Pain-Revised (SOAPP-R) are two validated opioid risk assessment tools that can help clinicians classify patients into low, moderate, and high risk for opioid misuse. The clinician should carefully describe the potential complications and risks of long-term opioid therapy and allow the patient to express his or her concerns. The clinician will need to explain the clinic's monitoring policies and the rationale for monitoring. It is strongly recommended to have explicit documentation of the patient's understanding of the risks of long-term treatment and the clinic's policies for safety monitoring in the form of a signed written opioid agreement or consent.

It is recommended to clearly establish and document the goals of treatment for each patient prior to initiation of opioids. This understanding enables the clinician to effectively measure the success of treatment and to justify discontinuing the treatment if there is no progress toward meeting the goals. Goals differ from patient to patient. For example, the patient with severe disability may simply want to be able to sit at a table long enough to have a family meal, whereas the patient who was previously fully functioning may want to return to work. Whether pain reduction without other improvement is an acceptable goal is debatable, but in view of the complex and broad effects of opioids, it would generally seem wise

TABLE 43.4 Identifying Risk of Abuse or Treatment Failure

- History of substance abuse or addiction
- Family history of substance abuse or addiction
- History of depression or anxiety
- Personality disorder
- History of abuse, especially childhood abuse
- Young
- Not working
- On disability
- Litigation pending
- Dysfunctional
- Poor interpersonal relationships
- Difficult personality
- Refusing other treatments or denying their efficacy

not to continue to prescribe especially if pain reduction is accompanied by functional deterioration.

B. Titration Phase

The titration phase aims to find an effective dose as quickly and safely as possible, enabling the patient to be maintained on a stable dose with known analgesic efficacy. It is recommended that therapy starts at a low standard dose (see Appendix VII: Drug Appendix) and increases as tolerated to achieve acceptable analgesia. If satisfactory analgesia is not achieved, or if the adverse effects are intolerable, the treatment should be discontinued. In the monitored inpatient setting, the titration phase can be achieved within days, but this process takes longer to accomplish safely in the outpatient setting. It should ideally not, however, take longer than 8 weeks, and it may be necessary to see the patient more often than usual or to monitor progress by telephone during the titration phase. Clinicians may want to consider a plan to titrate within reason, and not to escalate to substantial doses without rationale and safe judgment. Consultation with a pain specialist may be helpful when doses exceed 90 mg/day or oral morphine milligram equivalent (MME).

C. Stable Phase

Ideally, the patient should be maintained at a stable dose, which in addition to improved function is often an indicator of successful treatment. Scheduled long-acting opioid preparations are often chosen when treating long-term continuous pain to provide more stable analgesia, cause less disruption of normal activities, and reduce the need for frequent short-acting opioids that may increase the risk of opioid use disorder. The issue of long- vs short-acting opioids is discussed more fully in the chapter addressing substance use disorder, and drug choice is described in the chapter on opioids. During the stable phase of treatment, it is mandatory by law to provide individual prescriptions that do not exceed 30 days, and it is advisable to conduct regular comprehensive follow-up assessments. A critical component of these assessments is an evaluation of progress toward goals initiated at the start of therapy, a review of any signs of aberrant opioid-taking behavior, and a determination of whether it is appropriate to reduce or begin the process of weaning opioid therapy.

1. Monthly Refills

In the United States, prescriptions for schedule II controlled substances may not exceed 30 days for an individual prescription. Legally, providers may provide three individual 30-day prescriptions for a total of a 90-day supply; however, predating of prescriptions is discouraged in any patient who has not demonstrated longitudinal safe use of opioids. It is easier to conduct follow-up evaluations if the patient picks up the prescriptions in person, unless he or she is unable to do so for physical reasons. This is an opportunity for the prescribing clinician to assess and document the patient's state of health, pain level, and side effects, to treat side effects if necessary, to monitor for aberrant behaviors, and to arrange for more comprehensive follow-up if there are deviations or other problems.

2. Comprehensive Follow-Up

Periodically, preferably every 3 months, but at least every year, the patient should undergo a comprehensive follow-up. An assessment should be made of pain, the effect of pain on the patient's well-being, the achievement of treatment goals, the level of function, presence of aberrant opioid-taking behavior, and quality of life. The use of standard questionnaires such as the SF-36 can help the clinician assess function and quality of life and is encouraged.

3. Toxicology Screening and Identifying Aberrant Behaviors

The patient's presence at monthly clinic visits provides an opportunity to observe aberrant behaviors. Extra visits, requests for interim prescriptions, and frequent telephone calls to the clinic are included in the signs of prescription drug abuse listed in Chapter 44, Table 1. All of these behaviors should be documented. The clinician's regular comprehensive assessments also provide an opportunity to identify problems. Toxicology screening can be a helpful adjunct to monitoring for problematic opioid use, including for addiction and diversion. Many experts believe that all patients with CNTP who are treated with opioids should undergo random urine screening. In support of this view, 43% patients with CNTP who were treated with opioids in one pain clinic were judged "problematic," and of these, 49% were identified using toxicology screening, not behavioral parameters. The issue of toxicology screening is covered more fully in Chapter 44, Section VII. Most states now have electronic prescription monitoring databases, and these should be checked regularly to assess for aberrant behavior.

D. Dose Escalation

Sometimes an increase in dose will be necessary, but careful consideration should be given before each dose escalation. Tolerance to the analgesic effects of opioids can develop over time, but the more common experience is that tolerance levels out and most patients can be maintained at stable dose. Therefore, if a patient requests an increase in dose, it should always alert the clinician to the possibility that there may be other reasons for such a request. There may be a change in the patient's pain or underlying disease, which should be evaluated and treated if necessary. The need for a higher dose may also be a manifestation of psychological need or opioid use disorder, which should also be identified and treated if necessary. At high doses, apparent tolerance may be a sign of OIH, which will be made worse by dose escalation. Nevertheless, it may be reasonable to try a controlled dose escalation in an attempt to alleviate the pain and improve the overall status of the patient. The aim of each dose escalation is to reach a new, stable dose. For severe or new pain, it may be helpful to admit the patient to the hospital to aid in diagnosis and rapid titration.

The use of very high doses of opioids for CNTP is rarely helpful. It is hard to say exactly what dose should be considered a high one, and the issue of whether there is a clinical ceiling for dose is highly debated. The traditional teaching is that opioid dose can be increased in a limitless fashion and that dose increases are capable of overcoming pain. However, clinical experience suggests otherwise, especially with long-term treatment. This observation, together with the basic science observation that there are multiple splice variants of endogenous opioid receptors resulting in much cross-sensitivity between various opioids, provides the rationale for the clinical practice of opioid rotation. A switch to a different opioid can provide equal or better analgesia at a reduced equivalent dose of the initial opioid. Opioid rotation is a reasonable way to both optimize analgesia and avoid rampant dose escalation in a patient with fading therapeutic effect to a given opioid (opioid rotation is described in more detail in Chapter 11).

Current CDC guidelines recommend a maximum dose of 90 mg MME/day. That is not to say that some patients do not do well on higher daily doses, but rather that clinical experience suggests that most patients do better if the daily dose is maintained below this level. Consideration should also be given to alternative routes of administration, which include transdermal patches or continuous intrathecal delivery systems. One should also consider that some liabilities, including neurotoxicity, hyperalgesia, hormonal and immune effects, and problematic behavior, predominate at high doses. As noted, pain consultation may be helpful in guiding the decision to titrate higher than 90 mg MME/day.

E. Criteria for Success and Failure

There are no standardized guidelines that define the point at which opioid therapy is or is not considered a success. Pain scores, perceived functional status, emotional well-being, and lack of side effects are metrics commonly used to assess the efficacy of therapy. The World Health Organization Quality of Life Scale and the Flanagan Quality of Life Scale are useful tools for obtaining objective assessment of perceived quality of life in patients with chronic illness or disease. Indices of failure can include a lack of improvement in function, maintenance of poor quality of life, deleterious side effects, and the presence of substance use disorder. Ultimately the clinician must weigh the risks and benefits of chronic opioid therapy in the context of the pre-established goals that were determined with the patient prior to initiation.

F. Discontinuation

If the treatment fails, the patient should be weaned off opioids. It is important to wean cautiously to avoid the unpleasantness of opioid withdrawal, an experience that can make it hard for the patient to give up the medication again in the future. Weaning can usually be accomplished by stepwise reductions of 20%-25% of the total daily dose, but the exact weaning schedule will depend on dose, drug, and duration of treatment. Many patients, especially those who are not doing well on opioids, report an improvement in well-being and sometimes pain after an opioid wean. If necessary, opioid treatment can be restarted after a washout period has reduced the presence of opioid tolerance and yields greater benefit than before. If there is clear evidence of diversion, the clinician should cease prescribing immediately. If there is evidence of opioid use disorder, discontinuation may not be the appropriate course of action, but referral for medication-assisted therapy (MAT) with methadone or buprenorphine in addition to intensive counseling will be needed. Opioid weaning is not always straightforward, and it may be helpful or even necessary to undergo weaning in a rehabilitation setting if the process becomes complicated.

V. CONCLUSION

The clinical attraction of opioid therapy is understandable. Opioids are powerful analgesics capable of alleviating most types of pain at an adequate dose, at least in the short term. But when used as a long-term pain treatment, the complexities of opioid therapy begin to appear. The effects of opioids are more than just analgesic. Their euphoric effects present a double-edged sword and are intimately involved in the development and maintenance of opioid use disorder and its tragic consequences. Toxicities include neuroendocrine effects, immune effects, and hyperalgesia. Moreover, the long-term efficacy of chronic opioid therapy is not clear. Given this, long-term opioid therapy in patients with chronic, nonterminal pain should be reserved for those who have exhausted nonopioid therapies and who are not high risk for misuse. It is not inhumane—in fact, it is good practice—to restrict long-term opioid use to those who cannot obtain relief by other means and to those who are at the least risk of opioid harm. The risks and benefits should be discussed in detail prior to initiation, and a structured prescribing relationship with close monitoring should be implemented. Continued evaluation for safe progress toward predetermined goals should guide the decision to continue chronic opioid therapy.

ACKNOWLEDGMENT

We would like to acknowledge with great admiration the previous author of this chapter: Jane C. Ballantyne.

Selected Readings

Ballantyne JC, Mao J. Opioids for chronic pain. *N Engl J Med.* 2003;349:1943-1953.

Franklin G. Opioids for chronic noncancer pain: a position paper of the American Academy of Neurology. *Neurology.* 2014;83:1277-1284.

Katz NP, Sherburne S, Beach M, et al. Behavioral monitoring and urine toxicology testing in patients receiving long-term opioid therapy. *Anesth Analg.* 2003;97:1097-1102.

Lee M, et al. A comprehensive review of opioid-induced hyperalgesia. *Pain Physician.* 2011;14:145-161.

Mao J. Opioid-induced abnormal pain sensitivity: implications in clinical opioid therapy. *Pain.* 2002;100:213-217.

Morbidity and Mortality Weekly Report. CDC Guidelines for Prescribing Opioids for Chronic Pain—United States, 2016. http://www.cdc.gov/drugoverdose/prescribing/providers.html. Updated August 9, 2016. Accessed August 13, 2016.

Pergolizzi J, Böger RH, Budd K, et al. Opioids and the management of chronic severe pain in the elderly: Consensus statement of an international expert panel with focus on the six clinically most often used World Health Organization step III opioids (buprenorphine, fentanyl, hydromorphone, methadone, morphine, oxycodone). *Pain Pract.* 2008;8:287-313.

Trescot A, Helm S, Hansen H, et al. Opioids in the management of chronic noncancer pain: an update of American Society of the Interventional Pain Physicians' (ASIPP) guidelines. *Pain Physician.* 2008;11:S5-S62.

Zedler B, Xie L, Wang L, et al. Development of a risk index for serious prescription opioid-induced respiratory depression or overdose in Veterans' Health Administration patients. *Pain Med.* 2015;16:1566-1579.

44 Identifying and Mitigating the Risks of Long-Term Opioid Treatment

Chantal Berna, Ronald J. Kulich,
and Karsten Kueppenbender

Opioid prescribing and sales soared in the past 20 years in the United States of America, leading to a well known epidemic, and a large scale public health crisis. Given only limited, low-quality evidence for the benefits of long-term opioid treatment (LOT) for patients with chronic noncancer pain (CNCP) and documented risks of serious harm (Roger Chou et al., 2014), such treatments are increasingly questioned and regulated. Therefore, chronic opioid prescribing in general, and especially for patients with CNCP requires (1) a careful risk-benefit evaluation prior to initiation and (2) specific monitoring and reevaluation over the course of treatment.

I. WEIGHING BENEFITS AND RISKS

Components of the initial assessment involve a detailed diagnostic interview including medical and psychiatric history, review of prior medical records to assess past history of adherence or aberrancies, communication with current or recent other treating providers, prescription monitoring program checks, and urine toxicology. Including a family member may allow to assess levels of support and prior adherence to treatment.

A. Benefits

Anticipated benefits of opioid therapy should be clearly delineated before starting treatment and formulated in measurable functional outcomes. These allow for more objective tracking of the treatment response, compared to reliance on subjective pain scores alone. In fact, an isolated decrease by 1-2 points out of 10-point VAS (ie, the effect size demonstrated by short-term studies of opioids) is an unreliable indicator of patient well-being in the absence of functional improvement. It is important to note that functional impairment in chronic pain is determined by many psychosocial factors. Evidence for chronic opioids improving function or work performance is lacking (Dowell, Haegerich, & Chou, 2016). To the contrary, some investigations demonstrate a correlation between opioid dose and lack of function (Turner, Shortreed, Saunders, LeResche, & Von Korff, 2016). Yet, multidisciplinary functional restoration programs, which often include opioid tapering, may lead to increased function and in some cases are even associated with reduced pain scores (see review in Berna, Kulich, & Rathmell, 2015). Finally, expected benefits must be measured according to the literature. For example, certain conditions, such as fibromyalgia or headaches, lack data to support the use of chronic opioid therapy (Dowell et al., 2016).

B. Risks

Adverse course of treatment in the form of side effects and complications are summarized in Table 44.1. Patients on LOT need to be assessed for these regularly. Even before initiating LOT, risk factors for opioid-related harm should be evaluated (Dowell et al., 2016), as described below in Tables 44.2 and 44.3. Patients introduced to LOT despite a heightened risk for an adverse course might benefit from support by mental health specialists, and from more frequent monitoring.

C. Individual Risk Assessment

The concept of opioid "risk stratification" has been wrongly simplified to classify the patient into "low," "medium," or "high" risk of opioid use disorder (OUD).

The evaluation of the incidence of OUD in patients with chronic pain varies widely, partly due to methodological differences. Misuse of opioid pain medication occurs in approximately 1 of 5 patients and may have different causes, ranging from misguided attempts at self-medicating, persistent physical pain to emotional distress (Vowles et al., 2015). About 1 out of 10 patients on LOT develop OUD (Vowles et al., 2015). Of note, patients with OUD under long term methadone maintenance treatment experience pain at higher rates than the regular population, with multiple possible contributing factors (Eyler, 2013). Opioid-induced hyperalgesia may exacerbate pain. In addition, patients chronically treated with opioids in several studies exhibited increased fear of pain. Catastrophizing might contribute to a vicious cycle, in which pain and fear exacerbate each other,

TABLE 44.1 Side Effects and Adverse Events of Opioid Therapy

- Overdose and suicide[a] (Ilgen et al., 2016)
- Opioid use disorder[a] (Volkow & McLellan, 2016)
- Depression (Scherrer, Salas, Lustman, Burge, & Schneider, 2015)
- Constipation, serious fecal impaction
- Dry mouth and tooth decay
- Nausea, lack of appetite
- Sweating, itching
- Hormonal changes, which can lead to sexual dysfunction or osteopenia
- Fractures[a] (Saunders et al., 2010)
- Sedation, decreased concentration, impaired memory, drowsiness, dizziness
- Headaches
- Sleep-disordered breathing
- Risks for the fetus during pregnancy
- Reduced activity
- Opioid-induced hyperalgesia
- Tolerance
- Chemical coping: overreliance on opioids, discounting other sources of partial relief, use of opioids to self-medicate depression, anxiety, sleeplessness, or other symptoms

[a]risk shown to be dose dependent.

TABLE 44.2 Definitions

Physical Dependence: drug class–specific physiological adaptation resulting in withdrawal symptoms in case of abrupt cessation, dose decrease, or exposure to an antagonist
Tolerance: need for increased doses for similar subjective analgesic effects over the course of treatment
Opioid use disorder (OUD) (DSM-5): presence of any two or more of a cluster of nine signs and symptoms, indicative of craving for the medication, loss of control, and compulsive use despite harmful medical, psychological, or social consequences. This disorder is often informally referred to as "Addiction."

leading to more tension and focus on the pain, magnifying pain responses. This fear is compounded by potentially inadequate treatment, since not all clinicians appreciate that patients on methadone maintenance treatment typically require higher dosing of opioid pain medication to achieve an analgesic effect, and that methadone needs to be taken every 6-8 hours to treat pain (rather than the daily dosing, which suffices for maintenance treatment of OUD).

Nevertheless, patients with OUD benefit from less medical treatment for pain. This appears to be a consequence of clinician attitudes, insufficient knowledge, and regulatory burden, as well as reluctance of some patients with OUD to report pain, for fear of being labeled medication seeking. The

TABLE 44.3 Risk Factors for an Adverse Course (see Table 44.1) or Lack of Benefit with Long-Term Opioid Therapy[a]

- Prior or current substance use disorder with any substance, including alcohol, cannabis, and tobacco (self-reported, in medical history or indicated by relevant medical complications such as liver cirrhosis or history of overdose)
- Unclear or inconsistent medical diagnosis for pain
- Psychiatric comorbidity such as depression, anxiety, or posttraumatic stress disorder (PTSD)
- Sleep-disordered breathing
- Co-medication with benzodiazepines or other sedating drugs
- Renal or hepatic disease (risk of drug accumulation)
- Pregnancy
- Family history of substance use disorder or disability
- Chronic disability or work-related injury
- History of criminal behavior, eg, arrests linked to drugs, driving under the influence of substances, etc
- Refusal of nonopioid treatments
- High morphine dose equivalent, above 50 or 80 mg
- High levels of pain or disability despite opioid therapy
- Unrealistic expectation and goals for opioid therapy
- Trust issues: refusal to permit communication with other providers, refusal to supply medical records, or regularly missing appointments
- Inconsistent urine toxicology or prescription monitoring program

[a]*Note: No single risk factor is intended to predict an adverse course.*

complexities of prescribing opioids for pain in this population, including the higher required doses, implies the need for more frequent follow up visits with the clinician who treats the pain, a collaboration with addiction specialists, as well as specific overdose prevention with the patient and family members (Eyler, 2013). This unfortunately, compounds the stigma these patients encounter. Methadone clinics are typically not set up to dose more often than once daily. Yet, collaboration with a medical team and integrated electronic medical records are hindered by the administrative burden imposed by the current interpretation of the strict federal confidentiality law (42 CFR Part 2), which regulates methadone clinics and other addiction treatment facilities in the United States. A proposed revision of the interpretation of 42 CFR Part 2 promises fewer barriers to the sharing of clinical information between addiction and medical treatment professionals and settings (SAMHSA, 2016).

As summarized in Table 44.1, a problematic treatment course is seen here in a larger sense than OUD. Risk factors for an adverse course of LOT have been identified (Table 44.3) (Webster & Webster, 2005). No single factor should be assumed to be definitively predictive with any patient. Risk factors must be considered in the context of a thorough clinical assessment through review of multiple source of information. Multiple risk factors may suggest greater risk, although studies that classify the patient with respect to level of risk and relative contribution of each factor are lacking. Finally, it is important to consider that these risk factors are also predictors of poor outcome for many other psychosocial outcomes beyond opioid therapy. State-administered Prescription Monitoring Programs (PMP) are databases that reference controlled substances dispensed to patients. Checking them prior to prescribing an opioid is good clinical practice, and in some states required by law.

Standardized screening questionnaires such as the SOAPP-R, COMM, ORT, and PainCAS are useful, although specific cutoff scores should never replace clinical judgment (R. Chou et al., 2009). New computer-based applications have substantially reduced patient and clinician burden with respect to administration and scoring (Finkelman et al., 2015).

Within the context of LOT, definitions of "aberrant behavior" vary widely, and the underlying reasons for the behaviors always require exploration with the patient. Patient nonadherence with medical recommendations is common, with some studies showing that adherence rates may be 50% in the best of circumstances (McDonald, Garg, & Haynes, 2002). In part because of the potential risks, we place higher expectations on patients who use opioids. While substance use disorders or criminal behaviors such as diversion play a role in a significant minority of patients, other psychiatric comorbidities, cultural or language barriers, and cognitive or intellectual functioning factors can also be involved. Finally, disclosure of sensitive subject matters can be refused for many reasons, including impact on child custody, work status, or disability compensation.

II. RISK MITIGATION DURING LOT

Once it is established that the risk-benefit ratio for an individual patient is rather favorable, an opioid treatment agreement between clinician and patient should be signed, as a form of informed consent, before the first prescription (link to MGH contract, Appendix). It should specify obligations of the patient and clinician, and determine conditions that result in termination of opioid therapy. Once LOT is initiated, risk mitigation strategies should be applied.

A. Monitoring

Benefits of therapy, signs of an adverse course of treatment, and side effects need to be reevaluated periodically. This involves checking of the PMP, urinary or mouth swab toxicology screening, and possibly pill counts routinely in the course of treatment (R. Chou et al., 2009). Close monitoring of the patient in addition to reports from family members can help identify aberrant drug-related behavior, which requires evaluation to identify underlying causes and referral to specialized psychological or somatic treatment, as indicated.

Toxicology results negative for the prescribed opioid may indicate drug diversion, or nonadherence with the prescribed regimen (eg, cyclical intake of higher than prescribed doses, followed by withdrawal). Unexpected results may call for collaboration with a toxicologist to ascertain correct interpretation of the data and verification with more sensitive testing to assess for the possibility of false positive or negatives. Any incongruence with treatment requires a follow-up discussion with the patient, possibly leading to a change of the therapeutic plan, for example, referral to an addiction specialist. Irregular toxicology screen results may be part of a pattern of nonadherence, but may not be sufficient cause in themselves for termination in isolation.

B. Overdose Prevention

Specific factors associated with increased risk of overdoses include concurrent use of benzodiazepines, prescribed opioid doses >50 mg of morphine equivalents per day, sleep-disordered breathing, pregnancy, older age, concurrent mental illness, or a history of substance use disorders (Dowell et al., 2016). Formal overdose-risk screening questionnaires are now available (Zedler et al., 2015). Some of these factors can be eliminated or reduced, while others may be mitigated by more frequent monitoring. Finally, intranasal or intramuscular naloxone can be prescribed as a secondary prevention of overdose. However, its correct use requires education of the patient and family, which can be assisted by instructional videos available on the Internet (Multnomah County, 2016).

C. Managing a Difficult Course of Treatment

In case of nonadherence with the opioid agreement, more frequent visits (shorter prescriptions), pill counts, and toxicology screens can be proposed. Using opioids to treat other symptoms than pain is called chemical coping. If chemical coping is identified, more specific symptomatic treatments need to be offered, possibly in combination with a sleep or mental health specialist.

Psychological support or specific adherence-focused interventions combining education, motivational interviewing, and regular toxicology screens can help improve adherence (Jamison et al., 2010). If a suspicion of OUD rises, collaboration with a substance use disorder specialist is indicated. Continued opioid prescriptions may be made contingent on engagement in concurrent addiction treatment. The partial opioid receptor agonist buprenorphine, which is FDA approved for the treatment of OUD, carries a lower risk of fatal overdoses than do full opioid receptor agonists. There is preliminary evidence for its use to treat patients with chronic pain and OUD: studies have shown equal (Neumann et al., 2013) or, contrary to expectation, superior reduction of pain scores with buprenorphine compared to full opioid receptor agonists (Pade, Cardon, Hoffman, & Geppert, 2012; Roux et al., 2013). Finally, nonopioid pain management options should be optimized at all times (Volkow & McLellan, 2016).

D. Discontinuation of LOT

Given the frequent adverse benefit-risk ratio of LOT for CNCP, the option to decrease doses or to taper fully needs to remain on all prescribers' minds. While specific taper protocols are mostly empirical, a key to success is patient and clinician motivation (Berna et al., 2015). Hence, unless there is imminent danger to self/others or criminal behavior involved, tapers can usually be managed in the outpatient setting, and stretch over the course of months. This allows the patient to develop new coping mechanisms and limits the occurrence of withdrawal symptoms. During a progressive schedule, fluctuations in pain can be used as practice to manage pain exacerbations with less or without reliance on opioids. A pragmatic approach is to taper by 10%-20% of the original dose every 1-4 weeks, depending on the dose and duration of treatment (the higher the dose and the longer the course of treatment, the slower the taper). Withdrawal symptoms (including anxiety, hypertension, tachycardia, restlessness, mydriasis, diaphoresis, tremor, piloerection, nausea, abdominal cramps, diarrhea, anorexia, dizziness, hot flashes, shivering, myalgias or arthralgias, rhinorrhea, sneezing, lacrimation, insomnia, yawning, and dysphoria) can be managed by slowing down the taper or prescribing oral alpha-adrenergic agents such as tizanidine, (2-8 mg up to three times per day), or clonidine (0.2-0.4 mg per day). As anxiety and expectations play an important role in withdrawal symptoms, reassurance, a structured tapering protocol, and stress management techniques can also be helpful (Berna et al., 2015). Further, it should be emphasized that tapering is by itself a potentially effective treatment intervention, as many patients may report improved function, less pain, and reduced negative consequences from LOT.

III. CONCLUSION

The devastating effects of widespread opioid prescribing for CNCP have led to serious reconsiderations and progressive shifts in clinical practice. In addition to subjective pain reports, objective functional outcomes are receiving greater recognition. Physicians who optimize nonopioid therapies, perform baseline and follow-up risk-benefit assessments, use written opioid treatment agreements with their patients, and monitor toxicology screens as well as prescription databases routinely, are likely to prescribe less frequently and lower doses of opioids. Through this safer practice, they are likely to avoid the worst-case scenarios of LOT in CNCP.

Selected Readings

APS & AAPM. *Guideline for the Use of Chronic Opioid Therapy in Chronic Noncancer Pain: Evidence Review.* http://americanpainsociety.org/uploads/education/guidelines/chronic-opioid-therapy-cncp.pdf

Berna C, Kulich RJ, Rathmell JP. Tapering long-term opioid therapy in chronic noncancer pain: evidence and recommendations for everyday practice. *Mayo Clin Proc.* 2015;90(6), 828-842. doi: 10.1016/j.mayocp.2015.04.003.

Chou R, Deyo R, Devine B, et al. *The Effectiveness and Risks of Long-term Opioid Treatment of Chronic Pain.* Rockville, MD: Prepared by the Pacific Northwest Evidence-based Practice Center under Contract No. 290-2012-00014-I; 2014. www.effectivehealthcare.ahrq.gov/reports/final.cfm

Chou R, Fanciullo GJ, Fine PG, et al. Clinical guidelines for the use of chronic opioid therapy in chronic noncancer pain. *J Pain.* 2009;10(2):113-130.e122.

Dowell D, Haegerich TM, Chou R. CDC guideline for prescribing opioids for chronic pain--United States, 2016. *JAMA.* 2016;315(15):1624-1645. doi: 10.1001/jama.2016.1464.

Eyler EC. Chronic and acute pain and pain management for patients in methadone maintenance treatment. *Am J Addict.* 2013;22(1):75-83. doi: 10.1111/j.1521-0391.2013.00308.x.

FAIRHealth. *The Opioid Crisis Among the Privately Insured. The Opioid Abuse Epidemic as Documented by Private Claims Data.* 2016. http://www.fairhealth.org/servlet/servlet.FileDownload?file=01532000001nwD2

Finkelman MD, Kulich RJ, Zacharoff KL, et al. Shortening the Screener and Opioid Assessment for Patients with Pain-Revised (SOAPP-R): a proof-of-principle study for customized computer-based testing. *Pain Med.* 2015;16(12):2344-2356. doi: 10.1111/pme.12864.

Ilgen MA, Bohnert ASB, Ganoczy D, Bair MJ, McCarthy JF, Blow FC. Opioid dose and risk of suicide. *Pain.* 2016;157(5):1079-1084. doi: 10.1097/j.pain.0000000000000484.

Jamison RN, Ross EL, Michna E, Chen LQ, Holcomb C, Wasan AD. Substance misuse treatment for high-risk chronic pain patients on opioid therapy: a randomized trial. *Pain.* 2010;150(3):390-400. doi: 10.1016/j.pain.2010.02.033.

Kolodny A, Courtwright DT, Hwang CS, et al. The prescription opioid and heroin crisis: a public health approach to an epidemic of addiction. *Annu Rev Public Health.* 2015;36:559-574. doi: 10.1146/annurev-publhealth-031914-122957.

McDonald HP, Garg AX, Haynes RB. Interventions to enhance patient adherence to medication prescriptions: scientific review. *JAMA.* 2002;*288*(22):2868-2879.

Neumann AM, Blondell RD, Jaanimagi U, et al. A preliminary study comparing methadone and buprenorphine in patients with chronic pain and coexistent opioid addiction. *J Addict Dis.* 2013;32(1):68-78. doi: 10.1080/10550887.2012.759872.

Pade PA, Cardon KE, Hoffman RM, Geppert CM. Prescription opioid abuse, chronic pain, and primary care: a co-occurring disorders clinic in the chronic disease model. *J Subst Abuse Treat.* 2012;43(4):446-450. doi: 10.1016/j.jsat.2012.08.010.

Roux P, Sullivan MA, Cohen J, et al. Buprenorphine/naloxone as a promising therapeutic option for opioid abusing patients with chronic pain: reduction of pain, opioid withdrawal symptoms, and abuse liability of oral oxycodone. *Pain.* 2013;154(8):1442-1448. doi: 10.1016/j.pain.2013.05.004.

Saunders KW, Dunn KM, Merrill JO, et al. Relationship of opioid use and dosage levels to fractures in older chronic pain patients. *J Gen Intern Med.* 2010;25(4):310-315. doi: 10.1007/s11606-009-1218-z.

Scherrer JF, Salas J, Lustman PJ, Burge S, Schneider FD. Change in opioid dose and change in depression in a longitudinal primary care patient cohort. *Pain.* 2015;156(2):348-355. doi: 10.1097/01.j.pain.0000460316.58110.a0.

Turner JA, Shortreed SM, Saunders KW, LeResche L, Von Korff M. Association of levels of opioid use with pain and activity interference among patients initiating chronic opioid therapy: a longitudinal study. *Pain.* 2016;157(4):849-857. doi: 10.1097/j.pain.0000000000000452.

Volkow ND, McLellan AT. Opioid abuse in chronic pain--misconceptions and mitigation strategies. *N Engl J Med.* 2016;374(13):1253-1263. doi: 10.1056/NEJMra1507771.

Vowles KE, McEntee ML, Julnes PS, Frohe T, Ney JP, van der Goes DN. Rates of opioid misuse, abuse, and addiction in chronic pain: a systematic review and data synthesis. *Pain.* 2015;156(4):569-576. doi: 10.1097/01.j.pain.0000460357.01998.f1.

Webster LR, Webster RM. Predicting aberrant behaviors in opioid-treated patients: preliminary validation of the opioid risk tool. *Pain Med.* 2005;6(6):432-442. doi: 10.1111/j.1526-4637.2005.00072.x.

Zedler B, Xie L, Wang L, et al. Development of a risk index for serious prescription opioid-induced respiratory depression or overdose in Veterans' Health Administration patients. *Pain Med.* 2015;16(8):1566-1579. doi: 10.1111/pme.12777.

45

Geriatric Pain Management

Erin Stevens, Erin Scott, and
Mihir M. Kamdar

I. GERIATRIC OVERVIEW

A. Demographics and Prevalence

The world's population is rapidly aging, as adults 65 and older account for the fastest growing demographic age group. It is estimated that the population of people over 65 will double between 2010 and 2050 to nearly 90 million people in the United States. Pain is prevalent in the older adult but often unrecognized and underreported. The American Geriatric Society (AGS) Panel on Persistent Pain in Older Adults estimates that one in five older adults has pain. Studies show that 25%-50% of community-dwelling older adults and 45%-80% of nursing home residents have substantial pain. Complicating the diagnosis and management of pain in this population is the high prevalence of dementia, sensory impairment, and disability. Hence, it is imperative that clinicians gain expertise in the nuances of managing pain in geriatric populations.

B. Pharmacokinetics and Pharmacodynamics Considerations

It is very important to understand the physiologic changes that occur with normal aging that affect drug pharmacokinetics and pharmacodynamics. These age-related changes are summarized in Table 45.1.

C. Changes in Pain Processing and Perception With Aging

There are several significant neurophysiologic changes that occur with normal aging, which influence the experience of pain in the geriatric population. There is a decrease in the density of myelinated and number of unmyelinated peripheral fibers as well as an increase in damage of sensory fibers, resulting in a decrease in conduction velocity. There have also been impairments documented in peripheral Aδ fibers associated with decreased EEG amplitude and increased latency to acutely painful stimuli. Interestingly, these changes are not seen with C fibers.

TABLE 45.1 Pharmacologic Changes With Aging

Physiologic Component	Age-Related Changes	Clinical Consequences	Clinical Considerations
Pharmacokinetics			
Gastrointestinal Absorption	• Minimal change	• Gastric motility and blood flow affect bowel transit time	• Slow transit time may prolong effect of continuous release enteral drugs • More susceptible to drug-induced constipation
Distribution	• Reduced lean body mass • Increased body fat • Decreased serum binding proteins	• Increased volume of distribution and half-life with fat-soluble drugs • Increased unbound and active drug	• Consider obesity, fluid balance, and albumin with dose adjustments • Monitor free drug levels
Hepatic Metabolism	• Reduced liver mass • Reduced hepatic blood flow • Reduced cytochrome p450 activity	• Phase I metabolism (active metabolites) reduced • Phase II metabolism preferred	• Reduced drug metabolism and greater side effect risk • Caution with dosing • Monitor for drug-drug interactions
Elimination	• Reduced renal blood flow and mass • Reduction in functioning nephron • Decreased renal tubular secretion • Decline lean muscle mass	• Decreased elimination, increased half-life • Decreased glomerular filtration rate • Serum creatinine not an accurate reflection of creatinine clearance	• Estimated GFR may overestimate renal function • Cockcroft-Gault equation useful as initial estimate • Avoid drugs dependent on renal clearance • Monitor serum or plasma concentrations

(Continued)

TABLE 45.1 Pharmacologic Changes With Aging (*Continued*)

Physiologic Component	Age-Related Changes	Clinical Consequences	Clinical Considerations
Pharmacodynamics			
Baroreceptor Reflex	• Decreased response	• Postural and/or postprandial hypotension	• Caution with drugs that have orthostatic side effects
Respiratory Center	• Decreased sensitivity to hypoxia and hypercapnia	• Delayed/diminished ventilator response	• Caution with drugs that may cause sedation or respiratory depression
CNS	• More susceptible to CNS drug penetration • Decrease in μ-opioid receptors, binding affinity unchanged • Decreased endogenous opioids in dorsal horn	• Increased susceptibility and exaggerated response to drug interaction in peripheral and central nervous system • Decreased response to exogenous opioids	• Caution with medications that have CNS side effects

Clinically, this may result in a decreased ability to perceive acute pain, though elderly patients can still experience similar levels of chronic pain compared to the general population. Studies show that pain thresholds increase with nonnoxious stimuli, decrease with pressure, and do not change with heat. Though there are no definitive trials to validate this, clinically this implies that an older adult may require a higher stimulus before perceiving pain. Furthermore, loss of neurons at the dorsal horn has been documented with age, in addition to neural death and gliosis affecting the descending inhibitory tracts. These changes may result in decreases both in modulatory neurochemicals and in physiologic adaptation to painful stimuli with age. This suggests that older adults may be less tolerant of pain once it begins and experience pain for longer periods of time after tissue injury.

D. Consequences of Untreated Pain in the Older Adult

Persistent or inadequate treatment of pain in older adults has been associated with numerous adverse outcomes. Decreased activity from pain leads to negative cardiopulmonary effects, deconditioning, and gait disturbances. These changes impair rehabilitation and predispose to falls. Decline in function contributes to the well-established relationship between depression and pain in this population, as well as loneliness and social isolation. Older adults with pain are twice as likely to have sleep disturbances than those without pain. Pain can contribute to impairments in attention and cognition and can cause delirium. In those patients with existing cognitive impairment, pain is a common yet underrecognized cause of behavioral disturbances. Undertreated pain can be distressing for family and caregivers as well. The consequences of pain in the geriatric population result in greater health care utilization, increased cost, and an overall decrease in quality of life for patients and their families.

E. American Geriatric Society Position on Pain Management

The AGS Panel on Persistent Pain in Older Persons is a central resource on pain management in the elderly population. The recommendations in this chapter are largely based on the AGS's most recent updates on pain management in addition to clinical suggestions from the authors.

II. PAIN ASSESSMENT

A. General Overview

Pain assessment in the older adult can be challenging due to numerous factors. Compared to the younger population, older adults are more likely to present with dementia, delirium, confusion, fatigue, withdrawal, and/or depression. In addition, older adults may use language such as a "discomfort" or "not feeling well" to verbalize pain, which may be missed by medical professionals. There may also be a reluctance to report pain for fear of being a burden or due to the common misperception that pain is a normal consequence of aging. Another common reason for pain to be underreported in older adults is fear that pain may be a sign of a more serious illness. Some patients worry that reporting pain may result in undesirable hospitalizations, invasive testing, and even loss of independence. They may also be hesitant to take analgesics due to misconceptions that opioid medications are reserved for terminal pain or because of fear of becoming addicted or dependent. Others may worry that taking opioid medications now will render them less effective in the future when pain becomes more severe.

Similar to a generalized pain assessment, gathering a detailed description of the pain in the context of the patient's medical and psychosocial history is essential in diagnosing and effectively managing geriatric pain. An especially important part of the assessment of the older adult is understanding the functional and social impacts of their pain.

B. Addressing Misconceptions

A common misconception is that pain is a normal consequence of aging. While there is evidence of altered neural transmission that occurs with aging, it remains unclear how this may potentially affect an individual's experience of pain. Some older adults also falsely believe that enduring pain will lead to an increased tolerance. In general, the opposite has been found to be true, as poorly controlled pain often leads to functional decline. Some patients report that opioids are viewed as a sign of "weakness" by those around them. Lastly, the belief that treatment with opioids will definitively result in addiction in the elderly is false. This stereotype may be shared by patients, caregivers, and even clinicians. While the risk is not zero, older age is associated with lower risk of addiction.

C. Functional Pain Assessment

An assessment of how a patient is functioning in their normal everyday life can often fully reveal the impact of their pain. Ideally, clinicians would start with an assessment of functional activities using the Katz Activities of Daily Living (ADL) scale and the Lawton Instrumental Activities of Daily Living (IADL) scale. To achieve a greater understanding of how pain may be affecting function, it is important to discuss an individual's hobbies, ability to exercise and socialize, and elicit any changes that have occurred since the pain began. Validated scales that can assist in gathering this type of functional data include the West Haven-Yale Multidimensional Pain Inventory and the Pain Disability Index.

D. Pain Assessment in Dementia

The sensory aspects of pain remain largely intact in individuals with Alzheimer dementia as its typical neuropathology does not affect the somatosensory cortex. However, portions of the medial pain system (ie, the anterior cingulate gyrus and hippocampus) that are involved in an affective pain response can be severely affected by Alzheimer disease. This results in a diminished ability to interpret sensations as painful and, as a result, an underreporting of pain. Individuals with dementia, especially in the more advanced stages, may not be able to communicate when they are experiencing pain. They may instead show behavioral signs, such as moaning, irritability, increased agitation or confusion, and/or withdrawal from their normal social behaviors. In general, they likely will be unable to report memories of pain. Instead a thorough physical exam, assessing for pain with certain movements (active and passive), can be helpful in assessing for pain in patients with advanced dementia.

Self-report of pain remains the gold standard, and a pain assessment can and should be attempted at any stage of dementia. Short, directed questions with "yes/no" answer choices are the best approach, especially in more advanced dementia. Sometimes rewording questions may result in a different response for the patient and uncover pain. For example, a patient may deny "pain" but then endorse feeling "uncomfortable" or "sore" or having areas that "hurt." A pain scale that can be useful in advanced dementias is the Pain Assessment in Advanced Dementia (PAINAD) scale. The PAINAD scale assesses five different behaviors: breathing, negative vocalization, facial expression, body language, and the ability to be consoled.

Family- and caregiver-provided histories are key in obtaining a thorough and complete pain history, especially in the later stage of dementia. Caregivers can help clinicians understand what a behavior may mean based on past experiences. Caregivers are also likely to notice subtle changes in personality or behaviors that may signal pain, as well as help monitor for response to treatment.

E. Pain Assessment in Delirium

Pain in delirium can be particularly hard to assess, given the fluctuating level of cognitive impairment and behavioral disturbances that may be present. A standardized, consistent approach that can be conducted through the entirety of a patient's hospitalization is important. The Hierarchy of Pain Assessment Techniques is a stepwise guide to help providers evaluate pain in this population. The first suggestion is to try to elicit a self-report of pain from the patient. Second, identify any conditions or procedures that may be causing pain. Next, use a behavioral assessment scale, like the PAINAD scale discussed above. Use the same scale consistently with the patient throughout their admission. Involve family members in any discussions regarding changes in a patient's behaviors that may indicate pain. Finally, attempt a short-term empiric trial with an analgesic medication and assess response. Utilizing this systematic technique can help providers better assess and treat pain in the delirious, elderly patient.

III. PAIN THERAPEUTICS

A. General Overview

Pain management in the older adult should begin with identifying and treating reversible causes of pain. When treating pain, nonpharmacologic strategies should be optimized, and careful consideration should be given to the risks and benefits of analgesic therapies. Medications should be administered initially with the lowest possible dose and increased slowly based on response and side effects. Some pharmacologic agents have a delayed onset of action, and therapeutic benefits may be slow to develop. Adequate therapeutic trials should be conducted before discontinuing a seemingly ineffective treatment. While the use of multiple medications increases the risk of drug-drug and drug-disease interactions, one should be aware of the concept of "rational polypharmacy." Rational polypharmacy occurs when a combination of two or more drugs with complementary mechanisms works synergistically to yield better pain control and less toxicity than increasing doses of a single agent.

Any clinician prescribing medications to geriatric patients should be aware of the American Geriatric Society's Beers List for Potentially Inappropriate Medication Use in Older Adults. This guide was originally created in 1991 and most recently updated in 2015. The guide categorizes potentially inappropriate medications into the following groups: (1) medications to avoid in older adults regardless of disease or conditions, (2) medications considered potentially inappropriate when used in older adults with certain disease or syndromes, (3) medications that should be used with caution, (4) medications that should be dose adjusted based on renal function, and (5) medications that should be avoided due to drug-drug interactions. Each Beer's List medication recommendation is graded based on the level of evidence and strength of recommendations.

B. Pharmacotherapy

1. Nonopioids

Nonopioid therapy is appropriate for initial management of mild to moderate pain and/or as adjuvants in combination with opioid therapy. These agents must be carefully selected in the older adult given the prevalence of multiple comorbidities including renal, liver, and cardiac disease, as well as the risk for drug-drug interactions. Because of these complexities, the AGS has recommended earlier use of opioid therapy than what is typical for treatment of the younger population. Table 45.2 shows guidelines for nonopioid, adjuvant, and topical agents based on the AGS 2009 recommendations.

TABLE 45.2 Nonopioid Considerations in Geriatric Patients

Acetaminophen	• Absolute contraindications: liver failure • Relative contraindications and cautions: hepatic insufficiency, chronic alcohol abuse or dependence • Maximum daily recommended dose should not exceed 4 g/24 h
NSAIDs	• May be considered rarely, and with extreme caution, in highly selected individuals • Absolute contraindications: current active peptic ulcer disease, chronic kidney disease, heart failure • Relative contraindications and cautions: hypertension, history of peptic ulcer disease, concomitant use of corticosteroids or selective serotonin reuptake inhibitors • Older persons taking nonselective NSAIDs should use a proton pump inhibitor or misoprostol for gastrointestinal protection • Patients taking a COX-2 selective inhibitor with aspirin should use a proton pump inhibitor or misoprostol for gastrointestinal protection • Patients should not take more than one nonselective NSAID or COX-2 selective inhibitor for pain control • Patients taking aspirin for cardioprophylaxis should not use ibuprofen • Patients taking nonselective NSAIDs and COX-2 selective inhibitors should be routinely assessed for GI and renal toxicity, hypertension, heart failure, and other drug-drug and drug-disease interactions
Steroids	• Long-term systemic corticosteroids should be reserved for patients with pain-associated inflammatory disorders or metastatic bone pain • Increased risk of peptic ulcer disease and gastrointestinal bleeding when used in combination with NSAIDs or COX-2 selective inhibitors • Avoid in older adults with or at high risk for delirium
Tramadol	• Lowers seizure threshold; may be acceptable in individuals with well-controlled seizures in whom alternative agents have not been effective • Maximum daily dose should not exceed 300 mg/24 h • Maximum daily dose should not exceed 200 mg/24 h in ESRD • Avoid extended dose formulation in ESRD • Extended dose formulation should be titrated in 50-mg increments and no more frequently than every 3 d

TABLE 45.2 Nonopioid Considerations in Geriatric Patients (*Continued*)

Antidepressants	**Tricyclic antidepressants** • Should be avoided because of higher risk for adverse effects such as anticholinergic effects and cognitive impairment **Selective norepinephrine reuptake inhibitors** • **Duloxetine** ◦ Monitor blood pressure and cognition and for dizziness ◦ Has multiple drug-drug interactions • **Venlafaxine** ◦ Can have dose-associated increases in blood pressure and heart rates
Antiepileptics	**Gabapentin** • Monitor for sedation, ataxia, and edema • Titrate no more frequently than 100 mg every 3 d • Monitor for suicidality (FDA antiepileptic drug class warning) **Pregabalin** • Monitor for sedation, ataxia, and edema • Monitor for suicidality (FDA antiepileptic drug class warning)
Muscle Relaxants	**Cyclobenzaprine** • Should be avoided because of higher risk for adverse effects such as anticholinergic effects and cognitive impairment **Baclofen** • Starting low with gradual titration may minimize common side effects of dizziness, somnolence, and gastrointestinal symptoms • Tapering required after prolonged use to prevent delirium and seizure
Topical Lidocaine	• Minimal side effects, best for superficial pain such as postherpetic neuralgia
Topical NSAIDs	• Risk of GI complications but less frequent than with oral NSAIDs • Use with caution in patients with prior side effects with oral NSAIDs • Safe and effective for short-term use (<4 wk) in select populations
Capsaicin	• Repeated application needed before clinical effect may be apparent • Compliance issues due to burning at application site • Preadministration of lidocaine cream or coadministration of glyceryl trinitrate can reduce burning and enhance the analgesic effect

2. Opioids

Opioid therapy is appropriate analgesia for older adults with moderate to severe pain, functional impairment, or diminished quality of life because of pain or those patients at risk for gastrointestinal or cardiovascular adverse events with NSAIDs. For persistent, noncancer pain, opioid therapy must be balanced against potential adverse effects and the harm from unrelieved pain. Older adults have increased sensitivity to opioids due to normal effects of aging on the hepatic and renal system, as well as age-related brain atrophy resulting in decreased opioid receptors. Hence, monitoring and harm mitigation strategies should be employed when prescribing opioids in this population. Educating patients and families prior to initiating opioid therapy is essential to address barriers to successful pain treatment. Table 45.3 lists recommendations for starting opioid therapy based on the most recent guidelines published by the AGS.

TABLE 45.3 Recommendations for Opioid Therapy in the Geriatric Population

Route	• Use the oral route when possible • Intravenous route is preferred for acute pain if oral route is not feasible • Subcutaneous route is an option if unable to obtain intravenous access • Intramuscular should be avoided due to pain and fluctuation in absorption • Rectal, transmucosal, and transdermal routes are options, but the latter should not be used for acute pain
Dosing and Titration	• Start at a low dose and titrate slowly based on response and side effects • Start short-acting oral medications every 3-4 h as needed • For continuous pain or pain not expected to resolve shortly, consider around-the-clock dosing (4-6 h) with additional as-needed doses for breakthrough pain • Consider around-the-clock dosing for patients not likely to request medications due to reluctance or cognitive impairment • Continuous pain treated with long-acting or sustained-released formulations should only be started after an initial trial and dose estimation with short-acting agents • When long-acting opioid preparations are prescribed, breakthrough pain should be anticipated, assessed, and prevented or treated using short-acting immediate-release opioid medications • Unless patient is awakened by pain during sleep, continuous opioid infusion is not recommended due to risk of opioid accumulation and toxicity • For mild to moderate pain, consider low-dose opioid combination agents • For more severe pain, consider titratable short-acting opioid agents (nonopioid combination agents) with appropriate adjuvant drugs
General Considerations	• Maximal safe doses of acetaminophen or NSAIDs should not be exceeded when using fixed-dose opioid combination agents • Only clinicians well versed in the use and risks of methadone should initiate it and titrate it cautiously • Clinicians should anticipate, assess for, and identify potential opioid-associated adverse effects • Patients taking opioid analgesics should be reassessed for ongoing achievement of therapeutic goals, adverse effects, and safe and responsible medication use

C. Nonpharmacologic Interventions

A multidisciplinary and multimodal approach to pain is especially important in the older adult. There is a growing interest and willingness to adopt complementary and alternative (CAM) strategies for pain management. Existing evidence suggests that these therapies are reasonably safe and may improve pain and function.

Physical therapy and occupational therapy are mainstays in the treatment of multiple pain syndromes for older adults. Physical therapy can reduce pain, improve function, and decrease fall risk. Occupational therapists can observe a patient in their home environment and make recommendations about assistive devices that may help to improve ADL functioning. Both physical and occupational therapists can work with caregivers to reinforce concepts learned during treatment sessions.

Relaxation techniques (including deep breathing, self-control relaxation, biofeedback, progressive muscle relaxation, meditation) have been shown in geriatric randomized control trials to be helpful in treating headaches, low back pain, and rheumatologic pain. Hypnosis has also been shown to be an effective analgesic in the geriatric population but is limited to older adults with intact cognitive function. Yoga and tai chi have shown promise in the treatment of chronic pain in older adults, with positive trials in low back pain and pain from osteoarthritis. These exercises can also be tailored to the different physical limitations of geriatric patients.

Behavioral techniques are divided into two categories, cognitive behavioral therapy (CBT) and operant behavioral therapy (OBT), with both being effective in multiple different pain syndromes. Both therapies require intact cognition and the ability to sustain attention.

IV. CONCLUSION

As the population continues to age, it is important to have a good understanding of the nuances of pain management for the geriatric patient. In general, pain in the older adult is often overlooked and undertreated. Pain assessment and management is often challenging in the setting of comorbid conditions such as cognitive impairment and delirium. Older adults may have prior beliefs or misconceptions regarding pain management that if left unattended may become barriers to effective analgesia. Physiologic changes that occur with aging render the older adult more susceptible to side effects, and careful consideration must be taken when initiating and adjusting medications. Both polypharmacy and undertreated pain can have unintended consequences for older adults and their caregivers. Knowledge of these key differences can help the clinician provide safe, effective analgesia while maximizing the older adult's function and quality of life through a carefully designed multimodal approach.

Selected Readings

American Geriatrics Society Panel on Pharmacological Management of Persistent Pain in Older Persons. Pharmacological management of persistent pain in older persons. *J Am Geriatr Soc.* 2009;57:1331-1346.

Balducci L. Management of cancer pain in geriatric patients. *J Supportive Oncol.* 2003;1:175-191.

Bjoro K, Herr K. Assessment of pain in the nonverbal or cognitively impaired older adult. *Clin Geriatr Med.* 2008;24:237-262.

Bruchenthal P. Assessment of pain in the elderly adult. *Clin Geriatr Med.* 2008;24:213-236.

Deane G, Smith H. Overview of pain management in older persons. *Clin Geriatr Med.* 2008;24:185-201.

Management of pain in older adults. In: Chai E, Meier D, Morris J, Goldhirsch S, eds. *Geriatric Palliative Care: A Practical Guide for Clinicians.* New York, NY: Oxford University Press; 2014:159-169.

Semla T. Pharmacotherapy. In: Durso S, Sullivan G, eds. *Geriatric Review Syllabus: A Core Curriculum in Geriatric Medicine.* 8th ed. New York, NY: American Geriatrics Society; 2013:87-96.

The American Geriatrics Society 2015 Beers Criteria Update Expert Panel. American Geriatrics Society 2015 updated beers criteria for potentially inappropriate medication use in older adults. *J Am Geriatr Soc.* 2015;63:2227-2246.

46 Management of Noncancer and Chronic Pain in Children With Life-Threatening Illness

Jori F. Bogetz and Richard D. Goldstein

I. PRESENTATION OF NONCANCER AND CHRONIC PAIN IN CHILDREN WITH LIFE-THREATENING ILLNESSES

A. Epidemiology

Pain is a common symptom in children, warranting prompt recognition and appropriate treatment. Pain is multifactorial and can include sensory, physiological, behavioral, cognitive, emotional, and spiritual components. Children may experience acute pain or chronic pain. Chronic pain is often the consequence of an underlying complex chronic condition (CCC) that impacts function and coping. CCCs are defined as medical conditions where the child can reasonably be expected to survive for ≥12 months (unless death intervenes) and that involve either (1) several different organ systems or (2) at least one organ system severely enough to require specialty pediatric care and some period of hospitalization in a tertiary care center. Common pediatric CCCs leading to chronic pain include gastrointestinal conditions (eg, inflammatory bowel disease and chronic pancreatitis), sickle cell disease, cystic fibrosis, congenital heart disease/heart failure, genetic/chromosomal conditions, and neurological impairment. Children with these conditions represent an important category of pediatric patients experiencing pain, especially in the hospital setting, who have complex pain sources and require adequate pain assessment and management. Cancer pain, another common cause, is discussed in Chapter 41.

Although they account for <3% of the pediatric population, children with CCCs are frequently admitted to the hospital, accounting for 18% of hospital admissions and 23% of hospital inpatient charges. Pain symptoms

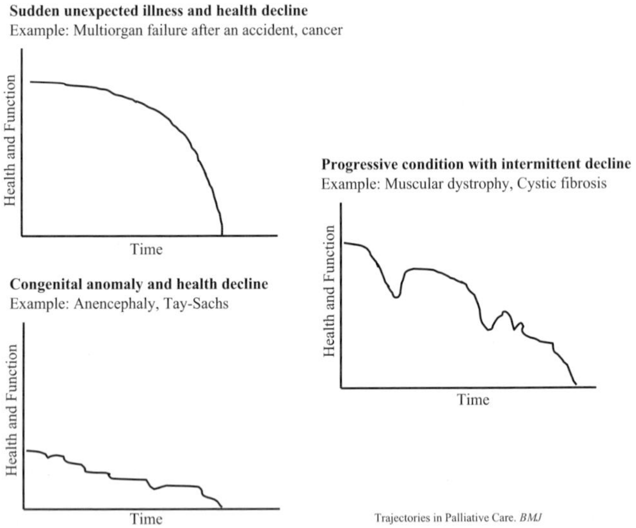

FIGURE 46.1 Illness trajectory. (Adapted from Murray S, Kendall M, Boyd K, et al. Illness trajectories in palliative care. *BMJ.* 2005;330:1007-1011.)

are extremely common in this population and especially in those with neurological impairment (eg, anencephaly, anoxic brain injury)—with 75% of parents reporting pain symptoms in their child at least once per month and with pain occurring weekly in 44% and daily in 24% of children.

B. Typical Trajectories

CCCs often follow typical disease trajectories, from conditions that are rapidly progressive to those that generally worsen with time (eg, muscular dystrophy). Many CCCs are marked by prolonged disability and subsequent deteriorations in overall health status leading to life-threatening illness. Figure 46.1 diagrams typical trajectories. Assessing pain symptoms in the context of these disease trajectories can aid understanding of a child and family's previous experience with pain and their anticipated future pain experiences.

II. GENERAL PRINCIPLES

A. Development and the Pain System

Pain transmission and sensation exists at birth. Myelination of pain communication tracts occurs as early as 22 weeks of gestation and are complete around 30 months after birth. Descending inhibitory pathways that modulate pain perception develop after birth.

B. Maturation of the Nervous System

The nervous system completes an enormous amount of development before birth and continues well into early childhood. Early pain experiences are imprinted and influence future pain behaviors. Recent research suggests that newborns and infants with undertreated pain can have behavioral changes and exaggerated pain responses that stay with them throughout their lifetime.

C. Developmental Aspects of Drug Metabolism

Changes in drug metabolism that occur as children age influence pain management. At birth, immature liver (hepatic cytochromes) and renal function (low GFR) impacts the metabolism and excretion of pain medications. Total body water is high in infants and decreases as children age, impacting the volume of distribution for drugs based on their water solubility. Gastric emptying and intestinal motility are also slower in neonates, delaying drug absorption and time to maximum plasma levels. Doses of opioid medications are often 25%-30% less than typical pediatric dosing for neonates due to their immature metabolism and excretion. However, for all practical purposes, equianalgesic opioid conversion ratios are the same for children as for adults.

D. Cognitive Development

A child's ability to report pain depends on their developmental stage and age. In children, cognitive development proceeds from "magical thinking" (ie, a belief that reality is influenced by their wishes and feelings) to a more rational cause and effect adult model. In young and school-aged children, their understanding of the context and meaning of pain is often limited (eg, a child may feel pain from a surgery but not understand why the surgery was necessary to make their body healthier in the future). For typically developing children, those as young as 18 months can usually report and localize pain. Children around 12 years can usually use pain descriptors such as quality, time, and aggravating and alleviating factors to describe their symptoms. Developmental progression of a typical child's understanding of pain is shown in Table 46.1.

E. Relational Aspects of Pain Presentation

A child's environment along with his or her own emotional and behavioral responses can influence pain. Children as young as 3 years will seek out parental support or play during painful events. A child and parents' past experiences with pain and the psychosocial context surrounding pain symptoms play a major role in pain perception. These complexities make comprehensive assessment using appropriate tools and effective management strategies critical.

III. ASSESSMENT OF PAIN

A. General Principles

Pain assessment for children often begins with a comprehensive history and physical examination, consideration of underlying causes, measurement of pain severity using an age/developmentally appropriate tool, and information

TABLE 46.1 Developmental Sequence of Children's Understanding of Pain

Age	Expression of Pain
6-18 months	Fear of painful situations, localization of pain
18-24 months	Use of simple words to describe pain such as "hurt" or "boo-boo"
24-36 months	Able to describe pain, able to describe what caused the pain
36-60 months	Able to describe vague levels of pain intensity and adjectives to describe type of pain
5-7 years	Able to describe clear levels of pain intensity
7-10 years	Able to explain why pain hurts
11 years and older	Able to explain the value of pain

about aggravating and alleviating factors. Pain assessment should also include a description of the pain's impact on function, coping, and daily routines. Noting information about previous pain treatments and their effectiveness is also important. School-aged children often can be asked about pain symptoms first and then parents can be involved for confirming and augmenting their descriptions. Older children and young adults are best approached as the primary sources for pain description and assessment.

Many pain assessment tools have been developed to facilitate pain scale rating and evaluation/reevaluation over time (Table 46.2). Observational pain scales are often used for children under the age of 7 years, and parents may be best suited to evaluate pain behaviors specific to children who cannot self-report symptoms or who have particular mannerisms. Participatory pain scales, such as the Wong-Baker Faces, can be used for older children. Children can typically use Numeric Rating Scales by the age of 12 years. Previous experiences with pain medications, nonpharmacologic pain management strategies, and psychological, emotional, and spiritual factors should also be assessed.

B. Pain Behavior and Physiologic Variables

Observation can be a helpful tool in assessing pain. Checking for general signs of distress/inconsolability, brow furrowing, facial grimace, activity

TABLE 46.2 Pain Assessment Tools

Name	Age/Indication	Scale	Notes
Face, Legs, Activity, Crying and Consolability (FLACC)	2 months to 7 years	0-10 scale for changes in Face, Legs, Activity, Crying and Consolability	Commonly used in hospitals
Wong-Baker Faces	3 years and older	0 for "no pain" to 5 for "worst pain you can imagine"	Uses 6 face pictures showing increasing levels of discomfort
Revised-Face, Legs, Activity, Crying and Consolability (R-FLACC)	2 months to 7 years, children with neurological impairment	0-10 scale for changes in Face, Legs, Activity, Crying and Consolability	Revised for children with neurological impairment
Individualized Numeric Rating Scale (INRS)	Children with neurological impairment	0-10 scale for pain behaviors, developed by family	Incorporated parent input, specific to individual child
Pediatric Pain Profile (PPP)	1-18 years with neurological impairment	20-item pain profile based on pain behaviors	Not often used in clinical practice
Visual Analog Scale (VAS)	8 years and older	0-10 shown on a line with equal spacing between numbers from "no pain" to "worst pain imaginable"	Also used for adults

level, and response to pain medication can be demonstrative. Physiologic variables such as heart rate, blood pressure, respiratory rate, and sweating can be helpful in evaluating for pain but should not be used exclusively nor relied upon for evidence of pain. Often these values are impacted by a child's underlying disease and are not reliable. Playfulness is also not a reliable indicator as many children will continue active play despite pain. Talking with the child directly whenever possible and asking parents and care providers about changes from baseline are often helpful.

C. Self-report

The ability very young children to express and participate in describing symptoms of pain can be remarkable. Preschool-aged children may use familiar terminology to describe pain (eg, a "boo boo"). When providers are able, they should keep these words and descriptors consistent when talking with the child. Older children will be able to be more precise, commenting on specific aspects of the pain (eg, sharp, shooting, stabbing). Older children and young adults will also be able to describe how pain changes after medications or how much pain is contributed to by anxiety, constipation, or other associated symptoms.

D. Conditions Presenting as Pain That Warrant Specific Attention

Pain assessment in children is often complicated by the difficulty of evaluating for other symptoms that can present as pain. Assessment for these symptoms is essential particularly in younger children and in those with neurological impairment. Symptoms commonly presenting as pain include:

- Gastrointestinal symptoms (gastroesophageal reflux, nausea, constipation)
- Musculoskeletal (spasticity, muscle spasm, dystonia)
- Psychosocial/affective (anxiety, depression)
- Neurological (seizures, dysautonomia)

These symptoms make pain discrimination difficult and can exacerbate pain. Talking with parents and care providers, reviewing the child's history/baseline, and determining patterns can be helpful.

E. The Assessment of Pain in Nonverbal Infants and Children

Children with neurological impairment can have complicated pain presentations, which make assessment and adequate pain treatment difficult. Pain inputs collected via the peripheral nervous system bring information to the dorsal root ganglion of the spinal cord, which then transmit via the lateral spinothalamic tract to the medulla, pons, and thalamus. Central inhibitory pathways from the periaqueductal gray area of the brain stem function in an inhibitory fashion to modulate pain perception. Children with impaired central nervous systems may have limited ability to modulate pain perception using central processes. These children often experience repetitive pain episodes, sometimes from benign sources, that can result in behavioral changes (eg, irritability, "acting out") and mood changes (eg, withdrawal). One helpful tool for pain assessment in children with neurological impairment is the Individualized Numeric Rating Scale (INRS) in which families work with providers to identify common pain behaviors indicating pain severity and then map them onto a reproducible numeric pain scale. This reinforces the parents' observations and involves them in adequately addressing their child's pain. These pain scales can also be used in the home setting and upon readmissions to the hospital. The revised-FLACC is another tool that has been validated in children with neurological impairment. Involving all members of the multidisciplinary team (ie, physical therapy, occupational therapy) can also be helpful to assess pain in this population of children.

IV. PAIN MANAGEMENT

A. Pain Presentations and Types of Pain

Mixed pain (ie, pain from multiple sources) is common in children. Adequate pain management requires selecting the appropriate pain medications (based on the type and level of pain day severity), dosing medications at regular intervals, using the least invasive effective route of administration, and modifying treatment plans to meet the needs of the individual child. Common pain presentations and types of pain are described below.

- Nociceptive: Nociceptive pain results from direct injury or inflammation to tissue areas sensed by C-fiber and A-delta pain nerve receptors. This type of pain typically has an inciting cause, such as a surgical incision or wound. Typically, nociceptive pain is self-limited with injuries often resolving within 5-10 days accompanied by pain relief.
- Visceral hyperalgesia: Visceral hyperalgesia, is increased pain from the gastrointestinal tract caused typically by distension or chronic stimuli. Visceral hyperalgesia is often triggered by gastroesophageal reflux or constipation. Children with chronic gastrointestinal problems (eg, inflammatory bowel disease, chronic pancreatitis) can have chronic nerve stimulation of pain receptors in the gut. Children with neurological injury (eg, cerebral palsy) can have increased sensitivity of pain receptors in the gastrointestinal tract from dysmotility, distension, and impaired pain modulation.
- Neuropathic pain: Neuropathic pain is caused by neuronal damage and dysregulation that occurs. Allodynia, or the sensation of pain in typically nonpainful circumstances, can be present. Often neuropathic pain is described as sharp, stabbing, or burning. Patients can also feel numbness, tingling, and changes in temperature.
- Central pain: Central pain, a type of neuropathic pain, often goes underrecognized in children. Children born with brain malformations or brain injuries resulting from anoxia or trauma can have pain caused directly from swelling and inflammation of the brain. Furthermore, decreased ability to regulate pain perceptions caused by brain injury can exacerbate pain symptoms generated from other sources. This can result in mild pain inputs being experienced and externalized as severe pain episodes.

B. Pharmacologic Treatment

Pain treatment often depends on the illness trajectory, developmental factors, and the type and severity of pain. Each type of pain will be described below with common treatment strategies.

- Nociceptive: Mild to severe nociceptive pain are treated according to World Health Organization (WHO) pain guidelines. These guidelines follow a stepwise approach to pain management utilizing lower-risk medications often adequate for mild pain and escalating through higher-risk medications often required for more severe pain (Fig. 46.2). Acetaminophen can be used in very young children, including infants, and can be given orally, rectally, or intravenously depending on the clinical situation. Risks with acetaminophen use include hepatotoxicity and acute overdose. Nonsteroidal anti-inflammatory drugs (NSAIDs) such as ibuprofen and naproxen can also be used in children >6 months once renal

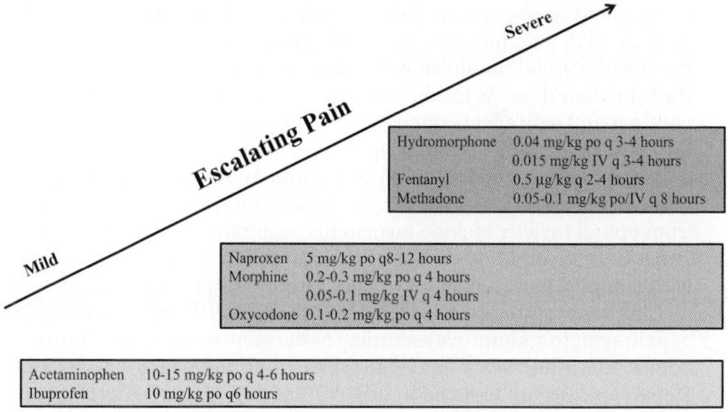

Pain Adjuvants

Visceral hyperalgesia	Gabapentin	2 mg/kg po q8 hours, titrate by additional 2 mg/kg per dose every 3 days
Neuropathic pain	Amitriptyline	0.2 mg/kg po QHS, titrate by additional 0.2 mg/kg/day every 3 days

Reference local formulary and maximum adult dosing

FIGURE 46.2 Stepwise approach to pain management with medications.

function is mature. NSAIDs should be used sparingly in children with thrombocytopenia, coagulopathy, or gastritis due to known side effects. Typically, medications used for mild pain are continued as stronger medications are added for more severe pain symptoms. For severe pain, opioids can be safely used in children of all ages. Weak opioids, such as codeine, are no longer recommended in children due to uncertainty about metabolism and bioavailability between patients. Tramadol has no analgesic advantage to other opioids and may cause undesired serotonergic effects. Meperidine is also no longer recommended due to its inferiority in pain management when compared to morphine and its risk for central nervous system toxicity. Careful dosing and close attention to side effects is necessary in any child but particularly important in children <6 months given their reductions in opioid clearance. Careful monitoring and diligence to use the lowest dose necessary for the shortest period of time is essential. Choosing the type of opioid based on the clinical situation is important, with morphine being effective in most situations. Hydromorphone or fentanyl may be used in settings of renal or liver injury. Long-acting preparations (eg, methadone) are available and can be used safely in children. Conversions between opioids should be done judiciously with careful attention to the clinical situation and resulting analgesia. Liquid formulations are available for children who cannot swallow pills. The unit doses of sustained release tablets may be too large for children <20 kg (eg, extended-release morphine or oxycodone). Extended-release tablets cannot be crushed, chewed, or cut. Opioid rotation should only be considered once medications have been adequately titrated, if there is poor analgesic response and/or if the child is experiencing side effects.

Children can also receive pain medications via infusions and patient-controlled analgesia (PCA) pumps. PCAs can be used successfully in children over 6 years depending on their cognitive, physical, and emotional abilities. Children who require opioids for extended periods of time due to prolonged recovery from severe pain or at end of life may need opioid doses escalated due to tolerance. Dose escalation is often performed in increments of 20% (mild pain) to 50% (moderate to severe pain) with careful monitoring. Breakthrough doses are often 5%-10% of the total daily dose. As in adults, there is no maximum dose for opioids in children and side effects often result in limitations in the use of opioids for escalating pain. Common opioid side effects include constipation, nausea, vomiting, sedation, and confusion. Active prevention of opioid-induced constipation is critical. Potentially life-threatening side effects from opioid toxicity include myoclonus, respiratory depression, and seizures. Careful attention should be given to children on high doses and/or with complex pain, which may benefit from multimodal management.

Children are often de-escalated ("weaned") off of their pain medications as pain symptoms improve according to the same stepwise fashion used in adults. This is necessary for children on opioids for longer than 7-10 days. Doses typically are reduced by 10%-20% of the original daily total every few days.

Other pain adjuvants for nociceptive pain include sucrose solution, which is thought to stimulate inhibitory corticospinal descending pain pathways in children up to 6 months. Topical eutectic mixture of lidocaine and prilocaine (EMLA) is also considered safe in infants and children and can be helpful before placement of intravenous catheters and injections.

- Neuropathic pain: Neuropathic pain is often treated with gabapentinoids (eg, gabapentin and pregabalin) or tricyclic antidepressants (eg, amitriptyline and nortriptyline). Side effects and drug-drug interactions must be considered, in particular QT prolongation and sedation. The use of topical treatments such as lidocaine patches over areas of superficial neuropathic pain can be helpful. When significant nociceptive and neuropathic pain occurs together, methadone is often the opioid of choice because of its impact on opioid and *N*-methyl-D-aspartate (NMDA) receptors. Low-dose ketamine can also be helpful due to its NMDA receptor blockade. Neuropathic pain can also be effectively treated with desensitization techniques involving nonpharmacologic pain management strategies. These are listed in Table 46.3 and include gentle physical therapy.
- Central pain: Central pain is often treated with mild pain medications such as acetaminophen as well as neuropathic agents such as gabapentin. Clonidine can also be helpful especially if children also have symptoms including autonomic dysregulation and/or storming.

C. Regional Anesthesia and Analgesia

For the majority of children with severe pain and life-threatening illness, systemic opioids will be the mainstay of management. Reasons to invoke regional techniques include (1) preprocedural or preoperative analgesia, (2) unacceptable side effects from opioid medications, and (3) ineffective pain management even at high doses of systemic medications. Regional anesthesia includes the use of local anesthetics to produce an area of numbness to limit pain sensation. Techniques such as neuraxial, plexus, and peripheral nerve blocks can be highly effective and safe in children when pain is localized after a surgery or in one area of the body that is easily treated with local blockade. Although there are limited studies in children, regional anesthesia and analgesia can be extremely effective. For children with life-threatening illness, those who most benefit tend to have an expected survival time of months or more. Complications include bleeding, infection, and catheter migration limiting pain control.

TABLE 46.3 Nonpharmacologic Pain Strategies and Support Staff

Strategies	Support Staff
• Massage • Acupuncture/acupressure • Transcutaneous electrical nerve stimulation (TENS) • Hot/cold packs • Positioning • Reiki • Guided imagery • Mindfulness • Hypnosis • Biofeedback • Deep breathing/stress reduction • Distraction • Art therapy • Music therapy • Pet therapy • Cognitive-behavioral therapy • Physical therapy	• Massage therapist • Acupuncturist • Clinical nurse with pain training • Child psychologist • Child life specialist • Chaplain • Art therapist • Music therapist • Physical therapist • Occupational therapist • Palliative medicine specialist

D. Other Techniques

There are a number of nonpharmacological therapies available to treat chronic pain and pain associated with life-threatening illnesses in children. Commonly employed strategies include acupuncture, acupressure, laser acupuncture, massage, and hypnosis. The use of behavioral therapy is another helpful approach especially for chronic pain. For younger children who may be unable to use cognitive coping strategies to help with pain (eg, relaxation techniques, guided imagery), often the comfort of a parent, distraction techniques, support from child life therapists, and games/toys to mimic calming strategies can be helpful. Although there is limited evidence to support these techniques, their risk of potential harm is low and are often worth discussing with parents and children. For children with chronic pain and/or life-threatening illness, spiritual and psychosocial issues often contribute to pain symptoms. Involving specialists such as spiritual care supports, psychologists, and palliative medicine providers may be helpful.

Cannabinoids are a growing area of interest in pain control in children. Cannabinoids act on the endogenous cannabinoid system, which has specific receptors in locations such as the prefrontal cortex, amygdala, hypothalamus, and the intestines. Synthetic tetrahydrocannabinol (THC) is now approved for nausea and appetite stimulation. While there is promising research on cannabidiol's effect on pain, there are no FDA-approved cannabinoids for pain control in children. With changing laws and policies, more research will likely improve our knowledge about cannabinoids and their impact on pain.

V. CONCLUSION

Children experience pain at all ages and can demonstrate signs of pain and self-report pain symptoms. Pain is approached similarly to adults, using pain scales and changes in behaviors to assess adequacy of pain control.

Medications are often used along with nonpharmacologic strategies to treat pain in children and can be very effective. In situations when pain is refractory or unacceptable side effects are being experienced, regional techniques can be helpful. Importantly, nonpharmacologic strategies can be fundamental to optimizing pain treatment in children.

Selected Readings

Ammerman S, Ryan S, Adelman WP. The committee on substance abuse and the committee on adolescence. The impact of marijuana policies on youth: clinical, research, and legal update. *Pediatrics.* 2015;135(3):e769-e785. doi: 10.1542/peds.2014-4147.

Anand KJS, Aranda JV, Berde CB, et al. Summary proceedings from the neonatal pain-control group. *Pediatrics.* 2006;117(suppl 1):S9-S22. doi: 10.1542/peds.2005-0620C.

Anand KJS, Hickey PR. Pain and its effects in the human neonate and fetus. *N Engl J Med.* 1987;317(21):1321-1329. doi: 10.1056/NEJM198711193172105.

Berry JG, Hall DE, Kuo DZ, et al. Hospital utilization and characteristics of patients experiencing recurrent readmissions within children's hospitals. *JAMA.* 2011;305(7):682-690. doi: 10.1001/jama.2011.122.

Chandok N, Watt K. Pain management in the cirrhotic patient: the clinical challenge. *Mayo Clin Proc.* 2010;85(5):451-458. doi: 10.4065/mcp.2009.0534.

Friedrichsdorf SJ, Kang TI. The management of pain in children with life-limiting illnesses. *Pediatr Clin North Am.* 2007;54(5):645-672. doi: 10.1016/j.pcl.2007.07.007.

Hauer J. Identifying and managing sources of pain and distress in children with neurological impairment. *Pediatr Ann.* 2010;39(4):198-205. doi: 10.3928/00904481-20100318-04.

Hauer J. Improving comfort in children with severe neurological impairment. *Prog Palliat Care.* 2012;20(6):349-356. doi: 10.1179/1743291X12Y.0000000032.

Hauer JM, Wical BS, Charnas L. Gabapentin successfully manages chronic unexplained irritability in children with severe neurologic impairment. *Pediatrics.* 2007;119(2):e519-e522. doi: 10.1542/peds.2006-1609.

Hechler T, Kanstrup M, Holley AL, Simons LE. Systematic review on intensive interdisciplinary pain treatment of children with chronic pain. *Pediatrics.* 2015;136(1):117-127. doi: 10.1542/peds.2014-3319.

Hechler T, Ruhe A, Schmidt P, et al. Inpatient-based intensive interdisciplinary pain treatment for highly impaired children with severe chronic pain: randomized controlled trial of efficacy and economic effects. *Pain.* 2014;155(1):118-128. doi: 10.1016/j.pain.2013.09.015.

Kearns G, Adbel-Rahman S, Alander S, et al. Developmental pharmacology—drug disposition, action, and therapy in infants and children. *N Engl J Med.* 2003;349(12):1157-1167.

Kitahata LM. Pain pathways and transmission. *Yale J Biol Med.* 1993;66:437-442.

Malviya S, Voepel-Lewis T, Burke C, Merkel S, Tait AR. The revised FLACC observational pain tool: improved reliability and validity for pain assessment in children with cognitive impairment. *Pediatr Anesth.* 2006;16(3):258-265. doi: 10.1111/j.1460-9592.2005.01773.x.

Meier PM, Zurakowski D. Lumbar sympathetic blockade in children with complex regional pain syndromes a double blind placebo-controlled crossover trial. *Anesthesiology.* 2009;111(2):372-380.

Mherekumombe M, Collins J. Patient-controlled analgesia for children at home. *J Pain Symptom Manage.* 2015;49(5):923-927. doi: 10.1016/j.jpainsymman.2014.10.007.

Murray SA, Kendall M, Boyd K, Sheikh A. Illness trajectories and palliative care. *BMJ.* 2005;330(7498):1007.

Postier A, Flood A, Friedrichsdorf SJ. Methadone conversion in infants and children: retrospective cohort study of 199 pediatric inpatients. *J Opioid Manag.* 2016;12(2):123-130.

Quibell R, Fallon M, Mihalyo M, Twycross R. Ketamine. *J Pain Symptom Manage.* 2015;50(2):268-278. doi: 10.1016/j.jpainsymman.2015.06.002.

Rork JF, Berde CB, Goldstein RD. Regional anesthesia approaches to pain management in pediatric palliative care: a review of current knowledge. *J Pain Symptom Manage.* 2013;46(6):859-873. doi: 10.1016/j.jpainsymman.2013.01.004.

Sharkey KA, Wiley JW. The role of the endocannabinoid system in the brain–gut axis. *Gastroenterology*. 2016;151(2):252-266. doi: 10.1053/j.gastro.2016.04.015.

Simon TD, Berry J, Feudtner C, et al. Children with complex chronic conditions in inpatient hospital settings in the United States. *Pediatrics*. 2010;126(4):647-655. doi: 10.1542/peds.2009-3266.

Solodiuk JC, Scott-Sutherland J, Meyers M, et al. Validation of the individualized numeric rating scale (INRS): a pain assessment tool for nonverbal children with intellectual disability. *Pain*. 2010;150(2):231-236. doi: 10.1016/j.pain.2010.03.016.

Stallard P, Williams L, Velleman R, Lenton S, McGrath PJ. Brief report: behaviors identified by caregivers to detect pain in noncommunicating children. *J Pediatr Psychol*. 2002;27(2):209-214.

Swiggum M, Hamilton ML, Gleeson P. Pain assessment and management in children with neurologic impairment: a survey of pediatric physical therapists. *Pediatr Phys Ther*. 2010;22:330-335.

Voepel-Lewis T, Merkel S, Tait AR, Trzcinka A, Malviya S. The reliability and validity of the face, legs, activity, cry, consolability observational tool as a measure of pain in children with cognitive impairment. *Anesth Analg*. 2002;95(5):1224-1229. doi: 10.1097/00000539-200211000-00020.

Wang CH, Bonnemann CG, Rutkowski A, et al. Consensus statement on standard of care for congenital muscular dystrophies. *J Child Neurol*. 2010;25(12):1559-1581.

World Health Organization. WHO Guidelines on the Pharmacological Treatment of Persisting Pain in Children with Medical Illnesses. 2012. http://www.who.int/about/licensing/copyright_form/en/index.html

47

Emergencies in Pain Medicine

Lucien C. Alexandre
and Christopher Gilligan

I. INTRODUCTION

Image guidance for interventional pain procedures with the use of fluoroscopy, ultrasonography, or computed tomography along with use of contrast dye helps to significantly reduce the risks of injection-related complications. Nevertheless, potentially serious, life-threatening complications may occur. These complications are compounded in settings of ill-prepared physicians and staff. The goal of this chapter is to highlight some of the potential complications that may be encountered and to offer insights to the signs, symptoms, and methods to best manage these emergent situations. Being cognizant of these emergencies, proactively training personnel, and having appropriate emergency equipment available are keys to preventing disastrous outcomes. Such measures include having resuscitation equipment, airway carts, oxygen tanks, and emergency medications available and readily accessible. Personnel should be trained in advanced cardiac life support, and patients should be appropriately monitored during all phases related to an interventional procedure, including adequate postprocedural monitoring. Lastly, it is essential that patients are educated with clear postprocedural instructions, made aware of critical red flags that may indicate a complication, and provided contact information to reach a clinician should a complication occur.

II. PROCEDURE-RELATED EMERGENCIES

A. Vasovagal Syncope

Vasovagal syncope is one of the most frequently encountered adverse events related to pain procedures. Severe emotion, such as anger and anxiety, and pain can serve as cortical triggers that act directly on the medulla leading to a vasovagal response. The resulting neural reflex causes a self-limited hypotensive state that is generally associated with bradycardia.

Reassurance is key for patients who appear anxious or who have a history of vasovagal syncope. While most cases of vasovagal syncope resolve spontaneously with conservative treatment, pre-emptive placement of an intravenous line may be considered.

1. Symptoms and Signs

Telltale signs of presyncopal vasovagal symptoms include feeling light-headed, nauseated, sweaty, generally weak, or experiencing tinnitus and blurry vision. The patient may appear pale and diaphoretic or may display no prodromal signs at all. Episodes of clonic movements, tonic posturing, and myoclonus may occur during vasovagal syncope and may erroneously be confused with seizure activity.

2. Treatment

If the patient displays any prodromal signs of vasovagal syncope, for example, light-headedness or nausea, the procedure should be halted and the following implemented:

- **a.** Place the patient in a supine position if previously seated or standing with legs raised, preferably in the Trendelenburg position.
- **b.** Begin physical counterpressure maneuvers: leg-crossing while simultaneously tensing the leg, abdominal, and buttock muscles and arm tensing (gripping one hand with the other while simultaneously abducting both arms).
- **c.** Administer oxygen.
- **d.** Monitor airway, breathing, and circulation.
- **e.** If the patient has persistent and worsening hypotension and bradycardia, place an intravenous line, start crystalloids, and administer a vasopressor, such as ephedrine (in 5-10 mg increments), or a chronotropic agent such as atropine (0.4-1 mg).
- **f.** Evaluate ECG tracing for other possible causes of bradycardia.
- **g.** Continue monitoring and maintain the supine position.
- **h.** Verify vital signs are stable prior to home discharge.

B. Systemic Local Anesthetic Toxicity

Though rare, systemic local anesthetic toxicity can result in devastating complications. Systemic toxicity may be secondary to excessive doses from local infiltration, rapid absorption, or intravascular administration. The upper limit dose of lidocaine is estimated to be 4.5 mg/kg and 7 mg/kg for lidocaine mixed with epinephrine. For bupivacaine, toxicity may occur with doses >2.5 mg/kg without epinephrine and 3 mg/kg with epinephrine. Prodromal symptoms can include perioral numbness, dysgeusia (distorted sense of taste), dizziness, tinnitus, dysphoria, confusion, and drowsiness. Neurotoxicity can lead to agitation, loss of consciousness, and seizures. Cardiotoxicity can cause dyspnea, hypertension, hypotension, tachycardia, bradycardia, ventricular fibrillation, ventricular ectopy, ST-segment changes, or asystole. Due to pulmonary clearance of venous blood, inadvertent intravenous injection poses less central nervous system or cardiovascular risks than intra-arterial injection. The risk factors that may potentiate toxicity include extremes of age, low/high cardiac output, hepatic dysfunction, pregnancy, or use of certain cardiac medications, such as betablockers.

1. Treatment (Primary Goal to Prevent Acidosis and Hypoxemia)

- **a.** Initiate ACLS protocol.
- **b.** Ventilate with 100% oxygen via a bag valve mask or endotracheal intubation.

c. Seizure suppression with benzodiazepines (midazolam 1-2 mg IV or diazepam 5-10 mg IV); avoid propofol.
d. 10-100-mcg epinephrine initially, with titration. Avoid vasopressin.
e. If the patient remains unstable, infuse 20% lipid emulsion as a bolus of 1.5 mL/kg over 1 minute followed by an infusion rate of 0.25 mL/kg/min. Consider repeat bolus.
f. If the patient remains unstable, double the infusion rate (upper limit 10 mL/kg over 30 minutes).
g. Monitor arterial blood gases.
h. If the patient does not recover, continue with the above protocol and consider cardiopulmonary bypass.
i. If the patient is stable, infuse the lipid for an additional 10 minutes and monitor for recurrence.

C. Complications of Epidural and Intrathecal Procedures

1. Epidural Hematoma

Significant epidural hemorrhage in the absence of coagulopathy is rare. Nevertheless, the sudden emergence of localized back pain that may or may not be associated with radicular pain along with motor and sensory deficits should prompt immediate suspicion of a progressing epidural hematoma. Unfettered expansion of a hematoma may lead to disabling myelopathy and cause spinal cord injury due to compression and/or infarction. Urgent and appropriate imaging is key to avoiding a diagnostic delay that could adversely affecting chances for functional recovery. Although CT scan can be diagnostic, it is not as sensitive as MRI. Therefore, an emergent MRI is preferred as it provides greater information regarding the presence and extent of the hematoma, as well as the severity of cord compression. In the vast majority of cases, treatment involves emergency surgical decompression and evacuation of the hematoma in patients with myelopathy. Conservative management may be an option in patients without cord compression and neurologic deficits, insofar as they are carefully monitored with serial neurologic exams and repeat MR imaging.

2. Epidural Abscess

The neurologic outcome of pyogenic spinal epidural abscess greatly depends on the promptness of diagnosis and treatment. Classically, the clinical presentation has four sequential phases: (1) spinal pain; (2) radicular pain; (3) muscular weakness, sensory loss, sphincter dysfunction; and (4) complete paralysis. The nidus of the abscess usually causes focal spinal pain and fever, and these findings should be considered red flags. However, it is important to appreciate that neuraxial infections may present in a more indolent fashion than infections in other areas of the body. Unfortunately, the diagnosis is often made after the onset of neurological dysfunction. Once myelopathic symptoms are present, permanent damage is likely if intervention does not occur within 24 hours. Diagnosis requires prompt suspicion and is aided by obtaining routine labs, which may reveal mild leukocytosis, elevated sedimentation rate, C-reactive protein, and possible positive blood cultures, though these are nonspecific. The cornerstone of diagnosis is neuroimaging; the gold standard is myelography; however, there is equivalent sensitivity seen in MRI with gadolinium. Treatment typically includes surgical decompression in conjunction with intravenous antibiotics. Like in epidural hematoma, some physicians advocate conservative treatment in patients who are neurologically intact with early identified organisms that allow for specific antibiotic therapy. Nevertheless, neurologic deterioration may still occur despite being on the appropriate antibiotic treatment, and close monitoring should continue until the infection is resolved.

3. High Spinal Anesthetics

The use of fluoroscopy and contrast media significantly reduces inadvertent intrathecal delivery of local anesthetics. However, on occasion, the needle tip may pierce beyond the epidural space to breach the subdural or subarachnoid space. The onset of blockade in subdural delivery of local anesthetic may have a slow onset (~15-20 minutes) followed by a full recovery. The sensory blockade is generally more pervasive with minimal effect on sympathetic and motor functions. Meanwhile, delivery of high concentrations of local anesthetic in the subarachnoid space occurs rather quickly and may lead to cephalad spread and cause high spinal blockade. This inadvertent blockade may cause sympathectomy (resulting in hypotension), inhibition of compensatory tachycardia, brainstem hypoperfusion (causing respiratory depression and nausea), dyspnea, diaphragmatic paralysis, loss of consciousness, and aspiration. Although the effects are self-limiting and will resolve with dissipation of the local anesthetic, the patient may require standard resuscitative measures that include airway protection, ventilation with 100% oxygen via bag mask or endotracheal intubation, and cardiovascular support with vasopressors and inotropes to maintain blood pressure. In a high spinal block, the patient may remain awake even though they are paralyzed. Reassurance that this is temporary is key, and use of an anxiolytic medication should be considered.

4. Accidental Overdose via Neuraxial Pump

Neuraxial pumps are used to deliver myriad medications directly to the intrathecal space. Morphine, ziconotide, baclofen, and clonidine have been FDA approved for this use although several medications are used as "off-label" agents. The neuraxial route allows for direct delivery of the medication to spinal receptors, allowing for greater analgesic potency with as substantially reduced medication dosages as compared to systemic delivery. The risk of accidental overdose remains a very serious potential complication. This may be due to a pump malfunction, dosing error, or injection of analgesics directly into the subcutaneous tissue or catheter access port. Clinical manifestations of opioid overdose can lead to respiratory or CNS depression and cardiac abnormalities. Overdose with ziconotide is not associated with cardiopulmonary compromise or death. In the case of baclofen, overdose may lead to cardiovascular abnormalities, respiratory depression, and CNS manifestations such as seizures and flaccid paralysis. Case reports of inadvertent clonidine overdose from softtissue injections during intrathecal pump refill have resulted in loss of consciousness, cardiovascular instability, and myocardial infarction.

5. Treatment

- Stop the injection.
- Ensure airway, breathing, and circulation.
- Establish intravenous access, high-flow oxygen, and setup monitoring.
- Intubate if necessary.
- Check the pump and stop the pump infusion.
- Opioids: Give naloxone 0.04-2 mg IV. Monitor the patient's vital signs. Repeat the dose of naloxone every 2-3 minutes. Naloxone infusion may be necessary.

- Ziconotide: Discontinue infusion. Begin supportive care and critical care monitoring.
- Baclofen: Pump may be stopped for a limited period of 48 hours, and in life-threatening cases, 30-40-mL CSF can be drained either by lumbar puncture or via the pump access port. Provide supportive care (intubation, intravenous fluids, ventilation support). For reversal of drowsiness and respiratory depression, consider physostigmine 1-2 mg IV over 5-10 minutes. May repeat every 10-30 minutes as required.
- Clonidine: Continue invasive blood pressure monitoring and advanced cardiovascular support; manage conscious state. Phentolamine, glyceryl trinitrate, metaraminol, or epinephrine may be employed.
- If subcutaneous injection is suspected, consider aspiration of injectate fluid pocket under ultrasound.

D. Hypotension

In the pain clinic setting, a significant drop in blood pressure (systolic blood pressure <90 mm Hg; a >40 mm Hg drop in systolic blood pressure from patient's normal baseline; MAP < 60 mm Hg; or a fall in systolic or diastolic blood pressure of >20 mm Hg or >10 mm Hg, with standing) may be due to vasovagal syncope, drug-induced reaction, anaphylaxis, myocardial ischemia, pulmonary embolism, or adrenal insufficiency. Iatrogenic causes can include intrathecal or subdural injection of local anesthetic, high neuraxial blockade, sympathetic blocks, or tension pneumothorax. Symptoms of hypotension may include generalized weakness, fatigue, anxiety, dizziness, dyspnea, syncope, chest discomfort, and confusion.

1. Treatment

- The patient should be oxygenated.
- Large-bore intravenous access should be established.
- If not contraindicated, an intravenous challenge with an isotonic crystalloid solution (normal saline or lactated Ringer solution) of at least 1-1.5 L or 20-40 mL/kg bolus should be administered.
- Accurate vital signs should be obtained and repeated frequently. ECG and cardiac monitoring are paramount.
- Place the patient in Trendelenburg position or elevate the lower extremities.
- Physical exam, including mental status evaluation, should be performed.
- Consider use of pressors if fluid resuscitation fails. May administer ephedrine 5-25 mg IV every 5-10 minutes; or phenylephrine 50-100 mcg IV bolus; or norepinephrine 8-12 mcg/min IV.
- Identify the specific cause of the hypotension and address it accordingly (eg, needle decompression of tension pneumothorax, treatment of anaphylaxis as below, etc.).

E. Hypertension

Acute pain or acute exacerbations of chronic pain may lead to significant increases in blood pressure. Pre-existing hypertension, agitation, anxiety, hypercarbia, hypoxemia, and hypervolemia are all known causes of hypertension. Additionally, treatments for chronic pain such as use of steroids for epidural injections, NSAIDs, or drug-drug interactions, for example, tricyclic antidepressants and ephedrine may also contribute to hypertension. Abrupt discontinuation of certain medications such as baclofen, opioids, α-blockers, or betablockers is also linked to possible significant increases in blood pressure secondary to withdrawal symptoms. Accidental intravascular administration of local anesthetic drugs or as a response during induction of anesthesia may also lead to hypertension.

1. Treatment

- Provide supplemental oxygen and ensure adequate ventilation.
- The procedure should be postponed for blood pressures above 180/110 mm Hg.
- Identify and treat the underlying cause. Assess for signs and symptoms of hypertensive emergency and organ compromise (stroke, ischemia, heart failure, etc.).
- Depending on the cause, treatment may entail reinstitution of a withdrawn agent (eg, restarting clonidine), use of labetalol 2.5-5 mg IV every 5-10 minutes if a betablocker was recently withdrawn, or nifedipine 10 mg sublingual.
- There must be careful attention to avoid lowering the blood pressure too quickly or too much (no >10%-20% in the first hour).
- Depending on the severity, the patient may need to be transferred to the emergency room, particularly if signs or symptoms of hypertensive emergency are noted.

F. Pneumothorax

Iatrogenic pneumothorax is a potential complication that may occur secondary to various interventional pain procedures. These can include thoracic sympathetic ganglion block, stellate ganglion block, interpleural catheter placement, supraclavicular block, intercostal nerve block, paravertebral block, trigger point injection, and celiac plexus block. Pneumothorax may also occur in thoracic transforaminal selective epidural steroid injections. The risk of pneumothorax is reduced greatly when the procedure is performed by an experienced interventionalist and with a proper imaging modality if indicated.

1. Symptoms

Iatrogenic pneumothoraces may progress to become a tension pneumothorax, which occurs when intrapleural pressure during expiration exceeds atmospheric pressure. Tension pneumothorax is a medical emergency. A patient with tension pneumothorax may develop dyspnea, decreased breath sounds, wheezing, unilateral chest hyperinflation, cyanosis, and hemodynamic instability. The clinical presentation of decreased breath sounds, hypotension, increased heart rate, distended jugular veins, and tracheal shift may suffice a presumptive diagnosis of pneumothorax. Diagnosis can be made with high specificity on chest x-ray in the upright position during inspiration. Chest x-rays in the supine and lateral decubitus positions, the latter being the most sensitive, can also be obtained. Imaging will reveal the presence of a pneumothorax with contralateral shift of the mediastinum and flattening or inversion of the ipsilateral hemidiaphragm. In an unstable patient, the decision to emergently decompress should be made on clinical grounds and should not be delayed to obtain an x-ray.

2. Treatment

- Treatment options include observation, inhaled oxygen range from observation, inhaled oxygen, needle aspiration, small-bore chest tube with unidirectional valve, and large-bore chest tube drainage with connection to water seal, pleurodesis, and thoracotomy.
- Patients with asymptomatic pneumothoraces or pneumothorax occupying <20% of the hemithorax may be managed conservatively as an

outpatient or in the emergency room with observation with or without supplemental oxygen (3 L/min nasal cannula or higher). X-ray may be repeated after 12-24 hours (or sooner if symptoms worsen) to determine that the lesion has not expanded.

- Guidelines for the management of symptomatic and large pneumothoraces vary.
- In symptomatic and unstable patients, needle decompression may be attempted by inserting a 14-gauge, 3-6-cm-long, or 18-gauge over-the-needle catheter inserted in the second intercostal space at the mid-clavicular line or a large-bore needle inserted into the pleural space through the second anterior intercostal space. Alternatively, a 17-guage 8.9-cm-long needle at the midhemithoracic line at the level of the sternal angle inserted perpendicular to the horizontal plane may be attempted.
- This should be followed by tube thoracostomy using either small-bore (10-14 French) or large-bore (20-28 French) connected to a water seal device without suction initially.

III. MEDICATION-RELATED EMERGENCIES

A. Anaphylaxis

1. Symptoms and Signs

Grade 2 and 3 hypersensitivity reactions, which correspond with anaphylaxis, are associated with multisystem disorder that may involve the cutaneous (80%-90%), respiratory (70%), cardiovascular (45%), gastrointestinal (45%), and central nervous (15%) systems. These may manifest as dyspnea, stridor, wheezing, chest tightness, presyncope, hypotension, cyanosis, hypoxemia, abdominal pain, headache, confusion, or loss of consciousness. Pruritus, erythema, and urticaria are present in most cases, though up to 20% of patients do not exhibit these characteristic cutaneous signs. Rapid identification of anaphylaxis is critical as respiratory or cardiac arrest and death can occur in minutes.

2. Treatment

- Stop the administration of the drug.
- Epinephrine (1 mg/mL) 0.3-0.5 mg intramuscular (mid-outer thigh) is the first and most important treatment to be administered and can be repeated every 5-15 minutes as needed. Concurrently, the patient should be placed in the recumbent position with elevation of the lower extremities; give oxygen 8-10 L/min via facemask; place two large-bore IV catheters (14-16 gauge); in hypotensive patients, 1-2 L IV normal saline should be given as a rapid infusion (normotensive patients may receive NS infused at 125 mL/h).
- Assess airway, breathing, circulation, and mentation. Immediate intubation should be performed if there is marked stridor or respiratory arrest.
- Continue monitoring of vitals, including cardiopulmonary status and oxygen saturation.
- For patients using betablockers, treatment resistance to epinephrine may occur. In this scenario, coadminister glucagon 1-5 mg IV over 5 minutes (may repeat dose; monitor for nausea and vomiting).
- Adjunctive agents may be used, but are not substitutes for epinephrine. May administer diphenhydramine 25-50 mg IV (max dose 400 mg/24 h) to relieve itching and hives and albuterol via facemask and nebulizer/compressor as needed for epinephrine-resistant bronchospasm; methylprednisolone 1-2 mg/kg/d for 1-2 days may be administered; however, this does not aid in the relief of the initial symptoms and signs of anaphylaxis.

B. Opioid Overdose

1. Symptoms and Signs

Patients with opioid intoxication may present with miotic pupils, decreased bowel sounds, respiratory depression, somnolence, and coma. Associated increased restlessness, agitation, hypothermia, aspiration pneumonia, myoclonus, and sudden onset seizures may occur.

2. Treatment

- Evaluate ventilatory status; patients with respiratory rates ≥12 breaths/min and oxygen saturation >90% on room air may be monitored.
- In patients who are breathing spontaneously but whose oxygen saturation is <90% on room air, give supplemental oxygen. Give naloxone 0.05 mg IV or IM, which may be repeated every 2-3 minutes until ventilation is adequate.
- In apneic patients, support ventilation with bag valve mask attached to supplemental oxygen, or consider endotracheal intubation. Administer naloxone 0.2-1 mg IV; may repeat every 2-3 minutes until ventilation is adequate. After 5-10 mg of naloxone, if there is no clinical effect, the diagnosis warrants re-evaluation.
- Due to its higher opioid receptor affinity, fast titration or large boluses may precipitate opioid withdrawal in patients on chronic opioid therapy and should be used judiciously, that is, no more than 0.04-mg naloxone every 2 minutes.
- Naloxone's high lipophilicity leads to significant adipose tissue redistribution within 10-15 minutes, thereby leading to diminished effect and recurrence of opioid toxicity in that timeframe. Therefore, naloxone infusion at 0.5-1.2 mg/h rather than repeated boluses may be required to clear a sufficient amount of the offending opioid to achieve adequate and sustained ventilation.

C. Opioid Withdrawal

1. Symptoms and Signs

Though rare, iatrogenic opioid withdrawal is potentially life-threatening due to hemodynamic instability that can occur with a sudden surge in catecholamines. Withdrawal symptoms may start 6-12 hours from the last dose of a short-acting opioid and last for several days, while withdrawal from methadone may occur 24-48 hours from the last dose and last up to 2 weeks. The symptoms experienced may include hypertension, nausea and vomiting, abdominal cramping, diarrhea, fever, chills, rhinorrhea, lacrimation, irritability, and muscle aches.

2. Treatment

- If the withdrawal is secondary to cessation of opioid, resumption of the opioid, even at 25%-40% of the original dose, will likely abort most of the symptoms. Methadone 10 mg IM or 20 mg oral is generally sufficient to mitigate withdrawal symptoms without producing intoxication in a patient with significant opioid tolerance. An additional option is supplemental use of diazepam 1-10 mg PO, IV, or IM every 5-10 minutes until stable blood pressure and sedation are achieved.
- Adjunctive nonopioid medications may be used for symptom management, especially in patients with iatrogenic opioid withdrawal. In severe cases, clonidine 0.1-0.3 mg orally every hour may be given until the symptoms of anxiety, restlessness, dysphoria, and hypertension are abrogated.
- For nausea, vomiting, restlessness, and insomnia, use promethazine 25-50 mg IM or diphenhydramine 50 mg IV, IM, or PO or hydroxyzine

50-100 mg IM or PO. Diarrhea and stomach cramps can be treated with loperamide 4 mg PO or octreotide 50 mcg subcutaneous every 6 hours or bismuth subsalicylate 524 mg PO. Pain and myalgia may improve with acetaminophen 650 mg PO or ibuprofen 600 mg PO. Muscle cramps may be aided by use of baclofen 5-10 mg PO.

- For a full description of opioid tolerance and withdrawal, see Chapters 11 and 44.

D. Steroid Overdose and Adrenal Insufficiency

Direct injection of glucocorticoids into the epidural space diminishes the likelihood of potential systemic effects of steroids. The hypothalamic-pituitary-adrenal (HPA) axis can be significantly altered leading to acute and chronic suppression. Transient adrenal suppression lasting 1-2 weeks may be evident even after a single dose of epidural glucocorticoid injection. Suppression of the HPA axis may be minimized or circumvented by limiting the dose and frequency of the glucocorticoid used. It is worth noting many medications used in the treatment of HIV alter adrenocortical function and in conjunction with exposure to exogenous steroids can lead to suppression of the HPA and Cushing syndrome.

1. Symptoms and Signs

Patients with adrenal insufficiency may present with diffuse myalgia and arthralgia, malaise, fatigue, anorexia, weight loss, hypotension, and rarely hypoglycemia. Adrenal insufficiency when acute presents as adrenal crisis, which is a life-threatening emergency and is characterized by hypotension and may involve hyponatremia.

2. Treatment

- Establish intravenous access with large-bore catheter.
- Obtain labs to measure serum electrolytes and glucose as well as plasma cortisol and ACTH. Do not delay treatment for the results of these tests.
- Administer isotonic saline or 5% dextrose in isotonic saline, at 2-3-L rapid infusion.
- Hemodynamic monitoring and measurement of serum electrolytes.
- Administer a bolus of dexamethasone 4 mg IV over 1-5 minutes, repeat every 12 hours, alternatively may use hydrocortisone 100 mg IV, and repeat every 6 hours.

IV. CONCLUSION

Adverse and potentially life-threatening complications may be encountered in the field of pain medicine. Though rare, it is incumbent upon the interventional pain physician to be aware of the potential complications associated with the procedures being performed and the medications used. Equally important is rapidly and correctly identifying potential emergencies while implementing lifesaving measures to prevent permanent disability or death. This can be achieved with appropriate training of personnel, availability and maintenance of necessary equipment, and development of safety protocols.

Selected Readings

Asadi-Pooya AA, Nikseresht A, Yaghoubi E. Vasovagal syncope treated as epilepsy for 16 years. *Iran J Med Sci.* 2011;36(1):60-62.

Baumann MH, Strange C, Heffner JE, et al.; AACP Pneumothorax Consensus Group. Management of spontaneous pneumothorax: an American College of Chest Physicians Delphi consensus statement. *Chest.* 2001;119(2):590-602.

Bellini M, Barbieri M. Systemic effects of epidural steroid injections. *Anaesthesiol Intensive Ther.* 2013;45(2):93-98.

Botelho RJ, Sitzman BT. Pharmacology for the interventional pain physician. In: Benzon HT, Raja SN, Liu SS, Fishman SM, Cohen SP, eds, Hurley RW, Narouze S, Malik KM, Candido KD, assoc eds. *Essentials of Pain Medicine.* 3rd ed. Philadelphia, PA: Elsevier Saunders; 2011:147-152.

Coffin ST, Raj SR. Non-invasive management of vasovagal syncope. *Auton Neurosci.* 2014;184:27-32.

Deer TR, Levy R, Prager J, et al. Polyanalgesic Consensus Conference—2012: recommendations to reduce morbidity and mortality in intrathecal drug delivery in the treatment of chronic pain. *Neuromodulation.* 2012;15(5):467-482; discussion 482.

Gilligan C, Stojanovic M, Rathmell JP. Emergencies in the pain clinic. In: Fishman SM, Ballantyne JC, Rathmell JP, eds. *Bonica's Management of Pain.* 4th ed. Philadelphia, PA: Lippincott Williams & Wilkins; 2010:1565-1576.

Groen RJ. Non-operative treatment of spontaneous spinal epidural hematomas: a review of the literature and a comparison with operative cases. *Acta Neurochir (Wien).* 2004;146(2):103-110.

Hacobian A, Stojanovic M. Emergencies in the pain clinic. In: Ballantyne JC, ed. *The Massachusetts General Hospital Handbook of Pain Management.* 3rd ed. Philadelphia, PA: Lippincott Williams & Wilkins; 2006.

Johnson ML, Visser EJ, Goucke CR. Massive clonidine overdose during refill of an implanted drug delivery device for intrathecal analgesia: a review of inadvertent soft-tissue injection during implantable drug delivery device refills and its management. *Pain Med.* 2011;12(7):1032-1040.

Osenbach RK, Pradhan A. Brain and spinal abscess. In: Rengachary SS, Ellenbogen RG, eds. *Principles of Neurosurgery.* 2nd ed. Edinburgh: Elsevier Mosby Publishing; 2005:415-428.

Paik NC, Seo JW. CT-guided needle aspiration of pneumothorax from a trigger point injection. *Pain Med.* 2011;12(5):837-841.

Pope JE, Deer TR. Intrathecal pharmacology update: novel dosing strategy for intrathecal monotherapy ziconotide on efficacy and sustainability. *Neuromodulation.* 2015;18(5):414-420.

Watve SV, Sivan M, Raza WA, Jamil FF. Management of acute overdose or withdrawal state in intrathecal baclofen therapy. *Spinal Cord.* 2012;50(2):107-111.

Wax DB, Leibowitz AB. Radiologic assessment of potential sites for needle decompression of a tension pneumothorax. *Anesth Analg.* 2007;105(5):1385-1388.

Weekes AJ, Zapata RJ, Napolitano A. Symptomatic hypotension: ED stabilization and the emerging role of sonography. *Emerg Med Pract.* 2007;9(11).

Zilberstein J, McCurdy MT, Winters ME. Anaphylaxis. *J Emerg Med.* 2014;47(2): 182-187.

APPENDIX

Dermatomes and Nerve Distribution

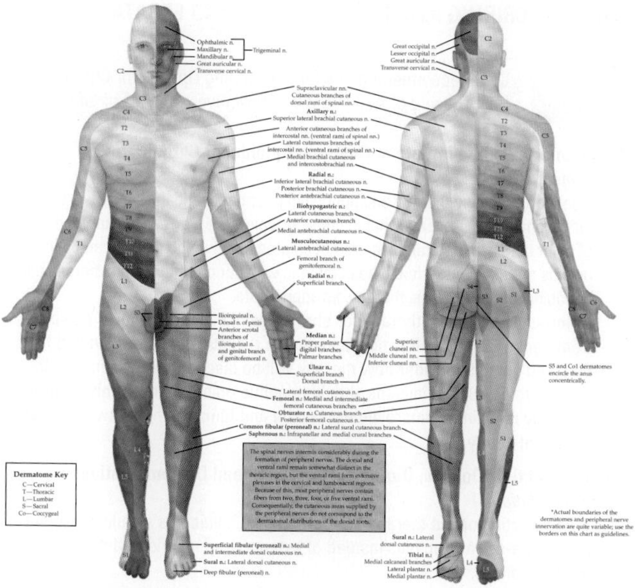

Courtesy Anatomical Chart Company. Dermatomes Anatomical Chart. Philadelphia, PA: Wolters Kluwer; 2004.

APPENDIX II

Prescription Guidelines

I. CDC PRESCRIBING RECOMMENDATIONS AND ERRATA

TABLE II.1 CDC Recommendations for Prescribing Opioids for Chronic Pain Outside of Active Cancer, Palliative, and End-of-Life Care[a]

Determining When to Initiate or Continue Opioids for Chronic Pain

Recommendation(s)

1 Nonpharmacologic therapy and nonopioid pharmacologic therapy are preferred for chronic pain. Clinicians should consider opioid therapy only if expected benefits for both pain and function are anticipated to outweigh risks to the patient. If opioids are used, they should be combined with nonpharmacologic therapy and nonopioid pharmacologic therapy, as appropriate.

2 Before starting opioid therapy for chronic pain, clinicians should establish treatment goals with all patients, including realistic goals for pain and function, and should consider how therapy will be discontinued if benefits do not outweigh risks. Clinicians should continue opioid therapy only if there is clinically meaningful improvement in pain and function that outweighs risks to patient safety.

Opioid Selection, Dosage, Duration, Follow-Up, and Discontinuation

Recommendation(s)

4 When starting opioid therapy for chronic pain, clinicians should prescribe immediate-release opioids instead of extended-release/long-acting (ER/LA) opioids.

5 When opioids are started, clinicians should prescribe the lowest effective dosage. Clinicians should use caution when prescribing opioids at any dosage, should carefully reassess evidence of individual benefits and risks when increasing dosage to ≥50 morphine milligram equivalents (MME)/d, and should avoid increasing dosage to ≥90 MME/d or carefully justify a decision to titrate dosage to ≥90 MME/d.

6 Long-term opioid use often begins with treatment of acute pain. When opioids are used for acute pain, clinicians should prescribe the lowest effective dose of immediate-release opioids and should prescribe no greater quantity than needed for the expected duration of pain severe enough to require opioids. Three days or less will often be sufficient; more than 7 days will rarely be needed.

7 Clinicians should evaluate benefits and harms with patients within 1-4 weeks of starting opioid therapy for chronic pain or of dose escalation. Clinicians should evaluate benefits and harms of continued therapy with patients every 3 months or more frequently. If benefits do not outweigh harms of continued opioid therapy, clinicians should optimize other therapies and work with patients to taper opioids to lower dosages or to taper and discontinue opioids.

TABLE II.1 CDC Recommendations for Prescribing Opioids for Chronic Pain Outside of Active Cancer, Palliative, and End-of-Life Care[a] *(Continued)*

Assessing Risk and Addressing Harms of Opioid Use

Recommendation(s)

8 Before starting and periodically during continuation of opioid therapy, clinicians should evaluate risk factors for opioid-related harms. Clinicians should incorporate into the management plan strategies to mitigate risk, including considering offering naloxone when factors that increase risk for opioid overdose, such as history of overdose, history of substance use disorder, higher opioid dosages (≥50 MME/d), or concurrent benzodiazepine use, are present.

9 Clinicians should review the patient's history of controlled substance prescriptions using state prescription drug monitoring program (PDMP) data to determine whether the patient is receiving opioid dosages or dangerous combinations that put him or her at high risk for overdose. Clinicians should review PDMP data when starting opioid therapy for chronic pain and periodically during opioid therapy for chronic pain, ranging from every prescription to every 3 months.

10 When prescribing opioids for chronic pain, clinicians should use urine drug testing before starting opioid therapy and consider urine drug testing at least annually to assess for prescribed medications as well as other controlled prescription drugs and illicit drugs.

11 Clinicians should avoid prescribing opioid pain medication and benzodiazepines concurrently whenever possible.

12 Clinicians should offer or arrange evidence-based treatment (usually medication-assisted treatment with buprenorphine or methadone in combination with behavioral therapies) for patients with opioid use disorder.

[a]All recommendations are category A (apply to all patients outside of active cancer treatment, palliative care, and end-of-life care) except recommendation 10 (designated category B, with individual decision-making required); see full guideline for evidence ratings.

See Table II.2 and Errata. 65(RR-1). *MMWR Morb Mortal Wkly Rep* 2016;65:295. DOI: http://dx.doi.org/10.15585/mmwr.mm6511a6externalicon for additional addendums and clarifications from the CDC regarding the guidelines.

From Dowell D, Haegerich TM, Chou R. CDC Guideline for Prescribing Opioids for Chronic Pain—United States, 2016. *MMWR Recomm Rep* 2016;65(RR-1):1–49. DOI: http://dx.doi.org/10.15585/mmwr.rr6501e1.

TABLE II.2 CDC Recommendations: Clarification Letter(s)[a]

April 9, 2019	• Guidelines are not intended for patients with cancer, sickle cell disease, or postop pain. • Guidelines are not designed to "deny any patients who suffer with chronic pain" the option of opioid medications. • Patients should not be denied coverage for their opioid.
April 10, 2019	*Per Robert Redfield:* • "CDC is working diligently to evaluate the impact of the Guideline and clarify its recommendations to help reduce unintended harms." • "The Guideline includes recommendations for clinicians to work with patients to taper or reduce dosage *only* when patient harm outweighs patient benefit of opioid therapy."

[a]In April of 2019, Robert Redfield released a statement that acknowledged that the 2016 CDC Guidelines were potentially causing patient harm.

From Errata. 65(RR-1). *MMWR Morb Mortal Wkly Rep* 2016;65:295. http://dx.doi.org/10.15585/mmwr.mm6511a6externalicon.

II. FSMB PRESCRIBING GUIDELINES

The goal of this Model Policy is to provide state medical and osteopathic boards with an updated guideline for assessing a clinician's management of pain, to determine whether opioid analgesics are used in a manner that is both medically appropriate and in compliance with applicable state and federal laws and regulations. The appropriate management of pain, particularly as related to the prescribing of opioid analgesics, may include (Table II.3).

TABLE II.3 FSMB Guidelines for the Chronic Use of Opioid Analgesics

	Guideline(s)	
ASSESS	**Adequate attention to initial assessment to determine if opioids are clinically indicated and to determine risks associated with their use in a particular individual with pain**	Not unlike many drugs used in medicine today, there are significant risks associated with opioids and therefore benefits must outweigh the risks.
MONITOR	**Adequate monitoring during the use of potentially abusable medications**	Opioids may be associated with substance use disorder and other dysfunctional behavioral problems, and some patients may benefit from opioid dose reductions or tapering or weaning off the opioid.
EDUCATE	**Adequate attention to patient education and informed consent**	The decision to begin opioid therapy for chronic pain is a shared decision of the clinician and patient after a discussion of the risks and a clear understanding that the clinical basis for the use of these medications for chronic pain is limited, that some pain may worsen with opioids, and taking opioids with other substances (such as benzodiazepines, alcohol, cannabis, or other central nervous system depressants) or certain conditions (eg, sleep apnea, mental illness, preexisting substance use disorder) may increase risk.
JUSTIFY	**Justified dose escalation with adequate attention to risks or alternative treatments**	Risks associated with opioids increase with escalating doses as well as in the setting of other comorbidities (ie, mental illness, respiratory disorders, preexisting substance use disorder and sleep apnea) and with concurrent use with respiratory depressants such as benzodiazepines or alcohol.

TABLE II.3 FSMB Guidelines for the Chronic Use of Opioid Analgesics (*Continued*)

	Guideline(s)	
AVOID	**Avoid excessive reliance on opioids, particularly high-dose opioids for chronic pain management**	It is strongly recommended that prescribers be prepared for risk.
UTILIZE	**Utilization of available tools for risk mitigations**	The state prescription drug monitoring program should be checked in advance of prescribing opioids and should be utilized for ongoing monitoring.

From Guidelines for the Chronic Use of Opioid Analgesics. April 2017. Federation of State Medical Boards (FSMB) website. https://www.fsmb.org/opioids/. Updated April 2017. Accessed October 7, 2019. With permission.

APPENDIX III

Drug Enforcement Administration (DEA) Drug Schedules

I. DEFINITION OF CONTROLLED SUBSTANCE SCHEDULES

Drugs and other substances that are considered controlled substances under the Controlled Substances Act (CSA) are divided into five schedules. An updated and complete list of the schedules is published annually in **Title 21 Code of Federal Regulations (C.F.R.) §§ 1308.11 through 1308.15**. Substances are placed in their respective schedules based on whether they have a currently accepted medical use in treatment in the United States, their relative abuse potential, and likelihood of causing dependence when abused. Some examples of the drugs in each schedule are listed in Table III.1.

TABLE II.1 DEA Controlled Substance Schedules and Definitions

Controlled Substances	Definition	Example(s)
Schedule I Controlled Substances	Substances in this schedule have no currently accepted medical use in the United States, a lack of accepted safety for use under medical supervision, and a high potential for abuse.	Heroin, lysergic acid diethylamide (LSD), marijuana (cannabis), peyote, methaqualone, and 3,4-methylenedioxymethamphetamine ("Ecstasy").
Schedule II/IIN Controlled Substances (2/2N)	Substances in this schedule have a high potential for abuse, which may lead to severe psychological or physical dependence.	*Examples of Schedule II narcotics include* hydromorphone (Dilaudid), methadone (Dolophine), meperidine (Demerol), oxycodone (OxyContin, Percocet), and fentanyl (Sublimaze, Duragesic). Other Schedule II narcotics include: morphine, opium, codeine, and hydrocodone. *Examples of Schedule IIN stimulants include* amphetamine (Dexedrine, Adderall), methamphetamine (Desoxyn), and methylphenidate (Ritalin). *Other Schedule II substances include* amobarbital, glutethimide, and pentobarbital.
Schedule III/IIIN Controlled Substances (3/3N)	Substances in this schedule have a potential for abuse less than substances in Schedules I or II and abuse may lead to moderate or low physical dependence or high psychological dependence.	*Examples of Schedule III narcotics include* products containing not more than 90 milligrams of codeine per dosage unit (Tylenol with Codeine), and buprenorphine (Suboxone). *Examples of Schedule IIIN non-narcotics include* benzphetamine (Didrex), phendimetrazine, ketamine, and anabolic steroids such as Depo-Testosterone.
Schedule IV Controlled Substances	Substances in this schedule have a low potential for abuse relative to substances in Schedule III.	Alprazolam (Xanax), carisoprodol (Soma), clonazepam (Klonopin), clorazepate (Tranxene), diazepam (Valium), lorazepam (Ativan), midazolam (Versed), temazepam (Restoril), and triazolam (Halcion).
Schedule V Controlled Substances	Substances in this schedule have a low potential for abuse relative to substances listed in Schedule IV and consist primarily of preparations containing limited quantities of certain narcotics.	Cough preparations containing not more than 200 mg of codeine per 100 mL or per 100 g (Robitussin AC, Phenergan with Codeine), and ezogabine.

From Controlled Substance Schedules. U.S. Department of Justice: Drug Enforcement Administration. https://www.deadiversion.usdoj.gov/schedules/. Updated August 2019. Accessed October 7, 2019.

APPENDIX V

Medications Commonly Used in Pain Practice

Paul Guillod and Gary J. Brenner

NOTE: This table provides a ready reference to the medications used in pain practice. The information provided is neither comprehensive nor complete and the reader is strongly encouraged to refer to the Physicians' Desk Reference (PDR), FDA labels, and other sources for a complete description of these medications.

Acetaminophen (**Tylenol**):

Description	Analgesic, antipyretic
Indications	Mild to moderate noninflammatory pain
Dosage	325-1000 mg PO every 4-6 h not to exceed 4000 mg total daily dose; generally, avoid or limit to 2000 mg/d in patients with liver disease or alcohol use disorder
Side Effects	Hepatotoxic in large doses causing severe, sometimes irreversible, acute liver failure
Precautions	Caution in presence of liver disease or alcohol use disorder; alcohol when combined with phenobarbital, may enhance hepatotoxicity; can interact with warfarin by prolonging INR

Acetylsalicylic acid, ASA (**Aspirin**) *see NSAIDs*
Almotriptan (**Axert**) *see Triptans*
Alprazolam (**Xanax**) *see Benzodiazepines*
Amitriptyline (**Elavil**) *see TCAs*
Baclofen (**Lioresal**):

Description	Skeletal muscle relaxant, antispastic; inhibits transmission of synaptic reflexes at the spinal cord level
Indications	Muscle spasticity, myofascial pain, trigeminal neuralgia
Dosage	Start at 5 mg PO 3 times daily; may increase by 5 mg every 3 d until adequate response; maximum of 40-80 mg/d Intrathecal administration used in cases of severe spasticity; if good, response to trial dose (usually 50-100 mcg) can be candidate for intrathecal pump
Side Effects	Drowsiness, confusion, hypotonia, nausea, headache, urinary retention
Precautions	Use with caution or avoid in elderly or patients with seizure disorders, respiratory disease, renal impairment (dose adjust), GI motility disorders; when used intrathecally, avoid abrupt discontinuation as will cause acute withdrawal symptoms

Benzodiazepines, BZDs:

Description	$GABA_A$ receptor agonist, sedative hypnotic, anxiolytic, amnestic, anticonvulsant, skeletal muscle relaxant

Indications	Chronic neuropathic pain with sleep disturbance, anxiety and restlessness, essential tremor, restless legs syndrome, burning mouth syndrome, palliative sedation Not a favorable drug class unless necessary and usually for short-term use
Dosage	Start at low dose initially given at bedtime; gradually increase dose and frequency every few days See **Table IV-4** for dosing of common benzodiazepines
Side Effects	Sedation, drowsiness, dizziness, memory impairment, change in appetite, constipation, xerostomia
Precautions	Avoid concomitant alcohol or other CNS depressant use; avoid or use with caution with elderly or patients with a history of substance use disorders, poor respiratory status, hepatic or renal disease (mostly hepatically metabolized); adjust dose gradually; counsel on risks for oversedation and dependence

Betamethasone *see Corticosteroids*

Botulinum toxin A (**Botox**):

Description	Neurotoxin, irreversibly blocks acetylcholine release at presynaptic neuromuscular junction
Indication	Migraines, cervical dystonia, spasticity, bladder dysfunction, cosmetic
Dosage	Given IM in various concentrations depending on indication and muscle site usually in 3-month intervals; limit to 400 units per 3-month period Migraine dosing: 5 units injected to 31 sites (155 units total)
Side Effects	Reaction at injection site, pruritus, muscle pain, stiffness, or weakness
Precautions	Potent neurotoxin, ensure proper application, spread of toxin can cause life-threatening respiratory compromise, diplopia, dysarthria, dysphagia; caution in patients with neuromuscular or respiratory disease

Buprenorphine, Buprenorphine/naloxone (**Suboxone, Belbuca, Subutex**):

Description	Opioid, partial μ-agonist with strong binding affinity, weak κ-antagonist
Indication	Acute and chronic pain, opioid dependence, opioid withdrawal
Dosage	Available in IV, IM, patch, SL spray, SL tablet, SL film, and buccal film with differences in bioavailability and dosing; when given PO usually combined with naloxone to reduce misuse by parenteral administration For chronic pain in opioid, naïve patients using buccal film (Belbuca) can start with 75 mcg once or twice daily and titrate up as needed up to 900 mcg twice daily
Side Effects	Drowsiness, dizziness, nausea, constipation, pruritus, headache, respiratory depression
Precautions	Can displace full agonist opioids precipitating pain or withdrawal symptoms; use with caution in elderly or in patients with hepatic disease, oral mucositis, respiratory disease, seizure disorders, or while on other CNS depressants; can cause QT prolongation

Bupropion (**Wellbutrin**):

Description	Antidepressant, norepinephrine, and dopamine reuptake inhibitor
Indication	Adjunct for neuropathic pain with depressive component, smoking cessation
Dosage	Start 150 mg PO daily, can increase after 1 wk to 300 mg daily (comes in immediate release and extended release forms)
Side Effects	Tachycardia, hypertension, CNS stimulation (insomnia, restlessness, agitation, and rarely seizures), headache, dizziness, xerostomia, constipation, nausea, blurred vision, weight loss
Precautions	Avoid use in patients with a history of seizure disorders or at high risk for seizures; adjust dose gradually

Butalbital-caffeine-acetaminophen (**Fioricet/Fiorinal**):

Description	Combination barbiturate (sedative), caffeine (stimulant thought to constrict cerebral blood vessels), and acetaminophen (analgesic)
Indications	Tension headaches, muscle contraction headaches, postdural puncture headaches (PDPH), mixed migraine headaches, menstrual and postpartum tension
Dosage	Take 1-2 capsules PO every 4 h up to 6 capsules per day; each capsule contains 50-mg butalbital, 300-mg acetaminophen, and 40-mg caffeine; some formulations also contain codeine
Side Effects	Dizziness, drowsiness, nausea, dyspnea
Precautions	Use with caution in elderly or patients with a history of alcohol or other substance use disorders, renal or liver disease, or porphyria; patients should track total acetaminophen dose; can cause rebound headaches with overuse; avoid concomitant CNS depressants

Capsaicin (**Zostrix, Bengay Heat, Capsugel, Qutenza**):

Description	Topical analgesic, antipruritic, antineuralgic
Indications	Arthritis, shingles, diabetic neuropathy
Dosage	Apply to affected areas (rub well) 3-4 times a day
Side Effects	Warm, burning feeling, stinging, redness
Precautions	Avoid contact with eyes or on other sensitive areas of the body (Note: Qutenza is not approved for home use)

Carbamazepine (**Tegretol**):

Description	Anticonvulsant, antineuralgic
Indications	Neuropathic pain, especially useful for trigeminal neuralgia
Dosage	Usually started at 100 mg PO twice daily, increased as needed by 200 mg/d up to a maximum of 1200 mg/d
Side Effects	Dizziness, drowsiness, nausea, blurred vision, pruritic rash, hyponatremia, rarely blood dyscrasias, LFT abnormalities
Precautions	Obtain baseline CBC and LFTs and subsequently monitor based on clinical judgment; use with caution in patients with history of bone marrow depression or liver dysfunction

Carisoprodol (**Soma**):

Description	Muscle relaxant (carbamate class), antispasmodic, central depressant, anxiolytic, sedative
Indication	Acute painful musculoskeletal conditions in conjunction with physical therapy
Dosage	250-350 mg PO up to 4 times daily, generally on a short-term (<1 month) basis
Side Effects	Drowsiness, dizziness, nausea, blurred vision, headache
Precautions	Caution in elderly, patients with a history of substance use disorders, renal or liver disease; can potentiate effect of opioids; slowly taper when discontinuing

Celecoxib (**Celebrex**):

Description	NSAID, selective COX-2 inhibitor
Indications	Pain with peripheral inflammatory component, arthritis, gout
Dosage	100-200 mg PO once or twice daily
Side Effects	Generally well tolerated with lower incidence of GI complications given selectivity; usual doses do not appear to affect platelet aggregation; renal toxicity similar to traditional NSAIDs
Precautions	Use with caution in elderly or patients with a history of GI bleeding, ischemic heart disease, fluid retention, renal impairment, or sulfonamide allergy; as with other NSAIDs, chronic use may increase risk of myocardial infarction or stroke

Chlordiazepoxide (**Librium**) *see Benzodiazepines*
Chlorpromazine (**Thorazine**):

Description	Phenothiazine derivative, 1st-generation antipsychotic, dopamine antagonist, antiemetic, sedative
Indication	Intractable hiccups, nausea, and vomiting
Dosage	10-50 mg PO or IM 3-4 times daily
Side Effects	Constipation, drowsiness, vision changes or dry mouth, extrapyramidal symptoms, rarely tardive dyskinesia
Precautions	Use with caution in elderly or patients with a seizure disorder or psychiatric illness, severe cardiovascular disease, renal or hepatic impairment, Reye syndrome, dementia

Chlorzoxazone (**Lorzone**):

Description	Muscle relaxant, antispasmodic, central depressant
Indication	Acute painful musculoskeletal conditions in conjunction with physical therapy, muscle contraction headache
Dosage	Start 250-500 mg PO 3 or 4 times daily; can increase dose up to 750 mg
Side Effects	Dizziness, drowsiness, nausea/vomiting, liver dysfunction
Precautions	Use with caution in elderly; discontinue for signs of liver impairment

Choline magnesium trisalicylate (**Trilisate**) *see NSAIDs*
Citalopram (**Celexa**) *see SSRIs*
Clomipramine (**Anafranil**) *see TCAs*
Clonazepam (**Klonopin**) *see Benzodiazepines*

Clonidine (**Catapres**):

Description	Central $\alpha 2$ agonist causing decreased sympathetic outflow; suppresses opioid withdrawal symptoms; adjunct analgesic
Indications	Neuropathic pain with sympathetic dependency, opioid withdrawal, nicotine withdrawal
Dosage	Oral, transdermal, and neuraxial formulations used for pain PO: Start at 0.1 mg 2-3 times daily and gradually escalate by 0.1-0.2 mg/d every few days up to a maximum daily 1.2 mg; Transdermal: Start 0.1 mg/24 h patch and increase strength by 0.1 mg in weekly intervals Epidural: 2-10 mcg/kg (150-800 mcg for a normal adult) bolus, and 10-40 mcg/h continuous infusion Spinal: 10-30 mcg bolus
Side Effects	Drowsiness, dizziness, headache, bradycardia, hypotension, xerostomia, abdominal pain, urinary incontinence, skin rash
Precautions	Use with caution in patients with cardiac dysrhythmias, renal impairment; abrupt discontinuation can cause rebound hypertension

Codeine *see Opioids*

Corticosteroids:

Description	Anti-inflammatory (referring to glucocorticoid activity)
Indications	Suppression of inflammatory and allergic disorders such as asthma, COPD, rheumatic diseases, and other inflammatory pain disorders; often used for epidural, intra-articular, or nerve root injections
Dosage	See **Table IV-7** for dosing
Side Effects	Dizziness, nausea, dyspepsia, increased appetite/weight gain, edema, heart failure, weakness/myopathy, headache, insomnia, agitation, skin atrophy, glucose intolerance, adrenal suppression
Precautions	Use with caution in elderly or patients with heart failure, poorly controlled hypertension, diabetes, GI disorders, hepatic disease, glaucoma, renal impairment, or osteoporosis

Cyclobenzaprine (**Flexeril**):

Description	Skeletal muscle relaxant; structurally and pharmacologically related to TCAs
Indications	Myofascial pain in conjunction with physical therapy, usually short-term effect
Dosage	Start 10 mg PO 3 times per day; gradually increase to maximum of 60 mg daily in divided doses
Side Effects	Drowsiness, dizziness, xerostomia
Precautions	Caution in elderly or patients with liver disease; monitor for anticholinergic side effects; like TCAs can precipitate serotonin syndrome when combined with serotonergic drugs

Dantrolene (**Dantrium**):

Description	Skeletal muscle relaxant (postsynaptic), antispastic, ryanodine receptor antagonist that inhibits calcium release from sarcoplasmic reticulum
Indication	Chronic muscle spasticity, malignant hyperthermia
Dosage	25 mg PO once daily for 1 wk, followed by 25 mg 3 times daily for 1 wk, then 50 mg 3 times daily, continuing up to a maximum of 400 mg daily in 4 doses of 100 mg; use lowest effective dose or discontinue if escalating doses not showing any benefit
Side Effects	Flushing, drowsiness, dizziness, weakness, dysphagia, dysphonia, dyspnea, hepatitis, blurry vision, photosensitivity
Precautions	Avoid in patients with active liver disease given hepatotoxicity risk

Desipramine (**Norpramin**) *see TCAs*
Desvenlafaxine (**Pristiq**) *see SNRIs*
Dexamphetamine (**Dexedrine**):

Description	CNS stimulant, sympathomimetic, stimulates norepinephrine and dopamine release and may block catecholamine reuptake as well
Indications	Excessive sedation due to opioids, especially in patients with cancer; primary indications: ADHD, narcolepsy
Dosage	Following a 2.5-mg test dose can start with 5 PO once to twice daily; can increase up to 20 mg/d
Side Effects	Nervousness, insomnia, anorexia, tachycardia/palpitations
Precautions	Tolerance and dependence may occur; caution with history of substance use disorder, seizure disorder, psychiatric disorder, or while already on a stimulant; contraindicated in presence of uncontrolled hypertension or other significant cardiovascular disease, hyperthyroidism, agitated states

Dextromethorphan (**Benylin, Robitussin**):

Description	Antitussive, weak analgesic, structurally similar to codeine; at high doses has NMDA antagonism producing dissociative effect
Indications	Combined with opioids to decrease the development of tolerance; second-line medication for neuropathic pain
Dosage	30 mg PO every 6-8 h; can increase dose up to 90 mg PO every 8 h
Side Effects	Dizziness, drowsiness, nausea/vomiting
Precautions	Not for use for persistent cough related to asthma, chronic bronchitis, emphysema, or smoking; when combined with serotonergic drugs increases risk of serotonin syndrome

Diazepam (**Valium**) *see Benzodiazepines*
Diclofenac sodium (**Voltaren**) *see NSAIDs*
Dihydroergotamine (**Ergomar, Ergostat**):

Description	Antimigraine, ergot alkaloid; activates 5-$HT1_D$ receptors causing vasoconstriction of intracranial vessels; also interacts with adrenergic and dopamine receptors

Indications	Abortion of severe, throbbing headaches including migraine (classic with aura and common without aura) and cluster headaches; orthostatic hypotension
Dosage	Intranasal: One 0.5-mg spray in each nostril; repeat 15 min later for total of 4 sprays (2 mg); can take up to 3 mg/d and 6 mg/wk IM, SC: 1 mg every hour up to 3 mg/d and 6 mg/wk IV: 1 mg every hour up to 2 mg/d and 6 mg/wk Often premeditated with antiemetic
Side Effects	Nausea/vomiting, dizziness, drowsiness, rhinitis, dysgeusia; rarely cerebrovascular events or pleural fibrosis with excessive use
Precautions	Avoid in patients with uncontrolled hypertension, severe liver or kidney disease, following vascular surgery, ischemic heart disease/history of MI; should not be taken within 24 h of a triptan as increases risk of coronary vasospasm

Diphenhydramine (**Benadryl**):

Description	Antihistamine (H_1) 1st generation, antiemetic, anticholinergic, sedative
Indications	Nausea, pruritus, rhinitis, motion sickness, insomnia
Dosage	PO: 25-50 mg every 4-8 h up to 300 mg/d IV/IM: 10-50 mg every 4-6 h up to 400 mg/d
Side Effects	Drowsiness, dizziness, xerostomia, urinary retention, constipation
Precautions	Use with caution in elderly given sedation and anticholinergic effects

Doxepin (**Silenor, Prudoxin**) *see TCAs*
Dronabinol (**Marinol**):

Description	Cannabinoid, CB_1 and CB_2 receptor agonist, antiemetic
Indications	Nausea associated with chemotherapy, anorexia
Dosage	2.5-5 mg PO twice daily or as needed for nausea
Side Effects	Flushing, tachycardia, nausea, multiple CNS effects including euphoria, dizziness, drowsiness, confusion, amnesia
Precautions	Caution given intoxication effects and for patients with significant cardiovascular disease

Duloxetine (**Cymbalta**) *see SNRIs*
Eletriptan (**Relpax**) *see Triptans*
Etodolac (**Lodine**) *see NSAIDs*
Fenoprofen (**Nalfon**) *see NSAIDs*
Fentanyl (**Duragesic, Actiq**) see Opioids
Fluoxetine (**Prozac**) *see SSRIs*
Flurbiprofen (**Ansaid**) *see NSAIDs*
Frovatriptan (**Frova**) *see Triptans*
Gabapentin (**Neurontin**):

Description	Anticonvulsant, adjunct antineuralgic
Indications	Neuropathic pain, postherpetic neuralgia, fibromyalgia, restless legs syndrome, chronic refractory cough, hiccups, alcohol withdrawal
Dosage	Start 100-300 mg 1-3 times daily, starting at night; gradually increase dose every few days up to a maximum of 1200 mg 3 times daily (3.6 g daily); beneficial effects can be delayed until after 1-3 wk of therapy

Side Effects Dizziness, drowsiness; generally well tolerated

Precautions Gradually taper at discontinuation; caution in patients with substance use disorders; dose reduce in renal disease

Haloperidol (**Haldol**):

Description Butyrophenone antipsychotic (D_2 antagonist), antiemetic, sedative

Indications Nausea/vomiting, behavioral disorders (agitation, delirium, psychosis)

Dosage Generally around 0.5-5 mg PO 2-3 times daily depending on indication

Side Effects Drowsiness, dizziness, headache, dry mouth, restlessness, extrapyramidal symptoms (rare in oral formulation), blood dyscrasias, orthostatic hypotension

Precautions Contraindicated in Parkinson disease; caution in patients with severe cardiovascular disease, dementia, thyroid dysfunction, or taking other CNS depressants

Hydrocortisone (**Cortef, Solu-Cortef**) *see Corticosteroids*
Hydromorphone (**Dilaudid**) *see Opioids*
Hydrocodone *see Opioids*
Hydroxyzine (**Atarax, Vistaril**):

Description Antihistamine (H_1) 1st generation, antiemetic, anxiolytic, mild analgesic

Indications Pruritus, nausea, anxiety, sleep disorder

Dosage 25-100 mg PO/IM up to 4 times daily

Side Effects Drowsiness, dizziness, xerostomia, urinary retention—generally lower frequency of anticholinergic effects relative to other 1st-generation antihistamines

Precautions Use with caution in elderly given sedating effects

Ibuprofen (**Advil**) *see NSAIDs*
Imipramine (**Tofranil**) *see TCAs*
Indomethacin (**Tivorbex**) *see NSAIDs*
Ketamine (**Ketalar**):

Description NMDA receptor antagonist (many other mechanisms postulated), modulates central sensitization; dissociative, analgesic, sedative, antidepressant; formulations include IV, IM, intranasal, oral

Indication Acute pain, chronic neuropathic pain such as CRPS, postherpetic neuralgia; depression, PTSD, phantom limb pain, chronic ischemic pain, fibromyalgia, depression

Dosage Chronic pain dosing protocol varies between practice, setting, and pain etiology; common starting outpatient IV infusion 0.2-0.5 mg/kg over 2 h

To reduce psychotropic side effects often coadministered with a benzodiazepine or an α2 agonist

Side Effects Psychomimetic (dysphoria, hallucinations), nausea, headache

Precautions Caution or avoid in patients with active substance use disorder, psychosis, or elevated ICP states; requires close monitoring

Ketoprofen (**Orudis**) *see NSAIDs*
Ketorolac (**Toradol**):

Description	Potent injectable NSAID
Indications	Acute postoperative pain, acute inflammatory pain; recommended for short-term use up to 5 d; IV, IM, and oral formulations
Dosage	IV/IM: 15-30 mg every 6 h up to 120 mg daily PO: 10 mg every 6 h up to 40 mg daily Lower dose for elderly, low weight patients (<50 kg), or in renal disease
Side Effects	Headache, nausea, dyspepsia, dizziness, prolonged bleeding time
Precautions	Contraindicated in patients with recent GI bleed/perforation; caution in patients with hematologic, cardiovascular, GI, or renal dysfunction

Lactulose (**Constulose**):

Description	Laxative, osmotic
Indication	Constipation; also used in hepatic encephalopathy for ammonia lowering effect
Dosage	Start with 10-20 g PO once daily and increase for effect up to 40 g daily in divided doses
Side Effects	Dehydration, abdominal cramps, nausea/vomiting, flatulence, hypokalemia, hyponatremia
Precautions	Caution in patients with diabetes (contains galactose and lactose) or with concern for intestinal obstruction

Lamotrigine (**Lamictal**):

Description	Anticonvulsant, antineuralgic; inhibits release of glutamate by acting on voltage-gated sodium channels
Indications	Neuropathic pain; beneficial effects may be slow to occur, as dose escalations are gradual
Dosage	Start 25 mg PO daily for 2 wk; can increase to 50 mg daily for 2 wk, continuing to increase by 50 mg each week if needed until a maximum dose of 200 mg PO twice daily
Side Effects	Somnolence, dizziness, ataxia, visual changes, nausea, serious skin rash (rarely SJS or TEN), blood dyscrasias; rapid dose escalation increases risk of rash
Precautions	Discontinue if rash develops; dose adjustment required with concomitant anticonvulsant medications; caution and reduce dose in renal or hepatic dysfunction; do not discontinue abruptly

Levetiracetam (**Keppra**):

Description	Anticonvulsant, antineuralgic; exact mechanism unclear, inhibits voltage-gated calcium channels, facilitates GABA transmission
Indications	Antiepileptic drug potentially useful for treatment of neuropathic pain

Dosage	Start 500 mg PO twice daily; can increase each dose by 500 mg every 2 wk to a maximum of 1500 mg twice daily (3000 mg daily) if needed
Side Effects	Drowsiness, fatigue, irritability, increased blood pressure (in children), nausea/vomiting, infection, and very rarely a serious skin reaction (SJS/TEN)
Precautions	Gradually reduce dose at discontinuation; caution and reduce dose in renal dysfunction

Levorphanol (**Levo-Dromoran**) *see Opioids*
Lidocaine (**Xylocaine, Lidoderm 5% patch**):

Description	Local anesthetic, class 1b antiarrhythmic Formulations include patch, ointment, oral gel, infusion, eutectic mixture
Indications	Itching and pain in disorders such as postherpetic neuralgia, diabetic neuropathy, burns; irritation and inflammation in the mouth and throat; can be diagnostic for neuropathic pain as an infusion; also used in joint injections
Dosage	Neuropathic pain diagnosis: prepare 1-5 mg/kg in 20-100 mL of saline and infuse over 20-60 min Patch: Apply 12 h on and 12 h off to avoid tachyphylaxis Topical: apply to affected areas 1-4 times daily
Side Effects	Stinging, burning, redness, tenderness, swelling, or rash
Precautions	Caution giving as infusion in patients with hepatic impairment, heart failure, respiratory depression, or with heart conduction abnormalities; generally well tolerated

Lorazepam (**Ativan**) *see Benzodiazepines*
Meclofenamate (**Meclomen**) *see NSAIDs*
Mefenamic acid (**Ponstel**) *see NSAIDs*
Meloxicam (**Mobic**) see NSAIDs
Meperidine (**Demerol**) *see Opioids*
Metaxalone (**Skelaxin, Metaxall**):

Description	Muscle relaxant, central depressant, antispasmodic
Indications	Acute painful musculoskeletal conditions in conjunction with physical therapy
Dosage	400-800 mg PO 3 or 4 times daily
Side Effects	Dizziness, drowsiness, paradoxical stimulation, abdominal pain, nausea, headache, nervousness, and rarely blood dyscrasias
Precautions	Use with caution in patients with impaired liver or renal function; contraindicated in patients with history of drug-induced anemias

Methadone *see Opioids*
Methocarbamol (**Robaxin**):

Description	Muscle relaxant, central depressant, antispasmodic
Indication	Acute painful musculoskeletal conditions in conjunction with physical therapy

Dosage	750-1500 mg PO 3 or 4 times daily; generally limit to 4500 mg/d after initial 3 d
Side Effects	Drowsiness, dizziness, nausea, flushing, vision changes
Precautions	Use with caution in the elderly and in patients with renal or hepatic impairment, seizure disorder, or who are taking other sedating medications

Methylphenidate (**Ritalin**):

Description	CNS stimulant; blocks reuptake of dopamine and norepinephrine similarly to amphetamines
Indications	Excessive sedation due to opioids, especially in patients with cancer
Dosage	5-10 mg PO in the morning; may increase by 5-10 mg weekly up to 60 mg/d in 2 or 3 doses
Side Effects	Nervousness, insomnia, headache, decreased appetite, nausea, xerostomia, tachycardia, rarely leukopenias
Precautions	Use with caution in patients with seizure disorders, psychiatric disorders, or significant cardiovascular disease; contraindicated in patients taking MAOIs, glaucoma, or significant anxiety/agitation; risk for dependence and tolerance; perform periodic blood counts during prolonged therapy

Methylprednisolone (**Medrol, Solu-Medrol, Depo-Medrol**) *see Corticosteroids*

Methyl salicylate-menthol (**BenGay, Icy Hot, Salonpas**):

Description	Topical analgesic, salicylate; available in balm, cream, spray, stick, foam
Indication	Mild to moderate superficial joint and muscular pain
Dosage	Apply topically to affected area 3 or 4 times per day; patches can be placed for up to 8 h
Side Effects	Skin irritation, rash
Precautions	Avoid when patient has allergy to aspirin or other salicylates

Metoclopramide (**Reglan**):

Description	Dopamine antagonist, antiemetic, peristaltic stimulant
Indications	Nausea and emesis
Dosage	10 mg PO up to 4 times daily; also has IV, IM formulations
Side Effects	Restlessness, drowsiness, anxiety, headache, extrapyramidal symptoms, rarely tardive dyskinesia
Precautions	Contraindicated in seizure disorders and in setting of GI obstruction, perforation, or hemorrhage

Mexiletine (**Mexitil**):

Description	Class 1b antiarrhythmic, sodium channel blocker
Indication	Adjunct medication for neuropathic pain
Dosage	Start at 150 mg PO nightly; gradually increase dose and frequency up to 3 times daily up to total 900 mg/d
Side Effects	Nausea, dizziness, tremor, nervousness, confusion, headache, fatigue, depression, tachycardia

Precautions	Use with caution in patients with cardiac disease, especially congestive heart failure, a history of seizures or with allergies to amide-type anesthetics (eg, lidocaine, tocainide)

Milnacipran (**Savella**) *see SNRIs*
Modafinil (**Provigil**):

Description	CNS stimulant, wakefulness promoting agent
Indications	Useful for excessive sedation due to opioids, especially in patients with cancer; commonly used for narcolepsy, sleep apnea, shift work sleep disorder
Dosage	Start at 100 mg PO every morning; may increase up to 400 mg as tolerated; usual dosage 200 mg daily
Side Effects	Headache, nausea, decreased appetite, anxiety, insomnia
Precautions	Caution with history of psychiatric illness or significant cardiac disease such as poorly controlled hypertension, mitral valve prolapse, or ventricular hypertrophy; reduce dose in renal or liver disease and in elderly

Morphine (**MS Contin, Duramorph, and others**) see Opioids
Naratriptan (**Amerge**) *see Triptans*
Naloxegol (**Movantik**):

Description	Peripheral acting μ-opioid receptor antagonist
Indication	Opioid-induced constipation
Dosage	12.5-25 mg PO daily
Side Effects	Abdominal pain, diarrhea, nausea
Precautions	Avoid use in patients with severe liver disease or gastrointestinal obstruction; discontinue other laxatives before starting

Naloxone (**Narcan**):

Description	Opioid receptor antagonist
Indication	Reversal of opioid effects
Dosage	IV 0.02-0.04 mg every 2-3 min titrated to effect; avoid high doses to prevent complete reversal of opiate effects; in emergency situations, use higher doses 0.4-2 mg every 2-3 min to a maximum of 10 mg; infusions may be required to prevent renarcotization Orally 1.2-2.4 mg every 4-6 h until the first bowel movement or to a maximum of 5 mg for reversing opioid-induced constipation Intranasal 4 mg per actuation. Can be repeated every 2-3 min, if desired clinical effect is not obtained
Side Effects	Acute cardiovascular and CNS excitability caused by rapid reversal of opioid effects, acute withdrawal symptoms
Precautions	Use low doses and titrate to effect; use with caution in the presence of opioid dependence as will precipitate withdrawal

Naproxen (**Aleve, Naprosyn, Anaprox, Midol**) see NSAIDs
Nortriptyline (**Pamelor**) *see TCAs*

NSAIDs (Nonsteroidal anti-inflammatory drugs):

Description Nonsteroidal anti-inflammatory analgesic; decreases synthesis of inflammatory prostaglandins by inhibition of cyclooxygenase (COX); divided into nonspecific (COX-1/COX-2) and selective COX-2 inhibitors (coxibs)

Indications First-line medications in mild to moderate pain, especially musculoskeletal; valuable adjunct in severe pain by modulating the peripheral inflammatory cascade; opioid sparing; CNS effects not clearly elucidated

Dosage See **Table IV-1** for dosing of commonly used NSAIDs

Side Effects Prostaglandin inhibition leading to decreased platelet adhesion, gastric mucosal damage with or without GI bleeding, and renal function impairment; coxibs are associated with less gastrointestinal risk given selectivity

Precautions Avoid or use with caution in elderly patients, in the presence of gastrointestinal ulcers or bleeding, cardiovascular disease (heart failure, coronary disease), coagulopathies, renal disease, or while concurrently taking blood thinners; NSAID use is associated with an increased risk of heart attack, heart failure, and stroke; use lowest effective dose

TABLE IV.1 Commonly Used Oral NSAIDs

Generic Name	Trade Name	Adult Oral Dosage		Max Daily Dose
Acetylsalicylic acid	Aspirin	325-975 mg	q4-6h	4000 mg
Celecoxib	Celebrex	100-200 mg	q12h	400 mg
Choline magnesium trisalicylate	Trilisate	500-750 mg	q8-12h	3000 mg
Diclofenac	Voltaren	25-75 mg	q8-12h	100 mg
Diflunisal	Dolobid	250-500 mg	q8-12h	1500 mg
Etodolac	Lodine	200-400 mg	q6-8h	1000 mg
Fenoprofen	Nalfon	200 mg	q4-6h	3200 mg
Flurbiprofen	Ansaid	50-100 mg	q6-12h	300 mg
Ibuprofen	Motrin	200-800 mg	q6-8h	3200 mg
Indomethacin	Indocin	25-50 mg	q8-12h	200 mg
Ketoprofen	Orudis	25-75 mg	q6-8h	300 mg
Ketorolac	Toradol	10 mg	q6-8h	40 mg
Meclofenamate	Meclomen	50-100 mg	q4-6h	400 mg
Mefenamic acid	Ponstel	250 mg	q6h	1000 mg
Meloxicam	Mobic	5-15 mg	q24h	15 mg
Naproxen	Naprosyn	250-500 mg	q6-12h	1000 mg
Naproxen sodium	Anaprox, Aleve	220-550 mg	q6-12h	1100 mg
Oxaprozin	Daypro	600-1800 mg	q24h	1800 mg
Piroxicam	Feldene	10-20 mg	qd	20 mg
Salsalate	Disalcid	500 mg	q4h	3000 mg
Sulindac	Clinoril	150-200 mg	q12h	400 mg
Tolmetin	Tolectin	200-600 mg	q8h	1800 mg

Ondansetron (**Zofran**):

Description	5-HT_3 receptor antagonist, antiemetic
Indications	Nausea and emesis commonly associated with chemotherapy, radiation, PONV, carcinoid syndrome, vertigo
Dosage	PO: 4-8 mg every 8-12 h IV: 4 mg every 6 h; higher doses used for patients undergoing chemotherapy or radiation treatment
Side Effects	Headache, fatigue, constipation, diarrhea; generally well tolerated and effective
Precautions	Rapid intravenous injections may increase the risk for headache

Opioids:

Description	Ligands at endogenous opioid receptors; opium constituents (eg, morphine, codeine, and thebaine) or their derivatives (eg, hydromorphone, hydrocodone, buprenorphine, and oxycodone) or synthetic (eg, levorphanol, methadone, meperidine, and fentanyl)
Indications	Potent analgesics for severe pain including postoperative pain and cancer pain; controversial and generally effective for limited time in chronic nonpalliative/noncancer pain
Dosage	See **Table IV-2** for dosing of common opioid medications Many formulations exist including PO, IM, SC, transdermal, IV, nasal, sublingual, epidural, intrathecal; start at lowest dose and gradually titrate to effect; add adjuncts for opioid-sparing effects; tolerance to analgesic effects and to side effects is common; use long-acting opioids for background analgesia and short-acting opioids for breakthrough or incidental pain Rotate opioid if excessive tolerance develops; new opioid can be started at half to one-fourth of the calculated equivalent dose of the new opioid because of incomplete cross-tolerance Approximate conversion ratio for intrathecal: epidural:IV:PO is 1:10:100:300; avoid rapid or frequent dose escalations in chronic nonterminal pain
Side Effects	Respiratory depression, sedation, euphoria, dysphoria, weakness, agitation, seizure, nausea, constipation, biliary spasm, urinary retention, sweating, flushing, bradycardia, tolerance, physical dependence, and addiction
Precautions	Use with caution in elderly patients, opioid naive patients, respiratory disease, infants, hepatic or renal disease, patients with history of drug abuse, patients performing tasks requiring high mental alertness, or with concomitant use of other CNS depressants such as benzodiazepines

TABLE IV.2 Standard Doses of Commonly Used Opioids

Generic Name	Formulation	Trade Name(s)	MME[a]	Duration	PO:IV	Starting Regimen[b]	
Buprenorphine	SL tablet[c]	Subutex, Suboxone[d]	30	~1 d	—	2-4 mg PO	q24h
	Patch (mcg/h)	Butrans	12.6	7 d	—	5 mcg/h	q7d
	Buccal film (mcg)	Belbuca	0.03	12 h	—	75 mcg	q12-24h
Codeine	Tablet, solution	—	0.15	4-6 h	2-3:1	15-60 mg PO	q4h
Fentanyl	Patch (mcg/h)	Duragesic	2.4	3 d	2:1	25 mcg/h	q72h
	Film, lozenge	Actiq	0.18	2-4 h	—	200 mcg	q4h
Hydrocodone	Tablet[e]	Vicodin, Lorcet, Lortab, Norco	1	3-6 h	—	2.5-10 mg	q4-6h
Hydromorphone	Tablet	Dilaudid	4	3-4 h	5:1	2-4 mg PO	q4-6h
Levorphanol	Tablet	Levo-Dromoran	11	6-12 h	2:1	1-2 mg	q6-8h
Meperidine	Tablet	Demerol	0.1	2-4 h	3-4:1	50-100 mg	q3-4h
Methadone	Tablet	Dolophine	4-12[f]	4-12 h	3:1	2.5-5 mg PO	q8-12h
Morphine	Tablet (IR)	MS-IR	1	3-6 h	3:1	5-10 mg PO	q3-4h
	Tablet (ER)	MS Contin, Kadian	1	8-12 h		15 mg PO	q8-12h
Oxycodone	Tablet (IR)	Percocet, Percodan	1.5	3-4 h	—	5-15 mg PO	q3-4h
	Tablet (ER)	OxyContin, Xtampza ER	1.5	8-12 h	—	10 mg PO	q8-12h
Oxymorphone	Tablet	Opana	3	3-6 h	10:1	5-10 mg PO	q4-6h
Tramadol	Tablet	Ultram	0.1	6 h	—	25-50 mg PO	q4-6

[a]MME = morphine milligram equivalents; conversion numbers adapted from CDC.
[b]For opioid naïve patients.
[c]Generally used for opioid withdrawal/dependence.
[d]Combined with naloxone.
[e]Combination formula with acetaminophen.
[f]Nonlinear, as dose increases so does equivalent morphine dose.

Orphenadrine (**Norflex**):

Description	Muscle relaxant, anticholinergic with central effect
Indications	Muscle spasms
Dosage	100 mg PO twice daily
Side Effects	Tachycardia, agitation, drowsiness, confusion, pruritus, nausea
Precautions	Avoid in elderly given anticholinergic effects and patients with significant cardiac disease, GI obstruction, glaucoma

Oxaprozin (**Daypro**) *see NSAIDs*
Oxcarbazepine (**Trileptal**):

Description	Anticonvulsant, antineuralgic
Indications	Neuropathic pain
Dosage	Start at 150 mg PO twice daily; may increase daily dose by 300 mg every 5 d up to a maximum of 900 mg twice daily (1800 mg daily)
Side Effects	Dizziness, drowsiness, headache, ataxia, diplopia, vertigo, nausea/vomiting, hyponatremia/SIADH; generally well tolerated
Precautions	Reduce dose in elderly and patients with renal impairment; monitor for fluid retention and sodium changes in patients with heart failure; discontinue gradually to reduce chance of a withdrawal associated seizure

Oxycodone (**Roxicodone, Norco, Xtampza ER, Oxycontin**) *see Opioids*
Oxycodone-acetaminophen (**Percocet**) *see Opioids*
Oxycodone-aspirin (**Percodan**) *see Opioids*
Oxymorphone (**Opana**) *see Opioids*
Paroxetine (**Paxil**) *see SSRIs*
Perphenazine (**Trilafon**):

Description	Phenothiazine derivative, 1st-generation antipsychotic, dopamine antagonist, antiemetic
Indications	Nausea/vomiting
Dosage	Start 4 mg PO 1-4 times daily; can titrate up to 24 mg daily; use lowest effective dose
Side Effects	Constipation, sedation, vision changes, xerostomia, extrapyramidal symptoms, rarely tardive dyskinesia
Precautions	Use with caution in elderly or patients with a seizure disorder, severe cardiovascular disease, renal or hepatic impairment, dementia

Phenoxybenzamine (**Dibenzyline**):

Description	α-Adrenergic antagonist, nonselective
Indications	Sympathetically mediated pain such as in CRPS; micturition disorders; commonly used in patients with pheochromocytomas
Dosage	Start at 10 mg PO 1-3 times daily; increase by 10 mg every 2 d, titrating to effect; maximum dose 120 mg/d
Side Effects	Hypotension, fatigue, congestion, headaches, tachycardia
Precautions	Use with caution in the elderly especially with a history of falls or significant cardiovascular disease

Phentolamine (**Regitine**):

Description	α-Adrenergic antagonist, nonselective
Indications	Diagnostic IV injection in suspected sympathetically mediated/maintained pain
Dosage	Infuse 35-70 mg over 20 min; preload with 500-mL crystalloid solution before infusion and pretreat with propranolol for preventing reflex tachycardia
Side Effects	Hypotension, dizziness, reflex tachycardia, syncope
Precautions	Monitor heart rate and blood pressure during treatment, pretreat as above, and have resuscitation equipment available

Phenytoin (**Dilantin**):

Description	Anticonvulsant, adjunct antineuralgic; voltage-gated sodium channel blocker
Indications	Neuropathic pain, trigeminal neuralgia
Dosage	100 mg PO 3 times daily
Side Effects	Constipation, dizziness, drowsiness, nausea, mood changes or confusion, slurred speech, rash, insomnia, headache, rarely blood dyscrasias
Precautions	Requires therapeutic drug monitoring; caution in patients with porphyria, liver disease, diabetes, hypothyroidism, renal impairment, or cardiac arrhythmias

Piroxicam (**Feldene**) *see NSAIDs*

Pregabalin (**Lyrica**):

Description	GABA analogue similar to gabapentin; anticonvulsant, anxiolytic, sedative; binds $\alpha_2\delta$ subunit of voltage-gated calcium channels in the CNS and inhibits release of excitatory neurotransmitters
Indication	Neuropathic pain such as in postherpetic neuralgia, diabetic neuropathy, or spinal cord injury; also used in fibromyalgia, neuropathic pruritus, restless legs syndrome, migraine prevention
Dosage	Start from 25 to 150 mg PO daily divided into 2 or 3 doses; based on response and tolerance can increase by 150 mg daily in 1 wk intervals up to a maximum of 600 mg daily; available in immediate and extended release formulations; adjust dose based on renal function
Side Effects	Dizziness, drowsiness, peripheral edema, headache, constipation, weight gain, xerostomia; rarely angioedema or rhabdomyolysis; generally well tolerated
Precautions	Gradually taper at discontinuation over at least 1 wk to avoid withdrawal effects; use with caution in patients with cardiovascular disease (especially heart failure), renal impairment (dose adjust), substance use disorders, or while on other sedating medications

Prednisolone see Corticosteroids

Prochlorperazine (**Compazine**):

Description	Phenothiazine derivative, 1st-generation antipsychotic, antiemetic
Indications	Nausea and vomiting
Dosage	5-10 mg PO or IM 3 or 4 times per day up to a maximum of 40 mg daily; IV 2.5-10 mg every 3-4 h up to 40 mg/d

Side Effects	Drowsiness, dizziness, constipation, xerostomia, extrapyramidal symptoms, rarely tardive dyskinesia
Precautions	Use with caution in elderly or patients with a seizure disorder, severe cardiovascular disease, renal or hepatic impairment, Reye syndrome, dementia

Promethazine (**Phenergan**):

Description	Phenothiazine derivative, antiemetic, antihistamine, sedative
Indications	Nausea and vomiting, motion sickness
Dosage	12.5-25 mg PO every 4 h up to 100 mg/d; also in IV, IM formulation
Side Effects	Dizziness, drowsiness, xerostomia, vision changes, extrapyramidal symptoms, leukopenia, obstructive jaundice
Precautions	Use with caution with cardiovascular or hepatic disease and in the presence of other CNS depressants

Propranolol (**Inderal**):

Description	Nonselective β blocker
Indications	Essential tremor, performance anxiety, migraine prophylaxis
Dosage	Start 10-20 mg PO every 4-6 h as needed; can titrate up to 240 mg daily
Side Effects	Bradycardia, hypotension, bronchospasm
Precautions	Caution in patients with asthma or significant heart disease with conduction abnormalities; can mask symptoms of hypoglycemia in patients with diabetes

Protriptyline (**Vivactil**) *see TCAs*
Rizatriptan (**Maxalt**) *see Triptans*
Ropinirole (**Requip**):

Description	Nonergot dopamine agonist, anti-Parkinson agent
Indications	Restless legs syndrome (RLS)
Dosage	0.25 mg PO once daily 1-3 h before bed; can increase by 0.25 mg every 2-3 d up to 4 mg maximum (3 mg maximum for patients with ESRD); average dose tends to be around 2 mg
Side Effects	Drowsiness, orthostatic hypotension, fatigue, nausea, constipation
Precautions	Use with caution in patients with cardiovascular, hepatic, or renal disease; evaluate iron stores before prescribing; can paradoxically provoke augmentation, or worsening, of symptoms with increasing doses; gradually taper at discontinuation

Salsalate (**Disalcid**) *see NSAIDs*
Senna (**Senokot**):

Description	Laxative
Indication	Constipation
Dosage	1-2 tablets once or twice daily; also comes as syrup; generally works within 1 d
Side Effects	Abdominal cramps, diarrhea, nausea, bloating
Precautions	Use with caution in patients with abdominal pain; generally well tolerated

Sertraline (**Zoloft**) *see SSRIs*

SNRIs, Serotonin and norepinephrine reuptake inhibitors:

Description	Antidepressant, potent inhibitor of serotonin and norepinephrine reuptake and weak inhibitor of dopamine reuptake
Indications	Antidepressant medication useful for migraine prophylaxis and potentially useful as adjuvant neuropathic pain medication
Dosage	See **Table IV-3** for dosing of commonly used SNRIs
Side Effects	Hypertension, insomnia, nervousness, gastrointestinal intolerance, anorexia, activation of mania, vivid dreams, acute angle-closure glaucoma, sexual dysfunction, sweating, cholesterol elevation
Precautions	Use with caution in patients with history of seizures; reduce dose in renal or hepatic dysfunction; check cholesterol with long-term treatment

TABLE IV.3 Commonly Used Antidepressants

Category	Generic Name	Trade Name	Starting Daily Dose	Max Daily Dose
TCA	Amitriptyline[a]	Elavil	10-25 mg	150 mg
	Clomipramine[a]	Anafranil	25 mg	100 mg
	Desipramine[a]	Norpramin	12.5-25 mg	300 mg
	Doxepin	Sinequan	25-50 mg	300 mg
	Imipramine[a]	Tofranil	10-50 mg	150 mg
	Nortriptyline[a]	Pamelor	10-25 mg	150 mg
	Protriptyline	Vivactil	10-20 mg	60 mg
SNRI	Desvenlafaxine	Pristiq	50 mg	400 mg
	Duloxetine[a]	Cymbalta	30-60 mg	120 mg
	Venlafaxine[a]	Effexor	37.5-75 mg	225 mg
	Milnacipran	Savella	12.5-25 mg	200 mg
SSRI	Citalopram	Celexa	10-20 mg	40 mg
	Fluoxetine	Prozac	10-20 mg	80 mg
	Paroxetine	Paxil	20 mg	60 mg
	Sertraline	Zoloft	25-50 mg	200 mg
Atypical	Bupropion	Wellbutrin	150 mg	450 mg

[a]Commonly used for neuropathic pain.

TABLE IV.4 Commonly Used Benzodiazepines

Generic Name	Trade Name	Starting QHS Dose	Max Daily Dose	Half-Life
Alprazolam	Xanax	0.25-0.5 mg	4 mg	0.5-1 d
Chlordiazepoxide	Librium	5-10 mg	40 mg	1-2 d[a]
Clonazepam	Klonopin	0.25-0.5 mg	3 mg	1-2 d
Diazepam	Valium	5-10 mg	40 mg	2 d[a]
Lorazepam	Ativan	0.5-1 mg	10 mg	0.5 d

[a]Has additional active metabolites with longer half-lives.

Sulindac (**Clinoril**) *see NSAIDs*
Sumatriptan (**Imitrex**) see Triptans
SSRIs, Selective serotonin reuptake inhibitors:

Description	Antidepressant, selectively inhibits presynaptic reuptake of serotonin (5-HT) with weak effect on norepinephrine and dopamine reuptake
Indications	Depression, general anxiety, OCD, PTSD, binge eating, body dysmorphia
Dosage	See **Table IV-3** for dosing of commonly used SSRIs
Side Effects	Dizziness, fatigue, insomnia, nausea, diarrhea, xerostomia, sexual dysfunction; rarely associated with SIADH/hyponatremia
Precautions	Avoid combination with other serotonergic agents to decrease risk of serotonin syndrome, especially MAOIs; caution with patients with history of seizure disorder or hepatic disease; may impair platelet aggregation

TCAs, Tricyclic Antidepressants:

Description	Norepinephrine (NE) and serotonin (5-HT) reuptake inhibitors, 1st generation; further categorized into secondary amines and tertiary amines, secondary being more NE selective and tertiary having mixed NE and 5-HT making them often more effective but less tolerated due to worse side effects
Indications	Depression, neuropathic pain such as postherpetic neuralgia and diabetic neuropathy, fibromyalgia, tension headache, migraine prevention, myofascial pain; evening dose may improve overnight sleep
Dosage	Usually given once daily at bedtime; increase dose every 3-5 d as tolerated to a maximum daily dose; beneficial effects may be noticed in 1-3 wk See **Table IV-3** for dosing of commonly used TCAs
Side Effects	Xerostomia, urinary retention, constipation, drowsiness, fatigue, paradoxical excitement, exacerbation of psychiatric symptoms, postural hypotension, cardiac arrhythmias
Precautions	Caution in patients with BPH urinary retention, closed-angle glaucoma, severe respiratory disease, seizure disorder, cardiac dysrhythmias, or other cardiac disease

Tiagabine (**Gabitril**):

Description	Anticonvulsant, antineuralgic, GABA reuptake inhibitor
Indications	Neuropathic pain
Dosage	Start at 4 mg PO daily; may increase by 4-8 mg PO in weekly intervals; maximum antiepileptic dose is 56 mg/d; however, 4-8 mg/d is usual effective dose for pain management
Side Effects	Dizziness, drowsiness, nervousness, fatigue, nausea, weakness, tremor, cognitive impairment; generally well tolerated at doses used for pain
Precautions	Do not discontinue abruptly; reduce dose in hepatic dysfunction

Tizanidine (**Zanaflex**):

Description	α2 agonist, antispasmodic
Indications	Myofascial pain (muscle spasticity), spasticity associated with cerebral palsy
Dosage	Start with 2-4 mg PO nightly; gradually increase dose by 2-4 mg up to 3 times daily; maximum dose 36 mg/d
Side Effects	Hypotension, drowsiness, dizziness, xerostomia, weakness, nausea, constipation, LFT abnormalities
Precautions	Caution in patients with hypotension, hepatic, cardiac, renal, or ocular diseases; gradually taper over weeks to avoid withdrawal associated hypertension, hypertonicity, or tremors

Tolmetin (**Tolectin**) *see NSAIDs*

Topiramate (**Topamax**):

Description	Anticonvulsant, adjunct antineuralgic, may act by inhibiting voltage-dependent sodium channels, enhancing GABA activity and antagonism of NMDA receptor
Indications	Second-line medication for neuropathic pain
Dosage	Start at 50 mg PO nightly and gradually increase by 25 mg each week up to a maximum of 200 mg twice daily; improvement may be noticed over weeks
Side Effects	Weakness, fatigue, drowsiness, dizziness, tingling sensation, loss of appetite, unsteadiness, speech problems, mental/mood changes, abdominal pain, vision changes
Precautions	Use with caution in patients with renal or hepatic disease

Tramadol (**Ultram**):

Description	Analgesic, weak μ-agonist with additional inhibition of norepinephrine and serotonin reuptake
Indications	Moderate pain, adjunct in severe pain; useful in patients who cannot tolerate opioids
Dosage	50-100 mg PO every 4-6 h as needed; start at low dose to minimize side effects and increase up to 400 mg/d; as with other opioids gradually taper at discontinuation
Side Effects	Dizziness, vertigo, headache, constipation, nausea/vomiting, dyspepsia, xerostomia, weakness
Precautions	Caution for use in elderly or history of seizure disorders as seizures may occur at high doses; risk of serotonin syndrome if used in combination with antidepressants; respiratory depression, constipation, and dependence rarer than with other opioids; can enhance warfarin causing increased INR; reduce dose in renal impairment

Triamcinolone (**Aristocort, Kenalog**) see Corticosteroids

Triptans:

Description	Selective 5HT-1 agonists
Indication	Migraine headaches
Dosage	See **Table IV-5** for dosing of common triptans Not to be used to treat more than 3-4 headaches in a 30-day period
Side Effects	Dizziness, drowsiness, flushing, fatigue
Precautions	Contraindicated in patients with history of stroke or TIA as increases risk; caution in elderly or patients with significant cardiovascular, renal, or hepatic disease

TABLE IV.5 Commonly Used Triptans

Generic Name	Trade Name	Adult Dose		Max Daily Dose
Almotriptan	Axert	6.25-12.5 mg PO	q2h	25 mg
Eletriptan	Relpax	20-40 mg PO	q2h	80 mg
Frovatriptan	Frova	2.5 mg PO	q2h	7.5 mg
Naratriptan	Amerge	2.5 mg PO	q4h	5 mg
Rizatriptan	Maxalt	5-10 mg PO	q2h	30 mg
	Maxalt-MLT	5-10 mg PO disintegrating	q2h	30 mg (MLT)
Sumatriptan	Imitrex	25-100 mg PO	q2h	200 mg PO
		6 mg SQ	q1h	12 mg SQ
		5-20 mg intranasal	q2h	40 mg intranasal
Zolmitriptan	Zomig	1.25-5 mg PO	q2h	10 mg PO
		5 mg intranasal	q2h	10 mg intranasal
	Zomig-ZMT	2.5 mg PO disintegrating	q2h	10 mg PO (ZMT)

Valproic acid (**Depakene, Valproate**):

Description	Anticonvulsant, adjunct antineuralgic
Indications	Seizure disorders, migraine headache prophylaxis, neuropathic pain
Dosage	For migraine prophylaxis, start at 500 mg PO daily in 1 or 2 doses; can increase daily dose by 250 mg every week up to 1500 mg daily; weight-based dosing in seizure management
Side Effects	Drowsiness, dizziness, headache, nausea, abdominal pain, dyspepsia, weakness, tremor, diarrhea, menstrual changes, dose-related thrombocytopenia, rarely pancreatitis
Precautions	Caution in patients with history of liver disease or bleeding disorder; perform LFTs before and during treatment given risk for hepatic dysfunction (more likely in patients with mitochondrial disease)

Venlafaxine (**Effexor**) *see SNRIs*
Zolmitriptan (**Zomig**) *see Triptans*
Zonisamide (**Zonegran**):

Description	Anticonvulsant, antineuralgic
Indications	Neuropathic pain
Dosage	Start at 100 mg PO daily; increase by 100 mg every 2 wk to a maximum dose of 400 mg PO daily
Side Effects	Drowsiness, dizziness, loss of appetite, nephrolithiasis, renal insufficiency, headache, nausea
Precautions	Caution in patients with history of sulfonamide allergy, discontinue use if rash develops; avoid in patients with significant hepatic or renal disease

TABLE IV.6 Commonly Used Muscle Relaxants

Generic Name	Trade Name	Pharmacologic Category	Type	Adult Oral Dosing	
Baclofen	Lioresal	Central depressant	Antispastic	5-20 mg	q6-8h
Carisoprodol	Soma	Central depressant	Antispasmodic	250-350 mg	q6-8h
Chlorzoxazone	Lorzone	Central depressant	Antispasmodic	250-750 mg	q6-8h
Cyclobenzaprine	Flexeril	TCA analogue	Antispasmodic	5-10 mg	q8h
Dantrolene	Revonto	RyR antagonist	Antispastic	25-100 mg	q6h
Diazepam	Valium	Benzodiazepine	Antispasmodic	2-10 mg	q6-8h
Metaxalone	Skelaxin	Central depressant	Antispasmodic	800 mg	q6-8h
Methocarbamol	Robaxin	Central depressant	Antispasmodic	750-1500 mg	q6-8h
Orphenadrine	Norflex	Anticholinergic	Antispasmodic	100 mg	q12h
Tizanidine	Zanaflex	α2 agonist	Antispasmodic	2-4 mg	q8-12

TABLE IV.7 Commonly Used Corticosteroids

Generic Name	Trade Name	Dosing and Administration	Equipotent Doses	Biologic Half-Life
Betamethasone	Betaject	1.5-12 mg[a]	0.75 mg	1-2 d
Dexamethasone	Decadron	1-4 mg[a], 0.5-9 mg PO	0.75 mg	1.5-3 d
Hydrocortisone	Solu-Cortef	20-240 mg PO	20 mg	0.5 d
Methylprednisolone	Solu-Medrol	20-80 mg[a]	4 mg	0.5-1 d
Prednisolone	Medrol	10-30 mg PO	5 mg	0.5-1.5 d
Triamcinolone	Kenalog	10-80 mg[a]	4 mg	0.5-1.5 d

[a]Injection dose—can refer to epidural, intra-articular, or nerve root administration.

APPENDIX V

Definitions and Abbreviations

Addiction a disorder characterized by compulsive use of a drug, resulting in physical, psychological, and/or social dysfunction to the user and in continued usage despite the dysfunction

Adjuvant analgesic a drug that has a primary indication other than pain but has analgesic effect in some painful conditions or is capable of decreasing the side effects of analgesics; commonly administered in combination with one of the primary analgesics (eg, opioids)

Allodynia pain associated with a stimulus, such as light touch, that does not normally provoke pain

Analgesia absence of pain; commonly used to mean pain relief

Anesthesia absence of sensation

Arthralgia pain in a joint, usually due to arthritis or arthropathy

Breakthrough pain pain that breaks through the analgesia achieved by long-acting medications

Causalgia see CRPS I

CNS central nervous system

Central pain pain that originates from lesions of the central nervous system, usually the spinothalamocortical pathway

Central sensitization a long-term potentiation of pain signals associated with NMDA receptor activation and with the induction of specific genes; a CNS response to prolonged painful stimulation

Chronic pain pain that persists a month beyond the usual course of an acute injury or disease; this definition varies between the various treating clinicians

CNMP chronic nonmalignant pain

CNTP chronic nonterminal pain embraces chronic nonmalignant pain and chronic pain due to cancer (not associated with terminal illness)

Complex regional pain syndrome (CRPS) a chronic neuropathic pain syndrome characterized by its association at some point with evidence of edema, changes in skin blood flow, abnormal sudomotor activity in the region of pain, allodynia, hyperalgesia, or hyperpathia

COX cyclooxygenase, an enzyme in the pathway from arachidonic acid to prostaglandin, prostacyclin, and thromboxane

Coxib collective term for a new class of selective NSAIDs known as COX-2 antagonists

CRPS I (formally known as reflex sympathetic dystrophy [RSD]); a painful condition that is associated with a continuous burning pain and sympathetic overactivity in an extremity after trauma but without major nerve injury; this condition is not limited to the distribution of a single peripheral nerve and is apparently disproportional to the inciting event

CRPS II (formally known as causalgia) a condition characterized by burning pain, allodynia, and hyperpathia, often accompanied by vasomotor, sudomotor, and late trophic changes, occurring after partial injury of a nerve (or one of its major branches) in part of a limb (usually hand or foot) innervated by the damaged nerve

CSF cerebrospinal fluid

DEA Drug Enforcement Agency

Deafferentation pain pain resulting from loss of sensory input to the CNS; the pain may arise in the periphery (eg, peripheral nerve avulsion) or in the CNS itself (eg, spinal cord lesions and multiple sclerosis)

Dysesthesia an unpleasant, abnormal sensation, spontaneous or evoked, that is considered unpleasant

Drug dependence (also known as physical dependence) this relates to the expression of a withdrawal syndrome upon sudden drug cessation; it occurs with the use of both addictive and nonaddictive drugs (eg, opioids, local anesthetics, and clonidine)

Drug tolerance this occurs when a fixed dose of a drug produces a decreasing effect so that a dose increase is required to maintain a stable effect; the effect occurs particularly with opioids

EMG Electromyography

EDX electrodiagnostic testing (also known as EMG)

FDA Federal Drug Agency

Fibromyalgia a pain syndrome that diffuses through the body and that is characterized by predictable tender areas within muscles

Hypalgesia (same as hypoalgesia) an increased pain threshold (a decreased sensitivity to noxious stimulation)

Hypesthesia an increased detection threshold (a decreased sensitivity to stimulation); the definition excludes the special senses

Hyperalgesia a decreased pain threshold (an exaggerated painful response to a pain provoking stimulus)

Hyperesthesia a decreased detection threshold (an increased sensitivity to stimulation); the definition excludes the special senses

Hyperpathia increased pain either after repetitive stimulation or due to decreased pain threshold

IASP International Association for the Study of Pain

Meralgia paresthetica a dysesthesia in an area of lateral femoral cutaneous nerve innervation

Myofascial pain pain stemming from muscles

Neuralgia nerve pain along a specific anatomically distinct nerve or nerves

Neuraxis the spinal cord and brain; the term neuraxial drug delivery is commonly used to encompass intrathecal and/or epidural delivery, although, strictly, the term should include intraventricular delivery

Neuritis inflammation of a nerve or nerves

Neuropathy a disturbance of function or pathologic change in individual nerves or groups of nerves; *mononeuropathy* involves a single nerve, *mononeuropathy multiplex* involves several nerves, and polyneuropathy involves several nerves bilaterally or symmetrically

Neuropathic pain pain initiated or caused by a primary lesion or dysfunction in the nervous system; these pain-producing lesions may involve the peripheral and central nervous systems and may include injury from chemicals, radiation, or trauma and involvement of nerves in disease processes such as tumor infiltration and inflammation

NMDA (*N*-methyl-D-aspartate) a synthetic agonist of the NMDA receptor. This receptor is involved in the wind-up phenomenon, in the central sensitization, and in the development of opioid tolerance

Nocebo a negative placebo effect; for example, undesirable side effects (eg, nausea); nocebo effects are thought to be the result of an individual's expectations of adverse effects from a treatment as well as from conditioned responses

Nociceptive pain pain arising from activation of nociceptors

Nociceptor a receptor that is preferentially sensitive to noxious stimuli or to stimuli that become noxious if prolonged; this term may also be used to refer to the entire nociceptive primary afferent

NSAID nonsteroidal anti-inflammatory drug

Opiate an opioid drug

Opioid a substance that is active at endogenous opioid receptors; it includes opiates (drugs) and endogenous opioids (eg, endorphins and enkephalins)

Pain an unpleasant sensory and emotional experience associated with actual or potential tissue damage or that is described in terms of damage

Pain threshold the lowest intensity of stimulus that is perceived as being painful

Pain tolerance level the greatest level of pain that a subject is able to tolerate

Paresthesia an abnormal sensation, spontaneous or evoked, that is not necessarily considered unpleasant; the term dysesthesia specifically refers to an unpleasant abnormal sensation

PCA patient-controlled analgesia

Peripheral neuropathy any disease of the peripheral nerves; the symptoms of a neuropathy may include numbness, weakness, pain (often burning), and loss of reflexes

Phantom pain pain felt in an anatomic structure that has been surgically or traumatically removed

Physical dependence see *Drug dependence*

Placebo a drug or therapy that simulates medical treatment but has no specific action on the condition being treated

Preemptive analgesia analgesic treatment provided before and during painful stimulation that aims to attenuate the development of hypersensitive pain states

Pseudoaddiction a phenomenon of drug-seeking behavior that results from undertreatment with analgesics; the condition resolves when the dose of the drug the patient seeks is increased appropriately; it should be distinguished from true addiction, where drug-seeking behavior continues despite adequate and appropriate dosing

Psychogenic pain pain inconsistent with the likely anatomic distribution of the presumed generator or pain existing with no apparent organic pathology despite extensive evaluation

Radicular pain pain that is evoked by stimulation of nociceptive afferent fibers in spinal nerves, their roots or ganglia, or by other neuropathic mechanisms; the symptom is caused by ectopic impulse generation; it is distinct from radiculopathy, which includes a focal neurological deficit

Radiculopathy a pathologic condition of the nerve root (or multiple nerve roots) that results in conduction blockade and produces sensory and motor changes and pain in the area of its distribution; distinct from radicular pain, but the two changes may arise together

Referred pain pain perceived as arising in an area remote from its source; this is thought to occur because the nerve supply to both areas (ie, the area pain is perceived and the area pain is produced) converge proximally in the CNS

Reflex sympathetic dystrophy (RSD) see *CRPS I*

Somatic pain pain that arises from stimulation of nerves in the skin and musculoskeletal system, including bone, ligament, joint, and muscle

TCA tricyclic antidepressant

Tolerance see *Drug tolerance*

Trigeminal neuralgia a condition that produces sharp pain in the face because of abnormal firing of the trigeminal nerve; also know as tic douloureux

Trigger point a focal loci of pain within a muscle or connective tissue. Prolonged stimulation of these areas can generate a pattern of pain that is referred distally

VAS (visual or verbal analog scale) pain assessment tools utilizing analogs (either a measured line [visual] or a numeric scale [verbal]) to represent pain

Visceral pain pain due to stimulation of nerve endings in viscera; these nerves characteristically respond to stretch more than to other changes (eg, cutting, inflammation, and crushing); pain is usually referred to other areas (eg, flank, skin, perineum, legs, and shoulders)

WHO World Health Organization

Wind-up sensitization of dorsal horn spinal neurons by persistent C-fiber stimulation. This neuronal sensitization progressively increases throughout the duration of C-fiber stimulation, and therefore, "wind-up," and is dependent on activation of NMDA receptors.

INDEX

Note: Page numbers followed by "*f*" indicate figures and those followed by "*t*" indicate tables.

D

G

H

O

T

U

V

W

X

Z